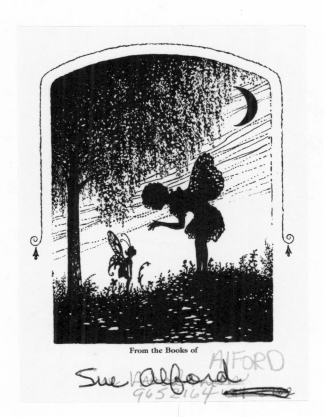

From the Books of

FOOD ALLERGY

Its Manifestations and Control
and the Elimination Diets
A Compendium

FOOD ALLERGY

Its Manifestations and Control
and the Elimination Diets
A Compendium

With Important Consideration of Inhalant
(Especially Pollen), Drug, and Infectant Allergy

By

ALBERT H. ROWE, M.S., M.D.

Lecturer in Medicine (Emeritus)
University of California
School of Medicine
San Francisco, California
Allergist, Samuel Merritt Hospital
Oakland, California

in collaboration with

Albert Rowe, Jr., M.D.

Department of Medicine
Highland Hospital and Samuel Merritt Hospital
Oakland, California

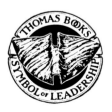

C H A R L E S C T H O M A S • P U B L I S H E R
Springfield • Illinois • U.S.A.

Published and Distributed Throughout the World by
CHARLES C THOMAS • PUBLISHER
BANNERSTONE HOUSE
301-327 East Lawrence Avenue, Springfield, Illinois, U.S.A.

© *1972, by* CHARLES C THOMAS • PUBLISHER
ISBN 0-398-02395-6
Library of Congress Catalog Card Number: 79-161182

With THOMAS BOOKS *careful attention is given to all details of manufacturing and design. It is the Publisher's desire to present books that are satisfactory as to their physical qualities and artistic possibilities and appropriate for their particular use.* THOMAS BOOKS *will be true to those laws of quality that assure a good name and good will.*

Printed in the United States of America
EE-11

Dedicated to Mildred Rowe

Foreword

This book confirms the causation of the many clinical manifestations of atopic allergy to inhalants and drugs and especially to foods, either alone or conjointly, which was reported in its first edition in 1931.

Realization of this major role of food allergy has largely depended on constant use of the elimination diets published in this book in 1931, with modifications thereof during the last forty years.

Experience, moreover, emphasizes the importance of such atopic allergy increasingly or anew in nasobronchial, cutaneous, neurocerebral, aural, ocular, urogenital, and other clinical manifestations of atopic allergy as reported in this volume. Its important role, especially of food allergy, in perennial bronchial asthma, perennial nasal allergy and nasal polyps, serous otitis media, abdominal allergy (especially in the allergic epigastric syndrome), chronic ulcerative colitis, regional enteritis, and in chronic bronchitis and particularly in obstructive emphysema has been increasingly realized since 1931.

The diagnostic fallibility of both positive and negative skin tests to determine atopic allergy, especially to foods, as is emphasized in Chapter 3, makes trial diet mandatory, even if allergy exists to only one to three foods. With the cereal-free elimination diets the causative foods are determined, and gradual control of the many manifestations of food allergy occurs. Where inhalant allergy, especially to pollens and less often to animal emanations and dust, and allergy to drugs are associated with food allergy or are sole causes, they are recognized and controlled as advised in Chapter 4 and throughout this volume.

Without the adequate, strict use of the cereal-free elimination diet and its advised modifications in 1931 and 1937, we are confident that many of these manifestations of food allergy would not have been recognized and controlled.

Proficiency in their use requires their strict and adequate maintenance, as advised in Chapter 3, in more than a few necessarily cooperating patients for at least three months and not in a few patients for three or even four weeks.

Therefore, since clinical food allergy is so frequent, since its recognition and control challenges all physicians including specialists, and because of the recognized fallibility of skin testing in determining food allergy, we opine that the strict, adequate use of the elimination diets whenever food allergy is possible to study and control such allergy by all physicians is most important.

Preface

This revision and amplification of *Food Allergy*, published first in 1931, confirms and emphasizes the importance of antigenic foods in the causation of clinical allergy. Other allergens participate but with a lesser role. Because of accurate and proper use of the elimination diets (with their modifications as indicated in this volume) over the last forty years, we can report ample confirmation and extension of the many recognized manifestations of food allergy.

Our work has assured the important and often major role of food allergy in nasobronchial, gastrointestinal, cutaneous, neurocerebral, joint, and muscle tissues. Failure of the majority of physicians and specialists, including most allergists, to recognize, study, and control such allergies is in our opinion one of the main deficiencies in medical practice today.

We have achieved excellent control with food allergy techniques of chronic ulcerative colitis, regional enteritis, allergic toxemia and fatigue, bladder inflammation, symptoms in all tissues of the eye, neurocerebral tissues, obstructive emphysema, bronchiectasis, chronic bronchitis, and bronchial asthma. Other physicians not using food allergy techniques but with use of the best other methods cannot report the kind of success we have achieved. Failure to recognize and control food allergy is, we maintain, a gross, preventable medical tragedy.

The challenge of study of atopic allergy, particularly to foods, in the causation of detached retinas and in glaucoma, as indicated by frequent improvement from our control of food allergy and as it appears in the literature, is discussed in Chapter 20.

Of great importance is general recognition of the pathognomonic history of bronchial asthma resulting from food allergy. When the patient's asthma comes in exacerbations every few weeks through the winter and slackens off in the summer, that asthma is caused by some food the patient is eating on a daily basis.

We also discuss the challenge of studying atopic allergy to foods in particular but also to some extent to inhalants, drugs, and chemicals in cardiac tissues, the parotid gland, enlarged lymphatic nodes in the abdomen, and such nodes in the omentum in regional enteritis. The periodicity of relapsing pancreatitis strongly suggests food allergy in its etiology. We show the importance of controlling dietary food antigens in diseases usually considered to be autoimmune. In many cases we believe they really are food allergy, but a combined action by antibodies to food and autoimmunity such that symptoms disappear on control of food allergy is not ruled out as yet.

Realizing the importance of diet trial in the 1920's and usual allergy to other foods than wheat, milk, and eggs which had been excluded in previous diet trials by other allergists, we first proposed the additional elimination of other foods which in our experience and that of other allergists had caused allergic symptoms in varying frequencies.

Emphasis in 1931 on the fallibility of positive protein skin tests and their frequent absence because of which trial diets (especially the cereal-free elimination diets) have become increasingly important in our continued daily study and relief of food allergy in the last forty years has been confirmed repeatedly in our practice. The usual dependence on skin tests to determine clinical food allergy with test-negative diets prevents its important mandatory recognition and control, establishing the tragedy of the skin tests in food allergy even today. The demonstration of serum antibodies to starches by Arthur Lietze, Ph.D., in the Merrill Food Allergy Research Laboratory in the Samuel Merritt Hospital is reported by him in Chapter 28.

Without these diets our increasing realization of the frequency and importance of food allergy would not have occurred. Failure to use diet trial, especially the cereal-free elimination diet, in the strict and adequate manner we have increasingly advised largely accounts for the unfortunate skepticism about the frequency of food allergy and resultant morbidity, absenteeism, frustration, and often, mortality.

The importance of trial diets (especially of the elimination diets) is realized primarily by the following failures which result if they are not used:

1. Failure to determine and confirm allergy to all or any causative foods by skin testing. This explains failure of test-negative diets to recognize and control food allergy.

2. Failure to recognize the frequent absence of dislikes or disagreements to food allergens responsible for clinical allergy.

The following paragraphs ending the Preface in 1931 convey even more important advice to all physicians including allergists today:

It must be emphasized very definitely that all physicians can obtain results in the treatment of food allergy who are willing to devote time and thought to the mastery of the methods of diagnosis and therapy described in this book. The appreciation of the many possible manifestations of food allergy is primarily important. The value of diet trial supplemented and aided by food tests must be understood. Of the two methods of diagnosis, I place diet trial ahead of testing, and as I shall explain in this volume, diet trial alone is justifiable and often productive of excellent results when a physician suspects food allergy to be a cause of symptoms and is not able to carry out food tests. For such diet trial, I have found my elimination method as mentioned above of ever increasing value.

But successful diagnosis and control of food allergy necessitates experience with a number of cases over a period of several months. The physician's assurance of the value of the method and his insistence on the cooperation of the patient and on the execution of the details of the elimination diets by the patient are of primary importance. With such an attitude, physicians will readily convince themselves of the frequency of food allergy and will be able to relieve their patients of many distressing symptoms which have resisted other attempts at control.

ALBERT H. ROWE, M.D.
ALBERT ROWE, JR., M.D.

Acknowledgments

We are greatly indebted to Carol Soma, Betty Prenter, and Sheila James for their devoted interest in the study and control of atopic allergy, especially to foods, and especially for their combined skills in the preparation and typing of this manuscript and Bibliography in its initial and its two subsequent revisions during the last three years, climaxing their appreciated secretarial assistance as required during three decades. To others of our office staff we are thankful. Without the loyal direction of our office manager, Helen Cable, with the help of her assistants, especially Peggy Hunt, during the last thirty years, our confirmation of clinical allergy, especially to foods, would have been greatly impaired. To Eva Court we express deepest appreciation, as in the books in 1944 and 1962, for her great help in our clinical laboratory and as a dietitian for her organization and testing of all of the recipes for bakery products and the important detailed menus in our elimination diets as published in Chapter 3.

We are indebted to Miss Marcella Allen for her important knowledge and cooperation in the preparation of allergens for testing and administering antigens with the aid of her assistants during the last twenty-four years. We express our deep appreciation.

We wish to thank Drs. Carl Mauser, E. James Young, Jack Berman, and Robert Tufft for their cooperation in the study and control of clinical allergy, especially to foods as well as inhalants, drug, and contactants in office and hospital and for their continued confirmation of the importance of trial diet, especially with our elimination diets, in their long established private practices. The present cooperation of Doctor Colin Sinclair is greatly appreciated.

Contents

FOOD ALLERGY

**Its Manifestations and Control
and the Elimination Diets
A Compendium**

Chapter 1

Characteristics of Food Allergy

Food allergy in man is a term which includes changes in the body tissues as well as the various manifestations and symptoms resulting from hypersensitivity in the body cells to specific foods. It explains the agelong realization that "what is one man's food is another man's poison." The resultant rejection of such foods by the sensitized tissues results in varying degrees of symptoms in the patient and even in death. It is generally accepted that allergic reactions are caused by the union of serum antibodies (allergins*) to proteins of foods attached to cells of the shock tissues with allergens of those foods entering the body. However, antibodies to starches and also to pectins (reported by Lietze) and possibly to other tissue substances, including ferments, must receive further study and recognition.

This book continues to evidence and emphasize the responsibility of every physician to recognize and control atopic allergy (especially to foods) as supported by Rinkel and Randolph in the last thirty-five years, whose study and control of clinical allergy to foods have long confirmed its importance.

This monograph, as it did in 1931, continues to discuss food allergy from the clinical, diagnostic, historical, and (in this edition) experimental viewpoints. Emphasis is placed on the greater frequency of clinical manifestations in various body tissues from food allergy than from inhalant, drug, chemical, or infectant allergies, which always must receive indicated and necessary study and control. In addition to the confirmation of its production of reactions and resulting symptoms in most tissues of the body, as reported in 1931, increased evidence that food allergy is the major cause of bronchial asthma; invaliding symptoms of chronic bronchitis and (according to our results) obstructive emphysema; gastric and abdominal allergy including chronic ulcerative colitis (CUC) and regional enteritis; perennial nasal allergy; eczema; urticaria; allergic headache and migraine; allergic toxemia and fatigue; urogenital and musculoskeletal reactions; and symptoms of other less frequent manifestations of allergy will be emphasized. Our opinion that food allergy is more frequent than inhalant allergy has depended on our open-minded consideration of clinical food allergy in the many tissues of the body and its daily study with elimination diets, especially our cereal-free elimination (CFE) diet, increasingly in the last forty years. Skepticism about such frequency would be justified only after real experimental evidence from the use of these elimination diets in a large number of patients for several months or better, from one to two years.

Because of the frequency of negative skin reactions to food proteins and other

---

*In order to avoid any implication that immunoglobulin E, or even atopic reagin, is necessarily the sole or principal antibody involved in allergic reactions to foods the term *allergin* is frequently used in this book to designate such antibody.

soluble allergens and the fallibility of positive reactions in indicating clinical food allergy, as emphasized in Chapter 2, the importance of the use of a trial diet eliminating the most common allergenic foods, especially the cereal-free elimination diet, has been progressively confirmed in our practice by the increasing relief of the many manifestations of food allergy.

The foods in these diets and the menus and recipes for bakery products, along with directions for the preparation of the diets with advice concerning their strict maintenance, manipulation, and development, are included in this volume and in previous publications. They are available to all physicians in this and other countries who are constantly challenged by the recognition of the many manifestations of food allergy with or without associated inhalant and drug allergies in the causation of clinical atopic allergy.

RECOGNIZED CAUSES OF CLINICAL ALLERGY

Though food allergy will receive major consideration, other causes of clinical allergy listed below will be considered as sole causes or concomitant with food allergy in our discussion of its various manifestations. All of these causes must be remembered by the physician if he is to be of maximum service to the allergic individual.

TABLE I

1. Ingestants
   Foods
   Condiments
   Ingredients in beverages
   Dentifrices and mouthwashes
   Drugs
   Water (mineral and organic content)
2. Inhalants
   Pollens
   Animal emanations
   Silk
   Spores of fungi
   House dusts
   Occupational and recreational dusts
   Flours and other dry foods
   Hay and feed dusts
   Cottonseed
   Kapok
   Pyrethrum
   Orris root
   Fly and other insect emanations
   Miscellaneous cosmetics
3. Bacteria, parasites, and products of diseased tissue
4. Contactants
   Vegetation
   Environmental
   Medicinal
   Recreational
   Occupational
   Cosmetics
5. Injectants
   a. Subcutaneous or intramuscular
      Drugs
      Sera
      Allergens
      Insect bites
      Vaccines
      Glandular and tissue extracts
      Hormones
   b. Intravenous
      Drugs
      Sera
      Vaccines
   c. Rectally
      Drugs
      Foods
   d. Nasal, aural, sinal, vaginal, urological, intra-bronchial, and cerebrospinal injections of drugs or allergens
6. Allergens transmitted through the placenta to the fetus
7. Rh or blood group reactions
8. Physical allergy (especially solar radiation or cold)

FREQUENCY OF POSSIBLE CLINICAL ALLERGY IN THE POPULATION

Indications of such allergy in four hundred unselected university students and nurses were published in 1931 from answers to the following questionnaire:

1. Has any one in your family—parents, siblings, aunts, uncles, grandparents—had asthma, hay fever, eczema, hives, headaches, or prolonged chronic indigestion?

2. Have you had any of the above symptoms?

3. Have any special foods ever produced such symptoms?

TABLE II

INDICATIONS OF POSSIBLE ALLERGY
IN 400 INDIVIDUALS

	%
Family history of probable allergy	43
Personal history of probable allergy	35
Foods as possible causes of symptoms	31
Food dislikes or disagreements	29
Questionable	14

Summary

	%
People with positive family or personal records of probable allergy	58
People with questionable evidence	16
People with negative evidence	26

TABLE III

	%
Frank or major allergy (cause not known to patient)	10.8
Minor allergy (cause recognized by patient)	48.1
Therefore, past or present history of allergy approximately in	59
Food sensitization	62.2
Inhalant sensitization	23
Contact sensitization	14.4
Gastrointestinal symptoms	50.7
Skin lesions	47.2
Nasal symptoms	26.4
Asthma	6.2
Migraine	9
Other less important manifestations of allergy	60

4. Are there any foods which definitely disagree with you or that you inherently dislike? (Name them.)

Since this information was obtained in only one conference in one age group, minimum probabilities of allergy are registered. Moreover, the history of headaches and chronic indigestion is not used as evidence of possible allergy, though the frequency of allergy (especially food allergy) in their causation has become increasingly evident, as summarized in Chapters 5 and 17 of this volume. In addition, many mild or subclinical manifestations of allergy are not elicited in answers to such a questionnaire.

Answers to our similar questionnaire by two thousand university students in 1936 also revealed the following:

1. A family history of probable allergy in 35 percent.

2. A personal history of probable allergy in thirty-three percent.
As in 1931, a history of recurrent headaches and chronic indigestion was not used to determine these percentages.

An important analysis of the histories of all 508 individuals in a small town by Vaughan in 1934 gave the information in Table III.

Vaughan concluded that over 60 percent of the population had present or previous clinical allergy and that 10 percent had active allergies requiring study and antiallergic control. Since such analyses cannot reveal all minor allergies or those allergies that become evident during continued study and cooperation of the patients, the above estimates of clinical allergy in the population undoubtedly are conservative. Vaughan stated that with long enough life, some clinical allergy would develop in practically every individual. Even greater than infection, allergy, according to Vaughan, may be the most common cause of human symptomatology.

COMMON OCCURRENCE OF FOOD ALLERGY

That food allergy is a more frequent cause of the many allergic manifestations in most tissues of the body than are inhalant, drug, and rare infectant allergies is indicated in the above statistics. The patient may be allergic to a single, several, or many foods. It is necessary to realize that mild and subclinical disturbances may arise from food allergy as they do from inhalant and other allergies. The mild or acute idiosyncrasies which have been attributed for centuries to various foods were probably examples of food allergy.

Most people during life suffer in varying degrees from allergy to foods. Such allergy occurs not only in childhood but, as our experience emphasizes, in adolescence, adult life, and frequently in old age. Such food allergy, especially, is responsible for allergic toxemia and fatigue; headaches; and gastrointestinal, nasobronchial and other symptoms specified above which will be discussed in later chapters of this volume. Overawareness of the body and its functions often results from atopic allergy, particularly to foods, making patients introspective; preventing proper use of their physical and mental powers; and causing depression, frustration, and inefficiency in occupations and in the home.

Clinical allergy to foods as well as to inhalants, chemicals, and drugs also occurs in patients suffering from other chronic disease. Thus it is imperative for general practitioners and all specialists to remember the manifestations of allergy and their usual origins from food as well as from inhalant and drug sensitizations. When food allergy exists, the diet must be manipulated so that foods causing both mild and severe sensitizations are excluded.

INDICATIONS FOR STUDY OF FOOD ALLERGY BY PHYSICIANS

1. History of manifestations of possible food allergy as is summarized in Table IV, Chapter 2.

When any of the possible manifestations of allergy in almost any tissue of the body is recognized by symptoms listed in this table by grades 1, 2, 3, and 4, the physician must adequately study food allergy. The possibility of inhalant or drug allergy must also be considered.

Our recognition of this importance of food allergy has resulted from the strict and adequate use of the elimination diets with their manipulation and supervision during the last forty years.

The role of food allergy in the causation of its many symptoms will be discussed in later chapters of this book.

2. Dislikes or disagreements for foods revealed in the diet history.

The importance of incorporating information from the patient which may indicate possible clinical allergies and the method of obtaining it from the history will be discussed in Chapter 2. That only 20 to 30 percent of food disagreements and dislikes are due to clinical allergy will be emphasized.

3. Recurrent exaggeration of symptoms with their absence or decrease between attacks.

This is a most important indication of food allergy, as was reported in this book in 1931 and as we have increasingly confirmed since then. It is most evidenced in cyclic attacks of bronchial asthma recurring every one to four weeks with interim relief or decrease of symptoms. These cyclic attacks occur especially in children and less often in young and older adults. Schloss was the first, in 1915, to report this important characteristic of food allergy. He suggested that it is best explained by refractoriness or relative desensitization which occurs after a severe attack of allergy similar to antianaphylaxis in guinea pigs after anaphylactic shock. He reported negative skin reactions to the causative foods during such periods. Other allergists, especially Rinkel and Randolph, have confirmed this cyclic recurrence for over thirty-five years.

This history is emphasized in Chapter 2 and especially in the chapter on bronchial asthma resulting from food allergy. Recurrent exaggeration of food allergy also explains recurrent allergic headaches and migraine, cyclic vomiting, recurrent serous otitis media, urticaria, and angioneurotic edema discussed in this volume. Its equivalent recurrent exaggeration of symptoms is also evidenced in carefully recorded histories of perennial bronchial asthma, chronic bronchitis, eczema, and at times in other allergic manifestations resulting from food allergy.

In 1933 in an important article, Cooke reported cyclic attacks of gastrointestinal symptoms including fever up to 104 F with interim relief resulting from allergy to cow's milk to which skin reactions were negative.

That regularly recurrent symptoms discussed by Reimann in 1963 arising in many body tissues, including fever even up to 104 F, recurrent abdominal pain, intermittent arthralgia, and other periodic diseases, justify study of food allergy as we advise requires consideration. Reimann's article contains many challenges of possible food allergy.

A detailed and carefully recorded history frequently reveals exaggeration of perennial symptoms every two to four weeks, especially in the fall, winter, and early spring months. Thus if the physician can elicit a history of recurrent intensification of definite or probable allergic symptoms, the possibility of food allergy must be studied as we advise.

We hypothesize that relief between attacks is due to a decrease or exhaustion of the antibodies to the allergenic foods in the tissues of the shock organs. Thus when foods responsible for the asthma or other allergic symptoms are eaten between the attacks, no allergic symptoms arise. With the assumed reaccumulation of the antibodies in the shock tissues above a reacting threshold, the attack or exaggeration of symptoms recurs. Such reaccumulation requires approximately the same number of days or weeks after each attack in any given individual. If the causative food allergies are not controlled, in one or two years the assumed antibodies apparently are not entirely inactivated during the attack and interim moderate wheezing or other allergic symptoms continue when the allergenic foods are eaten between the attacks.

4. Exaggeration of symptoms in the fall, winter, and spring with their absence or decrease in the summer.

This very important indication of food allergy has been reported by us for over forty years in four books and especially in two articles in 1958 and 1967. Failure to recognize and report this very important characteristic of food allergy would not occur if the cereal-free elimination (CFE) diet were adequately and strictly used as advised in Chapter 3. It explains the decrease or absence of recurrent attacks of bronchial asthma in children and young adults during the summer months as discussed in the chapter on bronchial asthma resulting from food allergy. Thus when there is a history of "winter eczema" or winter asthma or bronchitis in children often extending into adolescence or at times into adult life with relief or decrease in the summer, food allergy is a likely cause. Activation of chronic bronchitis, nasal or other bronchial symptoms, allergic headaches, fatigue and allergic toxemia, and gastrointestinal and other possible manifestations of allergy in the fall and especially in the winter and early spring always requires the mandatory study of food allergy as a definite possibility. Illustrative case histories are in the two articles noted above.

The frequency of chronic bronchitis or recurrent asthma in the fall to late spring requires the study of food allergy, particularly, as stressed in Chapters 8 and 9.

Though fever requires the consideration of primary or secondary infection, its origin from food allergy alone, as discussed below and especially in Chapter 24, must always be remembered.

The explanation of this decrease or inactivation of food allergy during the summer has been sought from various scientists, including physicists, meteorologists, and climatologists. The best available explanation is the beneficial effect of ultraviolet solar radiation, especially available during the summer. Patients can remain indoors most of the time during the summer months and receive this benefit.

This exaggeration of food allergy in the fall to late spring can explain the exaggeration of perennial bronchial asthma and chronic bronchitis in adults as it does in children and such exaggeration in the invaliding symptoms of some patients with obstructive emphysema in these seasons. Intensification of other manifestations of clinical allergy during the fall and winter can be explained by this cause. The increase in emergency-room treatments of bronchial asthma from October to June reported by Segal can be explained in large part by exaggeration of unrecognized or uncontrolled food allergy with or without associated inhalant allergy. This activation of food allergy explains the increase in symptoms of nasal and bronchial allergy in the fall to late spring months rather than the presence of often assumed infectious cold or respiratory infection. Though fever often is absent, it must be remembered that food allergy must be considered as a cause of such fever when present.

5. *Activation or exaggeration of symptoms in ocean areas with relief in inland areas suggests food allergy.*

This benefit has been reported by us for over thirty years. Though this inland relief has occurred in some patients with asthma and allergic bronchitis resulting from food allergy, it is less common than relief of such symptoms during the summer. Inquiry about such relief in inland areas and the activation near the ocean should be routine. This geographic benefit also occurs in some cases of perennial nasal allergy, allergic headaches, allergic toxemia, and other manifestations of food allergy. In those manifestations of allergy in which this beneficial effect of inland areas has been reported, inhalant allergens in or out of doors have been considered and ruled out. This inactivation of food allergy in inland, desert, or mountainous areas can explain the relief of manifestations of allergy, especially bronchial asthma, in areas away from the ocean, particularly in the Rocky Mountains, the Southwest, and in the desert areas in Nevada and California. Though relief may not be complete, symptoms of various manifestations of clinical allergy may be ameliorated with a definite decrease in body consciousness and discomfort.

The activation of food allergy in ocean areas must be adequately studied as a cause of marine asthma reported on the shore of the Caribbean Coast in Mexico when such symptoms were absent in Mexico City and those occurring on the Indian Ocean which were absent in Johannesburg. The opinion of Doctor Ordman that molds and house dust in marine areas are the only cause cannot be accepted unless food allergy has been studied and ruled out with trial diet as we advise.

6. *Large scratch reactions to foods often indicate clinical allergy.*

Lesser reactions, especially by the intradermal method, are of questionable significance. The clinical importance of both must be determined by provocation tests in the symptom-free patient, as advised in Chapter 2.

These large reactions usually occur to foods causing immediate asthma, nasal allergy, hives, localized edemas, vomiting, cramping, or other gastrointestinal symptoms which occur in a few minutes to an hour after eating the food. Their occurrence without evident immediate allergy justifies the study of possible delayed clinical allergy arising hours or even in one or two days. Provocation tests with the feeding of the reacting foods are not necessary when there is a history of immediate asthma, vomiting, or localized edema after ingestion of a reacting food. The clinical import of a large scratch reaction to a food to which immediate allergy is not evident must be determined by provocation tests, which are done according to the method described in Chapter 2. That smaller scratch reactions are undependable indications of clinical allergy, often being nonspecific or possibly indicative of past or potential allergy, is well known, as discussed in Chapter 2. This is especially true of intradermal tests with foods that have failed to give large scratch reactions. Because of the doubtful significance of these reactions and the occurrence of severe general reactions or even death when intradermal tests are done with foods having given immediate allergy and large scratch reactions, initial intradermal tests with foods are not done in our practice.

As emphasized in Chapter 2 and reiterated throughout this volume, much chronic or delayed food allergy cannot be demonstrated at all satisfactorily by skin testing. The specific antibodies responsible for the clinical allergy may be attached to the cells of the shock tissues, being absent in the blood, lymph, and skin. The demonstration by Doctor Lietze of serum antibodies to insoluble starch particles may also explain some of these negative reactions when tests are done with extracts containing only the soluble food proteins.

The limited information derivable from routine skin testing today is one explanation for the failure of nearly all skin test-negative diets to reveal and control clinical food allergy. The importance of trial diet, for which the elimination diets have been of established value to us daily for over forty years and to many other allergists and physicians, is emphasized.

7. Chronic, often recurrently exaggerated, and (at times) incapacitating symptoms unrelieved by long and varied medical and (at times) antiallergic therapy should be adequately studied and treated for possible allergy to foods.

This is particularly important before a diagnosis of psychoneurosis or some incurable malady is blamed, as so often occurs. Chronic, persisting, and (at times) recurrently exaggerated symptoms arising in the nasal, bronchial, gastrointestinal, urogenital, cardiovascular, and nervous tissues and fatigue and toxemia which cause longstanding body distress, varying degrees of incapacitation and invalidism, and frustration or depression justify the study of chronic allergy to foods with or without associated inhalant or drug allergy. It must be remembered that such an allergy can also occur concomitantly with diabetes, cardiovascular, gastrointestinal, hepatic, urogenital, or other diseases.

When cerebral, nervous, gastrointestinal, ocular, or other symptoms persist in spite of medical or antiallergic therapy, including the study of food allergy, it is important to remember the advice of our distinguished confrere and friend Doctor Walter Alvarez that an epileptic equivalent may be an associated or sole cause. The use of Dilantin®, as he has advised, has confirmed such convulsive states and has given resultant relief to the grateful patient.

ADDITIONAL CHARACTERISTICS OF FOOD ALLERGY

1. Food allergy arises and continues in any age.

Any of the manifestations of food allergy occur throughout life. The opinion of some allergists and many physicians that such a manifestation is rare or absent after childhood or early adult life is due to one or more commonly accepted misconceptions. Matsumura, for example, has shown that frequency of positive skin tests for egg and milk decreases with age among patients known to be sensitive to such foods. Thus overdependence on skin tests can produce an erroneous impression of decrease in food allergy with age.

Our increasing realization of the frequency and importance of food allergy has resulted from our consideration of it when its possible manifestations are evident in the detailed history we elicit and record from each patient together with the use of our strict elimination diets for the study and control of possible food allergy instead of test-negative diets. Our diagnosis of food allergy has been made only after symptoms have been controlled with the exclusion of allergenic foods determined with our elimination diets and the subsequent reproduction of symptoms with provocation tests. These tests are accomplished with the feeding of the allergenic foods when the patient has been free from symptoms.

In infancy, allergy to cow's milk is nearly always the cause of nasobronchial symptoms including croup; colic and other digestive symptoms; dermatitis and eczema; and unusual restlessness, irritability, and discomfort, especially when cow's milk

alone or supplemental to breast milk is given, as reported in Chapter 25. And throughout life, allergy to cow's milk requires consideration as well as to other animal milks. A varying degree of aversion for cow's milk may be indicative of food allergy. The relative frequency and age of onset of other food allergies and their continuation through life are discussed in Chapter 25.

To the frequent question "Why should I at my time of life (30 or 70 years) develop food allergy?" the answer must be "The only time one cannot develop such allergy is after death."

2. Food allergy occurs in most tissues of the body.

This is shown in Table IV, in which most manifestations and symptoms of allergy to foods are listed. The important challenge of its as yet unconfirmed occurrence with resultant tissue changes in the heart, kidney, and glands, including the pancreas, as occurs in the parotids is discussed in Chapter 26 and in the eyes, as summarized in Chapter 20. The relative frequencies of inhalant, drug, chemical, and of infrequent infectant allergies (and especially of food allergy) are also indicated either as sole causes or in association with other allergies. It will be seen that our good results have indicated that food allergy is the major or sole cause of these manifestations more often than inhalant allergy, drug allergy, and particularly infectant allergy.

3. Food allergy may cause its major manifestations in one tissue as in the lungs or skin, and lesser ones in the cerebral, gastrointestinal, ocular, urogenital, or other tissues.

It may be the sole cause, or inhalant, and/or drug allergies may be associated with food allergy to cause the major manifestation or one of the lesser clinical allergies in the patient.

4. It may be localized in a limited area of a body tissue, as on the fingers, ears, or even in the choroid of the eye.

This occurs especially in the skin, where eczema may be limited to one or both hands, the flexures, or neck. It may also be localized in the stomach, causing the allergic epigastric syndrome described in Chapter 5, or in the rectum or sigmoid or the entire colon, causing chronic ulcerative colitis. Nasal allergy resulting from pollens or foods may occur with no allergy in the pulmonary tissues. Thus allergy cannot be ruled out because there is no history of hay fever, asthma, or eczema.

5. Allergies to foods and other allergens tend to spread to other areas in the same tissue or to other body tissues.

This occurs most frequently in the skin. Eczema initially in the hands, flexures, or neck may gradually spread to the legs, thighs, and back or in varying degrees through the entire integument. The spreading tendency of CUC resulting from food allergy from an initial area in the rectum and sigmoid through the entire colon in days, months, or years is well known (Chapt. 6). Hay fever resulting from pollen originally involving nasal tissues alone often extends into the sinal and ocular tissues and if uncontrolled by desensitization therapy, extends into the lungs, often causing dominant bronchial asthma with a diminution of the hay fever.

6. Fever may arise from food allergy as it does from serum or drug allergies.

Fever from 100 to even 105 F as a result of food allergy occurs most frequently in children who have the pathognomonic history of attacks of bronchial asthma resulting from food allergy reported by us for thirty years, described in Chapters 8 and 25 and which was first reported in the

first edition of this book in 1931. This fever occurs in the first twelve to twenty-four hours when coughing, shortness of breath, and wheezing, often associated with gagging or vomiting, are maximal. Because nasal symptoms or an irritative cough and fever often precede the asthma, an infectious cold is incorrectly assumed by many physicians, and bacterial allergy incorrectly is diagnosed. The antibiotics or sulfa drugs usually given during these attacks often for months or years would be unnecessary if the causative food allergies are controlled by the elimination diet, as advised in Chapter 3. Antibiotics are not indicated unless fever does not decrease in two or three days or definite infection of the tonsils or pneumonitis shown by x-ray occurs. Infectant asthma, according to our experience, is rare or nonexistent.

Fever also occurs in recurrent serous otitis media (Chapt. 13) resulting from food allergy because of which antibiotics have been given with no relief for months or years until controlled with the cereal-free elimination (CFE) diet as reported in Chapter 3.

Further comments of fever resulting from food allergy in Chapters 6 and 7 discuss the daily fever even up to 104 degrees in CUC and regional enteritis relieved with the control of the causative food and (at times) pollen allergies.

This fever in patients with possible recurrent or chronic allergic symptoms justifies the study of chronic allergy, especially to foods, assuming that other possible causes are being studied.

The occurrence of high fever by our confrere Sherrick and of fever and vomiting reported by Carr from milk allergy was noted in the first edition of this book. In addition, fever in children from various foods, especially milk, and the occurrence of fever of 99 to 101 F for weeks or months from food allergy producing nasal symptoms at times associated with enlarged lymphatic glands has been reported by us for more than thirty years. Associated allergic fatigue and toxemia are discussed in Chapter 19.

7. Manifestations of food allergy may be activated or may continue if traces of allergenic foods are ingested or inhaled.

Since a maximum degree of allergy must be assumed when allergy to a food is being studied, its total elimination from the prescribed elimination diet is imperative. To accomplish this, patients must be given a list of allowed foods with suggested menus. The use of bakery products made by our recipes or by honest bakers who use our recipes, the necessity of eating no foods in restaurants or in friends' homes which may contain traces of disallowed foods, and other precautions necessary to exclude disallowed foods from the diet are emphasized in Chapters 3 and 8.

Bakery products containing disallowed wheat, milk, or cottonseed oil which are not in the prescribed diet must not be eaten. The use of butter or margarines containing disallowed cow's milk or milk solids instead of a prescribed milk-free margarine has reactivated recurrent asthma or eczema in children or adults which had been controlled with the cereal-free elimination (CFE) diet.

It must be remembered, moreover, that the inhalation of the dusts or odors of foods will activate manifestations of allergic symptoms. Patients often report such activation from the odor of fish, fruits, chocolate, coffee, peanuts, and other foods. Eczema or asthma often flares from the inhalation of airborne allergens at lunch counters or in the family kitchen when marked allergy to eggs is present.

When large scratch reactions to foods such as eggs, fish, and peanuts occur, their exclusion from the home, especially from refrigerators, may be advisable. Children should not be in the kitchen in high chairs when foods eliminated from their prescribed diets are being cooked. One of the corollaries to these preventatives is refraining from kissing a child or even an adult after eating a food which may remain on the lips and to which food the person has a marked clinical allergy.

8. It must be remembered that food allergens remain in the body for more than a few days and that the tissue pathology resulting from chronic food allergy requires entire elimination of the allergenic foods for days and even several weeks or longer before cellular structure and function approach normal.

This is illustrated in the gradual disappearance of eczema from the continued elimination of foods together with corticosteroid or adjunctive therapy in Figure 17 in Chapter 14. Volkheimer has, for instance, found starch granules in tissues of experimental animals 120 days after ingestion. The importance of this justifies its inclusion in this enumeration.

9. Finally, the variation in the degree of clinical allergies to foods, the time of onset after their ingestion, and the duration of the manifestations are of such importance that they receive special discussion below.

ONSET OF FOOD ALLERGY

Our studies show that allergy to milk and eggs is the cause of most clinical food allergy in infancy. It often continues to occur, with or without inhalant allergy, through childhood, adult life, and even in old age. Inhalant allergy is absent or very infrequent in infancy. It increases through childhood into adult life, possibly decreasing in old age.

Food allergy, especially to cow's and often to goat's milk, is the usual cause of colic, difficulties in feeding, abdominal distress, croup, bronchial and nasal symptoms, bronchial asthma, eczema, dermatitis, and irritability and restlessness in infancy. Human milk contains no beta-lactoglobulin, an established allergen, but all animal milks do contain it. Allergy to other foods, especially eggs, wheat, and cereal grains, may develop as they are added to the diet. As children grow older, these manifestations gradually decrease or may disappear by ten years of age. In many children, however, manifestations of food allergy continue into adolescence and adult life. Food allergy in early life is likely to occur when there is allergy to foods in both parents or their relatives. The role of food allergy in infancy and childhood is discussed more fully in Chapter 25.

It must be remembered that food allergy can start in any year of adult life, including old age, without evident occurrence in childhood or later years. This refutes the unfortunate assertion that clinical food allergy is infrequent in children and does not occur after the age of forty years. Patients are often told that allergy, including that to foods, fails to develop only after death.

When possible manifestations of allergy begin after the age of twenty, especially if they are perennial and recurrently exaggerated particularly in the fall, winter, and early spring, food allergy must be studied. It is the common cause of perennial bronchial asthma, chronic bronchitis, the bronchospasm and bronchorrhea in obstructive emphysema, recurrent headaches, perennial eczema, and other manifestations of allergy listed in Table IV. As emphasized throughout this volume, food allergy can be ruled out by diet trial, especially with the cereal-free elimination diet or its advised modifications.

ACQUISITION OF FOOD ALLERGY

Food allergy may develop *in utero* from the mother's overindulgence of specific foods during pregnancy. This fact was emphasized by Ratner *et al.* based on their experimental studies in guinea pigs in 1927. Volkheimer has more recently demonstrated the transplacental passage of particulate food allergens (and also their secretion in mother's milk.) This would help to explain croup or colic from allergy to cow's milk when first ingested after birth by the infant. Sensitization *in utero* may also occur to other foods eaten in excess by the mother even though she develops no clinical allergy to such foods.

O'Keefe, Shannon, and Donnolly, as reported in the 1931 edition of this book, presented evidence that nursing infants may develop allergy to allergens in the mother's milk from foods being ingested by the mother without previous ingestion of them by the child. If allergic symptoms develop in the breast-fed infant or from ingested milk in the first one to five days after birth, sensitization of the fetus to milk *in utero* by blood-borne allergens of ingested food by the mother during pregnancy is probable.

Sensitization by such infinitesimal amounts of food allergen which enter the body of the fetus *in utero* is supported by the severe sensitization to eggs established in a guinea pig with the preparatory injection of a 1/20 millionth of a gram of egg.

Excessive eating of a food may result in allergy thereto. Rosenau and Anderson, in 1909, established sensitization in animals by the overfeeding of specific foods. Ratner especially, in 1934, sensitized 50 percent of guinea pigs with massive ingestions of skimmed milk. He produced anaphylactic shock by subsequent oral feedings. One such guinea pig died in 1½ minutes after drinking 5 cc of milk. The rapid passage of undigested food protein through the intestinal mucosa is demonstrated by the Prausnitz-Küstner skin reactions. We have records of patients who have developed clinical allergy to foods after eating large amounts of oranges, apples, cherries, chocolate, coffee, honey, buckwheat, nuts, and others. Cooke, in 1933, suggested that allergy to foods such as shellfish, strawberries, mushrooms, or honey may result from intermittent eating of large amounts of them. Duke, in 1921, reported such development of allergy to shad roe and honey. Stuart and Farnham reported sensitization to fish continuing into adult life arising from drinking glue on a bet in youth.

Continued eating of a large amount of a food for weeks or months may sensitize the patient to it. New sensitizations occur especially frequently in patients who have severe allergy to many other foods. Thus trial rotation of tolerated similar foods in the diet from day to day, hoping to prevent new sensitizations, may be advisable. With or without such rotation, new allergies to foods may arise and may necessitate limiting the diet at times to a "minimal diet" including as few as four to ten tolerated foods. In one wheat-sensitive, rye-sensitive, and corn-sensitive patient with nasal and pharyngeal allergy, intolerance to rice and potato developed, leaving tapioca, oat, arrowroot, soy, and sugar as the only carbohydrates in the diet. Although it is usually impossible to prevent, development of allergy to new foods must be kept in mind.

As noted previously, clinical allergy tends to develop when there is a definite history of it in one parental side of the family and particularly when such a history occurs in both sides. Statistics show, moreover, that the tendency to develop a specific manifestation, such as bronchial asthma, eczema, or gastrointestinal allergy, may be inherited. Moreover, we have many records of allergy to milk, eggs, fruits, or other foods which has reappeared in several generations. In 1937 we reported eczema on the hands resulting from trout allergy in three generations.

Additional discussion of the origin of food allergy is found in later sections of this chapter.

TIME OF ONSET OF ALLERGIC REACTIONS TO FOODS

The allergic manifestation may arise in a few minutes after ingestion of an allergenic food if the allergy is severe. Severe allergy is often indicated by a large scratch reaction to the food. Ingested traces of or even the odor of such a food may cause a rapid or moderately delayed reaction. Immediate reactions in the lips, tongue, and oral mucosa may dissuade tasting, chewing, or swallowing allergenic foods such as eggs, fish, or peanuts. These reactions to foods can occur in a few minutes up to an hour from provocation tests such as that advised by Rinkel, Randolph, and others. Though indications of allergic symptoms from many ingested foods arise within one hour, they may not be realized by the patient for two to ten hours or at times only after the food has been eaten on two to three successive days.

Thus a boy with asthma resulting from milk developed a slight cough and nasal congestion three to four hours after the ingestion of 20 cc of milk. These symptoms increased slightly for four days, definite asthma developing in five to six days. Because of frequent delay of the reaction after ingestion of an allergenic food, we have always advised that provocation tests with a new food be done every two to seven days. The onset of symptoms, moreover, may occur only after the daily ingestion of a food for two to four days. This delayed allergy is not recognized when provocation tests are done two or three times a day as advised in Rinkel's method for determining food allergy.

Incorrect conclusions about the time of onset of a reaction to a food, moreover, occur if feeding tests are done during the refractory period after a severe attack of food allergy or during the summer, when inactivation of food allergy often occurs.

The time of development of a symptom from an allergenic food remains the same in each patient. One patient always developed dizziness, nausea, weakness, and semiconsciousness about seventeen hours after each ingestion of even traces of garlic.

DURATION OF ALLERGIC REACTIONS AFTER A SINGLE INGESTION OF A FOOD

Though symptoms and tissue changes arising from the ingestion of an allergenic food may last only a few hours, they usually continue for one to two and even up to seven to ten days. In addition to the body distress, visible evidences of clinical allergy develop, including eczema, hives along with physical evidences of asthma, hay fever, gastrointestinal allergy, and other allergic manifestations.

The duration depends on the time the food allergen remains in the body. Complete digestion of the food and its entire disappearance from the gastrointestinal tract require more than one to three days, especially if constipation is present. And the food allergen which begins to enter the blood and body tissues in a few minutes after ingestion, as shown by PK reactions, continues to enter the blood in

decreasing amounts as long as any food allergen remains in the gastrointestinal tract. The continuation of the allergic symptoms, be they bronchial asthma, eczema, hives, gastrointestinal, or other allergic manifestations, even up to seven to ten days after a single ingestion of even a minute amount of an allergenic food indicates that such allergens remain in the body up to seven to ten days or possibly longer, causing dysfunction of the shock tissues sensitized to them.

A second determinant of the duration of the allergic reaction is the time required for all of the specific antibodies to the foods attached to the cells of the shock tissue to unite and thus become inactivated by their union with the food allergen, especially in the blood. If this inactivation of the antibodies is active and rapid, then symptoms cease in hours or up to one to two days; if the union of antibodies and food allergens is slower or if antibodies are abundant, symptoms can continue up to seven to ten days. Such delay commonly occurs.

Allergic symptoms from a single ingestion of a food continue for more than a few hours and nearly always for one to seven days. Thus hives developed in one patient in three hours from two loganberries and continued for one week, similar to continued urticaria, erythema, and fever for one or two weeks arising from an allergic reaction to horse serum. Because of the delay of onset of such symptoms, we have always advised that provocation tests to determine the presence or absence of allergy to a specific food be done not oftener than every two to five days. Several tests a day, as advised by Rinkel for determination of possible food allergy, seem unwise, since symptoms arising from individual foods ingested every one to three hours may overlap and impair accurate deductions.

When a food productive of a definite allergic reaction is eaten at irregular intervals or at intervals from one to three months, symptoms arise in a few minutes, in hours, or in one to three days. And as already discussed, the reaction may continue unabated for one to three days, gradually decreasing in four to seven days as the food allergen leaves the body and the specific antibodies are inactivated or exhausted. Allergy to foods that are eaten occasionally such as shellfish, mushrooms, unusual nuts and fruits, and vegetables or condiments is responsible. This reaction usually recurs when the same allergenic food is eaten, with the following exception: refractoriness for one to six weeks may occur after a severe reaction from such an allergenic food, preventing a similar reaction if a food is eaten during the refractory period. In addition, the inactivation of food allergy in the summer in some patients may also prevent such a reaction if a food is ingested in the summer.

DURATION OF ALLERGIC REACTIONS TO FOODS EATEN EVERY ONE TO THREE DAYS

Food allergy often produces recurrent manifestations, usually with interim relief. As discussed previously, such recurrent attacks are best explained by the exhaustion of antibodies to the allergenic foods in the shock tissue. The attacks may last for hours or up to one to seven days. Recurrent exaggeration of perennial symptoms may occur and can be recognized in a carefully recorded history. Our recognition and control of food allergy causing these recurrent and also more perennial symptoms have depended on the use of the cereal-free elimination diet and its modifications.

SEVERITY OF ALLERGIC REACTIONS TO FOODS

The severity of reactions depends on the degree of the allergy to the allergenic foods and on the amount ingested.

Large scratch reactions usually occur to foods causing severe, immediate allergy in contrast to slight or negative reactions to foods producing delayed or chronic clinical allergy. To avoid marked or even fatal reactions from skin testing, initial intradermal tests are not done, as discussed in Chapter 2. The ingestion of a trace of the food or even the inhalation of the food allergen in the air, especially if the odor of the food is apparent, may cause severe symptoms. This largely explains our disuse of intradermal tests, especially to foods.

Fatal reactions resulting from food allergy have long been reported in infants and young children. Laroche, Richet, and Saint Girons, in 1919, cited Hutinel's report of three deaths from milk sensitization. Campbell, in 1926, reported such fatalities. Recent reports of crib deaths apparently from a variant of milk allergy are cited. Bowen reported fatal asthma in an egg-sensitive child. Talbot, in 1917, reported threatened death for several hours in such a child after biting into a cake. In 1936 we reported several attacks of severe vomiting and collapse in a wheat-sensitive child because of eating minute amounts of bread. Anaphylactic deaths ascribed to milk by several physicians were also reported by us in 1936. In adults, life-threatening allergy occasionally arises from laryngeal edema from an allergenic food or from extreme bronchial asthma arising from severe allergy. Severe anaphylactic shock also occurs from excessive doses of pollen or other inhalants. Deaths from parenteral drugs and hormones are recorded in the literature.

As emphasized in the treatment of food allergy, epinephrine 1:1,000, 0.1 cc hypodermically in infants, 0.1 to 0.3 cc in young children, and 0.4 to 0.5 cc in adolescents and adults, repeated every five to fifteen minutes, one to three times if necessary for relief, must be administered when severe and life-threatening allergic reactions occur. This and additional therapy is advised in Chapter 7.

Most allergic reactions to foods are not life-threatening, varying in degree from severe or moderate to slight in degree. They usually produce slight initial symptoms along with early localized vascular allergy, edemas, smooth muscle spasm, and hyperactivity of the mucous glands in the shock tissues. These physical results of the allergic reactions with consequent symptoms and body distress may reach a maximum in hours or in one or more days. The factors determining the duration of the reaction have been discussed previously in this chapter. These severe to slight reactions require relief with medications. Determination of the allergenic causes which are not apparent in the history requires study of allergy to foods, to possible inhalants, and to drugs, as advised in Chapter 2.

Until the allergenic causes are recognized and controlled by elimination or desensitization measures, the manifestations of clinical allergy continue, causing recurrent attacks or chronic perennial symptoms as listed in Table IV and discussed in the later chapters of this volume. Though food allergy especially causes such chronic clinical allergy, the less frequent role of inhalant and at times unrealized drug allergies must be remembered. Those symptoms arising from food allergy are especially chronic and persistent because of the continued ingestion of foods before their allergenicity is discovered. Thus recurrent

or perennial bronchial and nasal allergy, headaches and other cerebral manifestations, eczema, chronic urticaria, gastrointestinal allergy, and other less frequent manifestations of chronic allergy discussed in this volume always require study of possible food allergy.

In this discussion of the duration of allergic reactions, it must be stressed that the gradual relief and termination of recurrent or perennial chronic manifestations of food allergy require its study and control, especially with the cereal-free elimination diet and at times with its modifications. Such study has increasingly indicated the frequency of chronic food allergy in our practice.

PATHOLOGY OF CHRONIC FOOD ALLERGY

That chronic clinical allergy from foods eaten daily or even every two or five days produces chronic pathology in the cells and tissues of the shock organs causing persisting symptoms, body and mental distress, inadequacy, and varying invalidism must be remembered. These chronic changes are distinctly different from those of limited duration arising from the single and often infrequent ingestion of an allergenic food.

This chronic pathology is illustrated by a young man who had had perennial eczema all of his life. Its perennial occurrence justified the study of food allergy. With strict adherence to the cereal-free elimination diet, a moderate decrease in the skin pathology occurred in three months, definite improvement in six months, and complete relief in one year during which time the diet was strictly maintained. This relief occurred in 1946 with no corticosteroids and no desensitization therapy. With the availability of corticosteroids today together with the cereal-free elimination diet, evidence of relief and control of his eczema would occur in four to seven days.

That chronic food allergy may produce permanent tissue damage was stressed by Kline and Young in 1935 and has been realized by many allergists through the years. Chronic persisting allergy produces vasculitis with increased membrane permeability resulting in edema; infiltration of tissues with round, eosinophilic, and other cells; hyperactivity of the mucous glands; smooth muscle spasm; induration of the shock tissues; and when severe, necrosis, ulceration, and resultant scar tissue formation. These changes occur in varying degrees in the pulmonary tissues as a result of perennial bronchial asthma, chronic bronchitis, and as our experience indicates, in obstructive emphysema in which food allergy plays a major role. Perennial moderate bronchial asthma or bronchitis resulting from definite or unrealized food allergy, especially to milk and cereal grains, explains the occurrence of obstructive emphysema in patients who have never smoked tobacco. Food allergy also causes edema, cellular infiltration and thickening of the nasal and sinal mucosa, polypoid regeneration, and the formation of polyps in the nasal and sinal membranes. According to our experience such permanent tissue damage also occurs in the duodenum, causing allergic inflammation and often duodenal ulceration arising especially from food allergy (Chapt. 6 and 7). In chronic ulcerative colitis and regional enteritis, vasculitis, thromboses, cellular infiltration, edema, tissue induration along with necroses, and resultant ulcerations arise from chronic allergy, especially to foods and to a lesser extent to pollens, as we report in Chapters 6 and 7.

WAYS OF ESTABLISHMENT OF MANIFESTATIONS OF FOOD ALLERGY

Manifestations of food allergy are established through the ingestion of specific foods. The allergen enters the blood through the gastrointestinal mucosa, and sensitization to it develops in the pulmonary, nasosinal, cutaneous, gastrointestinal, or other body tissues. The shock tissue may depend on inheritance, as illustrated by the occurrence of asthma, gastrointestinal, or other allergic manifestations resulting from foods in relatives of the present or former generation.

Whether contact allergy to foods develops in the mucous membranes of the gastrointestinal tract similar to contact allergy to chemicals in the skin is uncertain. Allergic inflammation in the lips, bucchal, oral, and pharyngeal mucosa and canker sores arising from food allergy are frequent. When this allergy is localized in the mouth with no evidence of it in the rest of the gastrointestinal tract or any other tissue of the body, it is possible that the allergy might have developed from oral contact of the specific food. We have recognized oral allergy, for example, to cinnamon from the chewing of cinnamon gum with no evident allergy in other tissues. Allergy from foods in the stomach and small bowel might also arise from contact with ingested foods.

Blood-borne allergens, however, must be the assumed cause when allergy develops in the pulmonary, cutaneous, or other tissues as well as in the gastrointestinal tract, decreasing the likelihood of contact allergy even when oral allergy is the only manifestation.

Inhalation of dust and of airborne allergens of cereal grains, flours, various seeds such as flax and cotton seeds, coffee, and fish must be remembered. They can produce clinical allergy particularly in the nasobronchial tissues and in the skin. One woman whose severe migraine headaches were due to wheat, corn, chocolate, and especially fish developed an attack with vomiting for two days from inhalation of airborne fish allergens in fish meal fertilizer applied to the lawn. The inhalation of the odor of fish oil also caused severe nasal allergy in a man. Bakers especially develop bronchial asthma from the inhalation of the flours of wheat and other cereal grains. The inhalation of airborne dust from nearby factories manufacturing castor oil or cotton-seed oil or from the dusts of cotton gins has caused asthma in nearby residents. Osmyls of tomato in air blown from a cannery five blocks away caused asthma in one patient.

ASSOCIATION OF FOOD ALLERGY WITH INHALANT AND (AT TIMES) DRUG ALLERGY

Though food allergy is the sole cause of many manifestations of allergy, inhalant allergy and at times drug allergy may be associated or sole causes. In regard to inhalant allergy, positive reactions to inhalants do not necessarily indicate clinical allergy. Such reactions may be nonspecific or due to potential allergy. Their clinical significance must be determined by history, the results of their elimination from the patient's environment, or by the results of adequate desensitization therapy. Positive skin reactions to inhalants which cause no clinical allergy in children suffering with asthma resulting from food allergy alone are shown in Table V. In the same way the clinical importance of positive reactions to inhalants in patients suffering from other manifestations of food allergy must be determined. At times a positive history of allergy to pollens, animal emanations, or other inhalants may occur in the absence of positive skin tests.

Food allergy may be the sole cause of manifestations of allergy such as asthma, especially in the fall, winter, and early spring months, and pollen may cause hay fever or asthma in the pollen seasons. In the same way animal emanation allergy may cause nasal allergy or eczema in patients suffering with asthma because of food allergy. Thus food, inhalant, drug, or contact allergies may be concomitant causes of one manifestation such as dermatitis or each may cause a separate manifestation in the same patient.

INHERITANCE OF FOOD ALLERGY

That a positive family history of definite or very probable clinical allergy occurs in 60 to 70 percent of allergic patients has been reported for fifty years. Though this tendency to develop allergy is increased with a history of allergy in one and especially both parental histories, allergy can occur without any apparent inherited tendency. If the history of all transient or mild allergies were obtainable in both family histories, however, an inherited tendency to develop clincial allergy would be revealed in nearly 100 percent of patients, as stated by Vaughan and Ratner over thirty years ago.

In our study of a great many patients suffering with clinical allergy in the last forty years, the frequent occurrence of the patient's manifestation of allergy in his past and present family history has been evident. This familial occurrence is encountered especially in bronchial asthma, perennial nasal allergy, eczema, gastrointestinal allergy and cerebral allergy. When food is the demonstrated cause in the patient, such allergy as a cause of the same manifestation in the progenitors is quite probable. Along with this, the likelihood of inheriting the tendency to develop similar manifestations of food allergy and the occurrence of specific food allergy in two or more generations occur. We have many records of milk and egg sensitizations in two or three generations and also of allergy to fruits, vegetables, and fish, even to specific ones in parents and their progeny. Laroche, Richet, and Saint Girons reported egg sensitization in four generations. In a like manner, proclivities to develop sensitizations to specific inhalants, as to grasses or fall pollens, occur in parents, children, and forebears. Fantham, for example, reported seventeen cases of asthma in five generations, all arising from rabbit emanations and hair and even from ingested rabbit meat.

Therefore, heredity is responsible above all else for the tendency to become allergic. Predisposition toward specific manifestations in specific tissues and even tendency toward development of sensitization to specific allergens may occur. With a marked family history, clinical allergy tends to develop in infancy or childhood. Food, along with other allergies, however, develops at any time of life including old age with or without a family history of allergy.

WHY FOOD ALLERGY IS NOT BEING SUFFICIENTLY RECOGNIZED

Failure to recognize and control food allergy throughout life accounts for much unnecessary morbidity, invalidism, and even mortality. If physical examination, all indicated laboratory tests, and x-ray and other investigations are negative and allergy, especially to foods, is not considered, an unjustified diagnosis of psychoneurosis may lead to the use of tranquilizers, sedatives, or psychological therapy. If allergy is suspected and food allergy with or without inhalant or drug allergies is not controlled, patients may be given antihistamines, oral or inhalant bronchodilators, antispasmodics, antipruritics, and corticosteroids, which unfortunately may be continued without any adequate study of food allergy or of inhalant allergy.

Failure to remember the frequent occurrence of negative skin reactions to foods which cause delayed cumulative or chronic food allergy and the fallibility of moderate or slight skin reactions in determining clinical allergy, as discussed in Chapter 2, are largely responsible for failure to recognize the frequency of allergic manifestations of food allergy.

Food allergy therefore cannot be ruled out because of negative skin tests or because test-negative diets excluding skin-reacting foods only do not control symptoms arising from possible food allergy.

Failure to recognize and control food allergy is also due to failure to remember the seven indications for the study of food allergy and its additional characteristics discussed previously in this chapter.

Our increasing realization of this frequency of food allergy in the last forty years has been due especially to the routine use of the cereal-free elimination diet modified as advised in Chapter 3 rather than the use of test-negative diets in its study.

This important recognition and subsequent study of food allergy will be increased, moreover, if detailed histories as outlined in Chapters 2 and 8 record the presence or absence of the many manifestations of clinical allergy as listed in Table IV. The inclusion in the diet history of food dislikes or idiosyncrasies is important as possible indications of food allergy, as stated in Chapter 2.

This failure to adequately recognize food allergy will decrease when the patient's physician, be he general practitioner; internist; allergist or another specialist in private practice; or a professor or full-time member of the staff of a medical school, hospital, or clinic, records or critically evaluates the history and directs the study of possible food allergy with the indicated elimination diet, all the while being cognizant of the information about food allergy in this and other chapters of this volume. Most or even part of this task cannot be delegated to other physicians or assistants who have no confidence or successful experience in taking and analyzing histories of possible or definite allergy, in results of skin testing, and in the use and manipulation of elimination diets for the study and relief of food allergy along with the recognition and control of possible inhalant allergies.

Proficiency in obtaining available information about possible atopic allergy, the ordering and interpretation of skin testing, the prescribing and manipulation of elimination diets, and the recognition and control of inhalant and the less frequent drug allergies cannot be attained even by physicians with established and well-deserved reputations in private and institutional practice unless they have done all of this in a strict and adequate manner in many patients over a period of more than a few months. When this experience is attained, the frequency and importance of food allergy and of independent or associated inhalant and drug allergies will be realized. There is a definite need to incorporate instruction in the recognition, diagnosis, and treatment of the manifestations of food allergy in medical school curricula. Unfortunately this instruction occurs in a minimum of medical schools today.

EXPERIMENTAL ESTABLISHMENT OF FOOD ALLERGY IN ANIMALS

Rosenau and Anderson and also Wells over fifty years ago were able to sensitize guinea pigs by oral feeding of proteins of foods. Similar experiments were recorded in the monograph by Laroche, Richet, and Saint Girons (1919). They found that excessive feeding for a few days helped to induce such allergy. However, if the feedings were continued for thirty days, immunity rather than allergy at times resulted. Schloss (1920) reported similar results from guinea pigs. Ratner and Gruehl (1934) confirmed and extended their experiments. They found that 50 percent of all guinea pigs could be sensitized with the feeding of moderate amounts of skimmed milk. A small number were sensitized with a single small feeding. They found food allergens were absorbed through any part of the alimentary canal, most absorption occurring in the small intestine.

Sensitization to foods is readily established by their parenteral injection into rabbits, guinea pigs, monkeys, and other animals. With the usually recommended injection of doses every six days for three weeks, antibodies to the foods develop, especially in the animal serum.

Comparable to these experimentally produced antibodies are the antibodies to foods in human serum which are being increasingly demonstrated, especially by hemagglutination and Ouchterlony techniques in laboratories throughout the world. The occurrence of these antibodies to ingested foods in most people with a larger number usually in the sera of people allergic to the specific foods and the demonstration of antibodies to insoluble starches as well as to soluble proteins receive more discussion in Chapter 2.

FOOD ALLERGY—A CLINICAL STUDY

The study and control of food allergy today, therefore, as we stated in 1931, remain essentially a clinical problem. Of paramount importance is the recording of a detailed history of all possible manifestations of clinical allergy with indications not only of food but of associated inhalant and lesser drug allergies. The limited value of skin testing with foods in revealing clinical food allergies, discussed in Chapter 2, is more generally accepted than it was thirty-five years ago. The fallibility of skin tests explains the infrequency of diets eliminating skin-reacting foods (test negative diets) to reveal or relieve clinical food allergy. The value of the leukopenic index and the so-called pulse test advised at that time has not been confirmed. Moreover, the dependability and clinical value of the provocation feeding and injectant tests as proposed by Rinkel need carefully controlled confirmation, as stated in Chapter 2.

Therefore, trial diet remains the most dependable procedure for the study and control of possible food allergy. And for this purpose, the elimination diets have been of increasing value in our practice and in that of many other physicians. They are standardized trial diets which can be used by all physicians in private, hospital, clinic, or institutional practice. The clinical aspects of food allergy therefore remain a paramount challenge.

SUMMARY

1. Food allergy is a term for tissue changes and various manifestations and symptoms arising from hypersensitivity in body cells to specific foods. The allergy results from antibodies developed in the body to proteins, polysaccharides, and (as reported by Lietze), to starch, pectins, and possibly other insoluble tissue allergens in foods.

2. Symptoms arise from allergen-antibody reactions in all body tissues as reported in this volume.

3. The foods, inhalants, infectants, contactants, and oral and parenteral medi-

cations which may cause allergy are listed.

4. The frequency of food and inhalant allergy in the population indicated from questionnaires is reported.

5. Dislikes or disagreements for foods; the characteristic exaggeration of symptoms in the fall, winter, and early spring; recurrent exaggeration of attacks; and activation of symptoms near the ocean indicate possible food allergy.

6. Localization of the food allergy in any part of the body tissue, as in the skin of the face or hand, in the Eustachian tube, or in the cornea, is common.

7. Fever resulting from food allergy alone is emphasized in Chapter 24.

8. Traces of food, even by inhalation, will cause or reactivate a manifestation of such clinical allergy.

9. Acquisition, time of onset of symptoms after ingestion of food allergens, duration and severity of reactions to foods, and development of food allergy, especially in childhood or at any age, are discussed.

10. Pathology in tissues from acute and chronic food allergy is reported.

11. Reactivation of symptoms from inhaled osmyls of foods in the air from uncooked or cooking foods is discussed.

12. Association of allergies from foods, inhalants, and (at times) drugs in varying degrees occurs.

13. Inheritance in the establishment of food allergy must be understood.

14. The reasons why clinical food allergy is not adequately recognized by physicians are discussed.

15. Diagnosis of food allergy depends on clinical study primarily with trial diets, especially with the elimination diets and by provocation tests as advised in Chapter 3. This study is required in spite of negative skin reactions, especially to insoluble food allergens used in testing.

Chapter 2

Diagnosis of Allergy

The diagnosis of allergy first of all necessitates a carefully recorded family history and a personal history of past and present illnesses, a thorough physical examination, and all indicated laboratory and roentgen ray studies. The history must include detailed information about any major and minor manifestation of allergy and definite or possible allergenic causes. This history recorded according to our plan on page 23, as it has been routine in our practice for over thirty years, designates the challenge of the major and lesser manifestations of allergy which require recognition and continued study and control by the physician. Recognition and treatment of other associated diseases are mandatory. Duke, an important pioneer in the recognition of clinical food allergy, wrote in 1926 that "the diagnosis of food sensitivities is best made by history of the patient, observation of the patient, and by ingestion tests with foods eaten by the patient. Skin tests in food cases are often unsatisfactory."

ALLERGIC HISTORY

Allergy should be suspected if any of its possible manifestations listed below are found in the past or present history of the patient or in the family history of the parents, children, aunts, uncles, grandparents, or in former forebears. This constitutes a constant challenge and responsibility of all physicians in the specialties and general practice, as evidenced throughout this volume.

It must be stressed that although allergy is often responsible for these many symptoms in varying degrees and frequency, other disease states may be responsible. Allergy needs special study when its common manifestations such as bronchial asthma, chronic bronchitis, nasal allergy, eczema, urticaria, gastrointestinal allergy, or migraine are present rather than when separate symptoms such as nausea, abdominal distress, joint pains, or menstrual disturbances occur. However, the physician must keep allergy in mind as a possibility in all patients, as evidenced in our discussion of allergy in the average population in Chapter 1.

An adequate study of possible allergic causes is necessary when any of the symptoms listed above occurs. This is especially true of food allergy, which is a dominant cause in nine of the above listed manifestations of allergy compared with the dominance of inhalant sensitization in four.

HISTORY OF THE ALLERGIC PATIENT

This history has been recorded in our practice for over thirty years under the following headings.

1. Bronchial manifestations.
2. Nasal and sinusal symptoms.
3. Dermatoses.
4. Gastrointestinal symptoms.
5. Recurrent headaches, migraine, biliousness, fatigue, or "toxic states."
6. Genitourinary, cardiovascular, and

glandular disturbances.

7. Fatigue, tension, and nervous or psychoneurotic disturbances.

8. Dietary history.

9. Drug history.

10. Environmental history.

Information about the presence or absence of each possible manifestation of allergy along with the symptoms, their duration, frequency, variation, and degree must be recorded. The history is started with detailed information about the major manifestation followed by that about the lesser manifestations of allergy listed in Table IV.

TABLE IV

MANIFESTATIONS OF CLINICAL ALLERGY

Types of Allergy Responsible According to Probable Frequency (1 maximum, 4 rare)

	Foods	Inhalants	Drugs	Infectants
1. Bronchial asthma, allergic bronchiolitis, croup, chronic bronchitis, obstructive emphysema	1	1	3	4?
2. Nasal allergy (hay fever, recurrent colds, postnasal mucus, recurrent sore throats or laryngitis)				
a. seasonal (any season)	3	1	4	4?
b. perennial	1	2	4	4?
3. Atopic dermatitis	1	1	4	4?
4. Urticaria and angioneurotic edema	1	3	1	4
5. Acne (lipoidosis with or without infection the major cause) possible allergy	3	?	2	?
6. Contact dermatitis (epidermal cell sensitized)	None of these antigens			
7. Gastrointestinal allergy (canker and recurrent cold sores, oral and pharyngeal inflammation, distention, pyrosis, nausea, vomiting, cramping, pain, peptic ulcer, regional enteritis, diarrhea, constipation, mucus and chronic ulcerative colitis, irritable bowel, proctitis, and pruritus ani require study of possible allergy)	1	3	3	4?
8. Migraine, sick headaches, cyclic vomiting, bilious attacks (neuralgia, paresis, confusion and idiopathic epilepsy at times resulting from allergy)	1	3	4	4?
9. Allergic toxemia (fatigue, bodily aching, confusion)	1	3	4	
10. Arthritis (swellings of joints and tendons, rheumatic fever, rheumatoid arthritis, intermittent hydrarthrosis)	2	3	3	2
11. Ocular allergy (lid dermatitis, blepharitis, conjunctivitis, iritis, corneal ulcers, cataracts, retinal allergy, ocular pain, detached retina)	2	1	3	4
12. Aural allergy (dermatitis of ear and ear canal, edema of Eustachian tubes, deafness, tinnitus, vertigo, dizziness)	1	2	4	4?
13. Urogenital allergy (allergic cystitis, spasm in bladder and ureter, cankerlike ulcers, inflammation and dermatitis of vulva, menstrual pain, leukorrhea)	1	3	3	4?
14. Cardiovascular allergy (cardiac irregularities, pseudoangina, coronary thrombosis?, thromboangiitis obliterans, periarteritis nodosa, erythema nodosum and multiforme, glomerulonephritis)	3	4?	2	3
15. Allergic purpura, agranulocytosis and bleeding	2	3	1	4?
16. Allergic fever (recurrent or intermittent)	1	3	1	4?
17. Allergy to Rh substance (erythroblastosis fetalis, transfusion reactions)	None of these antigens			

The patient's answers to questions on an extended questionnaire (see Chapt. 30) will be of added help to the physician.

DIET HISTORY

Diet history must be recorded in every patient suspected of allergy. To do so would be wise in patients of all physicians, since food sensitization, at times of definite importance, may be revealed. The physician should first ask, "are there any foods that you definitely dislike or that disagree with you?" If an affirmative answer is given, details about such reactions should be recorded. Then specific questions about single foods should be asked. "Do you drink milk?" The answer may be, "I hate milk," "I never took it willingly since childhood," "It nauseates me," or "It is poison to me."

It must be remembered that many of these dislikes, aversions, and disagreements for foods are not due to clinical allergy. Fads or fancies established through habits of eating, psychic influences, or suspicions suggested by food faddists may be responsible. Gastrointestinal and other constitutional diseases may disturb digestion. We agree with Vaughan and other allergists that only 20 to 30 percent of these dislikes and disagreements arise from clinical allergy.

HISTORY OF DRUG ALLERGIES

A history of possible drug allergies should be routinely recorded in the study of all allergic patients. The drugs which most frequently produce allergy are noted on page 185. Direct questions such as "Does aspirin agree with you?", "Has quinine upset you?", "What physics do you take?", "Is phenolphthalein in any of them?", "Does codeine or morphine cause nausea or other distress?", "What other medications have you taken and have any of them disagreed with you?", "What ointments, salves, hair lotions, dentifrices, mouthwashes, or douching solutions do you use?", and "Do they cause irritation, burning or eruptions?" must be asked in order to assemble available information about possible drug allergies.

ENVIRONMENTAL HISTORY

The so-called environmental history is an important part of all records of allergic patients. Listing is desirable of all vegetations such as trees, shrubs, flowers, and even vines on the house as well as of all animals and birds inside and outside the house, including fowls that are encountered around the home or during the daily routine. One man had sixty pigeons and thirty-six chickens outside and two dogs, a cat, and two parakeets in the house! On a farm the type of work done by the patient or the kind of animals, hay, feed, and farm products to which he is exposed is important to record.

Causes of inhalant and contactant allergies, as discussed in Chapter 4, often can be suspected from a carefully taken history. Careful analysis of the patient's daily and weekly routine may suggest that such an allergen is encountered only in the house, in the office, on the train, in a friend's home, during recreation, or in special environments. Allergy may thus be found to cats, horses, or other animal hair; feed or grain dusts; spores of fungi encountered in damp houses; orris root or karaya gum at the hairdresser's; and various plant or pollen allergens in gardens or in the open country.

In the house the number in the family; the type of work each performs; whether the dust from work or recreation is brought into the home; the kind of mattresses, bedding, pillows, carpets, animals, or birds present; animal skins; fur; insect powders or chemicals in the rooms or closets; and similar information may be of great value. When contact dermatitis is suspected, the substances touching the skin or oils or resins as from poison ivy or other vegetations must be considered as possible causes. The effect of all types of inhalant and contact allergens encountered by the patient in his occupational routine also must be analyzed. Taking such a history has long been practiced by the writers according to the plan presented on page 169. Such a routine assures thoroughness of analysis and grouping of information.

FAMILY HISTORY OF ALLERGY

As already stated, a carefully recorded family history of possible allergy is important as a diagnostic aid. Although practically all persons during life are victims of one or another type of allergy, as noted on page 5, the propensity to develop allergy and the degree and type of allergic manifestations are definitely heightened and influenced by heredity. If allergy is present on both sides of the family, the progeny is predisposed to more definite allergy than when it is present in one parent or in other relatives. Analysis of family histories reveals that one manifestation such as asthma, nasal allergy, dermatitis, or migraine has a tendency to occur in a number of relatives and in successive generations. Many patients may have several manifestations of allergy simultaneously, one of which may be especially severe. Moreover, the tendency toward pollen, animal emanation, or food allergy frequently is determined by inheritance, and the susceptibility to allergy to one food, such as milk, eggs, fish, or fruit, occasionally recurs in family members of several generations.

FOOD ALLERGY INDICATED BY SKIN TESTING

That skin testing to determine food allergy is highly fallible has been emphasized in our work. This was stressed particularly in our detailed evaluation of skin reactions to allergenic foods in 1934 to which the reader is referred. This is evident in Table V. Much chronic cumulative food allergy is not indicated by scratch tests. When reactions do occur, they are often nonspecific or indicative of past or potential allergy. When, however, the immediate type of allergy to a food is indicated by the development of asthma or other manifestations of allergy shortly after ingestion, a large skin reaction often occurs. Such large reactions are frequently obtained to fish (fin and shellfish), eggs, peanuts, mustard, and at times to walnuts and other nuts, cottonseed, celery and other spices, as well as occasionally to milk. Such a reaction to soy is reported in this volume. However, all large scratch reactions to foods are not always indicative of such immediate severe food allergy. Clinical allergy to any food giving a positive reaction therefore must be determined by the reproduction of allergic symptoms by feeding the food to the symptom-free patient. That such large scratch reactions and some moderate reactions suggest possible food allergy is the reason for our routine scratch testing with most common foods eaten by patients, as listed in Chapter 30. When skin tests are negative to foods which produce cumulative or chronic or recurrent types of allergy, it must be assumed that allergy to soluble allergens in the foods are absent or that antibodies to allergenic foods are only in the cells of the shock tissues. Moreover, the antibody responsible for skin reactions may not be identical to that which causes the allergic reaction and the patient's symptoms. The demonstration of antibodies to starch and pectins by Lietze (see Chapt. 28) and clinical allergy to starches in cereal grains explain some negative reactions to foods. Thus the ruling out of food allergy because symptoms are not relieved by a test-negative diet excluding skin-reacting foods is unjustifiable and can be called "the tyranny of skin tests," especially to foods.

TABLE V
FALLIBILITY OF SKIN TESTS IN FOOD ALLERGY

	Bronchial Asthma				Migraine				Jacksonian Epilepsy Hay Fever			
	Clinically Sensitive	Scratch Test	Intradermal Co. 1	Intradermal Co. 2	Clinically Sensitive	Scratch Test	Intradermal Co. 1	Intradermal Co. 2	Clinically Sensitive	Scratch Test	Intradermal Co. 1	Intradermal Co. 2
Wheat	+				?					±	++	±
Eggs	?				+				+	±		
Milk	+		±		+	±					+	
Corn	+				+						+	+++
Rice	+		±	+	+						++	+
Rye	?		±	+++	?					±	++	±
Chicken												
Lamb		±								±		
Beef		±										
Peas		++	+				++			±	+	
Tomatoes						±	+					
Spinach		++	+				+				+	+
Pineapple			±			±	+					+
Lemon		+				±	+					+
Grapefruit			±									±
Pears			++			±						+
Apples			++		?	±	++					+
String beans			++									±
Potatoes		±			+							
Carrots		++					+			+		+

Note: Blank spaces mean negative reactions.

Though the writers have used food allergens prepared by various recommended techniques, as well as freshly prepared quick-frozen food allergens, this fallibility of the skin test in food allergy has not been altered. Demonstration of large reactions to fresh fruits in contrast to negative reactions to dry allergens was reported by Tuft and Blumstein in 1942. The clinical importance of such reactions, however, still has to be determined by individual provocation tests.

In spite of negative reactions and the fallibility of clinical information derived from moderate and especially slight reactions to foods, scratch or puncture tests with foods usually eaten by the patient should be done, hoping to reveal large reactions and less important moderate reactions to soluble allergens in foods.

Though dry allergens to foods are available for scratch tests, glucose or glycerine fluid extracts are generally used. Our tests are done with glucose extracts and only by scratch tests. The activity and stability of these extracts can be assured by demonstrating positive immediate (not the slight or delayed) reactions in patients who have proven clinical allergy to the specific foods.

Intradermal testing with foods has not been routine in our practice for over thirty years. When it was used for over fifteen previous years, it was never done with foods that had reacted to previous scratch tests because of the fallibility especially of intradermal tests and of deaths which have been reported from them. Because of this, if intradermal tests are done, they should only be executed by the physician or under his immediate supervision. In fact, allergists using this method must always have available epinephrine 1:1000 for immediate injection, a tourniquet to place above the site of injection in the arm, and an injectable corticoid to control constitutional reactions resulting from such intradermal tests. It is generally agreed, moreover, that such intradermal tests with cottonseed and flaxseed, even when negative scratch tests have occurred, are dangerous. Intradermal testing, moreover, often yields positive or indefinite reactions which cannot be correlated with any clinical allergy. These may be nonspecific or less often due to past or potential allergy. As with the scratch tests, negative intradermal reactions often occur to foods responsible for asthma or other clinical allergies. The fallibility of the scratch and intradermal tests is shown in Table V in this chapter and formerly published in "Food Allergy—Reasons for Its Delayed Recognition and Control," 1954, reading of which will be important to any doubting physician.

Unwarranted suspicions of foods from positive skin tests alone unfortunately is established in many patients today because of the failure of physicians to realize this fallibility of skin testing in food allergy. Too many patients are told to suspect or exclude in varying degrees foods which have given positive reactions, the clinical significance of which has never been proven by the reproduction of symptoms by the ingestion of foods in the symptom-free patient. Such test-negative diets infrequently control symptoms resulting from food allergy.

Too often the skin tests have been performed and interpreted by technicians not under the supervision of a physician or are done in a commercial laboratory or hospital. Tests are often conducted with many foods which are never eaten, too often to impress the patient with a thorough study or to justify a fee. Some patients carry copies of tests with foods and inhalants done in two or more laboratories which disagree with one another. They are told to eliminate some foods entirely and others to a partial degree! The many skin reactions obtained in many patients and the failure of relief of symptoms resulting from food allergy are emphasized in Table VI. Many patients told to eliminate milk continue to take sherbet, cheese, and butter, all containing allergens of cow's milk. Poor results lead to confusion, frustration, and lack of confidence in the role of food allergy not only in patients but also in physicians. In

TABLE VI

POSITIVE SCRATCH AND INTRADERMAL REACTIONS FROM COMMERCIAL LABORATORY

Failure of Test-Negative Diet and Relief from Elimination Diet

Milk	3+*	Crab	3+*
Arrowroot	3+	Oyster	3+*
Barley	2+	Sand dab	4+*
Buckwheat	1+	Shrimp	3+*
Rice	1+	Sole	3+*
Rye	1+	Chocolate	2+
Tapioca	2+	Cane sugar	2+
Bacon	2+	Brewer's yeast	4+*
Beef	3+*	Duck	3+*
Chicken	1+	Cow	3+*
Calves' liver	4+*	Goat (mohair)	3+*
Tea	4+*	Hog	4+*
Corn	3+*	Horse	1+
Cucumber	4+*	Cigarette smoke	3+*
Lettuce	3+*	Cottonseed	3+*
Lima Beans	1+	House dust	3+*
		Flaxseed	2+
Peas	3+*	Tobacco	2+
Sweet potato	2+	Bermuda grass	3+*
Pumpkin	3+*	Johnson grass	3+*
Yam	4+*	Rye	2+
Grapefruit	3+*	Annual saltbush	4+*
Peach	3+*	Russian thistle	3+*

*Intradermal reactions.
Our tests showed no scratch reactions to foods.
Symptoms: red, itching wheals 3-6 times daily for 2 years. Scaling eruption for 1-3 weeks every 1-2 months for 3 years.
Test-negative diet based on positive reactions from commercial laboratory failed.
The fruit-free and cereal-free elimination diet minus soy and beef gave relief. Symptoms recurred with ingestion of all fruits, beef, milk, chocolate, soy, and oats. Reacting inhalants caused no clinical allergy.

our practice the futility and nutritional damage resulting from these test-negative diets are often seen.

Because of this fallibility of skin testing in food allergy, some allergists omit it in their study of allergic patients. We, however, test all patients suspected of food allergy with the scratch or puncture method with commonly eaten foods and with other foods eaten by patients on occasions as suggested by the dietary history. With the scratch test this is done in fifteen to thirty minutes.

Before such testing we discuss its fallibility with the patient. To his question "Then why do skin testing at all?", we point out that unsuspected food allergy is at times indicated by moderate or especially by large reactions. Moreover, the scratch or puncture test is harmless and only requires one or two sittings of not more than forty-five minutes each, which includes the time necessary for the interpretation of the skin tests. Some patients object to skin testing because of the large number of tests done on friends not only by the scratch but also by the intradermal method often with an unwarranted number of foods, such testing requiring several office visits even up to ten or twenty in number, and also because of the expense of such testing. Such extended testing in our opinion is unjustifiable.

TEST-NEGATIVE DIETS—THEIR USUAL FAILURE TO DETERMINE CLINICAL FOOD ALLERGY

In spite of the vagaries of skin testing for food allergy, certain patients are relieved by diets in which skin-reacting foods are eliminated. Such diets have been well named by Rackemann as *test-negative diets*. The relief of a few patients unfortunately has encouraged many physicians to place unwarranted confidence in the test-negative diets. However, the fact that symptoms are not relieved does not by any means exclude the possibility that food allergy is a cause of the symptoms. It must be stressed that the allergenic effect of a suspected food can be determined only by the reproduction of the symptoms in a patient who has become symptom free through the elimination of causative foods. Thus the test-negative diets frequently exclude foods which are not productive of allergy. This is especially true if the intradermal test is used, since it often gives false reactions or those indicative of past or potential sensitization. Some allergists advise the exclusion of all foods which give even slight reactions by the intradermal tests. Retesting on several occasions is advised if relief does not occur. During this process additional reactions may occur and others may disappear, so that gradually most of the foods eaten by the patient may come under the suspicion of allergy. The possible allergenicity of such reacting foods is always in question and as stated above, can be determined only by feeding them to the symptom-free patient.

These test-negative diets often make the preparation of satisfactory meals difficult, especially when all foods that give slight or suspicious reactions, particularly with the intradermal test, are eliminated. It may be impossible to arrange balanced meals with the essential protein, minerals, vitamins, and calories with such nonreacting foods. The necessity of providing each patient with definite menus which protect nutrition and proper weight whenever a test-negative or the elimination diets are prescribed is discussed in Chapter 3.

Thus, if test-negative diets alone are used to diagnose food allergy, many patients will fail to receive relief and will be denied the benefit to be derived from the discovery and elimination of all allergenic foods. These test-negative diets are prescribed by the writers only when definite positive reactions obtained with the scratch test check with the patient's history of probable food idiosyncrasies. Moreover, in the majority of our patients who are suspected of food allergy, the elimination diets, modified by a history of probable food allergies and by definite skin reactions by the scratch method as described throughout this book, are used for the diagnostic study of possible food allergy as detailed and advised in Chapter 3. The elimination diets, moreover, may be used without the scratch tests if these are not available. This is further discussed in Chapter 30.

SKIN TESTING FOR INHALANT ALLERGY

Unless food allergy is the unquestioned sole cause of the clinical allergy, scratch tests with all important inhalants in the patient's indoor and out-of-door environments should be routine. If scratch tests are negative to inhalants that are suspect in the patient's history, intradermal tests are justified. In our practice such intradermal tests are not routine, since antibodies in the skin nearly always give positive scratch reactions when dependable inhalant allergens are used.

When the environmental history reveals animals or birds in the house of patients with perennial symptoms and scratch tests with such animal emanations are negative, intradermal tests with those allergens may be advisable. When scratch tests are negative and the history suggests clinical allergy to pollens, house dust, or fungi, intradermal tests thereto are justifiable. In our practice such intradermal testing with inhalants is infrequent. Negative skin tests to causative inhalants may occur.

That moderate and also large scratch reactions to pollens, animal emanations, and other inhalants are not necessarily indicative of clinical allergy must be emphasized. Pollen-sensitive patients quite often give moderate or large reactions to many or even practically all grass, tree, summer, and fall pollens and are allergic only to the grass or to the fall pollens. Many patients give definite reactions to house dust or to various fungi to which no clinical allergy exists. Desensitization to inhalants, especially house dust, because of positive skin tests without a definite history of clinical allergy thereto is unjustified. Provocation inhalant tests with a reacting inhalant allergen are usually necessary to prove its clinical importance.

The preparation of pollen and other inhalant allergens for testing, antigens for treatment, and the methods of desensitization used in our practice for forty years are summarized in Chapter 30.

Animal emanations, miscellaneous inhalants, and house and other dust allergens suggested for routine scratch tests are listed in Chapter 30. Important pollens of primary and secondary importance in all areas in the United States are listed on pages 80 to 81.

Children up to the age of one-half year are rarely allergic to pollens. If other inhalants in the house are suspected, strict environmental control is indicated for diagnosis and relief.

If inhalant allergy is suspected in older children, scratch or puncture tests with a limited number of pollens and other inhalant allergens in the patient's home and out-of-door environments are advisable.

No intradermal testing is justified in infants and young children.

Failure to realize that positive skin reactions to inhalants, as is the case with foods, do not necessarily indicate clinical allergy accounts for much ineffectual and often unnecessary injectant therapy. Unnecessary desensitization especially occurs when the allergic manifestations are due to food allergy which has not been studied and controlled as we advise and when the symptoms have been attributed to inhalant allergens based solely on positive skin reactions.

We have patients who have been injected one or two times a week for two to even twenty years with conventional inhalant antigens usually containing various pollens, animal emanations, and other inhalants; dusts; and fungi with no relief until the sole use of the cereal-free elimination diet has given excellent relief of symptoms resulting from causative food allergies in one to two months.

One woman with perennial asthma for thirty years resulting in moderate obstructive emphysema unrelieved by injections of a conventional inhalant antigen one to two times a week for twenty years was entirely relieved of her asthma and symptoms of emphysema in one month with control of previously unrecognized food allergy with our cereal-free elimination diet. Another young woman with perennial nasal allergy for twelve years unrelieved with the injection of a conventional inhalant antigen given every week for nine years was definitely relieved in one month and entirely relieved in three months by control of food allergy with adherence to our cereal-free elimination diet and with no injectant therapy.

FEEDING OR PROVOCATION FOOD TESTS

After relief from the advised use of the elimination diets published in 1928 and also in the first edition of this book, allergy to additional foods to those in the relieving diet was determined by feeding of single additional foods, each for one to three days every five to seven days, eliminating those reactivating the patient's symptoms. Determination of clinical allergy to such foods thereby has been made by the patient under the supervision of the doctor at home, obviating his and the patient's time in his office required by the method advised by Rinkel and modified by Randolph.

INDIVIDUAL FOOD TESTS (RINKEL AND RANDOLPH)

Though our long-advised use of elimination diets and additional provocation tests have revealed and controlled clinical food allergy as reported increasingly through the years and confirmed in this volume, additional information about allergy to various foods obtained from individual food tests as advised by Rinkel may be obtained, favoring the use of his method in our practice when a) possible confirmation of clinical allergy to single foods is desired in the office or hospital; b) when study of possible unrecognized allergy to individual foods in a minimal elimination diet does not control the symptoms in two to four weeks even though inhalant and drug allergies seem adequately controlled; and c) when possible allergy to cane, beet, or corn sugar and cottonseed or other vegetable oil, as discussed on pages 587 to 589, or when elucidation of allergy to unusual or even common foods seems advisable.

Resultant symptoms would require confirming evidence of clinical allergy, probably with additional feeding tests.

Since the technique of this individual food test advised by Rinkel and later by Randolph is or will be utilized by allergists and physicians with or without the use of the elimination diets, a summary of Rinkel's article on the indications for its use and his advised technique is printed below.

PROVOCATION INTRADERMAL FOOD TEST WITH COMMENTS

Rinkel also advised this test in patients with suspected food allergies who have required no medications for the control of symptoms when the tests are done. 0.05 cc of a 1:5 dilution of a 1:20 extract of a specific food is given in a superficial intracutaneous injection in two areas on the upper arm. If allergic symptoms develop in twenty minutes, probable allergy to the food is indicated. A local wheal is not required. According to Rinkel, neutralization of the symptoms usually occurs soon afterward from an injection of 0.1 cc of the number 8, followed if necessary by the number 7 dilutions. Such relief justifies performing similar tests with additional foods in one sitting during one to two hours.

Patients are required to omit all corticoids and other drugs for ten days and to avoid foods to be tested for four days before the tests.

If the patient is having symptoms, neutralization rather than provocation tests are advised by Rinkel, reference to which is omitted in Willoughby's article (1965). Rinkel states that subcutaneous injection of 0.1 cc of the number 12, followed if relief of symptoms does not occur by successive injections of stronger dilutions, may control the symptoms arising from the chosen food. If symptoms from two to eight or more foods are present, neutralization to one food obviously would not control the causative food allergies.

Comment

The good and excellent results from strict and adequate use of the elimination diets without which the important control of food allergy in its many manifestations reported by us in 1931 and increasingly confirmed by us and many other physicians during the last forty years has not encouraged our using Rinkel's technique.

Moreover, since more than one and usually several foods and at times even a larger number cause the patient's clinical allergy, individual tests to many foods would be required. This increases the time and effort by the physician for such studies.

The delay of the elimination of allergenic foods from the body tissues after ingestion for several days or longer and the slowness with which tissue changes resulting from chronic food allergy disappear even with meticulous complete elimination of all allergenic foods without the aid of corticosteroids are shown in Figure 16. These results occurred two years before such corticoid hormones were available.

Continued, precise effort is required by all physicians who are challenged with the control of the manifestations of foods by the elimination of all allergenic foods and not by corticosteroids. Such control of food allergy of course also necessitates the control of concomitant inhalant and contact allergies if they exist.

Necessary recognition of the various characteristics of food allergy reported in Chapters 1 and 2 of this volume emphasizes the total elimination of all allergenic foods.

The physician who wishes to evaluate the provocation test of Rinkel must be guided by the article of Rinkel *et al.* in 1964 and not by other articles since then.

Since the meticulous technique and use of his adjunctive recommendations require time to master by their use in many patients for weeks or longer periods, similar or even less time and effort in perfecting the use of our elimination diets will be preferable and rewarding. The successful utilization of our elimination diets, moreover, is available to all physicians and specialists, especially allergists, who desire to master the use of the elimination diets as advised in Chapter 3.

RANDOLPH FASTING TECHNIQUE

Initial fasting for four days with subsequent individual feeding tests to determine allergy to specific foods combined with the study of inhalant, chemical, and other factors detrimental to health in an ecologically controlled hospital unit was advised by Randolph. The disadvantages, including confinement in and cost of study in an ecologically controlled hospital unit, compared with the use of the elimination diets and environmental control usually at home, without which this volume emphasizing food allergy could not have been written, with considered use of Randolph's technique in some chronically ill, especially mentally disturbed patients are discussed in Chapter 30.

LEUKOPENIC INDEX IN THE DETERMINATION OF FOOD ALLERGY

Vaughan, in 1934 and 1936, utilized the reduction in the leukocytes in the blood as an indication of possible clinical allergy to an ingested food. Leukopenia during allergic reactions had been previously reported by French investigators. We evaluated this test for many months. Our conclusion agreed with that of other allergists that the counting of the leukocytes is open to possible error and that leukopenia is questionable or fails to occur to many foods productive of slight or recurrent allergy, so that its use was discontinued many years ago. As with positive skin tests, moreover, such leukopenia is only of clinical significance after the allergic manifestation has

been reestablished by the feeding of a food to the symptom-free patient.

SKIN WINDOW TECHNIQUE

Bullock and Deamer have shown that the skin window technique, for soluble allergens at least, has no advantage whatever over the conventional skin test.

BLACK'S CYTOTOXIC TEST

Bryan and Bryan have developed Black's cytotoxic test for finding the specificity of a patient's allergies. They place an allergen extract on a slide and add leukocytes and serum from the patient. If the patient is sensitive to the test allergen, the leukocytes cease producing pseudopods, become rounded, and if the reaction is strong, disintegrate. The test is reported by them only with allergen *extracts*, however, and thus cannot determine allergy to the great majority of food substances which are insoluble. The allergen extract concentration is usually kept down to 125μg per milliliter, so that it would seem to be technically very difficult to spread such small amounts of insoluble allergen over a slide. On the other hand, the thermodynamic activity of a solid is much less than that of a substance in solution. On purely steric grounds one would expect a substance with 50 Angstrom molecules to have about one thousand times the activity of a substance with 20μ granules. In any case difficulties may arise in ensuring contact between the leukocytes and the antigen granules.

For these reasons the cytotoxic method, while theoretically interesting, has not been shown to yield more information than scratch tests and is not as easy to perform. No proof that all soluble reacting antigens produce clinical allergy is available at the present time. Hence, provocation ingestion tests are required to determine clinical value of foods giving positive cytotoxic reactions. This information is obtained by any physician with the elimination diets without use of these tests which require the effort of specially trained technicians which in turn require provocation tests to obtain the same desired relief.

ACCELERATED PULSE TEST FROM FOOD ALLERGY

Coca, in 1943, reported an increased pulse rate above an established maximal normal after the ingestion of an allergenic food, especially in his book *Familial Non-Reagenic Food Allergy* in 1943, so named because of the usual negative skin test to causative foods, as we have long reported. Though this results from definite food allergies, its origin immediately after the ingestion of a food to which slight or recurrent or cumulative food allergy exists is questionable and also difficult to substantiate. The dependability of conclusions from testing several foods each day also is questionable, since allergic reactions are known to persist for hours and often for several days after the ingestion of even minute amounts of allergenic foods.

The value of this test has never been confirmed by carefully controlled clinical trial. Moreover, the use of our elimination diets is a more simple and standardized procedure for the study of possible food allergies.

PRECIPITIN HEMAGGLUTINATION AND GEL-DIFFUSION TESTS FOR ANTIBODIES TO FOODS

Evidence of possible food allergy is being increasingly reported by the demonstrations of specific γG antibodies with Boyden's tanned red cell hemagglutination (TRCH), and the gel-diffusion test of Ouchterlony. Taylor and Truelove have reported increased γG antibodies to milk in chronic ulcerative colitis relieved by its elimination. Gray also has found such an increase. Taylor, Thomson, Truelove, and Wright have also shown increased γG antibodies to wheat and milk in celiac disease and idiopathic steatorrhea.

Though positive precipitin tests to milk and other foods have long been reported, especially in children and recently by Diner, Kniker, and Heiner, the TRCH test is very much more sensitive. The bisdiazotized benzidene (BDB), hemagglutination test as discussed by Stavitsky and Arquilla gives similar information but is more complicated and only preferable when the TRCH test yields nonspecifically agglutinable cells. Complement fixation tests have not been so successful in showing antibodies to foods.

Thus the TRCH and gel-diffusion tests will be increasingly used to affirm food allergy. However, as with positive skin tests, the clinical importance of demonstrated antibodies depends on the reproduction of asthma or other manifestations of allergy by provocation ingestion tests with the foods in question.

TECHNIQUE OF SKIN TESTING
Scratch Tests

Since 1927 we have strongly advised initial scratch tests. This is done by making a superficial scratch one-third to one-half inch long with a dull, pointed knife or needle so that blood is not drawn. Dry or liquid food allergens are then rubbed into the scratches with clean toothpicks. Tests are made on the upper arms, forearms, or back, though the legs or abdomen are available if patients do not wish the scratches to show.

Patients other than infants and small children may be tested by the scratch method with 150 to 250 food, animal emanation, dust, and inhalant soluble allergens by experienced technicians in one to two hours. Infants and young children are tested with ten to forty ingested foods and if indicated, important inhalants occurring in their environments usually in one and at times in two sittings. Less important allergens should be reserved for future testing if symptoms are not relieved by therapy.

The reaction consists of an edematous wheal with varying peripheral erythema often associated with localized itching. The reaction varies from one-third to one inch in diameter. The edema may extend into the peripheral lymphatics, forming pseudopodia. The size of the reaction is indicated by one to six plus. The reactions usually disappear in one to four hours, though localized edema may persist or even increase for twenty-four hours.

General reactions have never occurred in our practice from even 250 scratch tests done in one sitting, providing the scratches do not exceed more than one-half inch in length.

Puncture Tests

This test is done by piercing or pricking the skin with a single-pointed or two-pointed sterile needle through a drop of liquid allergen. Though it is always used in infants two to four months of age, it at times replaces the scratch test even in adults. The positive wheal and surrounding erythema are usually smaller than that arising from the scratch test. This test is used in all ages by Doctor Frankland at St. Mary's Hospital in London.

Intradermal Tests

Though intradermal tests are not done with soluble food allergens even when negative reactions occur from previous scratch tests, they may be done with inhalant allergens that have not reacted by the scratch tests, with the exceptions noted in this chapter. Severe and even fatal reactions from initial intradermal tests with no previous scratch reactions do occur. These reactions have not occurred with the scratch test. In our office, when intradermal tests are indicated, they are done with 0.02 cc of a 1:1000 extract of inhalant allergens that have not given definite reactions by the scratch test.

Passive Transfer Tests

This test has been advised occasionally in patients so covered with dermatitis that skin testing is difficult. Prausnitz and Küstner, in 1921, discovered skin-reacting serum antibodies in most patients definitely allergic to food or inhalant allergens. If 0.2 to 0.3 cc of the serum is injected into many skin areas of a normal recipient, testing the injected sites in twenty-four hours with food and inhalant allergens usually gives positive skin tests to allergens when skin-reacting antibodies to the allergen are present in the patient's serum. This method of testing requires careful laboratory technique and must be reserved for specialists' use in selected cases. There is also the risk of transmitting hepatitis or other infections.

OCULAR AND NASAL TESTS

Since inhalants give negative scratch tests in 10 to 15 percent of sensitive patients, dry or liquid allergens dropped onto the palpebral conjunctiva may produce conjunctival erythema and watery discharge, sneezing, coughing, and wheezing in five to ten minutes, indicative of allergy. This ocular test is also used to determine the dilution of an inhalant antigen with which initial desensitization is indicated. When the allergen is blown into the nose or bronchial tract, resultant hay fever or asthma also indicates allergy to the allergen. Epinephrine 1:1500 dropped into the conjunctival sac will reduce the allergic reaction.

PATCH TESTS IN CONTACT ALLERGY

Erythema and itching may occur on the skin from contact with allergenic foods. For example, dermatitis may result from the handling of tomatoes, various fruits, fish, eggs, and other foods. Usually atopic allergy is also present, as indicated by scratch skin reactions and especially by history. The reaction occurs in a few minutes and is usually known to the patient. Contact allergy to various resins and vegetations or chemicals occurs in hours or one to two days after the allergen has been held in contact with the skin by a patch test. This test will be referred to again in Chapter 14.

WHEN TO DESENSITIZE

The clinical importance of positive reactions to fungi especially requires provocation tests. Whereas the importance of *Alternaria* is reported by many allergists, that of other fungi which give positive skin reactions needs clinical confirmation. Many slight or moderate and even large reactions to inhalants are not indicative of clinical allergy. Desensitization with allergens giving positive reactions and which cause no clinical allergy is not beneficial or justified.

ADVISED ROUTINE SKIN TESTING

1. *In children over the age of ten years, adolescents, and adults.*
Scratch tests with 100 to 180 soluble allergens of ingested food and inhaled allergens are indicated when perennial clinical allergy is present.
2. *In children five to ten years of age.*

Scratch tests with soluble allergens of 75 to 120 ingested foods and inhalants in the child's environment are advised.
3. *Infants after the age of one month.*
Puncture tests with the above allergens of ingested foods, often to cow's milk alone, are advised. If the child is on cow's milk, goat's milk, soybean, or beef-based or lamb-based formulas, tests with the respective proteins are indicated. As other foods are added to the diet, tests with them also are advisable.
4. *In infants older than three to four months.*
Scratch or puncture tests with the above allergens of ingested foods are advised. If inhalant allergy is suspected, scratch or puncture tests with environmental allergens which cannot be eliminated from the living environment and important pollens in the outdoor areas are advised.
5. *In children from the age of one and one-half to five years.*
Puncture or scratch tests with the soluble allergens of ingested foods and inhalants in the indoor and outdoor environment are advised.

This routine testing can be done by an experienced technician or physician in one-half to one hour on arms and back, as already advised. Though one sitting may suffice for the initial study, a second sitting may be advisable. Testing patients with three hundred to four hundred allergens even with the scratch test alone, doing twenty to thirty tests each day for ten or even twenty days, is unnecessarily expensive and time-consuming for the patient and physician.

As stated previously we do routine skin tests with nearly all ingested foods, hoping to reveal large reactions which indicate the immediate type of food allergy. Foods, however, which cause immediate symptoms are usually known to the patient. If the patient is not aware of immediate allergy to a food giving a large scratch reaction, its allergenicity has to be determined by a provocation test.

Lists of food and inhalant allergens for skin testing for adults and for children are given in Chapter 30. Methods for making food and inhalant allergens are on page 605. The botanical classification of foods is on pages 535 to 541.

WHEN SKIN TESTING IS NOT AVAILABLE OR NOT DEPENDABLE

If scratch testing with foods is not available, the possibility of food allergy can be studied with the cereal-free elimination diet as advised in Chapter 3. A detailed diet history must be recorded. If immediate or definite allergy is evidenced to specific foods included in the elimination diets, they should be deleted. Moreover, if skin testing must be done with food allergens of questionable strength and dependability or by one who is inexperienced in the technique, it may be best to omit skin testing and study food allergy with elimination diets alone as advised in this volume, especially in Chapter 3.

ALLERGENS AND ALLERGINS

The ingested or inhaled substance to which a patient becomes sensitized is called an allergen, to which reacting bodies, or antibodies, develop in the body. Evidence indicates that these antibodies arise especially in the plasma and probably in lymphoid cells in particular in the intestinal mucosa. They accumulate in the serum globulin. At the present time immunologists are demonstrating and hypothesizing hundreds of such serum antibodies (different specificities) to the proteins and probably to carbohydrates of ingestants, inhalants, infectants, and to the allergens of various body tissues, such as the thyroid, muscle, or colon.

Serum antibodies to foods are found by immunologists in all people. It is hypothesized that the antibodies (allergins) which are responsible for clinical allergy attach to the cells of the shock tissues, making them susceptible to an allergic reaction. After ingestion of the specific foods, the allergen passes into the blood and unites with the allergin on the sensitized cells, releasing histamine or other chemicals which disrupt the function of the cells causing allergic symptoms. Though these antibodies are found in all patients who ingest the foods, immunologists have reported increase in the allergins when allergy to the food is present.

Evidence indicates that the allergin responsible for the symptoms of clinical allergy is also responsible for the positive skin tests and the PK reaction. The common absence of skin reactions to foods which cause definite clinical allergy can be explained in part by the attachment of the allergin to the cells of the shock tissues along with its absence or the inability to demonstrate it in the skin by our present immunological techniques. Antibodies to insoluble carbohydrates, as demonstrated by Lietze, could also explain such negative skin reactions.

Antibodies to chemicals and drugs which cause manifestations of allergy, for example, aspirin, arise from their union with a body protein acting as a carrier. At present the demonstration of this antibody in the serum globulin fraction of sensitized patients has not been demonstrated.

Contact allergy to chemicals also depends on their haptenic union with a body protein to the combination of which an antibody arises. This is demonstrated by a patch test causing a delayed reaction.

Whether the antibody is present in the serum globulin as in atopic allergy has not been determined by immunologists.

SERUM ANTIBODIES TO FOODS

For over thirty years serum immuno-globulin antibodies to milk, wheat, and eggs have been demonstrated by immunologists with the Ouchterlony technique, by red cell hemagglutination technique, or by other precipitation techniques. Since then antibodies to other foods have been found. These antibodies are not directly involved in the allergy, but an abnormally large titer of any of them, particularly in children, indicates a probable high titer of allergin also.

At first, because of negative skin tests and the fallibility of positive reactions as indications of clinical allergy to foods, it was hoped that the presence of these serum antibodies might establish clinical food allergy. However, it was gradually found that these antibodies to ingested foods are present in the sera of nearly all people who have ingested the foods. The clinical significance of an antibody to a food therefore must be determined by a provocation test with a food in the symptom-free patient.

Recent investigations indicate that the antibody (allergin) responsible for the production of allergic symptoms as well as the positive skin test and the PK reaction to the food is in IgE, which is associated with IgA. Though precipitating antibodies to foods are increased in the patient allergic to the foods, the allergin responsible for the clinical symptoms and the skin test seems to be in IgE globulin and possibly other immunoglobulins.

EOSINOPHILIA AND OTHER CHANGES IN THE BLOOD

Eosinophilic cells also may be abundant in the tissues which harbor the main allergic reactions. The bronchial and nasal mucosae often are infiltrated with them in patients with bronchial asthma and with perennial or seasonal hay fever. The gastrointestinal tissues and the skin contain an excess of these cells when they harbor localized allergy. Thus the secretions from sensitized tissues may contain eosinophils, the presence of which offers diagnostic evidence of allergy, as noted on page 428.

Whether the eosinophilic cells are due to changes in the tissues themselves or whether they have been attracted to the tissues from the bone marrow through the bloodstream is not known, though the latter seems the more likely. Further discussion of eosinophils in allergy appears in Chapter 22.

DIET DIARIES

An analysis of the patient's accurate daily record of all foods he has eaten and of his various symptoms may enable him or his physician to discover specific foods which are responsible for various allergic manifestations. However, unless the patient is eating at home and every ingredient, including condiments, is listed, these diaries are of questionable value in ascertaining the foods, beverages, or condiments which in minute amounts cause allergy. When the patient eats away from home, he may not recognize traces of milk, butter, wheat, eggs, pepper, spices, or other ingredients. These foods therefore would not be listed in his daily record of ingested foods. Unless these diaries are accurate, the work incurred by their tabulation and the necessary time spent by the physician in their analysis are hardly justified. They are infrequently requested of our patients.

DIARY OF HOME, WORK, AND RECREATIONAL ACTIVITIES AND EXPOSURES

A patient's diary of his various activities, his routine of work, his social and recreational engagements, and a record of the various symptoms of possible allergic origin may be of considerable help in the determination of possible inhalant allergies. From such a diary the physician can ascertain possible contacts with household allergens (what animals are in and out of doors and what flowers, shrubs, trees, and vines are about the house) and the other possible origins of inhalant allergens. When inhalant or contact allergies are suspected as causes of the patient's symptoms, the physician must study the possibilities of all such allergens through careful questioning. Thus a diary of activities with a record of all possible inhalant and contactant exposures may aid in the solution of obscure or difficult problems.

DETERMINATION OF ALLERGENIC FOODS

It is noted in Chapter 3 that most patients either fail to react to all foods or often any to which allergy exists or give reactions which are nonspecific or which are not associated with any allergic manifestation. Thus diets only excluding skin-reacting foods usually fail to reveal or relieve food allergy. When positive skin reactions are present, their role in the production of clinical allergy can only be determined by the feeding of each reacting food to the necessarily symptom-free patient. Definite exaggeration or recurrence of symptoms, when confirmed, indicates probable allergy to the added food.

The unquestioned decision that a given food causes allergic reactivity often is difficult. Tolerance varies in every individual.

In some patients symptoms may recur immediately in a violent manner even from a trace of food or in very sensitive patients from inhalation of its osmyls; in others they may arise in a few hours or in two or three days; in still others they may not recur until the food has been eaten daily for one to three days. The tendency for allergic manifestations to recur in cyclic attacks with interim periods of freedom resulting from exhaustion of antibodies to the food with resultant refractoriness is emphasized in Chapter 8. The frequent decrease or absence of symptoms arising from food allergy in the summer, as emphasized in Chapter 1, always must be remembered. When the patient gives a definite history of intolerance or idiosyncrasy to individual foods, clinical evidence of allergy to those foods often is easily obtained.

Discussion of individual food tests as used by Rinkel and Randolph is in Chapter 30.

DIET TRIAL, ESPECIALLY WITH ELIMINATION DIETS

Because of the fallibility of skin testing and the resultant failure of nearly all test-negative diets to relieve chronic food allergy, trial diets, especially our elimination diets first advised in 1928, which exclude foods which most frequently cause food allergy, are advised in Chapter 3 for the study and relief of such clinical allergy.

Our realization of the role of food allergy as the sole cause of the many manifestations of clinical allergy or in association with inhalant or less often drug allergies has been increasingly affirmed with the adequate, strict use of our elimination diets for forty years.

When the published menus and recipes for bakery products are followed and the advised intake of proteins, minerals, and vitamins as well as calories is maintained, nutrition and weight are protected. All of this information and advice about the modification of these diets together with instructions for individual feeding (provocation) tests to determine other foods to which the patient is not allergic are published in Chapter 3. The elimination diets as we advise must be used to diagnose or rule out food allergy in the same way that other laboratory tests, x-rays, or diagnostic procedures are used in the investigation of other diseases.

The advantages of elimination diets compared with test-negative diets, other modified trial diets, and especially fasting for one week are discussed in Chapter 30.

SUMMARY

1. Food allergy is indicated by symptoms of possible atopic allergy, a history of food dislikes and disagreements, available information from scratch tests, and result of diet trial, especially with our elimination diets as advised in Chapter 3.

2. Routine scratch tests with important inhalants, including fungi and especially pollens, animal emanations, and dusts, are advised.

3. Limited use of scratch tests and their value are discussed.

4. The frequency of negative reactions and fallibility of positive tests make trial diet, especially with our elimination diets, mandatory. Confirmation of food allergy as indicated by history, trial diet, and even by large skin reactions, if they occur, usually requires provocation tests.

5. The methods of scratch and puncture tests and the disuse of intradermal tests in infants and children and infrequently in adults are advised.

6. Our advised Feeding (Provocation) Food Tests are discussed.

7. The Individual Food Test advised by Rinkel and Randolph is described.

8. Provocation Intradermal Food Tests of Rinkel and Lee are discussed.

9. Because of limited information from the leukopenic index, Coca's pulse test, and the necessity of expertized use of Black's cytotoxic test, as advised by Bryan and Bryan, with the necessity of confirming clinical allergy by provocation ingestion tests, the use of our elimination diets is favored. They afford a simpler and more dependable method of study and control of food allergy when they are strictly and adequately used as we advise.

10. Excellent results can be obtained by all physicians, including specialists and allergists, in the study and control of food allergy with or without inhalant allergy and drug allergy if elimination diets are used as we advise. Ability to study and control clinical allergy with these diets and efficiency and success in their use require accurate and adequate use in more than a few patients for more than a few weeks.

Chapter 3

Elimination Diets (Rowe)
in the Control of Food Allergy

The importance of the information in this chapter about our elimination diets for the study and control of the many manifestations of clinical food allergy justifies the following initial summary of its contents.

1. Evolution of elimination diets as we so named them forty-five years ago is summarized. Directions for their preparation and enlargement with additional tolerated foods, detailed menus, and recipes for prescribed bakery products are detailed.

a. The cereal-free elimination diet is of major importance for study of most clinical food allergy.

(1) It is modified for the study and control of food allergy in infants and children with soybean milk (Neo-Mull-Soy®) devoid of corn glucose or our lamb-base formula when allergy to soy and to cow's milk is possible.

b. A fruit-free, cereal-free elimination diet is advised when allergy to fruits also may be present.

c. Minimal elimination diet as necessary to study allergy to many or nearly all foods.

d. Rotary diet as suggested by Rinkel supplements minimal elimination diets. The following information is discussed:

1. Ordering of the elimination diets in hospital and home.

2. Important recipes for bakery products for the Elimination Diets (Rowe).

Note: These diets were revised in 1970.

3. The time necessary to determine role of food allergy.

4. The necessity of detailed menus.

5. Menus for meals away from the home and for lunches to take to work.

6. Necessary, strict, informed supervision of the diets by physicians.

7. Graphic Record of Manipulation of the Elimination Diets (Rowe).

8. Addition of foods after relief occurs (provocation tests).

9. The making of soy-potato bakery products.

10. Use of the CFE diet without bakery products.

11. Allergy to soy beans and lima beans.

12. The necessary delay in adding cereal grains.

13. Reasons for failure to obtain relief of symptoms with the elimination diets.

14. Development of tolerance to allergenic foods.

15. Necessary maintenance of weight and nutrition.

16. Directions of addition of cereal grains and beef to the cereal-free elimination diet.

17. Summary.

ELIMINATION DIETS (ROWE)

The elimination diets include foods which infrequently produce clinical allergy. Because of the frequency of negative skin reactions to foods which cause cumulative or chronic allergy and the fallibility of many positive reactions as indicators of present clinical allergy, diet trial, especially with our elimination diets, remains the most important diagnostic procedure, in our opinion, for the study and control of possible food allergy by all physicians and specialists, including allergists.

The clinical value of elimination diets, especially our cereal-free elimination (CFE) diet, for the study and control of the many clinical manifestations of food allergy, alone or associated with inhalant and (less often) with drug or chemical allergy, has been confirmed by us and other allergists for over forty years. Our good or excellent control of the many manifestations of food allergy with or without inhalant and (at times) drug allergy recorded in this volume, especially in recurrent or chronic perennial bronchial asthma, chronic bronchitis, and obstructive lung disease, have been reported only in patients who have cooperated with us for a minimum of three months.

The reported failure of several allergists to confirm our conclusion that food allergy is a major cause of atopic allergy especially in perennial bronchial asthma with our elimination diets is explained as follows:

1. Their diet was similar but not identical to our CFE diet.

2. Their diet was used for only "eighteen days" instead of a minimum of three months, according to our published advice, which we have always required to evaluate the role of food allergy.

3. Since developing facility in ordering and supervising our elimination diets requires their use in several cooperating patients for a minimum of three months, conclusions, especially from a trial diet in only one or two patients per physician for

a brief eighteen-day period by physicians are open to criticism.

Since 1926 when we first proposed the name *elimination diets* for those that omit foods which most frequently cause allergy, namely, milk, wheat, eggs, fish, nuts, chocolate, coffee, condiments, and a few vegetables and fruits, instead of previously advised elimination of wheat, milk, eggs, and other suspicious, usually skin-reacting foods, we have made several revisions in them:

1. By 1932 the frequency of allergy to one or all cereals in addition to wheat was recognized, and they were excluded from the cereal-free elimination diet which we have used most frequently since then.

2. It also became evident that allergy to several or all fruits, spices, and condiments required their total exclusion, leading to the formulation of our fruit-free, cereal-free elimination diet in 1942.

3. For the first time total elimination of beef is advised in the latest revision of our elimination diet. Previously beef has been allowed except when large skin reactions or probable symptoms arising to it have occurred. For several years frequent allergy to beef has been encountered, and its limited use one to three times a week has been advised. Now because of the increasing clinical and immunological evidence of frequent allergy to beef, it is entirely eliminated in our initial trial elimination diets. Advice about its later provocation feeding test is discussed on page 75.

4. Modification of this diet for infants and young children with the use of Mull-Soy, which contains no corn glucose, and also of our strained meat formulae as substitutes for animal milks has been established. Allergy to corn glucose when corn allergy is being studied or is present must

be taken into consideration, as discussed on page 468.

5. Realization that allergy exists to many or nearly all foods, comparable to allergy to nearly all pollens, also has required the use of minimal elimination diets. Therefore, in contrast to elimination diets 1, 2, and 3 published in the first edition of this book thirty-nine years ago, the cereal-free elimination diet has been in our daily use for over thirty-six years and its two modifications for over thirty years. This diet and its modifications have become standardized and are being used by many physicians today for the routine study of food allergy.

Before 1931 this diet was published as the cereal-free elimination diet 1, 2, 3. The numbers referred to Diets 1, 2, and 3 which were published in the first edition of this book, all of which contained one or more cereal grains other than wheat. Because of the increasing evidence of allergy to one and often to all cereals, initial use of diets containing cereals has been replaced by our cereal-free elimination diet to which the numbers 1, 2, and 3 no longer are appended. The initial use of Diets 1, 2, and 3 which contain cereal grains, published in 1928 to 1931, is no longer advised. Rinkel, Randolph, and other allergists have confirmed this frequent allergy to cereals as well as to wheat, especially to corn, not only in the United States but also in other countries as by Colldahl, in 1965, in Sweden and Kaplan in Johannesburg. Our diets are identified by "Rowe" in parenthesis to designate the diets with the routine use of which we have recognized the important characteristics and the clinical manifestations of food allergy reported in this volume.

The importance of the use of this standardized elimination diet and its advised modifications rather than various other similar but nonstandardized diets is discussed and emphasized in Chapter 30.

Food diaries and symptom records (see Chapt. 30) can be kept before use of our elimination diets to eliminate foods which may in the patient's opinion cause allergic symptoms.

The successful demonstration and confirmation of food allergy requires careful, adequate study of the discussion of our elimination diets, especially in this entire chapter, and not the casual use of lists of allowed foods usually without necessary recipes for allowed bakery products and little or no advice about the necessary strict preparation and supervision of the menus and gradual evolution of a final nonallergenic diet, all of which is impossible to impart in one to three pages of a medical article or textbook on clinical allergy. The physician's responsibility to recognize and control food allergy with or without inhalant and less often chemical allergy requires such adequate study and effort.

With their accurate, sufficient use as advised in this chapter, our diets have proved the "open sesame" to many explanations of unsolved and frustrating manifestations of atopic allergy challenging all general practitioners, specialists, and especially allergists.

Additional advice about the accurate preparation and strict maintenance of our elimination diets which is given to our patients after our personal instruction about the prescribed diet is in Chapter 30.

CEREAL-FREE ELIMINATION DIET (ROWE)—ITS PREPARATION, USE, MAINTENANCE, AND MANIPULATION

1. This diet includes foods which infrequently cause clinical allergy. If there is a history of definite disagreement or if a large scratch reaction occurs to a food,

it can be eliminated. Menus and recipes for bakery products must always be given to the patient.

2. No trace of any food not listed in the diet may be taken. Utensils and dishes must be clean.

3. Because the allergens of previously eaten foods remain in the body for one or more weeks and because slight traces of allergenic foods can produce symptoms, deviations from the diet must not occur. Maximum allergy must be assumed.

4. If relief occurs and continues for two to three times as long as previous periods of relief, other vegetables, fruits, and then cereals can be added one by one every two to five days. Directions for the addition of rice, oats, and corn are outlined later in this chapter.

5. When clinical allergy produces attacks or exaggeration, as in asthma, headaches, or other symptoms, every one-half to one month, the attacks should be relieved and be absent for at least one month before additional fruits and vegetables and two to three months before cereals are added. With continued relief, wheat, milk, eggs, and later other foods can be tried, eliminating any which reproduces symptoms.

6. If symptoms recur in hours or one to three days after the addition of a new food, it must be eliminated. This frequent delay in onset of symptoms after ingestion of a food suspected of producing possible allergy has made our use of Rinkel's technique of individual food tests unnecessary, as is discussed in Chapter 30.

The decrease of food allergy in the summer (Chapt. 1) and refractoriness often occurring after severe attacks of asthma or other clinical food allergy must be remembered in evaluating the effect of a new food. Foods tolerated in the sum-

mer may cause clinical allergy in the winter (Chapt. 1).

7. Soy-potato bakery products must be made at home or by honest bakers strictly supervised by the physician by our recipes or similar recipes. Muffins, cupcakes, and hotcakes can also be made by adding water to the self-rising Cellu-Grainless Mix.

Soy- or lima-potato bakery products sold in health food stores and food markets nearly always contain wheat or gluten of wheat, as demonstrated by Lietze (see Chapt. 28), and at times milk and other forbidden foods not listed in their labels. Serious recurrence of symptoms may result from their use.

Physicians who use this diet should ask women in the home to learn how to make these bakery products so that patients can be assured that it can be done.

The use of the cereal-free elimination (CFE) diet without soybean products if soy flour is not available, if soy produces allergy or disagreements, or if soy products cannot be made or obtained, as in foreign countries, is discussed later in this chapter.

8. A milk-free butter substitute made of soy oil should be used, such as Willow Run Margarine.* Milk-free butter substitutes in foreign countries are discussed later in this chapter.

9. After assured relief, cottonseed or sesame oil can be added. Large scratch reactions to cottonseed indicate possible allergy to its oil. Corn-sensitive patients often develop allergy to its oil, its starch, and to its sugar (glucose). Invert sugar must be given instead of corn glucose if required by vein.

After tolerance of cottonseed and its oil is established, other commercial milk-free oleomargarines containing cottonseed

---

*Obtained from Shedd-Bartush Foods, Inc., Detroit 38, Michigan.

and soy oil, such as Albertson's soft and Blue Bonnet soft, may be tolerated.

If a dislike, disagreement, or possible allergy exists to soy beans or lima beans, they and their bakery products should be eliminated.

If they are not available in foreign countries, other foods in the diet should be given in amounts to maintain nutrition and desired weight as advised later in this chapter.

10. Symptoms may result from the inhalation of airborne powders, molecules, or osmyls of allergenic foods, odors of which are apparent. This has been stressed by Feinberg in 1943 and Horesh in 1943 and 1944. Children should not be in the kitchens where foods eliminated from their prescribed diets are cooked. If allergy is marked, especially if large scratch reactions have occurred to allergenic foods, they should not be in refrigerators or in the house. If such allergy is moderate, total avoidance of odors is less important.

11. Initial and continued use of elimination diets requires maintenance of nutrition and weight. With adequate proteins, calories, synthetic vitamins, and minerals, maintenance of weight and nutrition can be assured. To increase weight, prescribed sugar or its syrup, potatoes, soy bakery products, tapioca, fruit or caramel pudding, milk-free margarine, and prescribed oil should be increased with and between meals and on retiring.

If soy milk or the meat-base formula is not taken, extra calcium in one-half teaspoonful of calcium carbonate in food or water daily is required. If children refuse it, Neo-Calglucon® 8 cc two to three times a day usually is accepted.

12. To produce tolerance to a food, its elimination for weeks, months, or years may be effective. Tolerance often increases

in children and adolescents but may decrease in adult life, especially in old age.

13. Inhalant, drug, and contact allergies associated with food sensitizations must be controlled.

14. The physician must supervise the diet and insist on strict adherence, remembering it must be assumed that it takes one to two weeks or even months for the tissue changes from food allergy to disappear (see Fig. 19 in Chapt. 14).

CEREAL-FREE ELIMINATION DIET (ROWE)

This diet is necessary to study and control possible food allergy in recurrent or perennial bronchial asthma, bronchiolitis, chronic bronchitis, and obstructive emphysema. It is especially important when the typical pathognomonic history of asthma resulting from food allergy characterized by recurrent attacks which are better in the summers occurs in infants, children, and young adults, as described in Chapter 8 and 25.

That most bronchospasm and bronchial mucus in obstructive emphysema are due to allergy, especially to foods, is stressed in Chapters 8 and 11. This diet is also required to investigate and control food allergy in perennial nasal allergy and postnasal mucus; in congestion in the pharynx, larynx, and sinuses; and in recurrent nasal polyposis.

Our CFE diet is also important to study food allergy in perennial allergic dermatitis and eczema, headaches, migraine, allergic fatigue, and other perennial manifestations of allergy.

The importance of the study of possible allergy to all cereal grains as well as to milk, beef, eggs, chocolate, coffee, fish, and other less common allergenic foods has been increasingly realized by us in the last forty years and importantly justified by the discovery of serum antibodies to starches, especially of cereal grains by Lietze reported in Chapter 28.

If fruit allergy is indicated by a history of definite or possible allergy to fruits, spices, or condiments, our fruit-free cereal-free elimination diet, as next detailed in this chapter, is important.

If soy beans and lima beans are disliked or cause allergic reactions, their products must be eliminated. If this occurs, modifications of the diet are necessary as discussed later.

The modification of this diet for infants and young children is also discussed in subsequent pages.

CEREAL-FREE ELIMINATION DIET (ROWE)

Tapioca	Apricots
White potatoes	Grapefruit†
Sweet potatoes or yams	Lemon
Soybean potato bread	Peaches
Lima bean potato bread	Pineapples
	Prunes
Soy milk (Mull-Soy)*	Pears
	Cane or beet sugar
Lamb	Salt
Chicken, fryers,	Sesame oil (not Chinese)
roosters and capon	Soybean oil
(no hens)	Willow Run oleo-
Bacon	margarine‡
Liver (lamb)	Gelatin (Knox's) with
	flavoring of allowed
	fruits and juices

*Mull-Soy (free of corn glucose) may be used. It may cause indigestion.

†The canned fruits should be preserved with cane sugar and not corn sugar. Water-packed fruits may be used and sweetened with cane sugar syrup.

‡A baking powder containing tapioca or potato starch instead of corn starch and no tartaric acid and also Willow Run oleomargarine can be obtained from Bray's, 3764 Piedmont Avenue, Oakland.

*Fruit may be peeled and be fresh or cooked with water or with cane or beet sugar (not with corn sugar, glucose).

Peas	White vinegar
Spinach	Vanilla extract
Squash	Lemon extract
String beans	Corn starch-free baking
Tomatoes	powder‡
	Baking soda
	Cream of tartar
Artichokes	
Asparagus	Maple syrup or syrup
Carrots	made with cane
Lettuce	sugar flavored with
Lima beans	maple

Note: This diet was revised in 1970.

Breakfast

Beverage: | Approximate Amounts
1. Fresh or canned grapefruit or tomato juice. — 4 to 6 oz
2. Pineapple, apricot, peach, or prune juice served singly or mixed with grapefruit juice.*
3. Neo-Mull-Soy (Borden's) is allowed as a drink or in cooking‡

Cereal Substitute:
1. Tapioca cooked with water or fruit juice or pureed apricots, peaches, prunes or pineapple with sugar or flavored with caramel. — ½ cup
2. If tapioca is unavailable, soy potato or potato starch cooked with prescribed fruits or caramel or vanilla and sugar or white or sweet potato may be served.

Bread:†
1. Soy-potato or soy-lima potato bread. — 2 slices
2. Soy-potato muffins, Grainless or Safe Mix may be used. — 2 muffins
3. Soy crackers.
4. Pancakes or waffles made of — 4 medium

†If a baker trusted and supervised by the physician is not available, it is best to make these bakery products at home by our recipes. Bray's, 3764 Piedmont Avenue, Oakland, California, has cooperated with us for over 35 years.

‡Other soy milks contain corn sugar. Neo-Mull-Soy contains sucrose. Neo-Mull-Soy is more palatable than Mull-Soy.

soy and potato flours or
Grainless Mix served with
maple syrup or sugar.

Meat:

1.	Bacon with fried potato if desired.	4 slices
2.	Lamb chops, patties, or tongue (unspiced).	2 med. pats
3.	Lamb liver (no calf liver) and bacon.	2 slices

Approximate Amounts

Butter Substitute:

Willow Run oleomargarine. If
unavailable, soy oil with salt,
bacon grease, jams, preserves
or jellies of specified fruits, or
maple syrup may be used.

Jams or Preserves:

1.	Jams made of pears, pineapple, peaches, apricots, and prunes, singly or in combination	2 tsps

Fruit:

1.	Fresh, cooked or canned* grapefruit, pears, pineapple, peaches, or apricots. Fresh peeled pears, peaches, and apricots may be eaten raw if allowed by the physician.	½ grapefruit, 1 peach or equivalent
2.	Cooked dried prunes. Lemon juice and sugar may be added as desired. No dried apricots, pears, or peaches unless allowed by the physician.	4 prunes

Note: This menu contains approximately 770 calories.

Lunch or Dinner

Approximate Amounts

Soup:

1.	Broth made of lamb or chicken (no hens) served clear with tapioca or cooked with vegetables as previously listed. (No	1 cup

pepper or spices, no canned
soups and no soups away
from home.)

2. Lima bean or split pea soup,
plain, salted, flavored with
bacon. (No milk, butter, or
any other food to be added.)

3. Tomato soup with soybeans.

Salad:

Any combination of vegetables or fruits listed in this diet, dressing only of sesame oil or soy oil, white vinegar or lemon juice, salt and sugar. (*Variations:* a) Lime or lemon flavored gelatin with grated raw carrots or crushed pineapple. b) Cooked, sliced beets pickled in white vinegar and seasoned with salt and sugar.)	½ cup veg. or fruit 1 Tbsp oil

Meat:

1.	Lamb—chops, tongue, or liver; ground plain lamb; roast (hot or cold)—cooked with salt in their own fats or with specified oil. No pepper, condiments, or sauces. Gravies thickened with potato starch.	Av. liberal serving
2.	Chicken, fryers, roosters, capon (no hens). Use prescribed flours and oil.	

Vegetables:

1.	Any listed in this diet, cooked with salt without pepper and served with soy oil or Willow Run oleomargarine.	½ cup
2.	White or sweet potato or yam, baked, boiled, or fried in soy oil or Willow Run oleomargarine. Salt may be used.	1 med.
3.	Sweet potatoes or yams candied with brown sugar or maple syrup.	1 med.
4.	Potato cakes.	

Approximate Amounts

Bread:

Choice of those suggested
for breakfast.

---

*Fruit may be peeled and fresh or cooked with water or with cane or beet sugar (not with corn sugar, glucose).

Butter Substitute:
As suggested for breakfast.
Jams, Preserves, or Jellies:
Choice of those suggested
for breakfast.
Desserts:
1. Fruits as suggested   ½ cup
for breakfast.
2. Tapioca fruit pudding   ½ cup
or Gerber's plum, apricot,
or prune tapioca pudding.
3. Soy-potato pudding.
4. Lemon, lime, or pineapple   ½ cup
flavored gelatin plain,
whipped, or with fruit added.
5. Pears baked with   1 whole
brown sugar.
6. Lemon, pineapple, or apricot
water-ice made with juice,
sugar, and water. (Com-
mercial sherbets and ices
contain milk, egg, or other
forbidden foods.)
7. Soybean, lima bean, potato
cookies, cakes, or cupcakes
or soy cookies made by
our recipes.
Beverage:
Choice of those suggested
for breakfast.
Candies:
1. Candied grapefruit or lemon
peel or glaced pineapple.
(Made at home.)
2. Dried prunes pitted and
stuffed with lemon flavored
fondant. (Made at home.)
3. Pure maple sugar candy.
4. Plain fondant may be made
at home and flavored with
the fruits on this diet.

Note: Between meals, if desired, the patient may have lime, lemon, or pineapple gelatin; potato starch or tapioca fruit pudding; canned fruits; cookies; cakes; cupcakes; or candy made according to recipes in these diets.
This menu contains approximately 1,227 calories.

Total for the Day:

Calories 3,225

Carbohydrate	368 gm	Ca	0.336 gm
Protein	112 gm	P	1.398 gm
Fat	145 gm	Fe	0.025 gm

FRUIT-FREE, CEREAL-FREE ELIMINATION DIET (ROWE)

Allergy to a few and not infrequently to most or all fruits, flavors, and condiments along with allergy to the other foods excluded from the CFE diet has been revealed by the adequate and strict use of our FFCFE diet. It should be modified according to directions for the use of the diet, and meals should be limited to the foods allowed. Fruit and condiment allergy must be suspected in urticaria, angioneurotic edema, urogenital and joint allergies, allergic toxemia and fatigue, and especially in gastrointestinal allergy (see Chapt. 5) and in other cases where fruit allergy is suggested by the diet history. This FFCFE diet and the minimal elimination diets have revealed the frequency of food allergy along with less frequent pollen allergy in the causation of chronic ulcerative colitis, regional enteritis and allergic (idiopathic) diarrhea, and in other manifestations of clinical allergy in which fruit and pollen allergies are causative.

This FFCFE diet requires elimination of all flavored bottled drinks and of other ingestants containing citric acid such as Canada Dry sparkling water and minute or other tapioca containing citric acid. Flavored dentrifices, mouthwashes, douches containing vinegar of fruit origin, denture adhesives and flavored chewing gums, candies and medicines are not allowed. Teeth must be brushed with a plain brush, water, and a little calcium carbonate or soda bicarbonate if desired.

If dislikes, disagreements, or possible allergy to soy beans or lima beans exist, they are eliminated as advised in the preceding diet.

Skin tests with fresh-fruit allergens when positive still require provocation tests for clinical evaluation, as noted in Chapter 2.

FRUIT-FREE CEREAL-FREE ELIMINATION DIET (ROWE)

Tapioca (pearl)°
White potatoes
Potato starch
Sweet potatoes or yams
Soybean-potato bread
Lima bean-potato bread
Neo-Mull-Soy (Borden's)

Cooked carrots
Squash
Artichokes
Peas
Lima beans
String beans

Lamb
Bacon
Chicken (no hens)

Cane or beet sugar
Willow Run oleomargarine†
Soybean oil
Gelatin (Knox)
Salt
Syrup made with cane sugar (no maple syrup)
Corn-free tartaric acid-‡
　　free baking powder§

Breakfast

	Approximate Amounts
Beverage:	
1. Water; tea with or without sugar (if ordered by physician).	5 to 8 oz
2. Neo-Mull-Soy milk (Borden's).	
Cereal Substitutes:	
1. Tapioca (pearl cooked with water and granulated or caramelized sugar or Neo-Mull-Soy).	1 large helping
2. Potato starch pudding.	
3. Pancakes or waffles made of soybean and potato starch flours, served with cane sugar syrup.	4 med. cakes
Meat:	
1. Bacon with fried potato or potato cakes.	4 slices
2. Lamb—chops, patties, or tongue (unspiced).	2 med. chops or equivalent
3. Lamb liver with bacon if desired.	
Bread:	
1. Bread made of any combination of soybeans, lima beans, and potato starch flours.	2 to 4 slices toasted
2. Muffins made of above flours.	2 muffins
Butter Substitute:	
Willow Run oleomargarine or soybean oil with salt, bacon grease, or cane sugar syrup.	1 Tbsp

°Minute tapioca contains citric acid (not allowed in this diet).

Jams or Preserves:

Carrot preserves (no lemon juice) or cane sugar syrup.	2 tsp

Note: This menu contains approximately 587 calories.

Lunch or Dinner

	Approximate Amounts
Soup:	
1. Broth made of lamb or chicken (no hens) served clear with pearl tapioca or cooked with the listed vegetables.	1 cup
2. Lima bean or split pea pureed, flavored with bacon.	1 cup
Salad:	
Any combination of the cooked, listed vegetables. Dressing may be made of soybean or sesame oil, salt, and a little sugar. (No vinegar or spices.)	1 cup mixed vegetables 1 Tbsp oil
Meat:	
1. Lamb—chops, ground plain lamb, roast (hot or cold) cooked with salt in their own fats or with specified oil. No pepper, condiments, or sauces. Gravies thickened	Av. liberal serving

†Kosher margarine is allowed if it contains no cow's milk or its products or if allergy is not present to its vegetable oil.

‡Tartaric acid is made from grapes (not in this diet).

§For corn-free baking powder, see preceding diet.

with potato starch or
soybean flour.

2. Lamb tongue and lamb or
   chicken liver cooked as
   above.

3. Chicken (no hens) may be   ½ broiler,
   roasted, fried, broiled, or   fryer,
   fricasseed, and sesame or   or equiv.
   soybean oil and salt may
   be used. Thicken gravy with
   potato starch or soybean flour.

Vegetables:

1. Any listed in the diet cooked 4 Tbsps veg.
   without pepper and served
   with sesame or soybean oil
   and salted to taste.

2. White or sweet potatoes or   1 med.-sized
   yams, baked, boiled, or fried potato
   in specified oil or butter
   substitute.

3. Sweet potatoes or yams
   candied with brown or white
   sugar and soybean oil if
   desired.

4. Potato cakes.

                                Approximate
                                Amounts

Bread:

Choice of those suggested
for breakfast.

Butter Substitute:

As suggested for breakfast.

Jams or Preserves:

As at breakfast.

Dessert:

1. Pearl tapioca cooked as at   Av. serving
   breakfast.

2. Potato starch or soy potato
   pudding (see breakfast
   menu).

3. Cookies, cake, or cupcakes   2 cookies or
   made of any combination of   1 cupcake
   soy, lima and potato starch
   flours and tapioca flour.

4. Soy ice cream.

Beverage:

Tea (if ordered by physician).   5 to 8 oz

Note: This menu contains approximately 1,263
calories.

Total for the day:

Calories 3,112

Carbohydrates 264 gm   Ca 0.370 gm

Protein	136 gm	P	1.459 gm
Fat	168 gm	Fe	0.024 gm

Comments: The directions for the use
of the elimination diets as summarized on
page 595 and discussed in this chapter
must be accurately followed. When weight
maintenance is important, special attention
to the proper intake of the calorie-carrying
foods included in this diet, as discussed on
pages 596 and 54 is necessary. Assurance
of the required intake of calcium, potassium, and other electrolytes, as advised on
page 54, is necessary.

When the allergic manifestation has been
absent for an adequate period, then various
foods, one every five to seven days, may
be added. The addition of fruits should be
delayed for one to three months. All fruits
may reproduce symptoms, or cooked fruits
only may be tolerated. At times tolerance
to allergenic fruits returns after their elimination for weeks or months. Fruit, including tomato, allergy may persist for years.
Allergy to various vegetables, especially
celery, occasionally may be present. The
use of additional calcium and vitamins is
discussed on pages 72 to 73. Vitamin C,
15 to 30 mg by mouth daily, is necessary
with fruit-free diets if white potatoes or
cooked vegetables containing vitamin C are
not tolerated. Occasional vitamin C allergy
occurs (see p. 72). No flavored mouthwashes or denture pastes or toothpastes
should be used.

Of interest was the use of the fruit-free,
cereal-free elimination diet containing potatoes, tapioca, beef, green beans, green
peas, carrots, soy oil, sugar, salt, tea, calcium carbonate, and vitamins by Colldahl in
Sweden with relief of food allergy and
symptoms of angioneurotic edema, bronchial asthma, migraine, and chronic ulcerative colitis (with no steroids). He con-

cluded that elimination diets should be used more often.

Modifications of our provocation food tests to determine allergy to additional foods suggested by Rinkel and Randolph are discussed in Chapter 30.

CEREAL-FREE ELIMINATION DIET FOR INFANTS (ROWE)

Food allergy must be studied in infancy, especially to animal milk and to the other foods added to the diet through childhood, as the probable cause of colic and difficulties with feeding, gastrointestinal symptoms, recurrent vomiting, dermatitis or eczema, hives, suspected nasal allergy, croup, recurrent so-called "colds," recurrent serous otitis media, bronchitis, bronchiolitis and bronchial asthma, unexplained fever, anorexia, nervousness, irritability, behavior and personality disturbance, fatigue, toxemia, restless sleep, and other less common possible manifestations of allergy, all of which are discussed in Chapter 25.

The elimination of foods to which allergy is suspected by the diet history or by large skin reactions as noted in this chapter for one to three weeks rarely relieves the symptoms.

Food allergy therefore is best studied with our CFE diet as advised below. If skin testing is not available, the use of this diet alone is justified.

When cow's milk only is ingested, relief of symptoms from its replacement with Neo-Mull-Soy milk (Borden's) or our lamb (not beef)-base formula emphasizes the importance of milk allergy in infancy. Its major importance may continue through life. Because of the presence of identical casein and beta-lactoglobulin in cow's milk and goat's milk, the latter is not used in our practice. The meat-base formula made of beef is not advised in the initial elimination

diet because of frequency of allergy to beef when allergy to animal milk (cow's) occurs.

Soybean milk usually replaces cow's milk. Neo-Mull-Soy (Borden's) is preferable because of its content of sucrose rather than corn glucose, since corn and its products are excluded from this diet. If intolerance or allergy to soy occurs in infants, our strained meat formula should be used. Though it can be made at home by our directions, an excellent canned meat-base formula is made by Gerber and Company. It is well tolerated and is diluted as is canned cow's milk according to age of young infants. When allergy to beef in the meat-base formula is suspected, then the lamb-base formula is advised.

Though allergic symptoms rarely develop when breast milk alone is ingested by the baby, as discussed in Chapter 25, their occasional development when such milk is the only food taken is usually due to food allergens in the milk from the mother's diet. Relief in the infant may occur if the mother adheres to our CFE diet. Breast-milk banks are available for breast milk.

Since allergy to cow's milk, raw, evaporated, and pasteurized is the usual cause of colic, gastrointestinal, and nasobronchial symptoms in infants, as emphasized in Chapter 25, it must be replaced by the following:

1. Mull-Soy or especially Neo-Mull-Soy (Borden's) which contains cane sugar instead of dextrose made from corn sugar. (We advise that cane sugar be substituted for corn glucose or its sugar in all other soy milks.)

If soy milk causes diarrhea, gastrointestinal, or other symptoms, we use the following:

2. A lamb-base formula made by Gerber's or by the mother with our recipes

(this page). Tender-cooked, small chunks of lamb may be homogenized in a Waring or other mixer as advised by Stuart. Both of these formulae contain required calcium and vitamins. A beef-based formula is added after tolerance to strained beef is assured.

If symptoms continue after ten to fourteen days:

3. Human breast milk from local or national breast milk banks may be advised. (further discussion in Chapt. 25).

Note: a) Since antigens of cow's and goat's milk are the same, goat's milk is not used. b) Nutramigen® (Mead, Johnson & Co.) is not advised. It contains traces of casein and pork. Its taste is repellant, except to infants. Substitute commercial products for cow's milk or cream are inadvisable, since they often contain a product of casein or lactose.

Salt and cane or beet sugar are allowed as are multiple synthetic vitamin drops. If fruits are eliminated, extra vitamin C up to 30 mg a day may also be given.

After symptoms are controlled for two to three weeks, the following foods in our CFE diet are added one every three to seven days according to the child's age, desire, and probabilities of allergy:

Grapefruit and tomato juice from the first to the third month. Pureed carrots, squash, peas, string beans, lima beans, and tomatoes from the third to fifth months. Trial of one every three to four days will allow determination of possible allergic reactions.

Pureed white or sweet potatoes, pureed cooked pears, peaches, apricots, prunes, and apples from the third to fifth months.

Tapioca cooked with sugar and a little salt or with pureed fruit and sugar from the fourth to the sixth months.

Strained meats (Gerber's or Swift's) from the third to the eighth months.

Scraped or finely minced lamb and bacon from the sixth to the tenth months. Beef is included when its addition causes no difficulty in the symptom-free patient. Soy-potato bread, muffins, cookies, and cake from the eighth to the twelfth months.

Salt, cane, or beet sugar and soy oil may be used.

SUBSTITUTE FORMULA FOR COW'S MILK CONTAINING STRAINED MEATS (ROWE)

	Wt. (grams)	Measure
Strained lamb 15.6% P, 4.5% F*	212.0	⅞ cup—7 oz
or		
Strained beef 17.7% P, 3.0% F*	186.0	¾ cup—6 oz
Sesame oil or soy oil		3⅓ Tbsps
Sugar		2 Tbsps
Potato starch flour 83% C		2½ Tbsps
or		
Tapioca flour 88% C	23.0	2½ Tbsps
Calcium carbonate	3.0	1 tsp
Salt		½ tsp
Poly-Vi-Sol (or comparable multivitamin)		0.6 cc
Water to make a volume of 1,000 cc		4¼ cups

Total for 1000 cc: Carbohydrate 50 gm, calcium 1.24 gm, protein 33 gm, fat 40 gm, phosphorus 0.31 gm, iron 0.005 gm. Calories 692.

All measurements are level, using standard measuring cups.

Heat water to boiling in top of double boiler. Add sugar, salt, and calcium carbonate. Mix the potato starch or tapioca flour to a paste in ½ cup cold water and stir into the boiling water. Cook for 10 minutes, stirring occasionally to prevent lumping. If necessary, add water to allow for evaporation. Add the strained meat oil, mix thoroughly, and cook for 10 minutes longer.

MINIMAL ELIMINATION DIETS

If food allergy is the probable cause of symptoms in various tissues as shown by their relief on the elimination of allergenic

---

*Strained meats can be prepared with a Waring mixer as advised by Stuart (1945).

foods in other patients and relief has not occurred after adequate use of the two foregoing elimination diets, allergy to foods in these diets may be responsible.

To study this possibility, use one of these minimal diets:

1. Lamb, white potatoes, pearl tapioca, carrots, peas, cottonseed or sesame oil,* salt, sugar, water, and Neo-Mull-Soy† may be tried. This eliminates beef, all cereals and fruits, soy beans and lima beans, and most vegetables which are in one or both of the preceding diets.

2. Chicken, turkey, rice, pearl tapioca, cottonseed or sesame oil, salt, sugar, water, and Neo-Mull-Soy,† which eliminates all cereals, legumes, meat, vegetables, fruits, or a similar diet may be used.

3. Fin fish, crab, eggs, pearl tapioca, soy tapioca bread, cake and cookies, Willow Run oleomargarine, sugar, salt, water, and Neo-Mull-Soy.†

Menus containing 50 to 75 gm of protein and 1800 to 2200 calories can be prepared with such limited foods. Final determination of a minimal elimination diet that controls symptoms requires the initial use of a few foods indicated largely by the patient's diet history. Subsequent manipulation of the diet is effected with additions and subtractions until a limited number of foods which are tolerated without resultant symptoms is determined. This manipulation requires cooperation of the patient and interest and supervision of the physician, usually for several weeks.

Prescribed meat, fowl, or fish three times a day and enough starches, oils, and sugar in the diet must be eaten to maintain desired weight. Inhalation of odors of fruits and other odorous foods off the diet should be avoided. Rice, tapioca, and white and sweet potatoes, if tolerated, take the place of bread in the CFE diet. Cube sugar can be eaten as desired to increase calories. Salted, prescribed oils can be used in place of butter.

Synthetic vitamins and indicated calcium are given as advised on page 72. Of great importance is the maintenance of mineral intake, especially potassium, sodium, and calcium. Determinations of serum electrolytes therefore are necessary. Assurance of sufficient vitamins, especially vitamin C (although occasional allergy to it exists), is very important if a minimal diet is long continued. This receives additional discussion in Chapter 29.

For over thirty-five years this diet has helped to study multiple food allergies in urticaria; localized angioneurotic edema; allergic toxemia and fatigue; possible allergic arthritis or cystitis and especially in possible gastrointestinal allergy particularly in the allergic epigastric syndrome and recurrent canker sores (in Chapt. 5); chronic ulcerative colitis (Chapt. 6); regional enteritis (Chapt. 7); and allergic diarrhea (Chapt. 5). It is used initially or after relief has failed with our FFCFE diet. No flavored mouthwashes or denture fixtures or toothpastes, gum, candies, medicines, lozenges, and so forth should be used. No trace of food, flavors, beverages, or condiments not in this diet is allowed.

Prescribed meat or fowl three times a day and enough starches, sugar, fats, and oils in the diet must be eaten to maintain desired weight. Occasional patients allergic to all meats and even fowl can tolerate fin fish.

---

*Chinese sesame oil is made from roasted sesame seeds and is not acceptable.

† Neo-Mull-Soy (Borden's) or other soy products, if tolerated, can be used in any of these minimal diets. Neo-Mull-Soy can be diluted with one-third water with cane sugar and salt added to taste and taken three times a day to increase calories if allergy to soy is absent.

Moderate relief in one to two weeks justifies the continued strict diet for the two or more subsequent weeks. When the patient is symptom-free, individual foods are added as already advised. In most cases approximately the same foods must be eaten three times a day with pearl tapioca or rice between meals if weight so requires. An illustrative diet follows:

Rice, oats*
    or
Soy- or lima-potato bakery products

White potatoes	Lamb
Tapioca (pearl)	Chicken
Soy oil	Salt
Wesson oil	Sugar (cane or beet)
Willow Run	Water

With relief, gradually try the following:

Rice bread	Carrots
or	Squash
Rice-potato bread	Peas

If relief fails, chicken may be suspected. Very rarely, cottonseed allergy, indicated usually by a large scratch reaction, occurs. Allergy to rice occurs less frequently in gastrointestinal allergy than in nasobronchial allergy. Rare allergy to potatoes occurs. Other individual foods can be added after relief is assured (page 66). In some patients allergy exists to most foods including all fruits or even to all vegetables. Adequate protein, calories, minerals, and vitamins to maintain weight and nutrition are discussed on page 72.

Comment: That some people have allergic reactions to many or even most foods, as many do to many or most pollens, must be recognized. That foods remain in the body for one up to four to five weeks requires their strict elimination before relief from their total elimination occurs.

---

*If rice or oats cause symptoms, soybeans and lima beans and their products as advised in the CFE diet may be tolerated or potatoes and tapioca in larger amounts as well as sugar can be given.

Routine diet histories in which are recorded dislikes, avoidances, disagreements, and distressing (at times invaliding) symptoms from specific ingested foods should be the routine of all physicians including specialists and (of course) allergists. And in all patients allergic to foods, concomitant inhalant allergy, especially to pollens as discussed in Chapter 4, and less common drug and chemical allergies must be recognized and controlled.

Disadvantages of initial total fasting for one to two weeks, as advised by Randolph, and of various modifications of my elimination diets are discussed in Chapter 30.

PREVENTION AND CONTROL OF ELECTROLYTE DEFICIENCIES FROM CORTICOIDS AND ELIMINATION OF FOODS

It is most important to prevent, recognize, and relieve electrolyte deficiencies in the allergic patient which arise from the following causes:

1. Long avoidance of many foods containing electrolytes required for nutrition eliminated because of distaste, disagreement, or allergic symptoms arising from the ingestion of such foods.

2. Long, continued minimal elimination diets ordered by the physician because of definite or possible multiple food allergies without prescribing electrolytes, especially calcium and potassium, to prevent deficiency in the nutritional requirements of such minerals.

3. Debilitating allergic or other chronic disease, especially in the gastrointestinal tract, causing anorexia, vomiting, diarrhea, and other symptoms particularly from esophagitis, gastritis, enteritis, and colitis, including the malabsorption syndrome and celiac disease.

4. Long-term corticosteroid therapy, causing hypocalcemia, hypokalemia, and

other electrolyte deficiencies.

5. Calcium deficiency from the use of long, continued milk-free diets.

6. Decreased ingestion of other minerals, including iron and iodine, usually supplied in iodized salt or enriched foods.

Advised relief of the above electrolyte deficiency follows:

If milk is eliminated, especially in infants and children and also in adults, the minimum daily requirement of one gram of ingested calcium is supplied preferably by one level teaspoonful of powdered calcium carbonate daily mixed in food or water.

This advice may prove of additional importance in man because of the possible beneficial effect of calcium, magnesium, and vitamin D on the parathyroid hormone, increasing the control of food allergy as discussed by Lietze in 1970 and in Chapter 28.

As well as the *nutritional* value of electrolytes, they may have a *therapeutic* effect also as suggested by Lietze in Chapter 28. The possibility that a parathyroid hormone may enhance the effects of the immune response and thus produce allergic inflammation suggests that the effect of high intake of calcium and magnesium may be a therapeutic one of causing the cessation of function of the parathyroid gland.

Deficiency in magnesium can be met by moderate, nondiarrheal-producing doses of unflavored milk of magnesia.

Deficiency in potassium results from continued, especially long-term corticosteroid therapy and also from minimal diets, especially when most or all vegetables, fruits, meats, or other potassium-containing foods are eliminated, producing thereby weakness or other symptoms. This must be suspected and relieved especially if the serum potassium is below normal.

For this relief potassium chloride 15 grains three times a day in capsules or sim-

ple elixir or the better tolerated potassium gluconate (Kaon) 5 mEq in tablets in doses as advised by the manufacturer are available. The necessary precautions and possible complications from its administration and the importance of preventing hyperkalemia as indicated by symptoms and confirmed by serum potassium determinations must be remembered.

The importance of maintaining normal intake of sodium chloride as assured by electrolyte determinations in the serum must be remembered.

ROTARY DIVERSIFIED DIETS PROPOSED BY RINKEL IN 1934

These rotary diets contain foods which can be eaten one to two days a week or only one time in ten to fourteen days without reactivation of the patient's symptoms resulting from food allergy.

After symptoms resulting from food allergy are relieved by one of our three elimination diets for an adequate period as already advised, provocation tests with additional foods not in the relieving diet are indicated, each food being ingested for three to seven days. A food which reactivates the allergic symptoms in a few hours to one or two days, indicating fixed sensitization according to Rinkel, should not be added to the original diet.

If symptoms, however, do not develop until an added food has been eaten for three to seven days, that food may be tolerated one to two times a week and may be included in a rotary diet for the patient. Such tolerance requires confirmation by additional feeding tests with the individual foods which, as Rinkel states, may entail a "long, drawn-out procedure."

The decrease in allergic reactivity to foods which we have long reported during the summer with activation of food allergy in the fall to late spring evident in some patients, even September or October or in others not until December or January, requires recognition by all physicians during their study and control of clinical food allergy. Thus, when foods are added during the late spring and summer with no activation of allergic symptoms, patients must be told that if allergic symptoms return in the fall and winter, such foods must be suspect and eliminated, remembering that it may be one, two, or even three weeks before such foods are entirely eliminated from the body with resultant relief of symptoms.

As reported in Chapter 8, such decreased allergic reactions to foods in the summer often occurs in bronchial asthma and atopic eczema in children, continuing at times into adolescence and adult life. It also explains the exaggeration of symptoms of chronic bronchitis and of obstructive emphysema in the fall and winter as a result of activated food allergy rather than bronchial infection, as emphasized in Chapters 9 and 11.

The use of foods in a rotary diet also requires realization that such foods may cause subclinical allergy in the body tissues resulting in symptoms which are not recognized by the patient but which disturb tissue function and may gradually produce pathological changes in the nasobronchial, cutaneous, cerebral, gastrointestinal, or in other involved tissues of the body. These disturbances may cause body consciousness and other symptoms of allergic toxemia and fatigue discussed in Chapter 19.

Thus the decision that a food can be included in a "rotary diet" requires confirmation that no activation of nasobronchial, cutaneous, gastrointestinal (as of allergic epigastric syndrome, allergic colitis, CUC, or others), or other controlled manifestation of food allergy in the symptom-free patient results from ingestion of such foods for at least two to three days. Control of

food allergy means that symptoms remain controlled with the elimination of specific foods without corticosteroids or other drugs.

In our practice the widening of the menus with foods in such a rotary diet frequently has not been possible. Corticosteroid therapy, even in small doses, must be the concerned physician's responsibility.

MULTIPLE FOOD ALLERGIES CONTROLLED BY A MINIMAL ELIMINATION DIET WITH A ROTARY DIET

A woman, forty-three years of age, was first seen in 1960 because of sore throats, postnasal drip, enlarged cervical glands, slight fever, fatigue, confusion, and abdominal cramping, especially from milk. These symptoms had occurred every three or four months from the age of fourteen to thirty-seven years. For five years they had been nearly continuous but markedly exaggerated every three to six months, being better in the summer. This history immediately suggested food allergy as an important cause. Pain and tenderness also occurred in the elbows, particularly after ingesting certain foods.

The diet history revealed abdominal distress, confusion, and increased fatigue from the ingestion of milk. Suspicion of allergy to many foods had restricted her diet to beef, chicken, cooked vegetables, white potatoes, tea, sugar, and water but without relief.

Drug, environmental, and family histories indicating possible allergy seemed negative.

Physical examination was also negative except for moderate enlargement of cervical glands and slight tenderness on pressure on the xyphoid process and upper epigastrium. Blood and urine analyses were negative.

Scratch tests with inhalant and food allergens were negative except one to three plus reactions to several fall and tree pollens.

X-rays of the lungs, sinuses, gastrointestinal tract, and gallbladder were negative.

Treatment and Results: With our FFCFE diet all symptoms were benefited in one month. During the next six months more improvement occurred with the gradual elimination of all vegetables, sweet potatoes, chicken, lamb, bacon, and chlorinated drinking water. Boiled white potatoes, rice, and tapioca gave no abdominal or other symptoms at that time.

With a final diet containing Grainless Mix and consisting of soy and potato starch flours,* beef, potato starch pudding, Wesson oil, sugar cubes, spring water, and a multiple vitamin, she gained weight from 106 to 122 lb in eight months. She was stronger, happier, and free from tension. She reported having "great strength and amazing energy." Small doses of triamcinolone had been of no benefit. Desensitization to a multiple pollen antigen even in a 1:5 billion dilution seemed to cause fatigue and epigastric distress. Premarin® and Stilbesterol® caused nausea.

In the last year in addition to the above foods, which she eats every day with no allergic symptoms, a rotary diet containing individual foods, one of which she can eat once a week, has been added to her minimal diet, which she takes every day. This rotary diet has helped to maintain her weight of 122 lb.

Thus a rotary diet may supplement a daily tolerated elimination diet as follows:

1. *Daily diet.*
Muffins and cookies made with Grainless Mix, water, salt, and sugar, beef, sugar cubes, salt, spring water, vitamin C 25 mg

daily. Neo-Mull-Soy (Borden's) as a drink or cooked with other allowed foods.

2. *Rotary diet.*
Each food being eaten one time a week: lamb, pork, bacon, fish, white potato, and rice boiled for one-half hour.

ORDERING ELIMINATION DIETS IN THE PHYSICIAN'S OFFICE

In office cases the physician or his assistant must give the patient or parents the list of foods in the prescribed diet with menus and recipes for soy-potato bakery products. These may be typewritten or mimeographed or are printed, as in our elimination diet booklet for patients' use. Changes required in the diet if soy bean or lima bean flour is not tolerated are discussed in subsequent pages. The patient must remember that ingested food allergens remain in the body for one to two or more weeks and that even slight breaks in the diet may prevent relief or reproduce symptoms in minutes, hours, or one to three days. Thus the patient must be told what foods to eat and never what foods not to eat.

ORDERING THE DIET IN THE HOSPITAL

1. In the hopsital it is easy to order our CFE diet or its modifications advised in this chapter. Most dietitians who have studied these diets and are familiar with them are anxious to cooperate.

The diet is ordered in the chart as follows:

Rx The Cereal-Free Elimination Diet (Rowe) at times minus some foods or plus others

2. If fruit and condiments also need elimination, the diet is ordered as follows:

Rx Fruit-Free Cereal-Free Elimination Diet (Rowe)

---

*Bray's, 3764 Piedmont Ave., Oakland, California.

3. If the diet is ordered for infants and young children, individual foods listed previously, according to age, are ordered.

4. If a minimal diet is required, the individual foods are ordered.

5. If anorexia or nausea is present, soft pureed, minced, or liquid prescribed foods are ordered. Daily weight should be recorded. Weight must be maintained. Extra feedings between meals and on retiring may be advisable.

IMPORTANT RECIPES FOR THE CEREAL-FREE ELIMINATION DIETS

Flour should be sifted only in an old-fashioned rotary sifter for these recipes.

TABLE OF ABBREVIATIONS AND MEASUREMENTS
tsp—teaspoonful
Tbsp—tablespoonful
cup—cupful
16 Tbsp—1 cup
8 Tbsp—½ cup
8 oz—1 cup
3 tsp—1 Tbsp

FRUIT TAPIOCA
2½ cups canned fruit juice and water
4 Tbsps Minute Tapioca°
½ cup sugar
¼ tsp salt
1 to 1½ cups chopped or pureed apricot, pears, or pineapple
1 Tbsp lemon juice

Combine fruit juice and water, minute tapioca, sugar, and salt in a sauce pan and mix well. Bring mixture to a boil, stirring constantly. Remove from fire. Do not overcook. Stir occasionally as it cools.

FRUIT-FREE TAPIOCA
3 cups water
⅛ cup Pearl tapioca
⅛ to ½ cup white sugar
¼ tsp salt
2 tsps caramel flavoring
Neo-Mull-Soy (Borden's) may be added if desired.

Combine all ingredients in a saucepan. Bring mixture quickly to a full boil over direct heat,

°If unavailable, use potato starch.

stirring constantly. Remove from the fire. Do not overcook. Stir occasionally as it cools. Mixture thickens as it cools.

LIMA BEAN OR SPLIT-PEA SOUP
1 cup split peas or lima beans
2 Tbsps bacon fat
Diced bacon, crisp
1 qt water
Salt

Cook the split peas or lima beans and salt until it forms a smooth puree. Before serving, add the bacon fat and crisp fried bacon.

TOMATO SOUP (WITH SOYBEAN FLOUR)
1 cup strained tomatoes or juice
1 cup water
2 Tbsps soybean flour
1 tsp salt

Mix the soybean flour thoroughly with some of the water and add to the hot tomato juice and water. Boil for ½ hour. This resembles a cream soup in consistency and flavor.

SOY-LIMA-POTATO MUFFINS OR BREAD
¾ cup potato starch flour
1 cup soybean flour°
¼ cup lima bean flour†
¼ cup sesame or soy oil
2 Tbsps sugar
1 cup water
6 tsps baking powder‡
½ tsp salt

Sift the flour, baking powder, and salt together three times. Blend the oil and sugar well. Add the sifted flour and the water alternately to the oil and sugar. Beat well and pour into muffin pans which have been well greased with sesame or soy oil. Bake at 375 F for 25 to 30 minutes. Makes 12 muffins. Or, bake in a loaf pan at 350 to 375 F for 1¼ hours.

°A full fat-processed soybean flour is advised such as Orange Blossom Soy Flour made by Archer-Daniels Midland Co., Minneapolis, Minn., or Soy Flour No. 1 made by A.E. Staley Manufacturing Co., Decatur, Ill.

†Lima bean flour can be purchased from wholesale grocers or local food stores or Bray's, 3764 Piedmont Avenue, Oakland, California.

‡Cereal-free baking powder can be obtained at F.A. Bray, 3764 Piedmont Avenue, Oakland, California. Grainless Cellu-Mix containing soy, potato starch flour, and leavening is sold by the above store. With added water and (if desired) extra baking powder, muffins, hot cakes, and waffles are easily made.

SOY-POTATO BREAD

Prepare a loaf pan 4 x 7 x 2 inches by oiling with soy oil and lining with waxed paper on bottom and sides. Use bright tin, aluminum, or aluminum foil pans but not glass, Pyrex, or darkened tin. The oven temperature regulator should be accurate or check temperature with an oven thermometer.

Preheat oven to 350 F.

Use standard measuring cups and spoons. All measurements are level and accurate. Sift the flours once before measuring and spoon lightly into measuring cups (use Mary Ann type cups).

Directions

Sift together *four times* . . .

1 cup soy flour
1 cup potato starch flour
½ tsp salt
2 Tbsps white sugar (or light brown sugar)
1 tsp baking powder (cereal-free)

To ½ cup of this mixture add . . .

5 tsps baking powder. Sift together *four* times and set aside to add later.

To the remainder add . . .

⅔ cup of cold water. Mix well and beat vigorously for 3 minutes by hand or with an electric beater at medium speed.

Add 3 Tbsps soy oil. Continue beating 3 minutes longer.

Add flour and baking powder mix which has been set aside—beat into the batter quickly for one minute. Batter will be thick and fluffy.

Pour into prepared pan. Bake at 350 F for 1 hour 10 minutes. Cool 5 minutes before removing from the pan. Do not slice until cold. To retain freshness, wrap in waxed paper, plastic food bags, or Saran wrap and keep refrigerated.

Notes

Moisture, temperature, and thorough mixing are important factors in obtaining a good product. Too much liquid or too high oven temperature are responsible for a soggy streak which may result. Full-fat soy flour and potato starch flour rather than potato flour must be used. Cereal-free baking powder is available at Bray's, 3764 Piedmont Avenue, Oakland, or from Chicago Dietetic Supply, 1750 Van Buren Street, Chicago, Illinois.

SOY-POTATO BREAD MUFFINS OR PANCAKES

1 cup soy flour
1 cup potato starch flour
1 tsp salt
¼ cup soy oil
3 Tbsps baking powder
2 Tbsps white sugar
⅔ cup water

Measure flour lightly to 1 cup level in measuring cup. Sift dry ingredients four times. Add water and beat 3 minutes. Add oil and beat one minute longer. Grease baking pan well with soy oil. Preheat oven to 350 F. Bake at 350 F for 10 minutes. Reduce heat to 285 or 300 F and continue baking for 1 hour, 20 minutes.

Bake muffins at 300 to 325 F for 25 to 30 minutes. Makes 12 muffins.

For pancakes or waffles thin this batter with ¼ cup of water.

SOY-POTATO CUPCAKES OR CAKE

1 cup soy flour
¾ cup potato starch flour
3 Tbsps baking powder
¾ cup sugar
½ tsp salt
¼ cup soy oil
3 tsps vanilla or
2 tsps vanilla and
1 tsp lemon extract
1 scant cup water

Sift soy flour once before measuring. Sift together all the dry ingredients well. Add water to sifted dry ingredients. Mix well. Add oil and vanilla and beat for 2 minutes. Pour into muffin or layer cake pans well greased with soy oil and bake at 350 F for 30 minutes. Makes 12 cupcakes or 2 small layers. Or bake in a loaf pan for 1½ hours at 300 F.

Variations: Flavor with lemon extract and grated lemon rind or with maple flavoring. Add chopped apricots, prunes, or pineapple. Substitute fruit juice for water. Use fondant slightly thinned with water or fruit juice for frosting.

For fruit-free diets eliminate lemon extract and all fruit and use caramel flavor.

COOKIES (CRISP)

1¼ cups lima bean flour
1½ tsps soda
¼ tsp salt
¾ cup sugar
¾ cup sesame or soy oil
½ cup water
1 tsp vanilla

Cream sugar and oil. Stir in flour which has

been sifted with soda and salt; add water and vanilla. After mixing well, shape dough into a long roll and let it thoroughly chill in the refrigerator. Cut into thin circles and sprinkle with sugar and bake in a hot oven for ten minutes.

SOY-POTATO COOKIES

Follow the recipe for soy-potato cake. Decrease the water to make a stiff dough. Force through a cookie press onto a cookie sheet well greased with soy oil. Or a thinner batter can be dropped from a teaspoon onto a greased cookie sheet. Bake at 375 to 400 F for 10 or 15 minutes. A thicker dough can be rolled and kept in a refrigerator. Cut into thin slices and bake as desired. If kept in an air-tight container, cookies will remain crisp.

SOY COOKIES*

1 cup soy flour	4 Tbsps soy oil
2 tsps baking powder	3 to 5 Tbsps water
¼ tsp salt	½ tsp vanilla or lemon extract
⅓ cup sugar	tract

Mix oil and sugar and add the flavoring. Sift soy flour once before measuring and sift twice more after adding baking powder and salt. Add flour to oil and sugar and sufficient water to make a stiff dough. Form into a roll and cut into cookies or force through a cookie press. With a softer dough, drop from a teaspoon onto a cookie sheet well greased with soy oil. Bake at 350 F for 15 minutes. Chopped prunes or apricots may be added or fruit juice may be substituted for water. Cookies will remain crisp if stored in an air-tight container.

SOY-POTATO PUDDING

4 level Tbsps soy flour
1 cup water
2 tsps potato starch flour
3 Tbsps sugar
¼ tsp salt
¼ tsp lemon extract
¼ tsp vanilla extract

Cook the soy flour and water for 15 minutes in top of double boiler. Stir potato starch, sugar, and salt into boiling mixture until it thickens. Continue cooking for 20 minutes. Flavor with lemon and vanilla extracts or with maple or caramel. May serve with fruit sauce or maple or caramel syrup if desired. More sugar may be

*May substitute lima flour for soy.

desired or a combination of white and brown sugar may be used.

For fruit-free elimination diets, caramel flavor instead of vanilla or lemon extract is necessary. Fruit sauce must also be omitted.

POTATO CAKES

Grate a medium-sized potato and add 2 Tbsps potato starch and ¼ tsp salt. Fry in soybean oil until brown.

CARAMEL FROSTING

⅔ cup water
2 cups brown sugar
3 Tbsps soy oil

Combine sugar and water. Stir slowly while bringing it to a boil. Boil hard, stirring constantly until the syrup has reached the "soft ball" stage (234 F). Remove from the fire, add soy oil, and allow to cool undisturbed until lukewarm. Beat mixture until it gets thick and loses its luster. Spread quickly over the cake.

PINEAPPLE FILLING

2 Tbsps potato starch flour
½ cup sugar
1 Tbsp lemon juice
2 cups crushed pineapple juice and fruit

Mix flour and sugar. Add pineapple and lemon juice and cook slowly until thick and clear. Cool slightly before spreading on cake. This may be used on top of cake as well as for the filling. Apricots or peaches may be substituted for pineapple.

BROILED FROSTING

4 Tbsps soy oil
⅔ cup brown sugar
¼ cup water
When flavors and fruits are allowed, add
½ tsp vanilla
¾ cup finely chopped dried
prunes or candied pineapple

Thoroughly combine all the ingredients and spread over warm cake. Brown lightly under the broiler.

SOY ICE CREAM

2 cups soy milk
¼ cup white sugar
2 Tbsps brown sugar

2 tsps gelatin
1 Tbsp potato starch
2 tsps vanilla or lemon extract

Dissolve the gelatin in a little cold water. Bring to a boil the soy milk and sugar. Mix the potato starch in ¼ cup cold water and add to the milk. Cook for 5 minutes. Remove from the flame and add the dissolved gelatin and flavoring. Cool and freeze in a mechanical freezer or refrigerator. If made in the refrigerator, remove from the trays after it freezes and beat well. Refreeze; serve with caramel sauce. Fruit or fruit juice may be added if it is in the diet.

POTATO CARAMEL PUDDING

2⅔ cups water
1⅓ cups caramel syrup
¼ cup white sugar
5 Tbsps potato starch

Bring to a boil 2 cups of water, caramel syrup, and white sugar. Mix the potato starch in the remaining ⅔ cup of cold water and add to the boiling syrup. Cook for five minutes, stirring constantly. Chill before serving.

CARAMEL SYRUP

1 cup sugar
1 cup boiling water

Place the sugar in a heavy pan, heat, stirring constantly until melted and light brown. Remove the pan from the fire and add the boiling water. Place over the heat again until the caramelized sugar is dissolved. This syrup can be kept in a jar and used for flavoring puddings and sauces.

FONDANT

2 cups sugar
¼ tsp cream of tartar
1 cup boiling water
¼ tsp salt
½ tsp vanilla

Measure sugar and cream of tartar into a sauce pan and add the boiling water. Stir over a low heat until sugar is dissolved. Do not let the candy boil until the sugar is dissolved and the sugar crystal wiped down from the sides of the pan with a clean cloth. When the boiling point is reached, cover the kettle and boil vigorously for 5 minutes. Remove the cover, wipe off crystals from sides of the pan and continue cooking without stirring until the medium ball stage has been reached (240 to 242 F). When done, pour the candy at once into a cold, wet platter and let it stand until lukewarm. Sprinkle salt over the surface, add vanilla, and beat until white and knead in the hands until smooth and creamy. Put fondant into a glass jar and cover. It will keep several weeks in a cool place.

PANOCHA

2 Tbsps sesame or soy oil
2 cups brown sugar
1 cup white sugar
1 cup water
⅛ tsp soda

Heat the oil in a kettle, stir in sugars. Add water and soda and mix well with sugar. Wipe down sugar from sides of pan. Heat slowly to boiling, stirring until sugar is dissolved. Boil to 240 F the medium ball stage (the ball holds its shape when lifted from cold water). Remove from stove, sprinkle a dash of salt over top, and set aside to cool undisturbed until lukewarm. Beat until creamy. Turn into greased pans and cut in squares.

MARSHMALLOWS

2 cups sugar
¾ cup water
2 Tbsps gelatin
½ tsp salt
1 tsp vanilla extract (if allowed)

Mix sugar and water and boil until the soft ball stage has been reached (234 to 238 F). Remove from the fire. Soften the gelatin in ½ cup of cold water. Pour the hot syrup over the softened gelatin and stir until dissolved. Let it partially cool, add vanilla and salt, and beat it until the mixture is thick and white and will hold its shape. Pour into straight-sided pans. When firm, cut into squares. Roll in sugar, or if corn is allowed, powdered sugar may be used.

BUTTERSCOTCH CANDY

1 cup sugar
¼ cup molasses
2 Tbsps boiling water
½ cup Willow Run oleomargarine

Boil together until when tried in cold water mixture becomes brittle. Turn into small buttered pan (Willow Run). When slightly cool, mark with sharp pointed knife into squares.

CARROT MARMALADE

Grind five large carrots and add 6 cups water. Boil for 30 or 40 minutes until very soft. Measure this mixture and add an equal volume of sugar. Boil again until quite thick. If allowed in the diet, the juice of four lemons may be added for flavor.

Additional recipes will be found in *Elimination Diets and the Patient's Allergies*, 2nd ed. 1944 (Philadelphia, Lea and Febiger) and in *Clinical Allergy—Manifestations, Diagnosis and Treatment*, 1937 (Philadelphia, Lea and Febiger).

TIME NECESSARY TO DETERMINE ROLE OF FOOD ALLERGY

The length of time during which the initial elimination diet should be used varies with the frequency of occurrence of symptoms.

1. If nearly daily symptoms disappear in two weeks of dieting and similar relief has not previously occurred for several weeks or months, it can be assumed that allergenic foods have been eliminated. Then individual foods can be gradually added, as suggested on the following pages.

2. When symptoms recur every two to six weeks with slight or no interim symptoms, as when the pathognomonic history of asthma resulting from food allergy occurs, relief from the elimination diet must continue for two to three months until there is adequate evidence that allergenic foods have been eliminated.

3. When symptoms recur only for one to two or three days irregularly one to five times a year, foods that may be responsible at times are ascertainable by listing unusual foods taken for one to four days before the symptoms develop. Drugs and inhalation of unusual inhalants also must be considered causes.

If the cause of such infrequent symptoms is not found and infrequent activation of allergy to a frequently eaten food is suspect, then our CFE diet or its modifications may be justified. Such diet trial should continue for three to six months because of the infrequency of the symptoms. Nutrition and weight must be maintained as advised in this chapter.

Thus the conclusion that foods are not the cause of clinical allergy when symptoms are not controlled with an elimination diet in a few days is not justified. Such insufficient use of elimination diets has led to the incorrect assumption of psychoneurosis or of other chronic maladies. These misassumptions account in part for the failure of some physicians to recognize clinical food allergy. When long-standing food allergy has produced marked tissue changes, as in perennial bronchial asthma with or without emphysema or in oozing, indurated atopic dermatitis, chronic ulcerative colitis, or regional enteritis, gradual restoration of cellular structure and function requires elimination of allergenic foods for weeks after the causative foods have been eliminated from the body. This decrease in pathological changes as a result of chronic allergy can be hastened by supervised, limited corticosteroid therapy. It must also be emphasized that the study of possible food allergy always requires study of possible inhalant and less frequent contactant drug and rare bacterial allergies before a conclusion can be reached that food allergy is the sole cause.

NECESSITY OF DETAILED MENUS AND MAINTENANCE OF NUTRITION AND WEIGHT WITH ELIMINATION DIETS

Since elimination diets usually have to be continued for more than a few days or even for weeks or months, detailed recipes for bakery products that allow satisfying menus and protection of nutrition including electrolyte and vitamin requirements must be given to the patient. This is accomplished with menus we have always published for the elimination diets.

DETAILED MENUS NECESSARY FOR ELIMINATION DIETS

The patient must be given a list of allowed foods with menus. If he is only told to omit suspected foods, strict elimination of possible allergenic foods rarely occurs.

Nutrition is maintained when meals are eaten according to our printed menus.

In infancy Neo-Mull-Soy (Borden's) or our meat-base formula (Gerber's) furnishes the protein, calorie, mineral, and vitamin requirements. In children and adults if these substitutes for cow's milk are not taken, proper amounts of prescribed meat or fowl furnish required protein. Calories are supplied by the prescribed starches, sugar, oil, and butter substitute. Assurance of adequate vitamin intake depends on the foods in the diet plus a supplemental dose of multiple synthetic vitamins A, B, C, and D if necessary to meet vitamin requirements. Calcium carbonate ½ tsp in food or water daily is cheaper and more concentrated than other calcium salts. Pregnant or lactating women on the CFE diet require 1 tsp daily. If children refuse calcium carbonate, Neo-Calglucon 2 to 4 tsps a day is usually accepted.

To increase weight, potatoes, tapioca, sugar, prescribed oil and butter substitute with meals, and extra feedings between meals and on retiring are required.

MENUS FOR MEALS EATEN AWAY FROM HOME—LUNCHES CARRIED TO SCHOOL OR WORK

When the CFE diet is used, the following lunch can be carried to work or school. Adequate similar lunches can also be prepared from our FFCFE diet and from foods in the minimal diets (pages 49 & 53).

1. Sandwiches of prescribed bread or muffins with jam or jelly of prescribed fruits if allowed.

2. Cold roast lamb, beef (no mixed meats), tongue, or chicken.

3. Jar of tapioca cooked with prescribed fruit and sugar or of soy-potato or potato starch pudding. (Caramel instead of fruit flavors must be used in the fruit-free diets). If the above puddings cannot be made, then 2 or more cold boiled or baked potatoes may be taken to be eaten with salt.

4. Prescribed cookies, cupcakes, or cake.

5. Jar of prescribed fruits or fruit juice (except in FFCFE diet).

6. Prescribed candy or cube sugar.

SIMPLIFIED MENUS FOR ELIMINATION DIETS (ROWE) AWAY FROM HOME

1. When cooking facilities are limited or difficulty in explaining the diet to the patient exists, these simple menus may be advisable. As with all elimination diets, accuracy and maintenance of nutrition and weight as advised in the directions in this chapter are necessary. If accurate bakery products are not obtainable in a bakery supervised for honesty by the doctor or cannot be made at home, they are omitted. Then, more potatoes, tapioca, sugar, and prescribed oil are required to maintain weight.

2. When meals must be eaten away from home, these simple menus can be followed in hotels, restaurants, or friends' homes. If traces of excluded foods may be in the foods served, they should not be eaten. Properly prepared foods can always be obtained a few hours later, that is, plain meat, plain potatoes, sugar, canned or fresh-cooked vegetables, and fruits in the diet. Cooks and waiters can be found who are willing to cooperate. Extra tipping usually is necessary. These diets, precautions, and care in their use are discussed further in the writer's previous books.*

*Elimination Diets and the Patient's Allergies, 2nd ed., Philadelphia, Lea and Febiger, 1944.
Bronchial Asthma—Its Diagnosis and Treatment. Springfield, Charles C Thomas, 1963.

Breakfast

1. Grapefruit or its juice with sugar or tomato juice, unspiced.

2. Tapioca or potato starch cooked with pears, peaches, apricots, prunes, pineapple, or grapefruit and sugar and/or white or sweet potatoes (baked or boiled, served with salt).

3. Bacon, lamb chops (no pepper, butter, gravy, or sauces).

4. Soy-potato starch bread or muffins brought in patient's pocket or bag if away from home. (If soy disagrees or is unavailable, it may be omitted.)

5. Pears, peaches, apricots, prunes, and pineapples—preserved, canned or fresh (peeled).

6. Water; tea (if ordered by physician).

Lunch and Supper

1. Broth (lamb, chicken), salted, no pepper or condiments; soup made with strained lamb (Gerber's or Swift's) thinned as desired, salted.

2. Salad of vegetables or fruits in this diet, served with vinegar, salt, and with prescribed oil (if it is available). This salad may be omitted.

3. Lamb (chops, roast, liver, or ground lamb) cold or hot with salt.

4. White or sweet potatoes (boiled or baked) served only with salt and soy oil if available.

5. Vegetables in diet (served only with salt).

6. Soy-potato starch bread or muffins (see Breakfast).

7. Tapioca or potato starch cooked with fruit, water, and sugar (if necessary, in a jar brought from home); fruits (see Breakfast).

8. Water; tea (if ordered by physician).

9. Neo-Mull-Soy (Borden's) milk diluted with ⅓ water plus desired cane sugar is allowed especially to increase weight.

SUPERVISION OF DIET TRIAL BY THE PHYSICIAN

Physicians must tell the patient that the diet excludes foods which most frequently cause the assumed or proven manifestation of food allergy, that he must not taste or eat a trace of a food not on the diet, that foods remain in the body for several days up to two weeks, that enough foods in the menus must be eaten to maintain weight and nutrition, and that even slight breaks in the diet will reactivate clinical allergy for two to ten days and prevent the physician's decision about the role of food allergy.

After the diet has been explained and given to the patient following his initial studies of possible allergy in the office or after discharge from the hospital, the physician must confer with the patient at his office or by telephone in two to five days. Questions about the preparation and cooking of the menus usually arise. To a usual question, "Can I (or my child) eat any food not on the diet?", the answer must be "If it is not in the printed list, do not take even a trace of it." Questions must be answered about the making of bakery products from soy and potato starch flours. The patient's wife, mother, or cook must be told to make muffins first, using half the recipe until reasonably good products result. Also, hotcakes or waffles (page 59) served with cane or beet sugar syrup made in the kitchen or pure maple syrup are agreeable, especially to children. Later, small loaves of bread can be baked. Bray's will mail a grainless dry soy-potato flour mixture devoid of all foods not on our cereal-free elimination diet with directions to make bakery products at home. Patients may write to Bray's for information. By adding water to Cellu-Grainless Mix muffins, hotcakes and cookies can be made. Honest bakers gradually will make these bakery products in many cities in our country, although because of difficulty in accurately baking these, they are reluctant to dispense with gluten. The patient is told that all meals must be prepared according to the printed menus. Lunches carried to work must be prepared as advised in this chapter. If meals must be eaten away from home, suggested menus with this diet must be ordered by the physician. If foods off the diet are served, they should not be eaten. Prescribed foods can always be obtained in the following two to eight hours. Missing one or even two to three meals rarely is a health hazard. If a vegetable, fruit, or other food seems to disagree, the patient is told to eliminate it.

After the first conference another, either in the office, by telephone, or by letter, is necessary in five to ten days. The physician must be certain that the diet is being maintained, that correct bakery products are available, and that protein, calorie, mineral, and vitamin requirements are being met.

As emphasized in this chapter, Chapter 8, and others, assurance that the diet is being maintained is important rather than analyzing an inaccurate list of all foods in a diet diary the patient has eaten at home, in restaurants, and in friends' homes. No candy other than that made by our recipes is allowed. As a substitute for bottled sweet drinks, refrigerated sparkling water to which cane sugar syrup and if desired, juice of a prescribed fruit are added can be taken. In place of ice cream, soy milk ice cream is allowed or water ice made of

TABLE VII
GRAPHIC RECORD OF MANIPULATION OF ELIMINATION DIETS

Date	1/10					Date	1/10		
Rice		2/10	0	3/15	0	Broccoli			9/8
Corn		2/24				Lemon	√		
Tapioca	√					Pear	√		
Rye						Peach	√		
Oats						Pineapple			
Wheat			4/1	0	5/15 0	Apricot	√		
Lamb	√					Prune	√		
Chicken	√					Plum	√		
Bacon				4/23		Grapefruit	√		
Beef	√					Orange		1/20	
Turkey					9/1	Apple		2/17	
Salmon		3/2				Banana		4/15	
Halibut		3/2				Cantaloupe		8/1	0
Cod		3/2				Watermelon		8/1	0
Lettuce						Grape		9/1	0
Spinach	√					Sugar	√		
Carrot	√					Maple syrup	√		
Squash			7/15	0		Sesame oil	√		
Asparagus	√					Soy oil	√		
Pea	√					Mazola oil			
Artichoke	√					Olive oil		5/1	
Tomato	√					Olive		5/1	
Beet	√					Salt	√		
String bean	√					Pepper		7/1	
Soy bean	√					Egg		2/1	
Lima bean	√					Milk		6/1	0
White potato	√					Butter		6/1	0
Sweet potato	√		0	3/2		Cream		6/1	0
Green pepper		4/15				Tea	√		
Eggplant		4/15				Coffee			3/24
Cauliflower		9/1							

frozen prescribed fruit juice, sugar, and water. All sherbets contain cow's milk and are forbidden. Cakes and cookies are made by our recipes.

Subsequent conferences in office, by telephone, or by letter are important every one to four weeks until the role of food can be determined. Thereafter, policing and supervision of the elimination diet is required every two to six months as tolerance for additional foods is determined by provocation feeding tests. The addition and exclusion of foods added to the initial diet, which has relieved the clinical allergy, are conveniently indicated on a Graphic Record of Manipulation of Elimination Diets (Table VII). Its use by all physicians who use and supervise these elimination diets is of great importance.

PROVOCATION FEEDING TESTS WITH ADDITIONAL FOODS AFTER RELIEF OF ALLERGIC SYMPTOMS OCCURS FROM THE CEREAL-FREE ELIMINATION DIET

When relief is apparent or assured, as discussed in previous pages, foods can be added, each one for two to four days. We first add cooked apples, then orange juice, a little melon, berry jellies, and in two weeks or so, individual vegetables except onion and garlic. Severe allergy has been seen to bananas and celery. Because of the frequency of allergy to cereal grains, they should not be added until daily recurring symptoms have been absent for two to three weeks or until attacks of asthma or headaches which have recurred every two to six weeks have been absent for six to twelve weeks.

As discussed previously, it is most important to remember refractoriness to food allergy after a) severe attacks of asthma or headaches and b) during the summer months in evaluating provocation tests with individual foods. Wheat, milk, eggs, fish, chocolate, coffee, condiments, and other foods can gradually be added to the diet after tolerance for the cereal grains has been determined. If symptoms are activated, one or more of the previously added foods must be suspected and eliminated.

Since allergic symptoms from a food added to those in an elimination diet which has relieved the clinical symptoms in the patient often develop in several hours or even two days rather than in one hour, we have never advised provocation feeding tests with single foods every hour as recommended by Rinkel and his associates. Moreover, allergic symptoms arising from a new food often persist for three to seven or eight days, and changes in tissues from allergy may persist for a longer period. It is always important that diet trials with a new food be done in a patient relieved by assured control of previous symptoms.

When recurrent or severe bronchial asthma with or without emphysema, perennial nasal allergy, headaches, allergic fatigue, longstanding cutaneous, gastrointestinal, genitourinary, or other manifestations of chronic allergy to foods have been relieved by an initial CFE diet or its modification, adults, children, and their parents willingly adhere to the strict elimination diet and cooperate in the trial of other foods. Indeed, they may hesitate to add other foods to the elimination diet which has given gratifying and at times long-sought-for relief. Since nutrition and necessary weight gain are assured with our standardized CFE diet plus vitamins and calcium and when necessary potassium, the addition of other foods, though advisable for convenience and satisfaction of the patient, is not necessary.

SOY-POTATO BAKERY PRODUCTS

It is important that someone in the physician's family or office or the dietitian in the hospital or medical clinic learns to make satisfactory bakery products with our recipes so that the patient or parent can be assured that such products can be made successfully at home. A baker also may be found who will honestly make these products for sale by our recipes under the physician's direction. Such a baker * has cooperated with the writers for over thrity years.

Our insistence that soy- or lima-potato bakery products advised in our CFE diet be made according to our recipes at home or by honest bakers * supervised by physicians is due to the inclusion of wheat or wheat gluten in such products made by many unsupervised bakers. Inclusion of wheat flour or wheat gluten which is not listed in the ingredients printed on labels has been detected in soy or lima or rice potato or other bakery products sold as being wheat-free in many health food stores in California as reported by us in 1967 † and in Chapter 18.

These products, moreover, can be made in homes in Britain and Germany where we have found soy flour and potato starch available, as they are in Scandinavia, and by importation, if necessary, in any country.

USE OF THE CFE DIET WITHOUT BAKERY PRODUCTS

One excuse for not studying food allergy, especially in foreign countries, is that the CFE diet is difficult or impossible to use. This excuse does not eliminate the responsibility of the physician to extend relief to the patient with the adequate use of the CFE

---

* Bray's, 3764 Piedmont Avenue, Oakland, California.
† Determination of wheat or wheat gluten has been done by the Ouchterlony technique by Arthur Lietze, Ph.D., in the Charles H. Merrill Immunochemical Laboratory for the study of Food Allergy.

diet. The objection that soy-potato bakery products cannot be made, especially in Europe or other foreign countries, is not justified, since soy and potato starch flours are available in England and Germany, as we have determined. If not, they can be obtained by importation.

If the physician decides that such procedures are too inconvenient, the CFE diet can be prepared in the hospital or home omitting such products and using an increased amount of white potatoes, yams, sweet potatoes, tapioca and sugar, and a vegetable oil rather than the milk-free butter substitute in order to increase calories and maintain a satisfactory weight. In England the kosher oleomargarine is milk-free. Along with increased amounts of these foods, the meats, fowl, vegetables, and fruits in the diet are given according to our menus. The excellent control of chronic asthma reported by Kaplan in South Africa and Colldahl in Sweden with our CFE diet without the use of soy-potato bakery products shows that the diet can be so used in any country as well as in the United States. Moreover, soy bean and lima bean flours can readily be imported if desired.

The phytohemagglutinin of soybeans, particularly, is known to be an immuno-inhibitor (Nishio and Lietze, unpublished results). This effect may be operative in relief of allergy on my diets.

ALLERGY TO SOYBEANS AND LIMA BEANS

Though nearly all infants relish soy milk, some children and adults dislike or are allergic to it and soy bakery products, or refuse them entirely. As already advised, our strained meat formula is an excellent replacement for soy milk in infants. In children and adults, fried, boiled, or baked white potatoes or sweet potatoes with the Willow Run milk-free soy margarine three times a day, our tapioca pudding made by our recipes with and between meals, and extra sugar as such will replace calories when the soy-potato bakery products are excluded. Children who refuse soy-potato bread and cookies may accept and relish hotcakes made from our recipe for muffins or bread or from Cellu-Grainless Mix served with the milk-free oleomargarine and maple or cane sugar syrup.

Occasional allergy to soy causes diarrhea and gastrointestinal symptoms, especially in infants. This is usually relieved by use of our meat-base formula. Asthma from soy which gave a large scratch test occurred in two of our adult patients, though allergy rarely occurs to soy oil in Willow Run oleomargarine or to the oil itself. If such allergy is suspected, sesame or cottonseed oil, if a skin reaction to cottonseed is negative, can be used. When salted, it can replace the butter.

Because of the frequency of allergic manifestations, especially bronchial asthma, to rice, corn, rye, and particularly wheat, the initial study of food allergy is best continued without bakery products from these grains when soy products cannot be used.

Though rice and oatmeal frequently cause asthma, nasal allergy, eczema, and headaches, they are often tolerated when gastrointestinal allergy is present. Then bakery products made with these flours can be eaten as advised in recipes in the Appendix.

IMPORTANT DELAY IN ADDITION OF CEREAL GRAINS TO THE DIET

Increasingly since 1930 the frequency of allergy to cereal grains other than wheat has been evident in our control of clinical food allergy. Next to milk and wheat, allergy to other cereals is most common in our patients. Allergy to eggs, chocolate, coffee, fish, nuts, and less frequently other foods follows in importance.

After relief of clinical allergy for two to three weeks, extra fruits and vegetables individually can be added each for two to three days. When symptoms have been absent for one to three months depending on the frequency of former symptoms, then rice, oats, corn, and later rye and wheat can be added. As reported throughout this volume, the refractoriness of food allergy after severe attacks of allergy and in many patients during the summer must be remembered in evaluating results from such additions. Thus, in infants and children who have recurrent bronchial asthma resulting from food allergy with interim relief of symptoms, cereal grains should not be added until attacks have been controlled by the CFE diet for two to even four months. And when they are added and tolerated in the summer, the patients or parents must be told that the CFE diet must be resumed if any former symptoms recur in September to January.

Confirmation of such allergy to cereal grains, especially to corn and its many products, has long been reported by Rinkel and Randolph, and its recognition and confirmation in our practice in these forty years are most important.

Many physicians, including pediatricians and allergists, do not realize the frequency of allergy to rice which we first recognized in 1930 and which Randolph, Johnstone, and the writers have emphasized. In spite of our emphasis of allergy to cereal grains because of which we have advised the initial study of most clinical food allergy with the CFE diet since 1934, our diets containing cereal grains published from 1928 to 1934 are still being advised in preference to the CFE diet, as in a recent textbook published in 1967 on clinical allergy. This failure to realize the frequency of allergy to cereal grains as well as to wheat, milk, eggs, chocolate, fish, and other foods accounts in part for the failure of much trial dieting to relieve perennial nasobronchial, cutaneous, cerebral, toxic, and other manifestations of food allergy.

It is unfortunate moreover that our CFE diet has been modified by some physicians not only by adding one or more cereal grains but by including cow's milk in the form of butter or margarines containing cow's milk and even 40 percent cream which contains 60 percent milk. The inclusion of rye, especially Ry-Krisp, as advised by commercial manufacturers also is unfortunate not only because it is a cereal but because of its close immunological relationship to wheat.

Realization moreover that many soy-potato bakery products sold in health food stores, as in our western states, contain wheat or the gluten of wheat, which is not listed in the printed labels, makes it necessary for such bakery products to be made at home by patients with our recipes or by an honest baker who uses our recipes. Bread which has risen well must be viewed with intense suspicion, as gluten is needed for rising. The use of these products containing unlisted wheat has reactivated allergic symptoms resulting from wheat allergy or has prevented initial relief of such allergic symptoms as well as of celiac disease resulting from wheat. It often is the sole reason for failure to control symptoms resulting from food allergy especially after clinical allergy causing bronchial asthma or obstructive emphysema has been well controlled with honestly made soy-potato bakery products.

The frequency of allergy to cereal grains is responsible for the study of antibodies in the sera of patients sensitized to cereals and in the sera of rabbits sensitized to individual grains in the Immunochemical Laboratory for the Study of Food Allergy in the Samuel Merritt Hospital in Oakland. In these studies Arthur Lietze, Ph.D., has not only studied the serum antibodies to the proteins of cereals but for the first time in 1969 has demonstrated serum antibodies to particulate starches of these cereals.

REASONS FOR FAILURE OF RELIEF FROM ELIMINATION DIETS

1. Failure of the physician to stress the importance of strict dieting and of avoidance of even traces of eliminated foods.

2. Failure to police children's adherence and that of young and older adults to the prescribed diet.

3. Failure to realize that inhalation of foods (that is, flours) including their odors (that is, fish, fruits, fried eggs, coffee, spices, peanuts, and other foods) cause allergic symptoms in very sensitive patients (page 45).

4. Failure to realize that relief is delayed for three to ten days or more until ingested allergenic foods are eliminated from the body or until antibodies to the foods are immunologically inactivated in the body tissues and even for one to two months or longer until the pathological tissue changes from chronic allergy decrease or disappear from the body.

5. Failure to realize that absence of relief may be due to unrecognized allergy to foods in the prescribed diet.

a) Definite or possible fruit allergy requires trial elimination of fruits and condiments (page 48).

b) Possible allergy to soy or other legumes requires their elimination (page 67). Though allergy to cereals, rice, and oats is common in asthma, nasal allergy, and other manifestations of clinical allergy, they may be tolerated in gastrointestinal allergy. They may also be tolerated after relief of other symptoms with the CFE diet as advised on page 46.

c) Allergy to potatoes, especially to its starch, occasionally occurs, requiring use of other starches—tapioca, arrow root, poa, sweet potatoes, or sago (page 548). Asthma from "minute potatoes" in a milk-sensitive patient was found to be due to powdered milk in the potato mixture rather than to potatoes.

d) Possible allergy to beef when definite milk allergy exists must be kept in mind.

6. Failure to remember that food allergy often decreases in the summer and after definite attacks of clinical allergy, especially of bronchial asthma and headaches. It also often increases in the winter. Thus, if foods are added in the summer with no resultant allergic symptoms, they may have to be eliminated in the fall and winter if symptoms recur. A liberal summer diet with a strict elimination diet in the winter may be necessary in the future.

7. Failure to realize that provocation tests (page 66) with additional foods to those in the initial diet which has given relief must be delayed until the patient is free of symptoms for periods of time as advised on page 66.

8. Failure to control inhalant allergy with environmental control or desensitization when symptoms are due to both food and inhalant allergy.

9. Failure to realize that symptoms resulting from severe food allergy may develop from minute particles of food (osmyls) in the air when their odors are recognized by the patient. Osmyls from animals and plants may cause symptoms in allergic patients, as reported by Feinberg and Avies, 1932, and Horesh, 1943, 1944.

10. Failure to recognize occasional allergy to nearly all foods as occurs at times to nearly all pollens. This necessitates study of some possible food allergy with our minimal elimination diets (page 53).

COMMENT

This control of food allergy as the important cause of its many clinical manifestations reported in this volume is best achieved with the adequate and strict use of the elimination diets as we have long advised. As emphasized in this book, ability to successfully use these diets necessitates their accurate, adequate use by the physician and the required cooperation of the patient for more than a few weeks. It is necessary to remember all of the above precautions so that failure will not occur. Patients with moderate and especially marked broad-based food allergy must face the fact that will power is necessary to adhere to the elimination diets required in the initial confirmation of such allergy and the necessary continued accurate elimination of the proven allergenic foods for several months or years and possibly throughout life. Antibodies to causative foods resulting from the body's rejection of foreign allergens associated with clinical allergy too often continues through life.

The time necessary to attain ability to study and control clinical food allergy is comparable to that required to learn methods to control diabetes mellitus or cardiovascular disease or for a surgeon to learn techniques required in gallbladder, gynecological, or other surgery. And as evidenced in this volume, the distress and morbidity with resultant inadequacies in work, body consciousness, tension, and frequent nervousness resulting from unrelieved food allergies make their recognition and control the challenge and indeed the responsibility of physicians in general practice and the specialties in their affected patients.

Failure to use these elimination diets because of being "difficult and cumbersome to apply" is unjustified, as is failure to do a necessary operation because the required technique is difficult. Moreover, the routine use of elimination diets becomes simple when the physician learns to use them as we have long advised.

DEVELOPMENT OF TOLERANCE TO FOODS

With total elimination of allergenic foods and relief of allergic symptoms, children often develop tolerance to most or all foods in one to five years. In some children, however, allergy to one or more foods continues through childhood into adolescence and at times throughout life. Unfortunately tolerance develops and continues infrequently in adults or in old age. Moreover, if tolerance develops and continues for even several years, sometimes with a general diet, food allergy may recur, causing the previous or other manifestations of allergy. Therefore, routine follow-ups by the physician or his secretary asking for a conference every few months is important. Policing these patients to relieve symptoms if they recur or prevent patients from inadequate cooperation is the physician's responsibility.

After a strict elimination diet has controlled bronchial asthma, eczema, gastrointestinal allergy, or other allergic manifestations, the patient may find that slight amounts of allergenic foods only produce slight symptoms. Because of the constant will power necessary to control symptoms, he accepts such discomfort, controlling it with bronchodilators, antihistamines, or unfortunately with corticosteroids which could be discontinued with strict adherence to the required diet. It is especially unwise to take corticosteroids for weeks or months when a strict elimination diet would make their use unnecessary.

After control of symptoms resulting from food allergy, a diet trial with additional foods may show that other individual foods may be taken one to two days a week and not every day. Thus a rotating diet as suggested by Rinkel, allowing additional foods on separate days each week, may be tolerated. If this produces slight or subclinical symptoms, especially in the fall and winter, the taking of such foods should be discontinued. It is far better to follow a diet containing a few nonallergenic foods providing weight and nutrition are maintained.

DESENSITIZATION TO FOODS

In spite of our attempted hypodermic and oral desensitization to allergenic foods for several years, no dependable evidence of relief of resultant allergic symptoms has resulted. It has not been utilized in our practice for over twenty years. Such failure has been reported by most allergists. It must also be remembered that desensitization to inhalants is successful when it protects against only a few milligrams of allergen. To foods it must protect against 100 gm or so.

In spite of this, some patients today are being injected with antigens containing foods as advised by commercial laboratories. Reported relief in our opinion is usually due to the use of antigens containing skin-reacting foods to which the patient was never sensitive. Positive skin reactions do not *a priori* prove clinical food allergy. Moreover, desensitization to foods with their propetans given by mouth has never been confirmed by well-controlled clinical studies. We reported their failure to control food allergy in 1931. The hope for increased tolerance to foods therefore depends on continued, usually prolonged complete elimination of the allergenic foods from the diet. This tolerance occurs most frequently in children and infrequently in adults.

MAINTENANCE OF WEIGHT AND NUTRITION

1. The necessity of maintaining nutrition with our elimination diets has always been emphasized since we first published the diets in 1928 and 1931. The nutritional requirements of protein, calories, minerals, and vitamins must always be satisfied. Normal serum electrolytes must be maintained. An adequate but not excessive intake of synthetic vitamins is especially important. If a carefully recorded diet history and laboratory studies indicate previous deficiency, especially in proteins, vitamins, and electrolytes, extra amounts must be given until remedied. Since eggs, milk products, and fish are eliminated from the CFE diet, maintenance of an adequate protein intake requires the eating of necessary amounts of the specified meat or fowl in the diet at least twice a day. If bacon is allowed, it also can be taken at breakfast. Canadian bacon may be preferable because of its higher protein intake. Soybeans especially are desirable because of their content of all amino acids essential for protein requirements. When soybeans and other legumes are refused by the patient, as previously discussed, or cause indigestion or occasional allergic reactions, more of the tolerated meat and fowl must be prescribed. The sparing influences of adequate carbohydrates on protein metabolism must be remembered.

2. The recommended amounts of the various foods in the menus of the CFE diet contain required amounts of vitamins A, B, C, D, and E, the partial exceptions being vitamin A because of the absence of cow's milk and its products and vitamin D. Therefore, if exposure to sun is not available, moderate amounts of synthetic vitamin D and synthetic vitamin A should be ordered. Such vitamin D is especially important during the fall, winter, and early spring months. Since fish is not in the original diet, fish oils or their concentrates for vitamins A and D cannot be used until fish is prescribed and tolerated. Occasional allergy to cod-liver oil occurs. Though the B vitamins are quite adequate when meat, vegetables and fruits are ingested, they are deficient in the infant's diet when these foods are not included. Therefore, an adequate amount of a liquid, multiple, synthetic vitamin preparation containing A, B, C, D, and possibly E vitamins is advisable in infants and young children to assure a sufficient intake of all these vitamins. Vitamin C is especially important in patients who are not fond of fruit, especially grapefruit, or if allergy to fruits, particularly to the citrus variety, requires their elimination. Whereas such fruit allergy is infrequent in bronchial asthma, it is a common cause in other manifestations of allergy, particularly urticaria, gastrointestinal, joint allergy, and allergic toxemia. Concomitant allergy to vitamin C in some of these very fruit-sensitive individuals might occur occasionally in bronchial asthma. The inclusion of extra cooked vegetables and potato containing vitamin C in such cases, particularly when parenteral vitamin C also produces allergic symptoms, is important. Occasional but definite allergy to vitamin C is discussed later.

3. The elimination of cow's milk results in a deficiency of calcium in the CFE diet. In infants and children until growth is achieved, one gram of calcium should be ingested daily. If children continue to take over 500 cc of a soybean milk (Mull-Soy

contains no corn sugar) or of our strained meat formulae, their calcium requirement will be satisfied, since calcium is present in other ingested foods and drinking water. If it is certain that deficiency is occurring, one-third to one-half teaspoonful of calcium carbonate in water or food daily will remedy the deficit. In children, moreover, when soybean milk or our strained meat formula is refused, one-half teaspoonful of calcium carbonate should be taken in water or in food during the day. Extra calcium is, of course, very important in pregnant and lactating women who are on these CFE diets or on an advised or enlarged elimination diet as long as milk and its products are excluded. In these women one teaspoonful of calcium carbonate in food or water should be a daily ration. Calcium carbonate is the cheapest source of calcium, 40 percent of its weight containing valuable calcium. A level, moderately packed teaspoonful weighs about 2.2 gm and contains 0.88 gm of available calcium. Dicalcium phosphate, on the contrary, only contains 24 percent calcium. One teaspoonful weighs 3.5 gm and contains 0.8 gm of calcium and 0.6 gm of phosphorus. Calcium gluconate is the most soluble salt but contains only 9 percent available calcium. One teaspoonful weighs 2 gm and only contains 0.18 gm of available calcium.

4. The prolonged use of soybean milk may at times lead to an iron deficiency. Soy milk also has led to enlargement of the thyroid gland in a rare child as reported by Wergeland and Mortimer. It is to be emphasized that desired nutrition and weight can be achieved with an animal milk-free diet, if necessary for years, providing required protein, calories, calcium, vitamins, and minerals are taken. This has been shown in our practice by the normal increase in weight and height and nutrition

in many children on milk-free diets for many years.

5. Parents as well as physicians must remember that the increase in weight for boys is between five and six pounds a year after the first year and up to twelve years, with only three pounds during the third year. This increase is slightly greater for girls. Increase in height is from two to three inches per year until the age of fourteen years. Thus greater increases cannot be expected when children are on an elimination diet. If increases in weight and height are slightly less, providing the child is eating the elimination diet in advised amounts along with proper vitamins and the family history reveals small statures and weights, concern may be unwarranted. Progeny of small dogs cannot be nourished into large ones.

6. If minimal elimination diets containing only three to ten foods are necessary, the physician must be certain that enough of the tolerated foods are ingested to maintain protein, mineral, and caloric requirements. Serum electrolyte determination and assurance of adequate but not excessive potassium are important. Supplemental synthetic vitamins including vitamin E and calcium carbonate or other calcium salts furnishing daily requirements must be ingested.

DIRECTIONS FOR THE ADDITION OF CEREAL GRAINS TO THE CEREAL-FREE ELIMINATION DIET (ROWE)

1. *Rice:* Recipes for the rice bakery products are found in *Elimination Diets* under the heading "Important Recipes for Elimination Diets 1 and 2." In addition, Cream of Rice, Puffed Rice, Rice Krispies, Rice Flakes, white rice, and brown rice may be used. Wild rice is not related to the ordinary rice, however. Rice flour may be used in the preparation of gravies and bakery

products according to the recipes.

Boiled rice can be served hot with cane sugar or maple syrup and may be cooked with fruit or if desired, with caramel flavoring and sugar. It may be served in place of potatoes. Cold, boiled rice can be fried in one of the oils specified in the diet and may be served with maple syrup or plain sugar syrup or with fruit juices allowed in the diet. Puffed Rice may be served with fruit juices and sugar or made into candy according to the recipe in our diet booklet. Rice Flakes and Rice Krispies may be served with any of the fruit juices allowed on the diet and sugar. It may also be eaten dry with cane sugar.

If corn or rye has been added to the diet, then bread, muffins, or cookies may be made by combining them with rice flour according to recipes in the diet booklet.

2. *Oats:* Oatmeal and other plain oat cereals may be used providing no other flavoring or adulterants are included. It may be served with the prescribed butter and sugar. If soy products are in the diet, Willow Run butter substitute is desirable.

3. *Corn:* Recipes for the use of corn appear in the diet booklet under the heading "Important Recipes for Elimination Diets 1 and 2." Corn on the cob, canned corn, cornmeal, corn starch, Mazola oil, and Karo syrup may also be used. If soy has been eliminated from the diet, Mazola or other prescribed oil with salt may be used in place of the Willow Run butter substitute, which is made of soy oil.

Corn meal may be cooked with water and a pinch of salt to make a mush. This may be served hot with fruit juices and sugar or maple syrup in place of cow's milk or cream. Cold cornmeal mush may be fried in sesame or Mazola oil and served with maple syrup. Polanta or coarse corn

meal may be cooked in the same manner. Corn Flakes and Corn Krispies may be served with any of the fruit juices allowed on the diet and also with sugar. Hominy may be boiled or fried in Mazola or sesame oil and served with maple syrup. Canned hominy is available. Cornstarch may be used in cooking, and cornstarch pudding may be made by substituting cornstarch for rice. Cornstarch may be used to thicken gravies. Corn syrup such as Karo may be used in candy recipes, in cooking, and as a substitute for maple syrup. Corn pone may be made according to the recipe in the diet booklet.

If rice and rye have been added to the diet, bread, muffins and cookies may be made by combining rice or rye flour with corn meal according to the recipes in the booklet and also according to other recipes, which we will be glad to furnish upon request.

4. *Rye:* Recipes for the use of rye appear in the diet booklet under the heading "Important Recipes for Elimination Diets 1 and 2." In addition, rye flour may be included as well as Ry-Krisp which is available packaged in all food stores.

5. *Wheat:* When wheat is added, white flour made of wheat may be used in cooking. Unadulterated wheat cereals such as Shredded Wheat, Puffed Wheat, Wheatena, and Cream of Wheat can be taken. Many crackers containing wheat can also be used, but possible inclusion of other foods, particularly of powdered milk, must be ascertained by careful reading of the ingredients on the carton or package itself. Graham crackers can be used if there is no other ingredient which is excluded from the diet listed on the package or label. Gluten flour is the protein of wheat flour, and therefore any gluten breads are not permitted when wheat is excluded from the diet. Sour

dough French bread usually contains no milk or other ingredients. Some of these breads, however, are glazed with egg. Low-calorie wheat breads such as Hollywood Bread contain no milk and are made of products of wheat. If other ingredients are listed on the package or label which are excluded from the diet, such bread is not allowed.

When wheat is added to the diet, bread and other bakery products containing wheat are not necessarily permitted. Most of these contain various ingredients which may not be in the diet.

ADDITION OF BEEF TO INITIAL ELIMINATION DIETS

As stated on page 42, beef for the first time is eliminated from our initial elimination diets. Previously it has been allowed except when large scratch reactions or probable previous symptoms to it have occurred.

Because of increasing clinical evidences of allergy to beef and of immunological evidence of frequent allergy to it in many patients sensitive to cow's milk, it is excluded in all of our initial elimination diets. Its initial elimination with dependence on lamb, chicken, and turkey is advised, since patients accept its exclusion in the initial diet.

After relief of the many and various symptoms occurs with the initial diet for one to two months, beef may be added one to two times a week with its more frequent use if reactivation of clinical allergy does not result in two to three weeks.

SUMMARY

1. A list of foods, menus, and recipes with directions for the preparation of our elimination diets are detailed in this chapter. These should be given the patient either in typewritten copies of the prescribed diet and of required menus, recipes, and other information or in an inexpensive booklet noted below.*

2. Emphasis on the time necessary to determine food allergy with elimination diets, the necessity of maintaining weight and nutrition, the necessary supervision of the diet by the physician, and directions for the additions of other foods after relief occurs are discussed.

3. The importance of cereal grain allergy and the delay in adding grains to the original diet are emphasized.

4. Elimination diets for diabetics and obese patients are in the Appendix in Chapter 30.

5. Successful use of our CFE diet without soy bakery products because of allergy to soy or when soy products are not available in foreign countries is discussed.

6. Our continued use of these diets and that of many other physicians and allergists emphasize their importance as the simplest available procedure for the study and control of clinical food allergy by physicians in general practice and in the specialities, including allergy.

The Elimination Diets (Rowe) is an inexpensive booklet which can be obtained from Sather Gate Book Shop, Berkeley, California, for patient's use, necessarily supervised by the informed physician.

Chapter 4

Control of Inhalant Allergies
and of
Allergy to Medications,
Animal Sera and Transfusions

CONTROL OF INHALANT ALLERGY TO POLLENS, FUNGI, ANIMAL EMANATIONS, AND HOUSE AND OTHER ENVIRONMENTAL AND OCCUPATIONAL DUSTS

Though control of this important cause of atopic allergy is discussed throughout this volume, more extended consideration and recommendations concerning inhalant allergy in this chapter are justified.

When inhalant allergy is indicated in the history, with or without positive skin tests, and when perennial symptoms are present, possible allergy to environmental allergens in the home warrants nonallergenic dacron rather than feather pillows; nonallergenic bedding, mattress, and floor coverings; and varying degrees of environmental control.

Control of Pollen Allergy

Pollen allergy is the usual cause of classical hay fever, with or without seasonal bronchitis and asthma in the pollen seasons, characterized by erythema and at times edema of the conjunctivae, and lacrimation with marked sneezing and itching of the nose and eyes and often of the palate, pharynx, middle ears, and eustachian tubes. These symptoms occur during the months when pollens of trees, grasses, and summer and fall weeds to which allergy exists are in the air.

Such pollen allergy causes seasonal ocular, cutaneous (evidenced by allergic dermatitis), urticarial, gastrointestinal including ulcerative colitis, cerebroneural, genitourinary, and other less frequent manifestations in other body tissues as reported throughout this volume.

Though scratch reactions usually are positive, they may be slight or negative in about 10 percent of the patients, placing a premium on history rather than on skin testing as the indication of pollen allergy.

Tests are done, as advised in Chapter 2, with all wind-blown pollens in the air when the symptoms are present as determined by published surveys of the patient's living and working areas and also by local surveys, especially of trees near the home or place of employment. The kind and number of trees, including fruit and nut trees, vary with each patient. Skin tests with pollens of cultivated flowers in gardens near the home and especially kept in the home are important. Likewise, pollens of flowers of insect-pollinated plants and shrubs require consideration if near the home or areas of employment or recreation, especialy if suspected by the patient.

In our practice intradermal tests with suspected pollens which fail to react by the scratch tests are not routine, though they are done by many allergists. Intra-dermal tests should only be done with pollens which have failed to react by the scratch method, using a 1:500 dilution of twenty to forty or more pollens, if indicated, in one sitting rather than with only sixteen or fewer pollens advised by some allergists who do no preliminary scratch tests.

The methods of determining and suspecting allergy to specific pollens have been described in Chapter 2. Confirmation of such allergy depends on the control of allergic symptoms resulting by the following procedures.

Summaries of pollen survey appear in Chapter 30.

Lists of pollens important for testing vary according to the patient's environment.

Environmental Control

Filters in rooms occupied by the patient which remove pollens and other inhaled allergens from the air yield relief according to their mechanical efficiency.

Electrostatic precipitators, which attract pollens and other particles from the air onto high-voltage plates, are most desirable, being nearly 100 percent efficient. Such electrostatic filters, made especially by Honeywell and Raytheon companies, can be moved about in the room while circulating and filtering the room air. However, the windows must be closed, and all cracks around them preferably should be sealed with painter's masking or similar tape so that no outside air containing pollen can enter the room. Ventilation should be from other rooms in the house. Efficient filters, moreover, should be on furnace pipes which conduct outside air into the room. In warm weather the temperature of such a room is only bearable when a water or electric cooling unit is also operating in the room.

Filters that remove pollen by blowing air through several layers of cellulose or of fiberglass installed in a window or which circulate room air reduce the pollen in the air in varying degrees of efficiency up to 85 to 95 percent.

A homemade pollen window filter can be made with little expense. The efficiency of this may be less than that of the commercial ones noted above.

The efficiency of any filter may be checked by the allergist or physician after installation in the patient's room by making counts of pollen on Vaseline-covered slides exposed in the room for several hours.

When any filter is installed in the window, all cracks between the filter and the window and its frame must be sealed with painter's masking or similar tape so that outside air will not enter the room except through the filter. In the homemade filter all cracks and apertures in the filter itself must also be sealed with such tape.

It must be emphasized that before any filter is placed in a room, the dust which contains varying amounts of pollens must be thoroughly removed from all the walls, furniture, floors, furnace pipes, and in the carpets, preferably with large, damp cloths or with a vacuum cleaner, to prevent the circulation of such dust and pollen in the room by the air currents created by the filter.

Air conditioning by a single unit throughout the house requiring the sealing of windows and doors is expensive and only justifiable if such filtration eliminates nearly 100 percent of the pollens from the air of all the rooms of the home. This efficiency must be determined by pollen counts in the various rooms occupied by the patient. Electrostatic filters should be utilized.

Changes of Location and Environment for Control of Pollen Allergy

Moving into areas where pollens causing the patient's symptoms are absent or infrequent may be desirable, especially if allergic symptoms are severe or invaliding. This is particularly helpful when desensitization has never been administered or is refused. In such patients the advisability of change of residence is decreased if the above-discussed air filtration removes pollen from the air of the home and working environments. It continues to be justifiable, however, if absence from the responsibilities of the home, family, and employment for one or two months is possible and the patient's finances permit.

Temporary or permanent residence in ragweed-free areas to prevent or relieve allergic symptoms has been resorted to for many decades. Dependable information about such areas is obtainable from the United States Public Health Service, the Allergy Foundation of America, and from physicians and allergists giving special attention to pollen allergy. Ragweed is absent in the coastal area of Northern California and of the Northwest, though Western Ragweed grows in Central and Southern California and in Eastern Washington, Oregon, and Idaho.

Changes of location to relieve allergic symptoms from grass pollens entail the following possibilities: Temporary residence in higher or more northern areas before the indigenous grasses bloom and while the allergenic grasses are blooming in the home area of the patient is of course beneficial. Moving into areas where species of grasses are different from those to which the patient is allergic also may give relief. Temporary or permanent changes of location benefit some patients from the coastal areas of Northern California where *Lolium perenne*, or rye grass, is most abundant and is a severe cause of hay fever and asthma during May and June. Such relief occurs in the mountains and in northern areas where freezing weather in the fall and winter months prevents growth of the *Lolium* species. Asthma and other symptoms resulting from Bermuda grass which pollinates from early spring to late fall in all areas where freezing weather is minimal are also relieved in such regions. Because of the specificity of grass pollens, residence in areas where grasses allergenic to the patient are absent or infrequent is usually beneficial. Thus patients who have experienced allergic symptoms from grasses of the Eastern or Northern states may be free of symptoms in the coastal or valley areas of California where entirely different species of grasses, especially Bermuda, grow. However, concomitant sensitization to many species of grasses is the rule. In one or more years, moreover, this potential susceptibility to grass pollens usually evolves as active sensitization develops to those in the new area.

Relief from allergy to pollens of trees needs special consideration. When the patient is allergic to the pollens of a tree which is abundant in the region where he lives, temporary residence in an area free of such pollens gives relief or prevents symptoms. Thereafter, desensitization to the causative tree pollens is important. Abundant mountain cedars (*Cupressus*) in the Southwest and various oaks, birches, or alders in other areas are examples. Pines and firs in great forests are similar problems when their pollens produce symptoms. Its fortunately rare occurrence has been reported by us. Further discussion of allergy to cedar and other conifers is in Chapter 8. The asthma and/or nasal allergy arising from allergens of Christmas trees is well recognized. Since the pine and fir trees are not pollinating when cut for the Christmas trade, the allergens must come from the leaves or bark or pitch of the trees. Desensitization with fir tree pollen has prevented usual symptoms from such Christmas trees in one patient, a result reported by other allergists. It has been suggested that a common allergen may be in the volatile oils of the trees and in its pollen. Since cedar pollinates in the winter, symptoms from such Christmas trees may also be due to its pollen.

Tree pollens usually can be avoided by a change of location to the windward side or out of a town or to areas in a city where the trees are absent. Trees of one type such as elm, sycamore, ash, olive, pecan, English and black walnut, or birch may line many streets or be around many or most homes. Or there may be one or several trees to the pollen of which the patient may be sensitive around the home, in adjoining yards, in squares, or in parks which are absent in another area, especially a newly developed area of the town or city. Acacia trees, for example, constitute such a problem around San Francisco Bay. Indigenous oaks in many areas and around and over patient's homes require recognition. Eucalyptus trees are also numerous throughout areas of California where freezing weather is absent. In areas where mountain cedar, especially large trees, are present around the home or in working areas, relief from symptoms resulting from its pollen may require moving to a location free of such trees until pollination ceases. Desensitization may be difficult or inadequate because of the mass of pollen falling from such trees. In California these cedars and enormous oaks in the Yosemite Valley and other areas of the Sierra Nevada Mountains are such hazards.

Of interest is the activation of nasal or bronchial allergy resulting from walnut pollens in some patients from the inhalation of dust during gathering of the nuts or of smoke from burning leaves or wood of walnut trees. Allergens in the dust or smoke similar to those in the pollens are suggested.

In California allergic symptoms from the pollens of fruit trees occur when the home or the working environment is in or in close proximity to such orchards. Though these trees depend largely on insect pollination, the pollens are also carried short distances in the air by the wind. Symptoms resulting from pear, apple, almond, cherry, apricot, and especially peach pollens have been encountered and successfully controlled with desensitization in our practice. One patient had severe asthma and some hay fever from peach pollen which gave a six plus scratch test and to which she was completely desensitized. Asthma resulting from walnut, pecan, and olive pollens may require moving away from homes surrounded by these trees during their pollination. When oaks extend around and over the home, the above also may be true. Desensitization to these pollens is difficult in some patients because of their abundance.

Asthma and nasal allergy from tree pollens therefore is a special challenge to the physician. Knowledge of all the trees around and especially over the patient's home, in his neighborhood, on the streets, and in the parks nearby is imperative. Trees in nearby agricultural areas as well as indigenous trees in forests or wooded areas in the surrounding regions must be known. Whereas published surveys for each state or special localities thereof are available, the number and variety of trees in and around the patient's home and area of occupation can only be determined by the physician, aided by the patient, or some person competent to identify such trees. Information from counts of airborne pollens is also valuable when done by trained workers.

Realization that asthma, nasal allergy, and other allergic manifestations arise from allergy to pollens of cultivated flowers and even to some insect-pollinated shrubs around the patient's home is important. At times their removal from the garden, especially under or around the windows of the rooms occupied by the patient, is necessary. One patient sensitive to pollens of chrysanthemums had asthma until they were removed from a small garden four stories below her apartment window. Pollens of cultivated flowers raised for seeds in some agricultural areas, especially in California, cause allergic symptoms not only in the workers but also in residents nearby.

Finally, pollens from agricultural products such as oats, rye, corn, wheat, hemp, and castor beans must be remembered as causes of manifestations of allergy. Allergy to sugar beet pollen (*Beta vulgaris*) in patients allergic to other Chenopodiaceae who live in areas where their cultivation is frequent must be remembered, as advised by Peck and Moffat in 1959. Temporary absence from areas where they are pollinating may be required.

Desensitization to Pollens

When the history of symptoms with or without skin reactions indicates pollen allergy as the sole or associated cause, desensitization usually is necessary. The exception is relief from environmental control in the home and working environments, maintained usually throughout the twenty-four hours or residence in a pollen-free area during the season as advised above. The good or excellent results, however, from

such adequate desensitization which will decrease or eliminate the necessity of environmental control in future pollen seasons are its justification.

Desensitization to pollens requires the hypodermic administration of combinations of pollens which predominate in the patient's living and working areas as shown by botanical surveys. If symptoms arise from one pollen such as ragweed, sagebrush, oak, walnut, or cedar, desensitization to it alone may be the challenge. If pollens of several trees, grasses, or weeds are probable causes, an antigen containing five to even fifteen such pollens can be administered. If more pollens are suspect, desensitization with two or even three antigens, each containing six to fifteen pollens, may be advisable.

Selection of Pollens for Desensitization

Desensitization must be done with the pollens which are in the air of the patient's home, occupational, and recreational environmental areas during the weeks or months that manifestations of pollen allergy are present. Though the causative pollens usually give reactions, they may be absent in 10 to 15 percent of cases, pollen allergy being indicated by a seasonal occurrence or exaggeration of symptoms. Those pollens which are most prevalent, especially if they give large skin reactions, should be in greater amount in the antigen than the less frequent and important ones.

The above information is obtained from published floras of pollens causing clinical allergy in the areas where the patient lives and works. Pollen counts (see Chapt. 30) also indicate the specific airborne pollens and their relative frequency. In addition, the physician's own observation of months of pollination of the trees, grasses, weeds, and cultivated flowers in the patient's environment is of definite help. As already discussed, such surveys by the physician or a qualified observer, especially of the trees around or in the vicinity of the patient's home or working area is most necessary. Published surveys and especially information in a brochure of a commercial laboratory must not be a substitute for this information concerning local trees. In view of the specificity of grasses, desensitization to representatives of the different species present in the area during the months of the patient's symptoms, instead of a single grass pollen like Timothy or Bermuda, is necessary. The exception is when asthma or other manifestations occur only during the pollinating season of a single pollen such as the *Lolium* pollen during May and June in our San Francisco Bay Area or of olive, walnut, peach, or other trees growing in profusion in the patient's environment and causing bronchial asthma or other allergic symptoms during their individual pollen seasons.

In the Eastern and Central states sensitization to ragweed pollen alone is the most frequent challenge. Whereas desensitization to Timothy apparently controls allergy to most grass pollens in the Eastern and Northern Central states, *L. perenne* is necessary where it is the major grass pollen in May and June in Northern California. Bermuda, moreover, may be the sole or major grass pollen in the summer and fall in California and also in the Southwest. That antibodies to Bermuda differ from those to other grasses was shown by us and other investigators.

In areas where bronchial asthma and/or nasal symptoms resulting from pollen allergy continue from early February to early December, as it does in some patients in the coastal and central areas of Northern California, three different antigens, one containing suspected trees and early grasses; another containing the late spring, early summer grass, and weed pollens, especially *Lolium* grasses; and a third containing the Bermuda, eucalyptus, Chinese elm if in the patient's area, and especially the weed pollens of the fall, are required, as indicated by the seasonal occurrence of asthma or other symptoms with or without positive skin tests, as discussed above.

In our practice, when perennial therapy with such antigens is required, pollens in all three antigens, even thirty in number, may be included in one single antigen for perennial therapy. After a maximum dose of its 1:50 dilution has been attained, an additional antigen containing a few of the most important pollens of the approaching season can be given up to maximum dose of its strongest dilution, combining it with similar maximum doses of the multiple antigen. Thus an extra antigen containing the most important tree pollens can be given before the tree season, the important grass or grasses before the grass season, and important fall pollens before the fall season. Thereby greater protection against the major as well as the secondary pollens responsible for the symptoms can be achieved.

In addition, when allergy to pollens of cultivated flowers is indicated by history and skin testing in patients living where flower gardens are abundant, working in floral shops or nurseries, or where flowers are grown commercially or in large acreages for their seed, desensitization to the important ones may be advisable. This is also necessary to pollens of agricultural vegetations such as wheat, corn, rye, and castor bean, when clinical allergy to them is evident, especially if they are grown around the patient's home or in his working environment.

In our administration of multiple pollens of various trees, grasses, fall pollens with at times those cultivated flowers, and fungi to which sensitization is indicated by history and usually by skin reactions, we have obtained no evidence of "immune paralysis" or so-called competition of antigens in the formation of antibodies arising in the tissues of the reticuloendothelial system. When sufficient allergens of specific pollen productive of severe hay fever or asthma have been given even when several other pollens in the same or separate antigens have been administered, symptoms arising from the individual as well as other pollens usually have been controlled.

The choice of pollens in the patient's antigen based on positive skin reactions alone with no utilization of the special information from published or local surveys or counts of airborne pollens about the actual pollens in the patient's areas is to be decried. This is emphasized by the negative or slight reactions to pollens and other inhalants in 10 to 15 percent of patients clinically sensitive to such allergens. This error occurs especially in antigens ordered by some physicians on the basis of skin reactions to extracts of pollens furnished by commercial companies, some of which pollens may not be in the patient's area at all. How unfortunate, for instance, it is to omit grass pollens such as *L. perenne* or Bermuda or tree pollens such as olive, acacia, oak, cedar, eucalyptus, or peach which may be the main or at times the sole causes of the patient's asthma and include pollens which are never inhaled by the patient and entirely absent in his environments because of skin reactions alone.

Determination of Initial Dilution and Increase of Doses of Antigen

Treatment must be started with 0.05 to 0.1 cc of a dilution which fails to react by the interadermal test, determined by titration of a 1:500, 1:5000, 1:50,000, and 1:500,000 dilution, and which does not produce or exaggerate the asthma, nasal allergy, or other allergic symptoms. It is never advisable to start with a less dilute extract than 1:5000 or a comparable dilution standardized in protein-nitrogen units in preseasonal therapy. In coseasonal therapy a 1:500,000 up to a 1:50 billion or a weaker dilution in very sensitive patients must be used. Weak extracts are required especially if only one to three pollens are in the antigen and if the patient's history indicates marked sensitivity to pollens. If the antigen contains four to ten or even twenty pollens, stronger dilutions of course are tolerated. Initial coseasonal therapy requires very dilute antigens, as discussed below.

The speed of increase of the antigen depends on the apparent degree of sensitivity and the size of the local reaction from the hypodermic injection. If erythema and edema greater than two inches in diameter occur within one-half to one hour after an injection, a slower increase may be advisable. If a greater swelling and erythema occur in six to twelve hours, the next dose should be repeated or reduced to a lower level. If asthma or hay fever develops in fifteen to sixty minutes after an injection, the next dose should be lowered to a previously nonreacting one. At no time during the therapy should injections increase or reestablish symptoms.

Desensitization is continued by Schedule I, II, III, IV, or V, as outlined in Chapter 30, the speed of increase depending on the degree of the patient's allergy to the pollens. In general, Schedules IV and V are utilized when weak dilutions in the 1:5 billion to 1:5 trillion dilutions are advisable. Schedule III and IV are used for the 1:5000 to the 1:50 million dilutions. Schedules II and III are for the 1:500 to 1:50,000 dilutions. If marked sensitization is not obvious, the 1:500 dilution may be given by Schedule II, especially if it contains a large number of pollens. In the treatment of marked pollen allergy, particularly if the antigen is continued after the season has started and especially if only one to three pollens are included in the antigen, Schedule I must be followed, repeating or reducing the dose if large local reactions or activation of allergic symptoms occur.

When the pollens are in the air, the amount or dose of the antigen often must not be increased or may be decreased if the local reaction is larger than four inches in diameter in six to twelve hours and especially if a moderate general reaction has occurred within one hour after an injection. Such a general reaction requires 1:1000 epinephrine 0.2 to 0.5 cc every ten to thirty minutes for relief according to age.

Control of pollen allergy requires desensitization hypodermically one to even two times a week for several months before the season of the causative pollens arrives, continued injections of tolerated doses during the season at five-day to seven-day intervals, and injections at first every week and in the winter every ten to fourteen days with large tolerated doses of the 1:100 or 1:50 dilution so that blocking antibodies to the allergenic pollens will be sufficient to prevent symptoms of pollen allergy in the pollen seasons of the following year. These large tolerated doses should be administered every seven to fourteen days thereafter until symptoms have been absent during at least two successive years.

If symptoms are gradually controlled by such pollen desensitization, the original one or two antigens are continued. However, if

symptoms develop in the later months or those of the succeeding year indicating pollen allergy, other antigens containing pollens in the air not included in antigens to which scratch reactions may or may not be present should be given along with the tolerated doses of the original antigens. Thus, in California symptoms occurring in January, February, and March are often due to the pollens of acacia, fruit trees, *Poa annua,* and at times to wild mustards which bloom especially in these months. Desensitization to these pollens may be required. In California, the Southwest, and the central states, allergy to late summer and fall pollens other than ragweed may become evident as treatment progresses. Such sensitization requires an extra antigen given in small doses in the season when symptoms are present and increased in the winter and following year to maximum tolerated doses into the fall.

Types of Therapy

Preseasonal Therapy

This must be started three to five months before the pollen season begins. If it is begun three months before, then injections should be given every two to three days to reach a maximum dose of 0.5 to 0.7 cc of the 1:50 dilution if possible at least three weeks before the causative pollens are in the air. This or other maximum tolerated doses of a weaker dilution should then be repeated every four to five days, reducing the frequency to once a week if tolerated during the pollen season. If symptoms then develop, the dose should be lowered to 0.1 to 0.3 cc or to similar doses of a weaker dilution as advised in coseasonal therapy discussed below, or treatment may be discontinued until the following year.

Preseasonal treatment in the following

years in most cases can be started at a later date and with stronger dilutions, and it can be increased more rapidly than during the initial year of therapy.

Perennial Therapy

This is favored by many allergists. It is started and continued as advised for preseasonal therapy, the maximum doses of 0.5 to 0.7 cc of the 1:50 or a weaker tolerated dilution being repeated at weekly intervals for six to twelve months and then every seven to fourteen days for one to two years thereafter. If symptoms develop during the pollen season, the dose is reduced into a weaker dilution, or possible allergy to pollens not in the original antigen may require consideration and their inclusion in an additional antigen, starting with 1:5000 to 1:500,000 dilution with as rapid subsequent increases as tolerated. Skin reactions may even be slight or absent to such suspected pollens. After maximum tolerated doses have been continued during the pollen seasons for two to three years with the control of allergic symptoms, skin reactions usually are reduced or may even disappear. After injections are stopped, freedom from symptoms may continue for one to several years or may be permanent thereafter. Without desensitization, skin reactions usually become as large as before treatment was given.

If symptoms of pollen allergy recur in the future pollen seasons, retesting with all pollens is necessary, and indicated desensitization must be reestablished again. If this is required in one to three years after stopping previous perennial therapy, treatment can be rapidly increased up to a maximum tolerated dose, usually of the 1:50 dilution. Perennial therapy for one to two years thereafter is again advisable.

Asthma, hay fever, or other symptoms from pollens controlled by dilutions of moderate or even weak strengths may be activated by the strong dilutions, such as the 1:500 or the 1:50. Temporary discontinuance is advisable with the resumption of weaker dilutions when and if the symptoms are controlled.

Until maximum or tolerated doses which control symptoms are reached, the injections can be given every two to four days. After relief is assured, treatment can be given every week and later, every ten days. The administration of maximum doses two times a week, even to children, for one or more years is unnecessary for good results and may increase expense of therapy which necessitates its discontinuance. Moreover, if symptoms persist when maximum doses are being repeated one to even two times a week, relief may occur with the cessation of therapy for one or even two months with the resumption of a weaker dilution at weekly intervals which controls symptoms thereafter.

Coseasonal Therapy

This is indicated for the control of symptoms during the pollen season. With no previous desensitization, extremely weak dilutions of one or more antigens containing all suspected pollens which then are in the air of the patient's environment are utilized. These doses may vary from 0.1 cc of the 1:50,000 or even 1:5 trillion dilution according to the number of the pollens in the antigen and the probable degree of sensitization. The initial dilution may be the one which fails to give a positive reaction by intradermal titration. Injections can be given every two to three days until relief occurs and then every three to seven days thereafter. Therapy can be continued by the perennial method.

Repository Type of Pollen Therapy

Though the oil-adjuvant type of pollen

antigen as advised by Loveless and especially by Brown is used, it has not supplanted our desensitization as reported in this chapter. When used, small booster doses of only 0.1 to 0.3 cc are given two to three times at weekly intervals subcutaneously after 0.1 to 0.4 cc of the 1:500 or 1:50 dilution have been tolerated two to three weeks before the onset of the pollen season.

Results of Pollen Therapy

Desensitization as utilized for many years by various allergists has relieved 80 to 90 percent of clinical allergy resulting from pollen sensitization, especially when perennial desensitization is given. Some cases require weaker dilutions for control than do the majority of patients with manifestations resulting from pollen allergy. This is especially so during the pollen seasons. Larger doses of the 1:50 dilution, however, may be tolerated with excellent results in many cases, especially as perennial therapy proceeds for two or more years. At no time should an injection intensify or reproduce the asthma or other allergic difficulty.

General Reactions and Their Control

Whether pollen therapy is administered by the physician or by a nurse, parent, or patient, the patient or parents must be informed about symptoms of a general reaction from too large doses given hypodermically or from the occasional entrance of the antigen into a blood vessel. Initial symptoms are itching and erythema of the palms and of the injected site and later in other skin areas. Thereafter, edema, hives, and itching around the injection and later of the eyelids, hands, face, and in other areas of the body; itching, congestion and sneezing, and watering of the eyes and nose; coughing; tightness in the chest;

wheezing in the lungs; and dyspnea may develop. These symptoms occur in five to sixty minutes, varying in severity according to the degree of the allergy and the increase of the dose above a previous nonreacting one. With severe reactions, abdominal cramping, hyperperistalsis, defecation, bladder spasm and involuntary urination, and even shock or death may occur. These reactions are most common during the pollen season, especially during the first year of therapy and particularly in very sensitive patients.

After an injection, therefore, the patient must wait in the physician's office from a few minutes up to twenty minutes according to the degree of his pollen allergy, especially if the stronger dilutions of the antigen are being administered. If any indication of a general reaction arises, then from 0.2 to 0.8 cc of 1:1000 epinephrine solution should be given hypodermically every five to sixty minutes until the reaction is controlled. The dose and the frequency of the injection depends on the patient's age and the degree of reaction. In severe reactions epinephrine may even be required, if necessary, every two to six hours during the subsequent twenty-four hour period after the immediate reaction has been controlled. To lessen and control symptoms within one to two or more hours thereafter, oral Prednisone, 5 to 20 mg or comparable doses of another corticoid can be given immediately when the reaction develops and repeated in 5 to 10 mg doses every two to six hours thereafter. If the reaction is severe, intramuscular therapy in similar doses is justifiable. As in the treatment of any anaphylactic reaction, vasopressors are indicated for the control of severe shock not responding to other therapy.

To lessen the speed of absorption of the injected antigen, a tourniquet can be applied on the arm or thigh above the injected site releasing it for one-half minute every two to three minutes. This is less helpful when injections are given in the lower lateral thigh because of the lesser efficiency of a tourniquet in the mid thigh, especially in an obese patient.

In addition, a patient may carry tablets of isopropylarterenol (Isuprel®) for sublingual use as well as ephedrine-aminophylline and corticoid tablets. If a reaction develops, an ephedrine-aminophylline and a corticoid tablet should be swallowed and an Isuprel tablet taken sublingually as he returns to the physician's office for the above parenteral therapy.

With the method of administration of pollen antigens advised in this chapter, general reactions are very infrequent, less than three or four occurring in the thousands of injections given by us every year. Their probability, however, always must be in mind, making accurate measurement of the increased doses out of the indicated dilution and not of a stronger, more concentrated one of paramount importance. As formerly stressed, at no time should pollen therapy exaggerate or reproduce symptoms.

Buck and Bryant have reported that reactions to desensitization injections occur when the patient has precipitating as well as reaginic antibodies to the allergen extract. High-risk patients may thus be detectable by Ouchterlony tests.

Self-Administration of Pollen Antigens

This is justified by the following circumstances:

1. If the patient lives many miles from a physician.

2. If work or school attendance prevents frequent visits to a physician.

3. If expense of such treatment is a fi-nancial problem, at times leading to discontinuance of necessary desensitization.

4. If the same frequent doses or gradually increasing doses of a single nonreacting dilution of an antigen is to be given with supervision at fortnightly, monthly, or at times less frequent conferences with the supervising physician.

5. If a maximum, nonreacting dose of an antigen is advisable every five to ten days for perennial therapy after the pollen season, providing the allergic symptoms are controlled.

When self-administration of any antigen is allowed, the physician must instruct the patient or person who will give the injections so that the syringe will be properly sterilized, the skin will be disinfected, and the antigen will be measured accurately in a tuberculin syringe and given subcutaneously in an area free from underlying large blood vessels, as in the outer lower thigh.

With self-administration the patient must be given ampules of sterile epinephrine 1:1000 or in bottles of 5 to 20 cc. Though adherence to the above directions leads to practically no general reactions, their onset occasionally occurs in five to sixty minutes after an injection. The patient therefore must be instructed in the hypodermic administration of 0.2 to 0.6 cc of the epinephrine in 1:1000, repeating it every five to thirty minutes depending on the patient's age and the degree of reaction as advised above. Hence, this desensitization should only be given when epinephrine will be available for one hour thereafter.

Control of Animal Emanation Allergy

Suspicion and determination of the many animal emanations that may cause perennial nasal allergy, bronchial asthma, atopic dermatitis, and other manifestations of allergy by history and skin testing have been discussed in Chapter 4.

Environmental Control

Environmental control in the home and working environment by removal of the incriminated or suspected animals and all of their emanations will control symptoms arising therein. This elimination, however, must be complete, since the inhalation of traces of such emanations will cause continued difficulty or reproduce symptoms. If the manifestation of animal emanation allergy is due to cats, dogs, rabbits, canaries, or other birds or unusual pets such as guinea pigs, mice, hamsters, or even monkeys in the house or basement, not only the animals but their emanations from carpets, furniture, drapes, walls, and other surfaces in the rooms in which they have been must be eliminated. The presence of such emanations in the pipes of a hot-air furnace and the possible cleaning thereof has to be remembered. When allergy to wool, feathers, goat or mohair, camel, rabbit, horse, cat, or other animal hair and emanations of silk are suspect, removal of carpets, pillows, blankets, fabrics, upholstery, clothing, furs, felt, and other materials made of or containing such animal products may be necessary to relieve the allergic symptom. Clothes on which animal emanations and feed and other dusts may be present should be changed to dust-free house clothes before entering the home of a person allergic to such inhalants. Cattle and other hair in Ozite and other pads under rugs and carpets must be kept in mind.

Complete removal of animals which are probable or definite causes of allergic manifestations from the working or recreational environments may also be necessary to relieve symptoms. In dairy farmers, cattle farmers, or horsemen; spinners of wool, silk, or fabrics containing rabbit, camel or other hair, wool, or silk; workers with animals in experimental laboratories, race tracks, rodeos, zoos, circuses, and certain sportsmen; and especially riders and tenders of horses, absence from such animals may become a financial as well as sentimental problem.

Desensitization

When occupational or recreational reasons make the absence of animals difficult or unacceptable to the patient, desensitization is justifiable, and antigens containing one or more animal emanations can be administered as we have advised with a pollen antigen. The initial dose and the gradual increase of subsequent injections is determined as advised for pollen therapy. Good relief from clinical allergy from such inhalants often occurs justifying this specific desensitization.

When marked sensitization to animal emanations as indicated by history and skin reactions exists, initial doses of the antigen in extremely weak dilutions, even in the billions or trillions, must be given to prevent serious general reactions. This is especially true in patients who have an inherited allergy to horse dander or serum. Such extreme sensitization emphasizes the wisdom of testing with the scratch or puncture method and only very weak antigens even in the billions or weaker dilutions with the intradermal method when the scratch test itself is entirely negative. As the dose of animal emanations is increased, especially into the stronger dilutions, the possibility of general, at times serious, reactions again must be emphasized. The precautions necessary in the administration of an antitoxic animal serum and the serious at times fatal reactions which may occur are discussed below.

Directions for environmental control of all environmental allergens are given in Chapter 30.

Control of Miscellaneous Inhalants

The role and detection of orris root and at times of rice powder in cosmetics and of karaya, acacia, tragacanth, linseed and quince seed gums in hair-setting solutions in producing allergic manifestations and symptoms from pyrethrum and occasionally from glue dust must be remembered. Elimination of these allergens from the environment of a patient who develops allergic reactions from them is of course required.

For many years we have desensitized patients allergic to orris root as with pollen antigens. At present its incorporation in cosmetics is less frequent than in former years. One beauty operator with nasal and bronchial allergy arising from the dust of karaya gum after it had dried on the hair was beneficially desensitized. Such treatment with antigens of other substances, especially flaxseed and glue, is not advisable and may be hazardous.

Clinical allergy from tobacco occurs from the inhalation of its smoke and by ingestion from cigarettes, cigars, or chewing tobacco. Nonsmokers sensitized to tobacco may develop nasobronchial or even cutaneous allergy from inhalation of smoke in the air from other smokers. Its possible role in causing obstructive emphysema is discussed in Chapter 11 and in Chapter 30.

Inhalant allergy to fish, castor bean dust, and other ingredients in fertilizers and sprays was reported by Small in 1952.

Control of Cottonseed and Kapok Allergy

Cottonseed allergy produces severe sensitization in certain patients. Relief occurs from the elimination of mattresses, pillows, and upholstery containing cotton and especially cotton linters from the living environments. Dustproof covers will also give relief. Sensitization may be so great that the minute amount of allergen from cotton fabrics, as in the air of a store selling them, will cause nasal or other allergic manifestations. Cottonseed meal in feeds for fowl or animals especially is deleterious if inhaled by the sensitized patient. Cottonseed allergy may prevent working in or around cotton gins, in cotton fields, in cottonseed oil factories, in mills weaving cotton fabrics, or in other industries handling cotton or its products. That the ingestion of cottonseed oil and shortening produces asthma and at times other marked allergic symptoms has been reported by us since 1937 and by other allergists.

Kapok allergen in dusts of its seeds and its floss also causes clinical allergy. This was first reported by Brown and later by Wagner and Rackemann. Removal of or the covering of pillows, mattresses, and upholstery containing kapok with dustproof slips relieves inhalant allergy therefrom. When its floss pulverizes and ages, increased allergy often results from its inhalation. Patients sensitive to cottonseed may also be sensitive to kapok.

Because of the severe fatal reactions which have been reported with even extremely dilute extracts of cottonseed, intradermal testing and especially desensitization are not done in our patients. Relief of symptoms must depend on elimination of these allergens from the patient's environments, whether in the house or in recreational or working areas, especially in cotton gins or where cottonseed meal or oil is processed or around fertilizers or feeds containing cottonseed.

Control of Fungus Allergy

Suspicion and identification of fungi which may cause bronchial asthma and nasal or other clinical allergy through the history and also by skin tests have been discussed in this chapter. If the patient has possible allergy to such molds, their meticulous elimination from rooms, closets, basements, and other areas in the house and the patient's working environment is most important. Avoidance of hay or feeds containing such molds is necessary.

When elimination of spores from the air is impossible, desensitization with antigens containing suspected fungi, according to the method described for pollen therapy, is indicated. Such an antigen may contain one or more allergens of such fungi. If symptoms do not respond to such stock antigens, an autogenous antigen can be made from all fungi grown on a Sabboraud media plate after its exposure for three to four minutes in the patient's rooms or areas of employment. Antigens for desensitization are especially effective, according to Prince, if prepared from a special broth used for the growth of fungi or according to Schaffer from the ground-up pedicle on his synthetic broth in which fungi are grown.

That asthma and hay fever may arise from allergy to airborne spores of fungi is reported by many allergists. These spores are increased in the air especially during certain pollen seasons. *Alternaria* is most important especially in the Midwest and Atlantic seaboard. Desensitization to fungi, especially *Alternaria,* particularly when definite skin reactions are present may be required along with that to the indicated pollens to obtain desired relief. Though dependable counts of airborne spores are difficult to obtain, they reveal the predominating fungal spores which may need inclusion in antigens used for therapy.

That allergy to fungi is a major or associated cause of symptoms is difficult to establish. Provocation inhalant tests to evaluate the role of specific fungi may be helpful. In California the lack of humidity and dampness discourages the growth of fungi. When evidence, however, points to clinical allergy therefrom, desensitization with stock or autogenous antigens is justified. Corroboration of fungus allergy, as in all causes of allergy, depends on results of such therapy. That a farmer's lung syndrome may be due to allergy to fungi and other allergens in moldy hay and grain is indicated by relief of early or moderate symptoms and pulmonary densities by removal of the patient from the causative environment, along with corticosteroid therapy as reported by Jackson and Yow.

Fungus allergy must not be assumed because of positive skin reactions alone, especially when allergic symptoms occur during months when large skin-reacting pollens are in the air. Adequate desensitization to such pollens usually yields excellent results without concomitant therapy with skin-reacting fungi. If symptoms are not satisfactorily controlled or continue beyond the pollen season when the reacting fungi remain in the air, then desensitization thereto is justified, as noted before in this chapter and in Chapter 8. Failure to study and control existent food allergy often encourages unnecessary desensitization to pollens, house dust, fungi, and animal emanations based on skin reactions alone. Such therapy, often empiric in type with so-called "conventional antigens," has continued for months or even years, at times combined with injections of stock or autogenous vaccine without satisfactory results, when on the contrary, our study and control of previously unrecognized food allergy proved the sole cause; in others it was a concomitant cause, and desensitization to one or more types of inhalants also has been required.

Control of Hay, Grain, and Feed Dust Allergy

This allergy has been discussed in Chapter 2. Asthma or other manifestations of allergy from these dusts can be relieved by avoidance of their inhalation. Around such dusts, the wearing of masks over the nose and mouth may reduce the degree of symptoms, though complete prevention of their inhalation is difficult. Unless glasses are worn with tight frames encircling the eyes, dusts enter the eyes and carried by the tears enter the nose. Absorption of such allergens from the conjunctivae and nasal mucosa may result in the allergic symptoms. Symptoms may be especially severe in workers in grain elevators and warehouses or around silos from dusts of machines harvesting any of the grains, legumes, castor beans, flaxseed, cottonseed, or other agricultural products to which allergy exists.

If the patient's business or livelihood entails inhalation of dusts which cause clinical allergy and relief from attempted protection against them fails, desensitization may be tried. Extracts can be made from the incriminated dusts or from ground-up feed or grain dusts, or stock extracts can be used. The exceptions are cottonseed and flaxseed. Treatment is conducted as advised for pollen allergy. When pollen allergy is evidenced by history and skin testing, desensitization to pollens is also important. In some patients allergy to the feed and grain dusts is controlled or greatly reduced with adequate pollen therapy alone. Excessive inhalation of these dusts unfortunately may produce asthma or other clinical allergy which is only partially controlled

with prolonged desensitization in contrast to excellent results from pollen therapy in hay fever resulting from pollens. Avoidance of their inhalation by change of employment may be necessary.

Control of House Dust Allergy

That clinical allergy may arise in whole or in part from housedust must depend on the patient's history and not on skin tests alone. Provocation inhalant tests may yield important information. We agree with Harris and Shure that mild reactions to house dust usually should be ignored. When the history indicates probable or definite house dust allergy, adequate environmental control in the patient's home and working environment often gives relief. If this cannot be complete or is inadequate and if (in addition) symptoms arise from the inhalation of house dust in other environments, desensitization is justified. The desensitization can be attempted with a stock extract of dust made in the physician's laboratory from the dusts of several homes or with commercial preparations. If results are not satisfactory, treatment with an autogenous dust extract may be effective, as we advised in 1928. Such an extract may also be used in the initial treatment. In our laboratory the strongest extract we prepare is empirically labeled 1:50 or the #1 dilution. If desired, the content of protein nitrogen can be determined. Weaker dilutions are made as advised for pollen antigens. The initial and increasing doses are given as advised for hypodermic administration of such antigens.

Since house dust allergy is infrequently the sole cause of symptoms, its administration alone without adequate study and control of food allergy and/or other inhalant allergies usually is ineffectual and is open to criticism. As already stated, much desensitization to house dust, even with weak dilutions, is given only because of a positive skin reaction without clinical evidence that allergy is arising from house dust.

The sole administration of stock house dust extracts usually in dilutions of 1:10,000 to 1:1 million one to two times a week for months or even years with little or no benefit and with no attention to possible or evident food or other inhalant allergies is too frequent, especially by physicians who are not specialists in the field of allergy. This is as reprehensible as the treatment of bronchial asthma or other clinical allergy with corticosteroids alone, ignoring the responsibility of recognizing and controlling all possible causative food or inhalant allergies before or when they are given.

Case 1: Thus a boy, four years of age, had had recurrent bronchial asthma preceded by nasal symptoms of 2½ years' duration. At first biweekly and later weekly injections of a dilute house dust extract had been continued for two years without any relief. Because of the presence of the pathognomonic history of asthma resulting from food allergy, our CFE diet was given with excellent relief in one month and with continued relief for two years, depending on the elimination of allergenic foods and with no desensitization to house dust.

Control of Allergy to Mites in House Dust

This recently recognized explanation of nasal and bronchial allergy as a cause of symptoms from house dust needs consideration, as summarized in Chapter 8, to which the reader is referred.

Inhalant Allergic Alveolitis

Inhalant antigens may produce an Arthus type response in the alveoli. This is not a disease of atopy and can occur in anyone. Many diseases have been described related to occupation or hobby which can all be relegated to inhalant allergic alveolitis: farmer's lung, pigeon breeder's lung, baggassosis, maple bark worker's lung, and so on. The initial formation of antibody may be caused by accidental introduction of the antigen below the skin, as by slivers of wood in maple bark worker's lung.

The clinical manifestations of inhalant allergic alveolitis can range from a sudden acute attack to the gradual development of pulmonary fibrosis. Typically there are attacks of dyspnea, tightness in the chest, and cough with or without sputum.

Diagnosis is by radiography (diffuse lung mottling), respiratory function tests, and in particular by detection of precipitating antibody in the patient's serum to the suspected inhalant. Delayed reactions are found on skin testing. Treatment consists of elimination of the inhalant from the patient's environment with steroid therapy for acute illness.

Control of Fly and Insect Allergy

When asthma is probable or definite to the airborne emanations of various insects, and their elimination from the patient's environment is not possible, desensitization with antigens of various incriminated insects is important, as advised by Thomas and others. Antigens for desensitization to various fleas and insects are made in the allergist's or in commercial laboratories.

Such desensitization has long been indicated for the control of asthma and other clinical allergies arising from the emanations of lake flies, as from the Great Lakes and also from Clear Lake in California. Such antigens made in our laboratory have controlled bronchial and nasal allergy in several patients. In recent years antigens of other insects giving positive skin reactions have been administered with varying success for the control of possible or demonstrated clinical allergy.

Moderate to fatal allergic reactions from bee, yellow jacket, or wasp stings especially justify desensitization with their antigens made in the allergist's or in commercial laboratories. Antigenic relationships between these insects were reported by Foubert and Stier in 1958. They are administered as advised for pollen antigens on pages 85 and 86. The size of the maximum dose depends on the age and the tolerance of the patient. A maximum dose should be repeated at weekly and later fortnightly intervals for one or two years. Until desensitization is terminated, the parent of a child or the patient and also a relative should be instructed in the administration of epinephrine 1:1000 and the use of other medications for the control of severe allergic reactions as discussed previously in this chapter.

The degree of protection is finally determined by allowing a vigorous bee or wasp to sting the patient on the forearm in the physician's office. A general reaction must be anticipated. If it occurs, it must be controlled immediately with epinephrine hypodermically, intermittent application of a tourniquet above the bite site, and other medications. Such a severe reaction has only occurred in one of the many patients we have treated when their protection was being tested with such provocative stinging. Our antigen, given to all other patients, had been replaced by a commercial extract a few months before this general reaction occurred. Treatment has been continued with our own antigen freshly made in our laboratory.

According to Loveless (1965), venom free of carcass proteins is to be preferred for desensitization.

Control of Tobacco Allergy

The possible development of bronchial and nasal allergy to tobacco allergen either by inhalation or absorption through the oral and gastrointestinal tissues and the irritating effects of its smoke and its other detrimental results in the body must be remembered.

When apparent clinical allergy is indicated in the history and by positive skin reactions, desensitization is justified not only to allergens in tobacco itself but as Swinny has reported, to those in tobacco smoke. He prepares the latter by drawing the smoke of four popular brands of cigarettes through 100 cc of extracting fluid in a flask with a vacuum pump. Possible irritants are removed by dialysis. He has relieved asthma and nasal allergy as well as ocular and pharyngeal irritation by desensitization with this extract.

Desensitization with Multiple Inhalant Allergens

Perennial bronchial asthma and other manifestations of clinical allergy are due at times to multiple inhalant allergy. Consideration of this is justified if an adequate study of possible food allergy, as advised in Chapter 3, fails to give relief and if environmental control and desensitization to allergens in one or two groups of inhalants has not benefited the symptoms.

Case 2: A woman, thirty-two years of age, had had perennial asthma for twenty-five years, especially in the autumn to the late spring. For twelve years she had been constantly desensitized to various inhalants, with questionable benefit. In one month after our CFE diet was started and desensitization was terminated, her asthma was entirely relieved and has continued to be relieved for the past five years except briefly after lapses in the prescribed elimination diet.

Summary

1. Inhalant allergy as an important cause

of nasobronchial allergy is discussed *in extenso* in this chapter.

2. Allergy to pollen and less so to fungi as the important cause of symptoms from early spring to late fall is emphasized.

3. In perennial nasal allergy, in addition to food allergy, inhalation of animal emanations, house dust allergens and mites, fungi, feed and grain and other occupational dusts, fly and insect emanations, and tobacco allergens must be remembered as possible causes.

4. Environmental control and indicated desensitization to inhalants that persist in the air in spite of environmental control are advised not only in nasal and bronchial allergy but also when indicated in other manifestations of inhalant allergy. Cooperation of the patient and modification of the desensitization therapy and environmental control are required according to results obtained.

5. Failure of relief requires reevaluation of evidence of possible food allergy. Many patients who have been receiving desensitization with conventional multiple antigens with no relief during months and years of therapy are rapidly relieved with the control of food allergy with our elimination diets as advised in Chapters 3 and 8.

CONTROL OF ALLERGY TO MEDICATIONS, ANIMAL SERA, AND TRANSFUSIONS
Control of Drug Allergy

After drugs have been recognized as causes of clinical allergy, relief is only possible with their entire discontinuance. Because of the persistence of such drugs in the body, symptoms may not disappear for several days or even for weeks. Desensitization is impossible.

When the history suggests allergy to a drug, determination of possible sensitization requires the trial of a minimal amount,

with gradual increase thereafter. Thus, if allergy to aspirin is suspected, especially in an allergic patient and particularly in bronchial asthma, a provocative oral dose of one-half to one grain should be given. Though asthma usually develops within an hour or so in the patient very sensitive to aspirin, resultant urticaria and localized edema may be delayed for twelve to twenty-four hours. If such occurs, aspirin must not be taken in any form whatsoever. Similar tests with other suspected drugs can be made. Cumulative allergy to drugs only after their administration for days or longer periods must be realized.

Penicillin is another medication in common use which produces immediate and even fatal allergic reactions and which frequently causes delayed and persistent manifestations of allergy, also discussed in Chapter 8. With a definite history of former clinical allergy to penicillin and especially if an anaphylactic reaction has occurred, it should never be given either parenterally or by mouth except as discussed in Chapter 8. When penicillin has been given previously with a resultant history of hives or other slight allergic reaction, then skin testing may be done, as advised in Chapter 8, if its use is adjudged necessary for control of some particular bacterial invader.

Even with such testing and careful administration of penicillin, resultant clinical allergy in one to three days and the serum sickness type of reaction in seven to twenty days, as discussed later, can occur. Moreover, in the penicillin-sensitive patient, foods such as milk and its products (because of the frequency of the practice of administering penicillin into the tits of cow's udders), cheese from such milk, and Camembert and Roquefort, containing the penicillium mold itself, and certain vegetables and fruits, especially citrus fruits on which penicillium may be growing, must be entirely avoided. Possible inclusion of penicillin in mixtures of drugs and especially in biologics such as polio vaccine must be remembered. Traces of penicillin may remain in syringes previously used for its injection. Though penicillinase may benefit some delayed persistent allergic reactions to penicillin, it should never replace immediate treatment with epinephrine, parenteral corticoids, and other measures to control immediate severe life-threatening reactions. Reported allergy to this enzyme, as reported by Caputi and others, discourages its utilization, especially after an initial injection.

Control of Chemical Allergies

The occurrence of clinical allergy from the various chemicals and products of petroleum is discussed in Chapter 9. Relief of such symptoms depends on the prevention of their inhalation, ingestion, and contact by the patient. As in drug allergy, desensitization is impossible.

Lists of allergens and possible symptoms therefrom are in Chapter 29.

Asthma or Other Clinical Allergy from Organ Extracts

Asthma is a rare result of allergy to these extracts compared with resultant urticaria and other cutaneous manifestations. It has occurred from liver extract. Moderate or severe anaphylactic shock has been reported from pituitary extracts. Such reactions to pituitary and liver extracts, however, are less frequent than a decade or more ago because of their greater purification. Reports of allergic reactions to ACTH are noted in Chapter 8.

Allergy to insulin usually occurs to the hormone rather than to the specific protein of the animal. This is evident in crystalline insulins from different animals and even from man, the allergic reaction occurring to the same crystalline insulin present in each source. Allergy to the protein of the animal also occurs, as illustrated by the relief of allergic reactions resulting from the substitution of beef insulin for pork insulin. The same relief also has been reported from allergic reactions from ACTH by substituting a product from beef for that from pork. Rare anaphylactic shock and asthma with more frequent urticaria and serum sickness in one patient and aplastic anemia from ACTH favor the use of corticoids when indicated for the control of manifestations of clinical allergy. Alexander estimated that clinical allergy from ACTH occurs in 0.3 to 0.5 percent of patients to whom it is given. Death may occur, as reported by Unger and Unger. Because of this and its more rapid action and also because of the absence of reports of symptoms of allergy and shock especially with intramuscular and intravenous administration of corticoids, they are used in our practice instead of ACTH. Further justification for the use of corticoids is the evidence that ACTH is not necessary to activate adrenal function when it is decreased by previous corticoid therapy.

Severe allergic reactions to trypsin and its questionable mucolytic effect contraindicate its use in the treatment of clinical allergy.

Clinical Allergy from Animal Sera

Allergic manifestations with or without anaphylactic shock and even death occur with the first injection of animal serum, especially of the horse, when there is an inherited or natural "sensitivity." For this and other reasons, intradermal testing is never done on a patient who gives a positive reaction to horse serum by the scratch method. Deaths after intradermal testing with horse serum were recently emphasized by a death from a 1:10 dilution reported in the *Journal of the American Medical Association*. Previous scratch and ocular tests would have contraindicated such intradermal injection. The outstanding discussion by Ratner of the anaphylactic and serum sickness type of reaction and the serious involvement of the nervous tissues from serum allergy must be remembered.* Therefore, immunization of everyone to tetanus toxoid every three to four years is imperative so that a booster injection of tetanus toxoid, rather than tetanus antitoxin, will suffice to stimulate immunity when penetrating wounds occur. This is especially important in allergic patients and particularly in those who have any suggestion of allergy to animal emanations. Serum allergy also develops when horse or other animal sera are given for the rare diphtheria of today where immunity has not been established by previous injection of diphtheria toxoid. It also occurs when animal serum is given to control botulism. Antipneumonic sera used over twenty years ago has been replaced by antibiotics. Sensitization to horse serum may arise from ingestion of horse meat or mare's milk.

Tetanus Prophylaxis

1. Without previous active (toxoid) immunization.

(a) Antibiotic prophylaxis—if wound is less than two hours old—administer tetracycline or erythromycin 0.50 gm every six hours for four doses, then 0.25 gm four times daily for three additional days.

(b) If wound is more than two hours old, administer antibiotics as above and 5000 units of tetanus antitoxin.

---

*If tetanus antitoxin is mandatory in a horse serum sensitive patient, human tetanus immune globulin is advised rather than rabbit or cow's serum antitoxin.

2. With previous active (toxoid) administration.

(a) Last injection within five years—administer 0.50 cc plain tetanus toxoid only for simple puncture wounds. If there is widespread tissue damage or possible infection, add antibiotic therapy.

(b) Last injection five to fifteen years previously—administer 0.50 cc plain tetanus toxoid plus antibiotic as above.

(c) Last injection over fifteen years previously—administer 0.50 cc plain tetanus toxoid plus 5000 units tetanus antitoxin plus antibiotic therapy.

The wound should be carefully cleaned if possible in all cases. Tetanus antitoxin should be administered.

Serum sickness, first described by Von Pirquet and Schick, occurring one to three weeks after the injection of horse serum also causes bronchial asthma and especially cutaneous, joint, gastrointestinal, and nasal symptoms; fever; and occasional death. It is due to the union of antibodies developed by the injection of the serum with the residual horse serum proteins still in the body. These antibodies, moreover, remain for several months or even for a longer period after an injection of horse or other animal serum. Thus the history of every allergic patient and indeed of all people should record any previous reactions to sera along with possible sensitization to horse or other animal emanations.

(Reactions from antirabies prophylaxis were discussed by Blatt and Lepper and Appelbaum *et al.*)

Allergy to Egg and Silk in Vaccines

Asthma with cutaneous edema at the site of the injection and also moderate anaphylaxis and even death have occurred in egg-sensitive patients after the injection of viral vaccines grown on egg media for immunization against typhus, yellow fever, Rocky Mountain spotted fever, influenza, and adenoviral infections. This has been discussed in Glaser's book. One severe allergic reaction with death, even on the nineteenth day, occurred after such an injection containing a trace of egg, a similar dose having been tolerated one year previously. Thus the possibility of allergy to egg must be determined before administration of such viral vaccines by a dietary history of possible egg allergy and especially by scratch testing. Though not necessarily present, a large scratch reaction often occurs when egg allergy exists. If a definite history of egg allergy is present, with or without a large scratch reaction, the vaccine should not be given. If the history and scratch test are negative, the vaccine can be administered.

Severe allergic symptoms have arisen from silk allergen in injected vaccines filtered through silk. With the increasing use of synthetic filters, such as Millipore, these reactions will disappear or decrease in frequency.

Clinical Allergy From Tetanus and Diphtheria Toxoid

Very rare asthma with cutaneous edema has occurred from allergy to diphtheria or tetanus toxoid. Anaphylactic shock in identical twins, with death in one, was reported after a second injection of diphtheria toxoid and pertussis antigen resulting apparently from unidentified degradation products. Other allergic reactions from toxoid have been reported. It has been suggested that possible allergy to toxoid should be considered. Immunization with tetanus or diphtheria toxoid and to pertussis vaccine, however, is not contraindicated in children with bronchial asthma or other allergic disease. It is especially important because of the possible danger of tetanus or diphtheria antitoxin in children and adults suffering with asthma or other manifestations of allergy. Vaccination against smallpox is not contraindicated unless uncontrolled eczema also occurs, which may result in generalized vaccinia and even death.

Clinical Allergy From Transfusions

Asthma with occasional shock and more often urticaria has occurred after transfusions from properly grouped donors who had eaten foods just before the blood was drawn to which the patient was allergic. Such clinical allergy to milk, eggs, berries, tomato, cabbage, fish, and other foods has been reported. Moreover, patients can be passively sensitized with antibodies to foods or other allergens present in the donor's blood. Asthma from the inhalation of horse dander because of antibodies in the patient after transfusion from a horse-sensitive donor was first reported by Ramirez in 1919. Evidence of such allergy to various foods and inhalants after transfusion of blood containing antibodies to such allergens has occurred in our practice. As Garver (1939) and Loveless (1941) have emphasized, possible allergic reactions in one to three hours after a transfusion must be remembered, especially when a high degree of sensitization to foods, inhalants, especially to pollens during the pollen season, is present in the patient. Fasting donors reduce the likelihood of transfusion reactions in food-sensitive patients or the elimination of specific foods from the donor's diet for one to two days to which the patient may be allergic may suffice to prevent such post-transfusion allergy. The transfusion of washed, properly grouped red blood cells in normal saline also reduces possible allergic reactions.

Summary

1. Symptoms of allergy to drugs require their entire elimination by mouth, inhalation, injection into body cavities and parenterally for weeks or for longer periods. Aspirin and penicillin especially are offenders. Allergy to other organic and chemical drugs, as discussed in Chapter 29, must be remembered.

2. Asthma, cutaneous, and at times other manifestations of allergy arise from organic extracts including those of liver and pituitary. Sensitivity to ACTH may be present, either to the animal protein or the pituitary hormone, causing varying degrees of clinical allergy as persistent generalized urticaria from daily injections of ACTH or in anaphylaxis and death, as reported by Unger.

Allergy may occur to the animal protein or fish allergens in protein insulin or to crystalline insulin. Allergy to trypsin given intrabronchially in asthma has also been recorded.

3. Allergy to animal sera may be inherited. Its possibility emphasizes immunization to tetanus with its toxoid to which rare allergy also has been reported.

The method of immunization with antitoxin in patients without previous immunization to toxoid is detailed.

4. The recognition and control of serum sickness is discussed.

5. Mild to severe or even fatal allergic reactions from egg in viral vaccines must be remembered.

6. Occasional asthma, urticaria, or other allergic symptoms in food-sensitive patients from foods or occasionally from inhalants in transfused blood must be remembered and indicates blood from fasting donors or transfusions of washed, properly grouped red cells in normal saline.

Chapter 5

Gastrointestinal Allergy

Gastrointestinal symptoms are due to food allergy more frequently than is generally appreciated. It is necessary for all physicians to consider such allergy in all patients with gastrointestinal symptoms.

The gradual evolution of information about gastrointestinal allergy up to 1937 was summarized in *Clinical Allergy* in 1937. In our early study of this allergy we received important encouragement from a lifelong friend, Walter C. Alvarez.

The information in this chapter deals entirely with adults. Gastrointestinal allergy is a special challenge in infants and children. It is extensively discussed in Chapter 25 on allergic diseases in children. The role of food allergy in colic, pylorospasm, hypertrophic pyloric stenosis, distention, belching, abdominal pain, recurrent vomiting, nausea, vomiting, diarrhea, and especially in chronic ulcerative colitis, according to our reports for over thirty years, must be recognized by all physicians and pediatricians, including allergists, abdominal surgeons, and proctologists.

As discussed in this chapter, inhalant allergy, especially to pollen, and drug allergy are at times also responsible. Mineral and organic allergens in drinking water and flavors in beverages must be suspect. Possible allergy to intestinal parasites always needs consideration.

Of all possible causes of gastrointestinal allergy, food allergy is by far the major cause, as increasingly indicated and confirmed by us in the last forty years. One can fully appreciate the possibility of such allergy by recalling the vomiting, retching, intestinal cramping, bowel tenesmus, involuntary defecation with gastric and intestinal bleeding, and marked hepatic congestion and enlargement which result from experimental anaphylactic shock in dogs. That allergic reactions can occur in intestinal tissues was evidenced by Gray, Harten, and Walzer, who obtained positive Prausnitz-Küstner reactions in the mucous membrane of patients with ileostomies and colostomies by feeding them a specific food within twenty-four hours after injecting the membranes with the serum of a patient giving large scratch reactions to that food.

It is also probable that more symptoms from food allergies occur in the gastrointestinal tract than in other body tissues because of the intimate and continued contact of foods with the gastrointestinal mucosa, especially in the mouth, stomach, duodenum, and small bowel. Thus localized allergy to foods in the mucosa is possible.

Failure to recognize the importance of food allergy in the gastrointestinal tract has led to much uncertainty of diagnoses not only of acute severe symptoms but of many mild obscure and chronic gastrointestinal disturbances. Many sufferers from food sensitizations have had chronic indigestion leading to consciousness of the alimentary tract and inefficiency in home, social, and occupational activities, with introspective and neurotic tendencies. Many patients, moreover, had had needless operations on the gallbladder, appendix, diaphragmatic herniae, and other abdominal surgery without benefit because of nonrecognition of food allergy. Thus it is imperative for all physicians and surgeons to consider food and other less frequent allergies in the differential diagnosis of all gastrointestinal symptoms. Such allergy was emphasized in our article* in 1932.

It must be emphasized that other causes of gastrointestinal symptoms (while atopic allergy is receiving study) must always be kept in mind. Though this needs constant consideration in the study of possible allergy in the causation of the many gastrointestinal symptoms discussed in this chapter, it will be assumed by us that it receives such attention. Peptic ulcer, gallbladder disease, intestinal parasites, adhesions, and especially cancer must be recognized. Heart, kidney, pancreatic, blood, nutritional, and other chronic diseases must be considered. All of these possibilities have been kept in mind in our study of gastrointestinal allergy.

That psychoneuroses and actual psychosis produce gastrointestinal symptoms, headaches, and fatigue has received important emphasis by Alvarez and others for over thirty years. Food allergy, however, may be the unrecognized major cause of such symptoms. With its control, some or all of the above symptoms may decrease or disappear. Moreover, food allergy may occur concomitantly with demonstrated gallbladder disease, appendicitis, diverticulosis, or even malignant disease. That food and at times pollen allergy are the major

causes of chronic ulcerative colitis and regional enteritis rather than psychoneuroses or unknown causes will be discussed in Chapters 6 and 7.

Most of our discussion of gastrointestinal allergy in this chapter centers about its many manifestations and control of symptoms in adults. Gastrointestinal allergy in infants and children will be discussed in Chapter 25. Though such allergy has been recognized for many years, its inadequate study and control by many pediatricians and physicians occur even today. That food allergy requires study in colic, pylorospasm, abdominal pain, diarrhea, mucous stools, constipation, croup, recurrent asthma, eczema, urticaria, anorexia, emaciation, malnutrition, vomiting, regurgitation, cyclic vomiting, fretfulness, irritability, crying, and (of course) food aversions in infancy and childhood will be discussed and emphasized.

A summary of the literature which increasingly evidenced gastrointestinal food allergy published in our book in 1937 is reprinted in Chapter 30.

CLINICAL STUDIES OF GASTROINTESTINAL ALLERGY

A series of 270 cases evidencing gastrointestinal symptoms which in our opinion were due to food allergy have received statistical analysis, as reported in Table VIII. As stated above, the frequent symptoms of gastrointestinal allergy in infants and young children are not analyzed in this table. A more detailed study of symptoms in 150 of these cases is shown in Table IX. These statistics, published in 1937,* are similar to those which would be obtained in our more recent patients studied in the last ten to twenty years. Since 1939, how-

*Since our study of atopic allergy, especially to foods, has confirmed the frequency of gastrointestinal and abdominal symptoms we reported in the first edition of this book in 1931 and in its first revision in *Clinical Allergy* in 1938, the reader is referred to our additional discussions and illustrative case histories of gastrointestinal allergy in these volumes, which are not included in this chapter.

Clinical Allergy, Philadelphia, Lea and Febiger, 1937.

TABLE VIII

STATISTICAL STUDY OF 270 CASES OF
GASTROINTESTINAL ALLERGY

	Percent
Male	30
Female	70
Ages:	
0 to 10	6
10 to 20	6
20 to 30	17
30 to 50	44
50 to 70	27
Family history of allergy	66
Other allergies in patients (past or present)	
Bronchial	18
Nasal	33
Urticaria or eczema	34
Angioneurotic edema	3
Migraine or headache	36
Ocular allergy	1
Bladder allergy	1.5
Symptoms:	
Canker sores	17
Gastric	79
Diarrhea	12
Constipation	43
Mucous colitis	14
Pruritus ani	4
Abdominal pain or soreness	60
Ulcer type of pain	5
Toxemia	25

Average duration of symptoms 11 yrs.

	No. Cases
Food dislikes or disagreements	232
Roentgen studies	
(1) Gastrointestinal:	
Normal	142
Abnormal*	36
(2) Gall Bladder†	4
Stomach Analysis:	
Normal	107
Hypochlorhydria	14
Achylia	13
Previous abdominal operations:	
Appendectomy	107
Gallbladder	10
Others‡	9
Drug idiosyncrasies	16

---

*Gastric retention in 4 cases; duodenal retention in 1; spastic antrum in stomach, decreased motility in small intestine, and hypermotility in the large bowel in 1; hyperperistalsis in stomach and upper intestine in 1; moderate duodenal stasis in 5 cases; marked dilatations of cap in 1; spastic bowel in 24.

†All normal except stones in 1 case, negative shadows in 1, questionable pathology in 2.

‡Four hysterectomies, 1 gastroenterostomy, 1 increase in gastroenterostomy opening, 2 for supposed intestinal obstruction, 1 for supposed perforation of ulcer.

Skin reactions:	Percent
Foods	19
Animal emanations	8
House dust	7
Pollens	18
Miscellaneous	7

TABLE IX

DETAILED ANALYSIS OF SYMPTOMS IN
150 CASES OF GASTROINTESTINAL
FOOD ALLERGY

Gastrointestinal Symptoms:	Percent
Canker sores	13
Coated tongue	18
Heavy breath	11
Distention	35
Belching	34
Epigastric heaviness	17
Sour stomach	21
Burning, pyrosis	20
Nausea	46
Vomiting	27
Diarrhea	16
Mucous colitis	14
Constipation	39
"Gas in bowels"	19
Pruritus ani	5
Pain and Soreness in:	
Epigastrium	27
Upper right quadrant	17
Lower left quadrant	3
Midportion of abdomen	19
Lower part of abdomen	22
Colonic soreness	17
Ulcer type of pain	6
General Symptoms:	
Toxicity	25
Weakness	27
Irritability	15
Nervousness	25
Mental dullness and depression	24
General aching	13
Fever	5

ever, cases of chronic ulcerative colitis and regional enteritis, which our studies have indicated are due to food and less frequent pollen allergies, would be included.

Statistics in Table VIII show that gastrointestinal allergy occurred more frequently in females than in males, that it was recognized more often in mid-adult life than in adolescence, that most patients had other manifestations of allergy, and that a positive family history of allergy was usual. The abnormalities in the x-ray findings of the gastrointestinal tract reported by us in 1934 had been confirmed and extended by other investigators. Because of previous gastrointestinal symptoms, operations, appendectomies being most frequent, had usually been done without relief, as emphasized in Chapter 27. Finally the negative scratch reactions in 81 percent of these patients in whom food allergy was the predominant problem emphasized the fallibility of such tests to reveal clinical food allergy. The importance of trial diet to study possible food allergy, especially our FFCFE diet, is emphasized. The fallibility of skin tests with soluble allergens and the role of antibodies to starches recognized and discussed by Doctor Lietze are presented in Chapter 28.

Eosinophiles often are found in stools, especially in children, as reported in Chapter 25.

FOOD ALLERGY IN THE ORAL AND PHARYNGEAL TISSUES—APHTHOUS STOMATITIS (CANKER SORES)

1. That food allergy is by far the most usual cause of canker sores in the mouth (aphthous stomatitis) in adults and children has been confirmed by us for over thirty-five years. These lesions occur in the lips; gums; on the edges, tip, and under the tongue; on the oral and pharyngeal mucosa; and on the palate. They often are associated with allergy in the stomach, small bowel, and colon, which are discussed in this chapter. They are best explained by minute, localized allergic vasculitis in the mucosa resulting in thromboses, ulceration, and necroses. Associated stomatitis resulting from the allergy may occur. Temporary refractoriness to the specific food allergen explains recovery and later recurrence of the canker sores. If the foods are not eliminated from the diet, the canker sores recur more often. Gradual healing and new lesions may constantly be present. In the first edition of this book, reports of canker sores resulting from food allergy were noted by Talbot, Andresen, Vaughan, and by us. Cooke (1935) reported this in a girl fifteen years of age who had urticaria; dermographia; recurrent abdominal pain; and vesiculopapular lesions on the lips, cheeks, tongue, with swelling of the tongue, and cervical glands apparently resulting from egg and milk allergy.

In a commendable article on aphthous stomatitis in sixty-two patients, Graykowski *et al.* described the resultant histological changes in oral tissues in one hour up to five days and noted the activating role of trauma, of food allergy in 22 percent and of drug allergy in 17 percent. We opine that food allergy would have been more evident, as it has been in our practice, if it had been studied and controlled with our FFCFE diet or at times with our minimal elimination diet. Favoring allergy is a reported benefit from corticosteroids and the activation of lesions at times during menstruation, as we report in our discussion of the manifestations of food allergy.

Case 3: A woman of thirty years had canker sores in the cheeks, gums, lips, and pharynx and also in the vulva for two weeks before and during periods for nine months. With our FFCFE diet, relief occurred. Mild canker sores recurred with slight breaks in the diet. Fruits, tomato, nuts, chocolate, eggs, milk, spices, and condiments were the offenders. In seven years occasional slight oral canker sores recurred with brief deviations in the diet. Vulval lesions have been absent for five years.

We have records of women who develop canker sores from food allergy only during or before menstruation resulting from the probable activation of food allergy by hormone activity.

Because of the importance of food allergy in the causation of canker sores, Behcet's triple symptom complex of oral and genital ulcers with conjunctivitis should be studied as a manifestation of allergy, especially to foods, as we advise.

Our study and control of canker sores during the past forty years have emphasized allergy to individual, many, or even all fruits, walnut, pecans, and at times to other nuts. Occasionally there is allergy to almonds and peanuts (which are not true nuts); chocolate; flavors and condiments, especially when allergy to most or all fruits occurs; and to flavors in chewing gum, candies, toothpastes, and mouthwashes. Less frequently, allergy to eggs, wheat, coffee, various vegetables, and drugs, as to phenolphthalein, has been responsible. That foods other than fruits, nuts, spices, flavors, and especially walnuts and pecans cause canker sores is illustrated by recurrent large lesions on the lip resulting from eggs as shown in Figure 1. The occurrence of canker sores requires the initial use of our FFCFE diet to study food allergy for at least three weeks. After assured relief, provocation feeding tests are indicated with separate foods, as advised previously (see Chapt. 3). Foods which reproduce canker sores are then excluded.

Realizing the frequency of allergy to fruits, including citrus fruits, the develop-

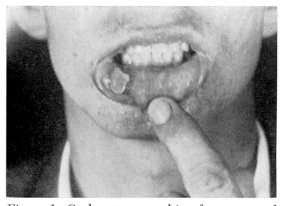

Figure 1. Canker sores resulting from egg and fruit allergy. This lesion explains peptic ulcers, especially in the duodenum, as reported in this chapter.

ment of canker sores by Tuft and Girsh in 1958 by the application of citric and tartaric acids to the oral mucosa in about 8 percent of patients with canker sores is of interest. This harmonizes with our advice that the strict FFCFE diet must exclude all foods containing citric acid and baking powders containing tartaric acid from grapes.

Pollen allergy as an unusual cause of canker sores occurred in the following case:

Case 4: A boy of thirteen years developed canker sores overnight on the mucosa of the cheeks, gums, lips, and tongue in May. These canker sores continued for only one month, necessitating hospitalization for eleven days. They recurred again during three successive Mays. Hospitalization was required for five days when we first saw him. The recurrence of these canker sores in May for four successive years and the prevention of them in the following Mays for two years from our continued pollen desensitization indicated pollen allergy as the cause. Only slight skin reactions to grass pollens had occurred.

Our documentation of the necessity of studying allergy, especially to foods and to pollens as illustrated above, in all cases of canker sores minimizes the role of viral infection as a cause. Many of our patients had had several vaccinations against smallpox with no help. Our results contradict the conclusion of Ship, Merritt, and Stanley in 1962 that food allergy is not a cause.

2. Soreness, burning, and stinging without canker sores may occur in the mouth from food allergy, as reported first by Schloss (1920) in children. Vallery-Radot (1930) reported prickling and burning in lips, tongue, and pharynx and erythema of the lips from contact with egg white. One of our patients had recurrent soreness on the left side of the tongue for years resulting from fruit allergy. Another patient had a raw, red tongue associated with gastrointestinal and severe bladder allergy to foods. One patient had burning

in the mouth and tongue with blisters on the lips from shellfish and peaches. It is interesting that botanically related apricots, cherries, and prunes gave no trouble. One mother and daughter had immediate sores in their throats from shellfish.

3. That riboflavin deficiency produces transverse fissures in the angles of the mouth with reddening and scaling of the lips extending at times into the oral mucosa and causing a red, denuded tongue must be remembered. These symptoms are at times associated with engorged conjunctival capillaries extending occasionally to the corneal limbus.

The marked inflammation from allergy to plastics and guttapercha in dentures and from nickel in dental appliances causes great and continued distress. Relief may require entire removal of dentures for weeks until the chemicals impregnated in the tissues of the gums and tongue and oral mucosa are dissipated. Then contact testing with other denture material may be helpful, as advised by Farrington in 1947, or actual wearing of a provisional denture, even of gold or other metal, may be advisable. Lain and Caughron, in 1936, and others reported lesions from electrogalvanic reactions between dissimilar metallic restorations, especially between mercury, silver, and gold.

Mucosal allergy, according to Fisher, to acrylic material in 90 percent of today's dentures occurs when the methyl methacrylate is not completely polymerized by heat. Patch tests with the liquid rather than scrapings of the denture is advised.

Erythema, vesiculation, and cracking of the lips and corners of the mouth arise from food allergy. Vitamin B deficiencies are important to rule out, as are contact reactions to chemicals, dyes in lipsticks, nail polish, and allergy to tobacco. Other in-

gredients, flavors, fruit juices, and paper in cigarettes rather than tobacco may be responsible.

4. Angioneurotic edema or localized swellings resulting from food allergy may involve the lips, tongue, pharynx, palate, esophagus, or larynx. Such swellings usually occur in other cutaneous areas, as in the eyes, extremities, or even the genitals. When they occur in the mouth and especially in the throat, laryngeal edema must be anticipated, and the patient must be taught to give epinephrine 1:1000, 0.3 to 0.5 cc hypodermically every five to fifteen minutes, until relief occurs and a physician is reached to prevent death from anoxemia. Severe, immediate food allergy is usually shown by large scratch reactions and causes rapid reactions in the lips and tongue which dissuade the patient from biting or chewing the food. Such immediate allergy may exist to peanuts, fish, chocolate, and some other foods. Other foods which produce cumulative or delayed laryngeal or oral allergy usually are not revealed by positive scratch tests.

Angioneurotic edema and its diagnosis and control are more fully discussed in Chapter 16.

5. Allergic gingivitis with or without inflammation of the buccal or pharyngeal mucosa may occur. Bleeding of the gums has occurred in three of our patients from food allergy, with bleeding in the mucosa under the tongue in one patient. Allergic inflammation in the mucosa in the cheeks (stomatitis), gums, and pharynx at times causes an adherent white membrane relieved by the elimination of allergenic foods. Healy (1934) presented evidence that gingivitis, stomatitis, and peridontoclasia, especially in children, were relieved by the control of existing food allergies. Gingival allergy to silk thread used to clean

between teeth was mentioned. From the dental viewpoint the necessity of orthodontia arising from narrowing of the upper jaw because of perennial nasal allergy, often resulting from food allergy, must be remembered.

Lesions in the oral mucosa from allergy to drugs, including iodides, phenolphthalein, Luminal®, bromides, and others must be remembered. Their elimination for several weeks to determine their possible etiological role may be necessary.

6. Pharyngitis resulting from food allergy often causes sore throats at times associated with croup, cough, "head colds," and fever which have been attributed to recurrent infection by most physicians. These symptoms may be recurrent with interim relief, as occurs in recurrent bronchial asthma resulting from food allergy in children and at times in adults. Their exaggeration or recurrence in the late fall and winter favors food allergy, as reported in Chapter 1. The sore throat may be moderately present most of the time but recurrently exaggerated every two to four weeks. These sore throats nearly always occur in patients with other nasal or bronchial symptoms or other manifestations of allergy because of food sensitization.

7. Postnasal mucus often associated with moderate or even severe perennial nasal allergy always requires study of food allergy, especially with our CFE diet. Mucous discharge from the posterior nasal passages causes an irritative and hacking cough. The cough is often persistent and may disturb sleep. Though it occurs in some patients with nasal allergy resulting from seasonal pollens or environmental allergens in home or working environments, the postnasal mucus usually is less in degree and frequency than when resulting from food allergy alone. The mucus often

contains eosinophiles. This cause of postnasal mucus is emphasized in Chapter 12 on perennial nasal allergy.

8. As stated in the first edition of this book, we continue to find food allergy as a common cause of heavy and foul breath. The occurrence of heavy breath is best explained by allergic edema or smooth muscle spasm in the intestines which results in disturbed and reversed peristalsis. One patient stated that milk produced a coated tongue, heavy breath, mucus in the throat, and constipation. Another had had heavy breath for many years not benefited by a smooth diet or later with large amounts of bulky foods. His distress was relieved with a diet eliminating wheat, milk, egg, chocolate, and coffee. Though eating of salads; meat; fish; and richly spiced foods, especially in excessive amounts along with cocktails and wines before and during meals, causes much indigestion and resultant heavy breath, allergy to foods taken even in moderate amounts is a common cause.

The recognition of gastrointestinal food allergy and its control as advised in this chapter would diminish the sale of the multitude of antacid nostrums being advertised and sold with much profit and questionable or brief relief.

FACIAL AND DENTAL DEFORMITIES FROM PERENNIAL NASAL ALLERGY

Marked facial, nasal, and dental deformities from perennial nasal allergy and resultant mouth breathing are realized. These cases are further discussed in Chapter 7.

ESOPHAGEAL ALLERGY

Substernal pain, aching, or burning suggests allergy in the esophagus, especially in patients who have symptoms of oral, gastric, and abdominal allergy discussed below. It is often a part of or associated with symptoms of the allergic epigastric syndrome next discussed. The visualization of localized edema and erythema with an esophagoscope by Jackson and others supports such localized allergy. The sensation of a "lump" under the sternum, especially in its upper area, called globus hystericus for several decades, can be explained by a localized spasm or edema in the esophagus. This spasm or edema has been relieved with the control of food allergy with our elimination diets in many patients during the last forty years. The presence of striated muscles in the upper two-thirds of the esophagus and of smooth muscle in the lower third must be remembered. The tight sensation high in the epigastrium suggesting cardiospasm resulting from allergy is relieved by elimination of allergenic foods. The absence of an actual sphincter at the cardia may account for the absence of esophageal retention resulting from allergy. We have failed to demonstrate a possible role of food allergy in achalasia.

Distress under the sternum, at times relieved by elimination diets, may radiate laterally, especially into the precordium, suggesting cardiac angina. The patient's history, physical examination, laboratory tests, and EKG, however, exclude angina pectoris or coronary artery disease. Relief from our elimination diet supports food allergy as the cause. The possibility of cardiac allergy always must be kept in mind. Gallbladder disease must be excluded. Withers reported esophageal allergy in 1939.

Chronic esophagitis with thickening of the layers of the wall, especially the increase in fibrous tissue from edema and at times ulceration in the mucosa, usually in a limited distal area justifies the study of possible atopic allergy, particularly to foods

as a cause. It may arise from localized allergy which our evidence indicates is responsible for regional enteritis (Chapt. 7) and necessarily duodenal ulcer. Regional enteritis involving any area of the small bowel, including the duodenum, indicates its possible occurrence in the esophagus. Andresen, in his excellent book *Office Gastroenterology*, 1958, advised study of food allergy not only in esophagitis but as a possibility in achalasia.

ALLERGIC EPIGASTRIC SYNDROME (EPIGASTRIC PRESSURE, DISTENTION, PYROSIS, NAUSEA, VOMITING, AND ANOREXIA)

These symptoms attributed especially to gastric allergy reported in the first edition of this book were emphasized in our book published in 1937. They have been increasingly recognized in our practice in the last forty years, being relieved by the elimination of allergenic foods. This recognition is an important responsibility of all physicians.

Because of their frequency they have been grouped into the "allergic epigastric syndrome," which we reported in 1954.

This syndrome is characterized by epigastric pressure and fullness, aching and pain in varying degrees, burning, soreness, and xiphoid tenderness. The pressure, fullness, and to a lesser extent burning are present in most cases. Nausea, vomiting, belching, and sour stomach occur less frequently. Burning, pressure, and aching may also occur under the sternum, radiating into the neck, throat, shoulders, or even the arms, suggesting cardiac angina (pseudoangina), neuritis, or arthritis.

Occasionally, buccal and/or pharyngeal burning, erythema, and even white patchy eruptions, including canker sores on the mucosa, are due to food allergy. Globus hystericus relieved by elimination diets may occur. Soreness, pain, or cramping in the abdomen; allergic diarrhea; or constipation result from allergy. Headaches, mild to severe and at times migraine, may also be present. Fatigue, dullness, drowsiness, irritability, aching, and other symptoms of allergic toxemia and fatigue (Chapt. 19) resulting from food allergy may occur in such patients. Manifestations of allergy in other body tissues may be present, though the gastric and other abdominal tissues may be the only shock tissues of allergy.

Symptoms usually last in varying degrees for long periods as for one-half to fifty years, with an average of thirteen years as noted in Table X. Although the symptoms are usually persistent with irregular variations, they may be cyclic with interim relief.

Car sickness causing nausea, often vomiting, and usually associated with dizziness and vertigo may be relieved by strict adherence to our CFE diet, or if fruit and condiment allergy is suggested in the diet history, to our FFCFE diet. One of the many patients relieved of car sickness with such control of food allergy was a woman of forty-two years whose recurrent sick headaches also were controlled. She had disliked milk all of her life.

TABLE X

ALLERGIC EPIGASTRIC SYNDROME
IN 50 PATIENTS

Age: 22 years to 64 years (average 45 years)
Male: 20
Female: 30
Duration of symptoms: ½ year to 50 years (average 13 years)

	Percentage of Cases
Epigastric pressure or tightness	94
Epigastric distention	58
Epigastric burning	72
Substernal burning and aching	30
Precordial distress	14
Mid- and lower abdominal distress	18

Sour stomach	32
Heartburn	20
Belching	20
Cankers	22
Oral burning	6
Diarrhea	20
Constipation	40
Hemorrhoids	12
Pruritus ani	10
Headaches	38
Fatigue	42
Dullness and confusion	24
Nervousness	25
Depression	22
Nasal allergy	44
Bronchial allergy	14
Food disagreements	56
Food dislikes (usually milk)	18
Positive skin tests	
Foods	10
Pollens	18
Other inhalants	4
Family history positive for allergy	24

Stomach analysis:
Normal — 15 patients
Achylia — 2 patients
X-ray of upper gastrointestinal tract:
Negative — 32 patients
Slight or inactive duodenal ulcer — 2 patients
Pyloric spasm and irregular segmentation of small bowel — 1 patient
Duodenal diverticulum — 1 patient
Hypertrophic rugae — 1 patient
Negative in previous studies — 13 patients
X-ray of colon:
Negative — 25 patients
Diverticulitis — 2 patients
X-ray of the gall bladder:
Negative — 24 patients

Physical examination, laboratory studies, and x-rays of the upper gastrointestinal tract, colon, and gallbladder are usually negative. As indicated in Table X, possible slight duodenal ulcer occurred in two cases, and pyloric spasm and irregular segmentation of the ileum and possible hypertrophy of the gastric rugae were minor in degree. One patient had had gallstones. Their removal, however, gave no relief to her symptoms until the allergenic foods were eliminated.

The diagnosis of psychoneurosis which has been made in several patients is never justified unless allergy, especially to foods and other possible pathological causes, have been adequately studied.

Because of the frequency of relief of symptoms of the allergic epigastric syndrome by the elimination of allergenic foods, trial diet with our FFCFE diet is important to study probable food allergy. Scratch tests with ingested foods infrequently indicated any or all causative foods. The few reactions listed in Table X did not indicate the causative foods. No large reactions were obtained to suggest immediate food allergy. The diet history of dislikes or disagreements for foods suggested food allergy, especially to milk, in a limited number of patients. When soybeans and at times other legumes cause indigestion or possible allergy, rice and later oats are substituted. If evidence of relief fails in three weeks, a minimal fruit-free elimination diet should be tried before ruling out food allergy. The supervision and maintenance of the diet with the addition and deletion of additional foods after relief has occurred are advised in Chapter 3.

These epigastric symptoms are best explained by allergic inflammation and smooth muscle spasm causing disturbed peristalsis in the stomach, esophagus, duodenum, and possibly in the jejunum. Gastroscopy in two patients revealed moderate erythema and edema and in one patient, enlarged gastric rugae. Abnormalities in the x-rays of the gastrointestinal tract are discussed on page 128. These symptoms of the allergic epigastric syndrome, especially in the burning, distention, and belching because of which antacid tablets and liquid forms are purchased over the counter and by prescription by thousands of people daily, can be controlled when the causative allergic foods are eliminated, thus rendering such medications unnecessary. If they persist, a physical and roentgen ray study must rule out other causes.

CASE SUMMARIES

Case 5: A man fifty-one years of age had had pressure and burning in the epigastrium for fifteen years, one to three hours after meals, recurring every two to three days, keeping him abed recently for four weeks. Former severe nuchal headache occurred. Milk, fruits, and tomato had caused sour stomach. The father had abdominal pain and nausea. With our minimal fruit-free elimination diet, milk, fruits, tomato, celery, sweet potatoes, and beets were found to be responsible.

Case 6: A woman forty-nine years of age had had tightness and knotting in the epigastrium for twenty-five years associated with soft stools and abdominal cramping after meals. She had had aching in her joints for several years. Depression, irritability, and frustration because of failure from medical therapy had been present. With our FFCFE diet minus soy, plus rice and cottonseed oil, all symptoms were relieved in two weeks. Beef, milk, oats, and fruit reproduced symptoms. Wheat especially caused pains in the joints.

PAIN IN THE UPPER RIGHT QUADRANT SIMULATING HEPATIC AND GALLBLADDER DISEASE

We called attention in 1928 to pain and discomfort in the upper right quadrant from food allergy and confirmed the importance of such etiology as a cause of such symptoms in the first edition of this book in 1931, again in 1937, and in publications since then.

That the liver along with other organs and body tissues are involved in experimental anaphylaxis and chronic allergy in animals has been reported in the literature for over sixty years. Weil and Manwaring especially emphasized the rapid, marked congestion and swelling of the liver with later congestion of the gastrointestinal tissues and intestinal bleeding from canine anaphylaxis. The rapid damage of the hepatic parenchyma and resultant cloudy swelling of the cytoplasm and final central lobular necrosis, the stasis of blood in the hepatic sinuses, and vascular thromboses and phagocytosis of the Kupffer's cells were described by Weatherford. Simonds and Brandes attributed congestion of the liver with blood to allergic spasm in the smooth muscles of the hepatic vasculature. The localization of anaphylactic reactions in other animals may depend, according to Manwaring, on the location of increased smooth muscle, as in the bronchi of guinea pigs and in the pulmonary artery in rabbits. Gray, Harten, and Walzer produced allergy in the gallbladder (1940), experimentally yielding edema, hyperemia, and increased mucus. Recently, evidence has accumulated that the pathogenesis of certain acute and chronic liver diseases involves immunological mechanisms including autoimmunity as discussed by Tomasi in 1965. Such hepatic changes in experimental animals require consideration of comparable reactions in varying degrees of severity or chronicity from clinical allergy in man.

Symptoms in the upper right quadrant have suggested probable hepatic-biliary disease for many years. Rolleston stated in 1927 that many abdominal symptoms formerly attributed to liver disease were due to food allergy. Graham *et al.*, in 1928, reported several patients with symptoms suggestive of gallbladder disease resulting from food allergy, studied and controlled by Alexander and Eyermann.

The following statement on page 177 of Graham's book is pertinent. "Intestinal allergy is probably frequently confused with cholecystitis. . . . In one case the patient had been operated upon for supposed chronic cholecystitis. . . . The surgeon found a normal gallbladder. . . . Later the old symptoms recurred. He was found . . . sensitive to wheat, the ingestion of which

produced his supposed gallbladder symptoms." Graham listed intestinal allergy as the third possibility in the differential diagnosis of cholecystitis as follows:

1. General visceroptosis, giving gallbladder stasis.
2. Spastic constipation or mucous colitis (food allergy must be a considered cause).
3. Intestinal allergy.
4. Cancer.
5. Chronic appendicitis.
6. Disease of liver.
7. Lesions of spine.
8. Intrathoracic inflammatory lesions.
9. Lesions of stomach and duodenum.
10. Lesions of kidney.
11. Hemolytic icterus.
12. Other less frequent causes.

Lichtwitz, in 1934, observed sudden swelling of the liver with angioneurotic edema or anaphylactic shock with or without jaundice. Generalized hemorrhagic urticaria; ocular, nasal, laryngeal and bronchial congestion; and remarkable swelling of the liver with jaundice and high fever occurred in a girl from allergy to milk. Eiselberg (1933) found biliary colic from allergy to milk, eggs, and tomatoes. Haritantis (1933) observed hepatic hypertrophy and intermittent fever for three months attributed to milk allergy. Lintz (1934) relieved seven patients of symptoms suggesting gallbladder disease with the control of food allergy. Our confrere had severe pain simulating gallbladder spasm with pylorospasm and gastric retention within twenty-four hours after eating citrus fruits on several occasions. Eyermann told us about a patient with upper abdominal colic from eggs because of which a cholecystectomy and two subsequent abdominal operations were done.

Hepatic and biliary allergy or the allergic epigastric syndrome probably accounts for many symptoms failing to respond to medical and surgical therapy. Such allergy at times is probably responsible for unsatisfactory relief from removal of stoneless gallbladders in 40 percent of patients, as reported by Graham and Macky (1934) and emphasized in Chapter 28 of this volume. Blackford, King, and Sherwood (1933) warned against cholecystectomy in the presence of mucous colitis, irritable indigestion, and migraine in all of which food allergy must be a considered cause, as noted in this chapter. Alvarez (1934) reported "pseudocholecystitis" resulting from food allergy. Actual pathology in the gastrointestinal and urogenital tracts, liver and gallbladder, and spleen and vertebral column must not be overlooked. Alvarez for years has stressed the frequency of pseudocholecystitis and reported three cholecystectomies in a patient whose symptoms later were found to be due to allergy to foods. The demonstration by Auer (1919) and Valy Menkin (1930) that antigens and subsequent allergy tend to localize in inflamed tissues suggests that this may occur in infected biliary tissues in man. Thus allergy and infection may coexist.

CASE SUMMARIES

In some of our patients food allergy has caused symptoms simulating hepatic and biliary disease. In Table IX pain or soreness in the upper right quadrant occurred in 17 percent of 150 patients with gastrointestinal allergy. Cholecystectomy had been done in eight patients. One woman had had pain in the upper right quadrant associated with sour stomach and belching for thirty years relieved by elimination of allergenic foods.

Case 7: A young woman had had two attacks of colic in the upper abdomen associated with slight jaundice. Roentgen rays revealed shadows misinterpreted as gallstones. Toxemia, fatigue, and recurrent headaches were present. Another x-ray showed no stones. All symptoms were relieved for over two years with elimination diets. Recurrent soreness and rigidity in the upper right quadrant with nausea, vomiting, and fever led to cholecystectomy in another woman. Symptoms recurred every three weeks thereafter, suggesting possible food allergy. They were entirely relieved with the elimination of allergenic foods.

Case 8: A man thirty-nine years of age had had increasing pain in the right side of the abdomen, especially in the upper right quadrant and to a lesser extent over the lower quadrant, for fifteen years. Associated with this pain there had been marked distention and belching, a tendency to sour stomach, recurrent canker sores, a heavy breath in the mornings, and a coated tongue. As a boy he had frequent bilious attacks. Six years ago an appendectomy was done because of the pain, a congested cecum being found, but no definite pathology in the appendix or gallbladder was present. After this the pain persisted, with a tendency to dysentery for several months. Since then a spastic type of constipation with frequent mucus had been present. Three years ago a sudden severe abdominal pain in the lower left abdomen associated with great tenderness, increasing fever, and leukocytosis indicated an emergency operation for possible obstruction, and again a diffuse congestion of the intestinal coils in the lower abdomen with considerable gray sterile fluid was found. No abnormalities in the gallbladder, stomach, or duodenum and no adhesions were discovered, and later an idiosyncrasy to crab was found to produce mild but similar attacks of abdominal pain. In one month roentgen ray studies of the gastrointestinal tract, including a colon enema as well as stool analyses, were negative. For two years the pain in the upper right quadrant and the spastic constipation have been entirely relieved by the elimination of apples, bananas, oranges, lettuce, and pork, which were gradually found responsible by diet trial. Skin reactions to all foods were negative. The taking of a little apple or banana in a fruit salad or cake, a little apple cider, jellies made with Certo (an apple product), oranges, or lettuce brought back the upper right abdominal pain in about one-half hour, and recently the eating of liver fried with bacon produced the same distress. After these infringements on the diet, there was a return of spastic constipation for about two days. It is interesting that all his life he had eaten many apples, bananas, and oranges, especially in childhood. The recent ingestion of oranges and lettuce in larger amounts than usual in an effort to put vitamins and bulk into the diet apparently reestablished an old sensitization from childhood and possibly sensitized the patient to lettuce.

CYCLIC VOMITING

This occurs in children and adolescents often because of allergy, the interim relief being similar to that between recurrent attacks of bronchial asthma and migraine resulting from food allergy. This recurrent vomiting as well as recurrent bronchial asthma resulting from food allergy is further discussed in Chapter 25. Bilious attacks are the equivalent of cyclic vomiting in children.

DUODENAL AND GASTRIC ULCERS

Since 1928 and the first edition of this book in 1931, we have opined that food allergy can produce ulcers in the duodenum which are similar to canker sores in the mouth, which we have found are usually due to such allergy (see Fig. 1). Creazzo (1935) opined that canker sores in the duodenal and gastric mucosa best explain peptic ulcer. Lintz (1934) also suggested that cankerlike lesions could occur in the duodenum. Kern and Stewart (1931) stated that allergy, especially to foods, needed study in the causation of duodenal ulcer. Allergy, food allergy in particular, needed study as a possible cause of duodenal ulcer. Such study was advised especially when ulcers recur after surgery. The fallibility of skin testing to determine food allergy was noted.

Further discussion of the ulcer-type of pain including that in the literature appears in *Clinical Allergy*, 1937.

Allergy, especially to foods, also needs study in the causation of gastric ulcers. Be-cause of the necessity of ruling out cancer in gastric ulcers and the importance of surgical removal if medical therapy does not heal the gastric ulcer in six weeks and the necessity of immediate surgery if cancer is definitely indicated by x-ray, study of allergy as a possible cause should not continue for more than one month or not at all if operative cancer is likely unless gastric cancer has been excluded by x-ray and other indicated studies. If possible study of gastric ulcer is justified, our FFCFE diet is advised instead of the usual, bland nonresidue diet.

Since our study of allergy in canker sores has revealed a frequency of allergy especially to fruits and condiments, walnuts, and to a lesser extent cereal grains, eggs, chocolate, coffee, and at times other foods, our FFCFE diet has been used to study the role of possible allergy in duodenal ulcer. A minimal elimination diet at times is required if the above diet does not give relief in two or three weeks. Since it usually takes two or more weeks for foods to leave the body and a longer time for tissue changes from chronic food allergy to decrease, strict adherence to the diet has been required until relief has continued for one to two months. Prolonged use of our FFCFE diet is justified in studying duodenal ulcer because of the infrequency of cancer in the duodenum in contrast to the stomach. Associated with or without canker sores, duodenal enteritis requires such study of food allergy which is not suggested in the article by Wilder and Davis (1966) and in other articles in their references. There may be evidence of regional enteritis resulting from atopic allergy, as noted in Chapter 7.

It is important to remember that massive eosinophilic infiltration and hypertrophy of the pylorus in an adult might be due to food allergy as in infants.

The frequency of allergy to fruits, condiments, chocolate, coffee, and less frequently to other foods explains in part the benefit from the diet advised by Sippy nearly fifty years ago. Starting with milk and cream, other foods were gradually added after relief occurred. Reactivation of the duodenal ulcer often developed after fruits, condiments, chocolate, coffee, and at times other foods were added, indicating that the benefit of the Sippy diet arose from the possible control of food allergy.

In our patients manipulation of our FFCFE diet is continued until a diet is found that maintains relief for at least two months. Thereafter, individual foods are gradually added. Because of the reactivation of duodenal ulcers and of other manifestations of allergy in some patients resulting from milk allergy, its exclusion from the initial elimination diet is justified. If symptoms develop with its later addition, its continued elimination is required.

When the elimination of soybean and lima bean bakery products is necessary because of distention, indigestion, or possible allergy to legumes, rice, and oatmeal, extra potato and sugar are ordered to maintain nutrition and weight. Though rice and oats are common causes of bronchonasal allergy, eczema, and cerebral allergy, they are less frequent causes of gastrointestinal allergy. We have also found that brushing teeth with water or with soda and water to prevent the swallowing of flavors in toothpastes and the elimination of flavored denture fixers or creams and the substitution of water and soda for flavored mouthwashes are advisable when fruits and condiments are eliminated from the diet. Paraffin can be chewed instead of flavored commercial gum. Antacid medications are

not required as relief from my diet occurs. If they are used, the unflavored tablets and fluid preparations should be used. The use of pearl instead of instant tapioca and carbonated bottled water containing no citric acid also is important while relief of distress from the ulcer is established and maintained. The possibility of allergy to vitamin C in fruit-sensitive patients discussed in Chapter 29 is important to remember.

In addition to actual ulcers, duodenitis with induration or edema and even scar tissue formation may arise from food allergy. This would cause an irritable and contracted duodenum or even pyloric edema or spasm. Oozing of blood from the mucosa may arise. Such inflammation may be one cause of ulcerlike pain in the upper right quadrant already discussed.

EXPERIMENTAL EVIDENCE OF ALLERGY IN THE DUODENUM

Experimental support for the development of duodenal ulcers was the production of duodenal ulcers by Demel (1923), Ivy and Shapiro (1925), and Vallone (1930). An Arthus type of reaction was suggested. Culmone (1933), in Italy, produced such ulcers. He reviewed ten theories of ulcer formation and concluded that Demel's anaphylactic theory suggested in 1923 best accounted for duodenal ulcer. He felt that localized Arthus lesions may arise in the mucosa of the duodenum and stomach in areas sensitized to ingested foods. Experimental evidence was published. We are not aware of other evidence from animal experimentation supporting the role of allergy especially to foods, which in our opinion best explains duodenal ulceration.

Our FFCFE diet seems preferable to the Sippy diet for the healing of duodenal ulcers, especially in patients who give a history of large scratch reactions to milk, suggesting milk allergy. Carr, in 1926, reported headaches, nausea, urticaria, painful joints, and fever of 101.2 F when milk and cream were given because of a duodenal ulcer. Relief occurred in three days after milk was stopped. In 1934 O. H. Brown recorded duodenitis resulting from food allergy, causing thickened mucosa infiltrated with leukocytes and eosinophiles. Allergy to milk has prevented its use in several of our patients with duodenal ulceration, as in one patient who had symptoms of duodenal ulcer for fifty years. Moderate deformity of the cap was found by x-ray. Milk intolerance had occurred since childhood. A Sippy diet mainly of milk exaggerated the distress.

Study of possible food allergy with our FFCFE diet or a more minimal elimination diet as advised in Chapter 3 is justified if pyrosis, epigastric pain, and pressure or other symptoms persist after surgery for duodenal ulcer. Or such strict diet trial for three to four weeks may relieve allergic inflammation and pyloric spasm, making surgery unnecessary. Subsequent addition of individual foods in provocation tests (see Chapt. 3) will gradually reveal one or more foods responsible for the pathology and symptoms.

CLINICAL NOTES

For more than thirty years we have studied many patients with various symptoms relieved with our elimination diets, suggestive of duodenal or gastric ulcer which had not been revealed by x-ray as shown in our statistics on 270 cases of GI allergy in which upper GI x-rays in 172 showed no ulcer and duodenal statis in only seven. The symptoms were only suggestive of possible peptic ulceration. Rinkel (1934) noted the "mimicry of the ulcer syndrome" resulting from food allergy and

reported five operations for recurrent symptoms of duodenal ulcer late relieved by elimination of wheat, milk, and egg. Friedenwald and Morrison (1934) and Alvarez made similar reports. Ulcerlike symptoms were reported by Brown and Brown in 1942. One of our patients had ulcerlike pain from egg and milk. Another, seventy years of age, had had such pain for fifty years. Several x-rays showed no ulcers. His daughter had perennial coryza, toxemia, and recurrent fever resulting from food allergy. His pains were also relieved by the elimination diet.

Holmes, in 1941, stated that seven of seventy-five patients with duodenal ulcer had gastrointestinal allergy relieved with elimination of allergenic foods.

Case 9: A man forty-one years of age had had epigastric pain, burning, sour stomach, and substernal discomfort constantly for two years. Oral canker sores had recurred for ten years. Duodenal ulcer was confirmed by x-ray. Medical therapy had only given partial relief. For constipation, extra fruit had been taken. With our FFCFE diet, unflavored Amphojel® and no cigarettes, relief occurred in two months. Gastric resection had been advised. With gradual addition of all foods, symptoms did not recur except for exacerbations after ingestion of fruits. After the sixth year moderate amounts of fruit could be taken one to two times a week. X-ray still showed a deformed cap.

Case 10: A woman twenty-nine years of age had had gnawing epigastric pain and nausea relieved by eating for three years. X-ray showed a moderate duodenal ulcer. Eczema of the hands had been relieved for eight previous years by a milk-free diet. With our FFCFE diet minus soy plus rice, her pain disappeared. Eight years later she reports that pain recurs with any fruit or condiment in her diet.

Other patients with symptoms of duodenal ulcer confirmed by x-ray have been relieved with modifications of the FFCFE diet, allergy to all fruits and condiments being the sole cause or of major importance.

ALLERGY IN THE SMALL INTESTINE

In spite of our increasing realization of gastrointestinal food allergy for several years, its occurrence in the small intestine except in the duodenum had not been recognized when the first edition of this book was published in 1931. In 1937 evidence of its occurrence, however, had increased, so that we wrote the following comments:

Allergic reactions undoubtedly occur in the small intestine and may explain the colic, cramping, hyperperistalsis, congestion, soreness, and at times bleeding arising therein. Severe pain from obstruction by varying amounts of localized edema may occur as noted in my discussion of angioneurotic edema. Hyperperistalsis and reversed peristalsis may be due to allergic reactions in the mucosa and smooth muscle, as suggested by roentgen rays studies noted on page 130. With the technique of study of small intestine there noted, more definite information about the effects of specific allergies will be forthcoming. Jonckheere (1935) described infarction of the small intestine of probable anaphylactic origin. It is probable, moreover, that the hemorrhagic allergy of Sanarelli-Schwartzman also occurs in the intestine, stomach, and colon. Allergy as a likely cause of duodenal ulcer has already been discussed, and the occurrence of intestinal purpura from food allergy is indicated on page 427. Many of the symptoms described in subsequent pages may arise from allergy in the small bowel.

The abdominal pain, vomiting, and melena of Henoch-Schonlein purpura, long reported by many investigators in the last one hundred years, are best explained by allergy, especially in the small bowel and particularly to foods. These symptoms together with the others in the cutaneous, urogenital, and ocular tissues and the occasional abdominal surgery in these patients, as reported in the literature, receive important consideration in Chapter 22.

Along with our study and control of atopic allergy in CUC evidence soon occurred and has steadily increased in the last twenty-five years that similar allergy best explains the pathology including the enlarged peritoneal glands (see Chapt. 6) and the resultant and associated symptoms of regional enteritis (RE).

We first reported this in 1948 and again in 1950 and 1951 and especially in *Gastroenterology* in 1953. Previously probable food allergy in the causation of RE had been stated by Collins and Pritchett even in 1938. This importance of atopic allergy in RE justifies its emphasis and elucidation in Chapter 7.

In the decades after 1937 as our study of chronic ulcerative colitis increasingly indicated that food and at times pollen allergy causing an allergic eczematouslike inflammation with resultant vascular thromboses and ulceration was the major cause, allergy to foods and at times pollens increasingly became evident as the cause of regional enteritis and ileocolitis. This etiology was discussed in 1948 and was supported by the excellent control of three cases of regional enteritis first relieved in 1948 and two in 1950 and 1951, as reported in *Gastroenterology* in 1953. Previously, only one case of regional enteritis, reported by Collins and Pritchett in 1938, had been relieved by elimination of allergenic foods. The importance of allergy to foods and less often to pollens in regional enteritis justifies the more detailed discussion in Chapter 7.

CONSTIPATION AND ABDOMINAL CRAMPING

Constipation has been reported by many students of gastrointestinal allergy for over forty years. The colonic smooth muscles are subject to allergic contractibility from food and less often from pollen and probably from other allergens. The mucosa is subject to allergic edema and as noted on page 111 to bleeding because of allergy. That mucous colitis always requires study of allergy especially to foods as the major cause is noted on page 119.

Rectal and sigmoid spasm often arise from allergy. It is possible that diverticulosis at times may arise from chronic constipation resulting from long-standing food allergy which could also produce minute areas of weakness especially in the muscular layers of the colon.

The spastic type of constipation occurred in 58 percent of our 270 cases of gastrointestinal allergy in Table VIII. Many of these and many more adult patients since then have been definitely or entirely relieved of constipation with our elimination diets, especially with the initial use of the FFCFE diet. The frequent colic, cramping, abdominal distress, constipation, or diarrhea in infants and young children resulting from food allergy will be discussed in Chapter 25.

Food allergy needs study as the possible cause of constipation because of which many patients eat large amounts of bulky fruit and vegetables and take mineral oil and bulk-producing medicaments.

Constipation is rarely the only result of gastrointestinal food allergy. Usually it is associated with mucous colitis, abdominal soreness, and pain, especially in the right lower abdomen. Symptoms of the allergic epigastric syndrome, chronic headaches, allergic toxemia and fatigue, bronchial asthma, and other clinical allergies also may be present.

As in most manifestations of possible gastrointestinal allergy, food allergy is studied with the initial use of our FFCFE diet as advised on page 132. To obtain results or rule out food allergy, the diet must be maintained strictly for one to two or more weeks, remembering that allergens of ingested foods remain in the body for one to two or more weeks and that tissue changes require one to two months to definitely decrease or disappear. The degree of allergy in shock tissues may be so great that a trace of an allergenic food once every few days will prevent recovery from allergic constipation or other symptoms resulting from allergy to the specific food.

ALLERGIC DIARRHEA

Food allergy as a cause of colic and diarrhea in infants and young children with or without gastrointestinal symptoms has been recorded by many physicians since 1917. The causative foods and the varying symptoms will be discussed in Chapter 25.

Fewer reports of diarrhea resulting from food allergy in adults have been published. Eyermann, in 1927, reported five cases of diarrhea with other gastrointestinal symptoms arising from food allergy. In the first edition of this book in 1931 and again in 1937 we reported such diarrhea in 15 percent of fifty cases of gastrointestinal allergy.

As emphasized through this volume, a detailed history and all indicated physical, laboratory, and x-ray examinations are required to reveal pathology and other diseases which may be causing the diarrhea. Intestinal parasites; achylia as an occasional cause, especially with pernicious anemia; and the gram-positive bacterial flora resulting from too prolonged use of the mycin antibiotics must be remembered. Thus stool examinations for ova, parasites, predominate gram bacteria, as well as for other pathogenic bacteria, are necessary. This is discussed below.

Though allergy to many foods justifies the use of our FFCFE diet or its modifications, allergy to milk as well as to fruits is especially frequent. One patient with milk allergy had taken 1 tsp of milk as a laxative for a number of years. A few drops of milk produced five to fifteen loose movements in another patient. Piness and Miller (1933) recorded diarrhea, incontinence, swellings, emaciation, and chronic invalidism resulting from milk or other food allergies in a patient who had had a cecostomy without relief. Friedenwald and Morrison (1934) reported diarrhea from milk in a woman twenty-four years of age.

Most physicians including gastroenterologists fail to recognize allergic diarrhea in their patients. Because of its continued occurrence in our patients, we reported, in 1956, cases of diarrhea in 30 children and adults even in old age in a group of approximately 220 patients with probable gastrointestinal allergy studied in the preceding seven years.

Diarrhea resulting from chronic ulcerative colitis and regional enteritis was noted in this 1956 article. This is discussed in Chapters 6 and 7. The frequency of diarrhea in infants and children, as reported in Chapter 25, is not shown in these statistics.

The occurrence of allergic diarrhea in adults and especially in old age is not generally recognized without chronic ulcerative colitis or regional enteritis (see Chapts. 6 and 7). Its long average duration of 7.7 years with its rapid control with our elimination diets is noteworthy. That intermittent constipation occurs in about one-third of the patients is shown in the statistics. Other GI symptoms relieved by elimination of allergenic foods occurred in about one-half of the patients, as did varying symptoms of allergic fatigue and toxemia. The diarrhea resulting from milk in three generations in the family history of one patient exemplifies the inheritance not only of a predisposition to specific manifestations of food allergy but also allergy to specific foods, as noted in Chapter 1.

Milk was the most common cause, disagreeing in eighteen and disliked by seven patients. It was always vomited by two

TABLE XI

STATISTICS ON DIARRHEA RESULTING FROM ALLERGY IN 26 ADULTS AND 5 CHILDREN

	No. of Cases
Age of onset:	
0 to 6	5
20 to 40	9
40 to 50	10
50 to 60	6
Age at first visit:	
0 to 5	4
20 to 40	7
40 to 50	7
50 up	12
No. of daily stools:	
1 to 3	4
3 to 6	12
6 to 10	10
10 up	4
Duration of diarrhea:	
¼ to 50 years (av. 7.7)	
Intermittent relief	16
Abdominal cramping	20
Intermittent constipation	6
Constipation with mucus	4
Other gastrointestinal symptoms:	
Epigastric pressure, distention, and burning	6
Nausea	6
Vomiting	2
Belching	6
Sour stomach	4
Canker sores	1
Additional symptoms:	
Fatigue	6
Body aching	4
Toxemia (allergic)	7
Nervousness	7
Depression	5
Personal history of allergy:	
Bronchial	8
Nasal	7
Dermatitis	6
Hives	2
Headaches	6
Family history of allergy:	
Gastrointestinal symptoms	3
Diarrhea resulting from milk in mother, grandmother, and patient	1
Bronchial allergic symptoms	7
Nasal symptoms	7
Cutaneous symptoms	6

and known to cause diarrhea before our study by three patients. Eggs were disliked by eight patients, being the sole cause of diarrhea in one case. Fruits, including tomato, caused diarrhea or gastrointestinal symptoms in fourteen, fish in two, chocolate in three, tomato in one, wheat in one, all cereals in one, and eggs in one child. Cottonseed allergy as a cause is discussed in a case summarized below. That food dislikes and disagreements are not always due to clinical allergy must be remembered.

Positive skin tests to foods occurred in four cases, but they did not correlate with causative food allergies. A few reactions to inhalants were of no clinical significance except for pollen reactions in three patients suffering with seasonal hay fever.

Other laboratory studies including stomach analyses, stool examinations for ova and parasites, and x-rays of the upper GI tract in sixteen cases, small bowel in five, colon in twenty-two, and gallbladder in fifteen were negative, as was proctoscopy in twenty cases except for slight erythema and edema in the rectum with no ulcerations, blood, or pus in five cases.

Illustrative of the importance of stool examinations was the man twenty-eight years of age who had marked nasal allergy and was referred because of possible allergic diarrhea. Stools contained Giardia, and the diarrhea disappeared after Atabrine® was given for ten days.

Case 11: Another man sixty-five years of age had had severe diarrhea with some blood in the stools for five months. Ulcerative colitis had been diagnosed, but conventional therapy had failed. X-ray of the colon did not confirm CUC. Predominant gram-positive bacteria were found in the stool explained by continued oral tetracycline for three months. Rectal injections of a watery extract of normal stool reestablished the normal gram-negative flora, with relief of the diarrhea.

Abdominal surgery because of diarrhea was infrequent. Cholecystectomy in one

case and removal of ten inches of the descending colon containing diverticulae had not helped the diarrhea, which was rapidly relieved, however, with our elimination diet.

Psychogenic diarrhea had been diagnosed in twelve cases, with no benefit from suggested therapy. Allergic diarrhea was incorrectly attributed to CUC in three hospitals.

Protein-losing enteropathy and intestinal bleeding justified study of atopic allergy, especially to foods, as advised in this chapter as a possible major or complicating cause, as is indicated in severe diarrhea in children discussed in Chapter 25.

CASE SUMMARIES

Case 12: A woman of fifty-six years of age had diarrhea for two to three days every ten to fourteen days for seven years. Bloating and gas were frequent. Studies and treatment by two internists failed. Tension was blamed. Skin reactions to foods did not correlate with those causing the diarrhea. With our FFCFE diet relief occurred in three weeks. It was found by provocation tests that milk caused diarrhea in 2 to 8 hours, onion and mustard in 1½ hours, walnuts in 1 hour, coffee in 1 hour, and cottonseed oil in 2 hours.

Case 13: A one-year-old child had loose, odorous stools of eight months' duration. Paratyphoid from canned egg yolk had been suspected. Fever was absent. There were hives in the mother, asthma in an uncle, eczema in the father, and hay fever in a grandmother. Scratch tests gave eight plus reaction to egg, two plus to beef, two plus to peanut, and three plus to chicken. These foods were eliminated with relief. Only egg, however, reactivated the diarrhea.

APPENDICEAL TYPE OF PAIN

Food sensitization not infrequently produces colonic irritation, congestion, and probably spasm in the ascending colon, first suggested by Duke in 1921 and confirmed by him in 1931. Such reactions are also probably present in the appendix and may predispose to secondary infection in the same way that allergic congestion in the nasal passages or the bronchial tract encourages bacterial infection. Lintz, in 1925, reported the frequency with which appendectomies are done because of allergic reactions. He also thought that a family history of appendicitis usually indicated an allergic cause. We feel that his emphasis of such a cause of lower right abdominal distress is justified. Acute allergic reactions can even produce a mild fever and a leukocytosis of twelve thousand to eighteen thousand, with a moderate increase in the polymorphonuclears, especially shown in many asthmatic children, as reported in Chapter 25.

This pain in the right lower abdomen may be due to allergic inflammation in the appendix which may predispose to infection, causing rigidity and justify appendectomy. It may also be due to allergic inflammation and spasm in the cecum, with varying involvement of the peritoneum, relieved especially as we now advise with our FFCFE diet with gradually decreasing corticosteroid therapy.

The association of chronic constipation, a tendency to a coated tongue, a heavy breath, and a right-sided abdominal aching and soreness without rigidity or fever have occurred in several patients in our experience and are due to food allergy. The following case record illustrates these possibilities very strikingly. The patient felt she had a chronic appendix which was causing her constipation, pain and soreness, coated tongue, and lack of appetite. The relief of her painful menstruation suggests that allergic spasm was also responsible for this symptom.

Case 14: Pain in the lower right quadrant, constipation, painful menstruation, and urticaria occurred in a girl eighteen years of age. Attacks of pain in the lower right quadrant at times radiated down into the right thigh. These attacks had recurred for three years and usually lasted three or four days, occurring two or three times a month, especially before her periods. Her bowels had been constipated all her life but especially in the last three years, and she had to take physics or enemas every day. Enemas gave some relief to right-sided pain. She had no nausea or vomiting but much belching and heaviness after eating. Her periods were extremely painful, especially in the first four hours, and were associated with pain in her lower right quadrant. As a baby she was unable to tolerate milk and ever since had always disliked it. Hives around the abdomen had been frequent since childhood, especially when she was nervous or excited. Her father had severe constipation and hay fever, and his father had asthma. Her mother and the patient's sisters were unable to take milk—"was like rat poison." Otherwise she had always been well except for severe intestinal influenza three years previously.

Her physical examination was negative except for her underweight and small stature and some tenderness over the lower right quadrant. No rigidity was found. Her urine, blood examinations, and metabolic rate were normal. Her roentgen ray studies of the gastrointestinal tract were normal except for retarded motility in the ascending colon and some lack of mobility in the cecum. The barium enema showed no other abnormalities.

Cutaneous skin reactions were negative to foods, animal emanations, dusts, pollens of all kinds, and miscellaneous allergens. On January 8 she was placed on our elimination diet. On January 13 she stated she had had no pain since going on the diet and her appetite had improved. Her diet history indicated that she had never cared for milk, although she had taken many chocolate milkshakes. Since then for nine months her pain has been entirely relieved, her bowels have moved normally, and her periods have been free from pain except on two occasions when she had overstepped her diet. She has gradually added rye, potato, butter, and several vegetables and fruits. Wheat was found to disagree. Her weight has increased from 101 to 107 pounds, and her appetite has been greatly improved.

Comment: The rapid relief of the appendiceal type of pain, the life-long constipation, and the anorexia indicates that an allergic spasticity and congestion in her colon were probably present.

ALLERGIC COLITIS

Allergic colitis increasingly has been recognized in the last fifty years. In the first edition of this book, diarrhea, mucoid stools, cramping, and abdominal pain resulting from food allergy in the colon along with other symptoms of gastrointestinal allergy reported by various students during the preceding twelve years were discussed. In adults, diarrhea resulting from allergy, particularly to foods, was noted in the colon. Increasing evidence of allergic colitis since that time has accrued in our practice. The necessity of studying allergy, especially to foods, as the major cause of mucous colitis was advised in 1931 and continues to be necessary. Abdominal pain arising from allergy to foods in the colon as well as in the stomach and small bowel was reported and receives confirmation later in this chapter.

Proctitis and pruritus ani from food allergy, reported in 1931, has been confirmed during the last thirty-six years.

That food and less frequently pollen and drug allergies always need consideration as the sole initial cause of chronic ulcerative colitis (CUC) had not been realized in 1931. In our book six years later, evidence of this recognition was not recorded. However, we did write: "Whether bacterial and at times food allergy plays a role in the etiology (of CUC) is difficult to determine in the present state of knowledge of its causes. . . . Allergy to milk, wheat, specific fruits, and less often to specific vegetables and fish is not infrequent. . . ."

Since 1939 the evidence that the initial and continued importance of food and at times pollen allergy as the cause of the eczematous-type of colonic inflammation in CUC has so increased that the role of atopic allergy, especially to foods, in the causation and control of CUC is presented

in a separate chapter (Chapt. 6) of this volume. And in Chapter 7, the role of atopic allergy especially to foods in the causation and control of regional enteritis (RE) in the small bowel will be reported. Reasons for present failure to confirm food and less frequently pollen and at times drug allergy as the underlying cause of CUC and RE are stated in Chapters 6 and 7.

ABDOMINAL PAIN

Abdominal pain, as indicated in Table VIII, often occurs in patients with gastrointestinal allergy. Duke, in an article on "Food Allergy as a Cause of Abdominal Pain," in 1921, first interested us in such pain, which we have confirmed in several contributions. The necessity of ruling out other possible causes of abdominal pain while food allergy is being considered was emphasized in our article "Food Allergy in the Differential Diagnoses of Abdominal Symptoms" in 1932. Paroxysmal abdominal pain as reported by Moore in the *JAMA* in 1945 may be an epileptic equivalent relieved by Dilantin. It requires study of allergy, especially to foods, as a possible cause, as discussed in Chapter 18 on cerebral and neural allergy.

That allergy is a frequent cause of abdominal pain in infants and children has been noted and receives further discussion in Chapter 25. Ratner, in 1945, wrote an important article on abdominal pain in children resulting from food allergy worthy of study. In adult life too frequently allergy, especially to foods, has been overlooked. Many abdominal operations have been performed needlessly on patients because of allergic pain. Such pain can occur in any part of the abdomen and be diffuse or localized. Pains in the upper right quadrant suggesting gallbladder disease or peptic ulcer have been discussed. Pain from food allergy in our patients has occurred in the upper left quadrant usually associated with other gastrointestinal symptoms, including those of the allergic epigastric syndrome, allergic colitis, or constipation. Such pain may be due to localized spasm resulting from allergy in the spenic flexure. One patient had been awakened regularly at 2 to 3 AM for months with such a pain relieved with an elimination diet. Pain resulting from food allergy may occur in the midlateral or lower abdomen.

Case 15: One patient had pain in the lower and mid-left abdomen, especially at 3 to 4 AM relieved by elimination of allergenic foods.

Case 16: A woman had been abed for six weeks with pain across the upper and mid-abdomen until wheat was excluded from the diet.

Case 17: A confrere had aching across the upper abdomen in an hour, lasting eighteen hours, after the ingestion of a slight amount of egg, as in two pieces of candy containing eggs.

An interesting localization of severe pain resulting from food allergy in a small area below and to the left of the umbilicus occurred in several patients, as evidenced in the dramatic case recorded below.

Pain in the right lower abdomen from allergy in the cecum or appendix requiring surgery has already been discussed. Pain over the mid-lower abdomen with urinary symptoms resulting from bladder allergy to foods is discussed in Chapter 21.

Severe acute pain resulting from food allergy and producing the signs of intestinal obstruction may be due to angioneurotic edema of the intestinal tract, as reported by Harrington (1905), Briggs (1908), Crispin (1915), and Bogart (1915). Many years ago Osler, and more recently Christian (1917), described this type of case and warned against unnecessary surgery.

Several of our patients afflicted with gastrointestinal allergy have had emergency surgery because of symptoms suggesting intestinal obstruction. Efron (1932) reported such attacks of pain resulting from wheat allergy.

Case 18: A child had abdominal pain and a recurrent apple-sized tumor resulting from localized edema in the bowel. Pain simulating appendicitis and frequent gastrointestinal bleed-ing, as discussed later in this chapter, resulting from food sensitization may occur. It is important to realize that food allergy may also produce kidney and ureteral pain and abdominal pain suggestive of such distress. This topic will be discussed in the chapter on bladder allergy (see Chapt. 21).

MUCOUS COLITIS

Duke, in 1921, and Vaughan, in 1922, first called attention to the role of food allergy in mucous colitis. Vaughan (1928) reported seven such cases of mucous colitis resulting from food allergy, and Hollander (1927) had formerly published a similar paper. Chiray and Baumann (1933) also discussed allergic colitis and recalled confirmatory articles by other French students, including Gutmann, de Loeper, Tzanck, and Vallery-Radot. In other older literature mucous colitis has been called "asthma of the bowels" by von Strümpell (1910) and Wiener (1912), as noted by Kammerer (1934). Hurst (1929) also commented on the analogy between mucous colitis and asthma and on the fact that both conditions at times occur in the same family. Beecher (1929) reported four cases resulting from food sensitization, two being sensitive to coffee and two to wheat. A. Cohen (1934) had a patient with mucous colitis of years' standing treated in a tuberculosis sanatarium with heavy milk ingestion, which later proved the cause of her colitis.

In various publications since 1928 we have affirmed our opinion that food allergy must always receive consideration as a cause of mucous colitis. When allergic in origin it is often associated with other gastrointestinal, cutaneous, or nasobronchial manifestations of allergy, which may be due to food or possibly inhalant allergies.

Case 19: One physician fifty years of age had nasal congestion, marked tenesmus and diarrhea and bowel mucus for many months. Because of slight fever, infection and parasites had been considered. Stool examinations were negative, and food sensitizations were found to be causative.

Case 20: Another patient had mucous colitis, right-sided abdominal pain and soreness, weakness, fatigue, generalized aching of the body, and palpitations, all relieved by our elimination diet.

Case 21: Another patient had had mucous colitis for many years with obstinate constipation and colonic soreness. With elimination of allergenic foods, these symptoms, together with a facial eruption, disappeared. Her stools became large and well formed.

The literature has long emphasized the neurotic tendencies in these patients and gives little or no consideration to the part food allergy may play in this condition. Thus Bastedo (1917) described the neurotic tendencies and the mental and physical fatigue. The persisting pains had led to exploratory operations. He recognized the semblance to bronchial asthma. There was a familial tendency to both intestinal allergy and bronchial asthma in certain patients.

Continued symptoms with the frustration resulting from failure of relief from medical advice and from many medications, including tranquilizers and sedatives, are usually responsible for the nervousness, tension, and irritability which decrease or disappear when the allergy is controlled. Existent hormone deficiency, especially in women, always must be recognized and controlled.

Eggleston, in his article in 1928, did not mention food allergy and felt that nervous instability was the main cause. Though much emphasis was laid on the abnormal spasticity of the smooth muscle of the colon, no mention of allergy as a possible cause was made. Mallory, in 1928, considered food allergy as a possible cause of colonic distress but said that foods which gave skin reactions often produced no

bowel disturbance. He was not aware of the localization of allergic reactions, of the necessity of trial diets to study food allergy, and of the frequency of negative reactions in food allergy.

A case record of mucous colitis resulting from allergy will be found on this page. A case of colonic polyposis with constipation, mucus, and occasional blood recorded by Gay (1936) was entirely relieved of symptoms with elimination of allergenic foods. Thus allergy as a cause of colonic polyposis must receive attention.

PRURITUS ANI AND PROCTITIS

Localization of allergic reactions in the anus and rectum must be recognized, especially in patients who have an allergic history. Rectal pain and spasms are commonly due to food sensitizations, frequently awakening patients in the early morning and causing marked tenesmus with the possible expulsation of a little mucus, at times blood stained, and usually a little gas. Bramigk (1935) described high rectal pain relieved by elimination or test-negative diets and noted the frequency of wheat as a cause. Tumpeer (1934) noted anal spasm from food allergy in infants. The pruritus ani may or may not be accompanied by an eczematous type of perianal eruption which may become severe and associated with cracking, oozing, and induration. M. B. Cohen (1931) reported pruritus ani resulting from pork to which a two plus reaction by skin testing occurred. Andresen (1925) pointed out food allergy as a cause of this condition. We have studied cases greatly benefited with accurate use of the elimination diets. One physician determined that marked itching in the anus and pains in the rectum result whenever egg and cantaloupe are ingested. Drueck (1935) has recognized the allergic etiology in many cases of pruritus of the anus, genitalia, and perineum.

It is certain that pruritus ani is frequently a localized allergic reaction to food and possibly to airborne allergens.

Case 22: A recent patient with pruritus ani which had resisted all types of therapy for over one year gave large reactions to many spring, fall, and cultivated flower pollens as well as to many foods. Several foods to which known idiosyncrasies existed failed to give reactions. With an elimination diet and pollen therapy, the pruritus disappeared in two months.

Another patient had severe pruritus of the anus relieved by the elimination of pineapple. Strawberries produced vaginal itching. The sister had itching of the forehead and temples without rectovaginal distress from other foods. The importance of studying patients with pruritus ani in the same complete way required in patients with eczema is emphasized. Vaughan, in 1930 and other contributions since then, reported cases of pruritus ani resulting from food allergy. One of our patients had pruritus ani from shrimps three-fourths of an hour after ingestion, but crab was taken without difficulty. Gay described the red anal canal with excessive mucus or a grayish mucosa in patients with such allergy. The rectum and sigmoid undoubtedly are frequent sites in the so-called idiopathic cases of anal pruritus. Examination of the mucous secretions for eosinophiles will aid in the determination of such allergic membranes. Other causes of pruritus ani are epidermophytosis, especially if present on the feet; leukorrhea; diabetes; fissures or external hemorrhoids; irritants such as toilet paper; intrarectal pathology; seborrhea; and other chronic diseases or necrosis.

Through the last thirty-five years, food and at times pollen allergy have continued to be confirmed as frequent causes of pruritus ani, as reported in the first edition of

this book in 1931. Being an eczematous reaction, it may be localized in the anal and perianal tissues or be associated with eczema in other cutaneous areas, as reported in Chapter 14. One patient with pruritus ani which had resisted other therapy for 1½ years was relieved of the eruption in 2 months with elimination of allergenic foods determined with our elimination diet along with the control of pollen allergy. The latter was indicated by seasonal exaggeration of his perennial pruritus and by large scratch reactions to pollens.

Allergy to caine drugs may be the sole cause of pruritus ani or may be a complicating factor in its causation. Allergy to other medication in ointments or rectal suppositories, to cathartics (especially phenolphthalein), and to oral or parenteral medications which produce eczema in other skin areas may cause pruritus ani or proctitis. Contact allergy to fabrics, especially nylon and silk; to chemical finishings of fabrics, especially formaldehyde; and to perfumes, deodorants, and chemicals in douches and other vaginal medications and contraceptives, including rubber, must be ruled out.

Symptoms from allergy in other gastrointestinal tissue often are present, and other manifestations of clinical allergy especially to foods are present. Severe allergic vulvitis, vaginitis, and involvement of the perineum may occur, as discussed on page 415.

When pruritus ani is present, possible allergic proctitis must be investigated by sigmoidoscopy. Cancer must be excluded.

If proctitis is found, especially if diarrhea with blood and mucus occurs, possible localized chronic ulcerative colitis may be present, especially if the mucosa is inflamed, friable, and granular even if ulcerations are not found. Stool examinations for ova, parasites, and pathogenic bacteria are necessary. Further discussion of the important role of atopic allergy in chronic ulcerative colitis and also in regional enteritis follows in Chapters 6 and 7.

CASE SUMMARIES

Case 23: A man fifty-seven years of age was seen in 1958. He had had pruritus ani for one year with itching but no eruption. A hivelike eruption developed on the scrotum three months before we saw him. This eruption extended eight to ten inches down the adjacent thighs. No oozing or crusting occurred. He gave marked reactions to pollen, and desensitization was started beginning with a 1:10-12 dilution. The injections were gradually increased up to the 1:10-10 dilution over a period of eight months. He never reached a dilution stronger than the 1:10-10. During this time he took Prednisone at intervals, and he reported three years later that good results had been obtained.

Case 24: A man twenty-six years of age was seen in 1947. He had had pruritus ani for six months. A rectal and anal fistula had developed. Two months before we saw him, itching had developed on the scrotum, the penis, and the gluteal areas associated with redness of the face, eyes, neck, wrists, and feet. He gave no reactions to any pollens, but pollen allergy was the assumed cause, and desensitization beginning with a 1:10-12 dilution was gradually increased up to a 1:50 dilution over a period of three years. Relief occurred in four or five months. His difficulty recurred slightly at intervals but was absent for sixteen years after the last injections were given.

ALLERGIC PERITONITIS

In the first edition of this book we reported upper right abdominal pain, distention, belching, sour stomach, canker sores, heavy breath, coated tongue and constipation for fifteen years in a man thirty-nine years of age. After removal of a normal appendix six years previously, intermittent diarrhea with his former constipation occurred. Finally, sudden severe abdominal pain in the left abdomen indicated an emergency operation for possible obstruction. Fever of 103 F and a leukocyte count of 18,200 with 83 percent polymorphonuclear cells were present. Diffuse erythema of the ileum and cecum along with considerable gray sterile fluid was found with no pathology in the gallbladder, large intestine, or small intestine. Streptococcal peritonitis was suspected, large drains were placed into the sigmoidal area, and the wound was partially closed. With intravenous fluids, serous drainage stopped in four days, and a liquid soft diet was given excluding milk, wheat, fruits, and spices to which allergy had been suspected in previous months. The drains were removed in four days, the patient returning to work in twelve days. Culture of the peritoneal fluid was negative. Recovery occurred in spite of no sulfonamides or antibiotics, this case having been encountered long before the discovery of the above drugs.

During the last forty years symptoms have been well controlled with the strict elimination of all fruits and condiments, nuts, wheat, rye, milk, corn, chocolate, coffee, bacon, and beef. The pain, fever, increased leukocyte count, and free abdominal fluid were best explained by allergy to foods to which skin tests were negative.

Various surgeons have informed us about simliar free abdominal fluid and congested intestinal tissues with no other pathology or with palpable lymph nodes in the peritoneum. It is possible that food allergy in these patients could be demonstrated today with the accurate use of our elimination diets.

UNSTABLE OR IRRITABLE COLON

For many years we have pointed out that the irritable or as Kantor (1932) terms it, the unstable colon, may often be due to food allergy. To us it seems evident that the large bowel becomes a frequent site of allergic reactions to foods because of its long retention of food residues containing undigested food proteins. This is especially true of the ascending colon. Until the early thirties the literature had contained little recognition of this possibility. Thus Emery (1925) stated that nothing was known of the cause of irritable bowel. According to Singer (1928) the irritable colon was a diagnosis made when no definite cause could be found for the patient's symptoms. Subsequent to the first edition of this book, Kantor suggested allergy as one possible cause. Hurst (1934) and Jordan (1932) drew attention to allergic reactions in the colon. Lintz (1934) in particular stated that allergy, especially to bacteria, is the outstanding cause of such colonic distress and dysfunction, and Kruse in part substantiated this idea.

It must be remembered that the unstable colon has been attributed to many causes more commonly than to allergy. However, Alvarez (1931) wrote in *Oxford Medicine* that he has often observed such colons at operation and that no evidences of pathology or inflammation have been ascertainable. Jordan, Kantor, and Kruse have discussed the unstable colon in articles. Spasticity, atony, dilatation, stretching, hypermotility, and the other disturbances in peristalsis are present in varying degrees. Kruse (1934) especially emphasized the poor coordination of the nervous system and the frequency of neuroses, fears, and phobias in such patients. Distention, belching, colonic soreness and pain, exhaustion, fatigue, constipation or diarrhea, cramping, and mucus in the stools are frequent complaints. Colonic consciousness is constant in many such patients. Most of these symptoms might arise from allergic reactions in localized or large sections of the colon. It is

possible that long-continued allergic reactions lead to slight but definite pathological changes which require prolonged elimination of the causative allergens for relief. The pathology may never completely disappear. Patients with unstable colons should be given the opportunity of prolonged and careful study with balanced and adequate diets based on the concept of food allergy as a cause. At times an allergic status requires months to counteract. Allergy in the etiology should not be discarded until several weeks or even months of trial dieting have been continued. A few months are not too many to devote to this important study. The fact that Mateer *et al.* (1935) have reported relief from vaccines of stock coli bacilli indicates the possibility that bacterial allergy may be at times causative. Mogena (1935), from the Diaz Clinic in Madrid, reported his experience with allergic colopathy. Food allergy was often causative. Elimination diets were of value and skin reactions of little help in diagnosis. The possibility of products of tissue disease acting as allergens was discussed. Particularly favorable results were obtained with desensitization with specific bacteria from the stools in certain patients whose bacterial allergy caused colitis. At times more than one stool culture was required to obtain the causative bacteria. Colon bacilli were often at fault. After such study these patients may have to be treated with various therapeutic procedures recommended especially by Kantor, Jordan, and Kruse. Such allergy has not been confirmed in our practice possibly because of our earnest study of food and possible inhalant and drug allergies.

It is our conviction, however, that allergy often of a chronic type is frequently at fault. That food allergy is a common cause of the so-called unstable or irritable colon which was a frequent diagnosis by Sippy around 1920 and by other internists in the ensuing twenty years has been repeatedly evidenced in our practice. The colonic soreness and pain, cramping, mucus, constipation, or diarrhea can best be explained by food allergy in view of the failure of physical findings, laboratory studies, and x-ray studies to reveal abdominal pathology and because of the relief often arising from our FFCFE diet or one of our minimal elimination diets.

The distention, belching, and burning in the upper abdomen in some of these patients can be explained by epigastric food allergy, as reported in this chapter. The exhaustion, fatigue, fears, tension, and "toxic feelings" can also be explained by the allergic toxemia and fatigue syndrome which we discuss in Chapter 19. It is possible that long-continued allergic reactions lead to slight but definite pathological changes which require prolonged elimination of the causative allergens for relief. Patients with unstable colons should be given the opportunity of careful and if necessary prolonged study with balanced and adequate elimination diets to control possible food allergy. Allergy in the etiology should not be discarded until trial dieting has been continued for an adequate period of time.

APPENDICEAL TYPE OF PAIN

Food sensitization not infrequently produces varying degrees of colonic congestion, inflammation, and probably spasm in the ascending colon causing soreness and pain in the right lower quadrant.

Allergic reactions may often occur in the cecum and even in the appendix because of the comparative rapidity with which ingested foods reach this region and the long period that food is retained while bacterial

digestion and fluid absorption are occurring. Such reactions are also present in the appendix and may predispose to secondary infection in the same way that allergic congestion in the nasal and sinal tissues or the bronchial tract encourages bacterial or viral infection. This colonic irritation, inflammation, and probably spasm in the appendix was first suggested by Duke, in 1921, and confirmed by him in 1931. Lintz, in 1925, reported the frequency of appendectomies because of unrealized allergic reactions. He also thought that a familial "predisposition to appendicitis" usually indicated an allergic cause. We favor his emphasis of such a cause of lower right abdominal distress. Acute allergic reactions can produce mild or even moderate fever, as in recurrent attacks of bronchial asthma (Chapt. 25). Leukocytosis of 12,000 to 16,000 with moderate increase in polymorphonuclear leukocytes may even occur.

This pain in the right lower abdomen may be due to allergic inflammation in the appendix, which may predispose to infection, causing rigidity and justifying appendectomy. It may also be due to allergic inflammation and spasm in the cecum with varying involvement of the peritoneum, relieved especially as we now advise with our FFCFE diet with gradually decreasing corticosteroid therapy.

This area, therefore, as Ratner (1945) and other allergists have confirmed, becomes a logical site for the development of frequent localized reactions to food allergens. Allergic vasculitis, edema, and smooth muscle spasm can arise from food allergy. Secondary infection may require surgery. Such reactions might be more common in patients with low cecums which are often associated with stasis and with attacks of vomiting and headaches which may be of allergic origin. Fresh fruits seem to produce cecal reactions quite frequently, possibly because of the tendency to overeat, the hypermotility they produce, and the fact that they are likely to remain only partially digested for a long time in the ascending colon. Moreover, fresh fruits may be more allergenic than cooked ones. Overeating of any food, however, may lead to the same result. If allergy develops to such foods, minute amounts of them will precipitate allergic reactions and symptoms.

Cooke (1942) opined that allergy to foods could result in appendicitis. Friedenwald and Morrison (1934) observed a patient fifty-five years of age who had had constant distress in the lower right quadrant for thirty-four years. The family history was positive for allergy. The distress was found to be due to chicken, tomatoes, turnips, and cabbage. Gay found definite rigidity, fever, and leukocytosis resulting from food sensitizations in the abdomen.

Most of the appendectomies which had been performed in 107 of our 270 cases of gastrointestinal allergy had failed to relieve abdominal symptoms. With such symptoms, however, if definite rigidity is present, appendectomy is warranted even if the allergic status of the patient is quite definite, since, as stated above, allergic edema may predispose to infection.

McIntosh (1930) found eosinophilic infiltration in 310 appendices. Excessive mucus and Charcot-Leyden-like crystals also occurred. Such pathology was very different from that of actual infection and often occurred in patients who gave a history of recurrent attacks. Many so-called chronic appendices are removed because of probable allergic reactions, especially in the cecum and ascending colon. The Shwartzman reaction of hemorrhagic allergy in the appendix may explain necrosis, infection,

and rupture. In 1934 Dutton discussed inflammation of the appendix resulting from probable food allergy predisposing to infection.

In 1959 acute allergic colitis resulting from lobster led to a diagnosis of acute appendicitis by Karpman. At operation, the ascending colon was thickened and edematous, with bullae on the mesenteric border. The abnormalities were relieved by injection of 0.3 cc of 1:1000 epinephrine. The pathological study of the appendix was normal.

The association of chronic constipation, a tendency to a coated tongue and heavy breath, and right-sided abdominal aching and soreness without rigidity or fever has occurred in several of our patients because of food allergy.

CASE SUMMARY

Case 25: A boy twelve years of age had had recurrent attacks of pain in his right lower abdomen, nasal congestion, sore throats, and a hacking cough without fever every one to two months for several years, indicating food allergy. With the control of his nasal allergy with our CFE diet, his abdominal pain was relieved. As other foods were added to his diet, his abdominal pain reappeared. Rice, especially, in three trials caused the pain. The pain had suggested chronic appendicitis for years.

HEMORRHOIDS RESULTING FROM ATOPIC ALLERGY

That hemorrhoids can arise from allergic inflammation in the anal canal has long been evident in our practice. Their development is explained by vascular dilatation in the mucosa and spasm in the anal muscles from localized allergy. Straining at stool engorges and protrudes blood vessels and mucosa, resulting in initial, acute, inflamed hemorrhoids which gradually become fibrotic and organized into hemorrhoidal tags. The inflammation and muscular spasm in the anal canal produce a pain, soreness, and continued discomfort, especially in the sitting position. Such allergy explains many internal as well as external hemorrhoids. Allergy may be a predisposing cause of hemorrhoids in pregnancy, since they do not occur in all pregnancies.

Allergy to fruits, at times to most or all of them, and to flavors and condiments is commonly responsible. Allergy to other foods excluded from our FFCFE diet and occasionally to foods in the diet itself must be suspect. To study such food allergy as in all possible gastrointestinal manifestations of food allergy, the diet must be strictly maintained, as advised at the end of this chapter and in Chapter 3. After relief of the burning, spasm, itching, and a recession of the hemorrhoids has continued for one to two months, other foods can be added according to our directions. To relieve the initial inflammation, burning, and itching, hot Sitz baths, large doses of corticosteroids by mouth with their gradual discontinuance in seven to fourteen days, and local application of corticosteroid ointment are advisable. This control of frequent allergy has made surgery unnecessary in many patients. If large, organized hemorrhoids indicate surgery, this antiallergic therapy for two to three weeks preceding surgery may reduce postoperative discomfort and encourage healing of the tissues.

As in allergic eczema in other cutaneous areas, pollen allergy alone or with food allergy may occur and require desensitization therapy. And possible localized allergy to caine ointments or suppositories or to other medications must be remembered.

GASTROINTESTINAL BLEEDING

Because of increased vascular permeability which characterizes the allergic reaction, as first stressed by Manwaring (1921),

capillary hemorrhages are not uncommon. Auer and Lewis previously had demonstrated this in many animal experiments, as summarized in 1910 in their excellent article "Experimental and Clinical Anaphylaxis."

Bleeding from the mucosa in various areas in the gastrointestinal tract and in other tissues from allergy to foods has been reported in the literature and encountered in our practice. Bleeding in the lung parenchyma, reported elsewhere, even from traces of milk for fourteen years exemplifies bleeding in other tissues than the gastrointestinal tract. Gastrointestinal bleeding from pollen allergy is discussed in Chapter 6. Rubin, in 1940, reported allergic intestinal bleeding with colic in infants usually resulting from allergy to cow's milk after its ingestion for three to four weeks, which is further discussed in Chapter 25.

Case 26: One woman, sixty-two years of age, who has had distention, burning, and soreness in the epigastrium; headaches; fatigue; and toxic symptoms from multiple food allergies also has bleeding from the gums, pharynx, and sublingual tissues from eating meat, eggs, chicken, and rice. The latter two also cause nausea, epigastric tightness, and pain. Inflammation, vesiculation, and bleeding of the lips occur in a boy from biting into oranges or grapefruit.

Case 27: A woman forty-six years of age had had vomiting of dark blood and black stools for four days in 1946 and again in 1948 requiring two transfusions from a previous physician. X-rays of the stomach and small bowel were negative. Oral canker sores had recurred in childhood. Since 1948 previous epigastric distress and blood in the stools have been absent from the elimination of fruits, condiments, wheat, corn, and milk except for slight blood in 1954 after eating pears and peaches. In 1963 hematuria continued for three weeks. Cystoscopic examination revealed thirty to forty areas of 1 to 2 cm in size of dilated, congested capillaries in which slight bleeding was seen. For one month a moderate amount of fruit had been taken for the first time in several years. No blood in the stools or urine and no digestive or urinary symptoms have occurred since then with the exclusion of fruit, flavors, milk, wheat, and corn from the diet. Though a gastroscopy was not done in 1948, gastritis with bleeding areas similar to those seen in the bladder can explain her former gastric hemorrhages, since x-rays revealed no ulcers.

In the differential diagnosis of gastric bleeding, aspirin as a cause at times associated with marked painful gastritis must be remembered. That food allergy especially to fruits is a logical cause of duodenal ulcers has been discussed on page 110. Duodenal inflammation and bleeding even without ulceration may also arise from food allergy. When the control of the symptoms and healing of the ulcer occur from the control of assumed or proven allergy to foods, previous superficial bleeding and even severe bleeding from large blood vessels can be attributed to the localized allergy.

Bleeding in the small bowel in cases of Henoch-Schonlein purpura resulting from food allergy reported by Alexander and Eyermann in 1927 and 1929 has occurred in two of our patients, as discussed in Chapter 22 of this book. Hematemesis, hematuria, and ocular hemorrhages may also occur with more usual urticaria, abdominal pain, and even fever. In the small bowel bleeding can occur from any area of regional enteritis, especially in the distal ileum and also in the rest of the ileum and occasionally in the jejunum. Since regional enteritis in our opinion is due to atopic allergy, especially to foods (see Chapt. 7), the bleeding must be attributed to rupture of allergically inflamed capillaries or small blood vessels in the mucosa. Golden (1945) reported gross and occult bleeding from inflamed and edematous mucosa from ileal allergy resulting from foods. He also reported gross bleeding from the sigmoid and rectum from milk allergy. Proctoscopic ex-

amination showed hyperemia with small areas of oozing blood.

The bleeding of CUC may be attributed to atopic allergy to foods and at times to pollen allergy because of our confirmation for nearly thirty years of atopic allergy as the sole initial cause of this disease (see Chapt. 6). Andresen reported profuse bloody diarrhea from ten drops of milk in one case of CUC (1958). In those cases in which atopic allergy is the cause of hemorrhoids, as discussed on page 125, allergy is responsible for bleeding.

GASTROINTESTINAL SYMPTOMS FROM POLLEN ALLERGY

Nausea, vomiting, epigastric distention, pressure, cramping, soreness, tenderness in various abdominal areas, diarrhea, anal soreness, and spasm may result from pollen allergy alone or concomitant with food allergy. Pollen allergy as the sole cause or associated with the more common food allergy as the major cause of chronic ulcerative colitis and also of regional enteritis is discussed in Chapters 6 and 7. In our book on *Clinical Allergy* in 1937, we wrote: "Duke's original observation that pollen allergy occasionally causes abdominal symptoms has been confirmed. Eyermann reported two such manifestations accompanying general reactions during pollen therapy and called attention to the experiment of Freeman, who showed that pollen taken with food might give nausea, vomiting, indigestion, and diarrhea. I have seen inhalant allergy due to pollen produce a toxic sensation, dizziness, nausea and even vomiting."

Pollen allergy is indicated especially by occurrence or exaggeration of gastrointestinal symptoms during the pollen seasons from early spring until mid-fall or late fall. When symptoms continue through the winter, food allergy must be considered.

Though a history of hay fever, asthma, or allergic dermatitis may be present and positive scratch reactions to pollens may occur, neither is necessary to justify pollen therapy. History of seasonal occurrence or exaggeration of symptoms is more important than skin testing (see Chapt. 2). The gastrointestinal symptoms may be the only manifestation of pollen allergy. Diagnosis of pollen allergy and its control are discussed in Chapter 4. Corroborating pollen allergy is the relief of gastrointestinal symptoms especially in the subsequent pollen season from adequate desensitization with antigens containing all of the allergenic pollens in the patient's area. Initial doses of weak dilutions (that is, 1:5 million or even 1:500 billion) usually are prudent with a gradual increase, if possible, into the 1:500 or 1:50 dilutions. If symptoms are increased by doses of any dilution, their repetition may be sufficient for control of pollen allergy. An attempt to decrease pollen in the air of the living environment with electrostatic filters may be advisable. If associated with food allergy, the latter must be controlled, as advised in Chapter 3.

CASE SUMMARY

Case 28: A woman fifty-five years of age had had cramping in the lower abdomen with nonbloody loose stools from early spring to November with no winter symptoms for fifteen years. For five years severity of symptoms had kept her abed from May to September. Abdominal distention, nausea, and slight hemorrhoids had occurred with the diarrhea. Hay fever and asthma had not occurred. Scratch tests gave one plus reactions to grass, plantain, alder, oak, and ash pollens. All laboratory tests and x-rays of the GI tract were negative. Desensitization was started with pollens present in her area of residence. Treatment was begun with a 1:50 million dilution and gradually increased into the 1:500, repeating the tolerated dose every week for two years. In two months desensitization gave relief which has continued through five subsequent pollen seasons.

ROENTGEN DEVIATIONS IN THE GASTROINTESTINAL TRACT BECAUSE OF FOOD ALLERGY

Roentgen deviations from the normal in the gastrointestinal tract in forty of two hundred patients with proven gastrointestinal allergy were reported in the first edition of this book in 1931.

Roentgen ray studies of the gastrointestinal tract were made in 66 percent of 270 patients subsequent to the initial report in 1931. The following deviations from the normal were visualized in 20 percent of the patients: gastric retention in four cases, duodenal retention in one case, spastic antrum in one case, decreased motility in small intestine and hypermotility in the large bowel in one case, hyperperistalsis in stomach and upper intestine in one case, moderate duodenal stasis in five cases, marked dilatations of cap in one case and spastic bowel in twenty-four cases. These findings occurred in patients with definite gastrointestinal symptoms relieved by elimination diets, and it is probable that they resulted from allergic reactions in the alimentary tissues.

Four patients who were especially egg and milk sensitive revealed gastric retention and other marked disturbances in muscular tone and motility. These patients were selected for careful study (1933) because of their prolonged gastric symptoms which had been relieved by the elimination of specific foods. Careful physical examinations and laboratory studies had ruled out other causes. The elimination of definite foods had relieved the symptoms, and the reintroduction of the same foods in the diets had reproduced the symptoms on more than one occasion in each patient. Roentgen observations consisted of fluoroscopic examinations and roentgenograms made immediately upon ingestion of barium and thereafter at three hours, six hours, and twenty-four hours. Such studies were first made when the patients had been free of symptoms for several weeks as the result of their strict adherence to their elimination diets. The barium was administered in a corn meal gruel. About two or three weeks after this initial study, a second series of observations was made after the patient had taken milk or milk and eggs for one or two days. The barium was administered in malted milk to which each patient was sensitive.

We reported in 1933 the following deviations from the normal roentgen ray findings when the patients were on elimination diets which controlled their symptoms and subsequent additions of milk or eggs were made to their diets:

1. Gastric retention was observed in each of the four patients. This was marked in three hours and very definite in six hours. In Case 1 there was definite evidence of pylorospasm. In the other cases it could have been present to a degree difficult to visualize. In all the cases and especially in Case 3, in which gastroenterostomy was present, some disturbance in peristalsis interfering with the gastric or intestinal gradient best explains the gastric retention. Such disturbance could be the result of localized or generalized mucosal edema or smooth muscle spasm arising from allergic reactions resulting from milk or eggs.

2. In each patient barium was present in the duodenum and jejunum in three to six hours. This was to be expected with the gastric retention and was due to the same causes that were responsible for the residues in the stomach.

3. In Case 1 definite hypermotility was observed in three and six hours. It is impossible to say that allergy was definitely responsible. However, diarrhea is not an infrequent manifestation of food allergy in children and adults.

4. A spastic colon was observed in Cases 1, 2, and 3 during the second studies. Such spasm could readily be explained by an allergic reaction of the smooth muscle in the colon. It is our opinion that constipation is frequently due to food allergy resulting from colonic spasm and that when it is accompanied by a mucosal reaction, mucous colitis or an irritable bowel may result.

It is interesting that long-standing constipation in Case 1 and especially in Case 2 was relieved by elimination diets only to return when milk and eggs were taken again.

It is our opinion that these conditions with their accompanying symptoms are probably due to food allergy for the following reasons: (a) They were absent when milk and eggs were excluded from the diet. (b) The symptoms reappeared when milk or egg had been added for from one to three days. Case 3 had definitely determined before consulting us that these two foods along with a few others invariably produced nausea, vomiting, and gastrointestinal soreness for which gastroenterostomy had been done without relief. (c) Such relief and reproduction of symptoms in each patient had occurred on two or three occasions by the withdrawal or inclusion of these specific foods.

In comparison with these marked disturbances, many mild ones undoubtedly occur which are more difficult to demonstrate roentgenographically. This of course is especially true of reactions in the small intestine, evidence of which we have found. Crispin (1915) reported a patient who had angioneurotic edema associated with severe abdominal pain and hematemesis for many years. Roentgen ray examination of the stomach just before an attack showed a lesion near the pylorus which was recognized to be due to visceral swelling, this being confirmed at an exploratory operation. Duke (1931) also reported the roentgen ray observations on a case with hyperperistalsis resulting from food allergy. Such hypermotility resulting from food allergy would be simple to demonstrate in the many children and adults suffering from diarrhea arising from food allergy. Spastic colons observed in our studies occurred in many patients relieved of constipation by elimination diets.

A unique report of roentgen ray studies made on the gastrointestinal reactions to food allergy was published by Eyermann in 1927. The patient, a woman thirty-five years of age, had had urticaria, epigastric burning, regurgitation of all foods, frequent hiccough, alternating constipation and diarrhea, abdominal colic, upper right quadrant pain, and excessive abdominal gas and bloating for eight years because of wheat sensitization. When wheat was ingested by the patient, no definite abnormalities were shown by roentgen ray study in the stomach or small intestines, but the colon was definitely spastic compared to its condition when the patient was on a wheat-free diet. A roentgen ray film taken when pain was present following ingestion of whole wheat showed a colon of disharmonic tonus, being hypotonic in the cecum and ascending portions and hypertonic in the transverse and pelvic portions. Adrenalin chloride, 0.5 cc of 1:1000 solution, given hypodermically produced subjective relief in a few minutes, and fluoroscopic examination revealed less spasticity of the transverse and descending colon. These findings were in direct contrast with those observed when no abdominal pain was present, for then the colon showed normal haustra and a tendency to be hypotonic in the ascending portion. Serio (1932) reported roentgen ray demonstration of spasticity in the stomach and colon with intestinal hyperperistalsis resulting from ingested foods to which sensitization existed. Gay (1936) also reported localized spasm in the colon resulting from food allergy.

Cooke, in 1942, recorded a six-hour residue and hypermotility with barium in the small intestine after the ingestion of milk in a milk-sensitive patient.

In 1942 Fries and Mogil reported roentgen ray changes from the ingestion of allergenic foods in thirty children. Gastric retention which we had reported in 1933 occurred in eleven of the thirty cases. Though gastric hyperperistalsis was usually decreased, it was increased in two cases. Peristalsis in the small bowel was disturbed in five of the thirty cases. In two cases barium reached the cecum in one hour.

In 1949 Schloss reported spastic contractions superimposed on elevated intralumenal pressure in the jejunum when an allergen-barium mixture was instilled through a Miller-Abbott Tube. These disturbances were reported graphically and by x-ray associated with a moderate increase in transit in one and a slow transit through the small bowel in another.

Tallant, O'Neil, Urbach, and Price in 1949 reported many narrow segmented areas with segmentation and scattering of barium in the distal small bowel after ingestion of an allergenic food. The transit time was increased in one third of the cases and decreased in another third.

Buffard and Crozet, in 1952, reported six cases of GI allergy showing wide edematous mucosal gastric folds, hypotonia, and slow transit in the small intestine. Dilution of barium in one case suggested hypersecretion. Hyperperistalsis in transit into the cecum occurred in fifteen minutes in one case.

Golden, in 1945, in his chapter on allergy in the small bowel emphasized hypertonicity and segmentation in the lower half of the small bowel for the first time. The lumen of the bowel was decreased, and hypermotility or a slow transit of the barium at times occurred. Edema of the mucosal folds in the lower jejunum was found in two patients. This at first suggested regional enteritis, but other roentgen ray indications of regional enteritis were absent. X-rays showing these changes published in the first and second editions of his book are worthy of study. Golden described hyperperistalsis after the ingestion of milk, calling it "the milk reaction." It was likened to "rhinorrhea in nasal allergy." Whereas allergy can cause hypermotility with the absence of other roentgen ray abnormality, the deficiency of intestinal lactase requires study as a possible cause.

Lepore, Collins, and Sherman, in 1951, reported roentgen ray findings in the small intestine from food allergy, showing hypermotility and hypertoxicity, especially in the lower half with segmentation of the barium column. Informative photographs of abnormal x-ray findings in the small bowel with symptoms resulting from ingested allergenic foods emphasize the results of food allergy. Rapid transit occurred in fourteen, compared with a slow transit in the small bowel in four.

ORIGIN OF GASTROINTESTINAL ALLERGY

Our opinion in 1936 that "It is probable that more mild, moderate, and severe symptoms from food allergies arise in the tissues of the gastrointestinal tract than in any other structures of the body . . ." has been supported in our practice of allergy since then. Though the manifestations of food allergy may occur only in the gastrointestinal tract, they are usually associated with minor or major symptoms arising in the nasobronchial, cutaneous, central nervous, urogenital, eye, ear, or other body tissues. This frequency in the GI tract may be explained by the intimate and long-continued contact of foods with the alimentary mucosa especially in the upper gastrointestinal tract and also in the cecum, where foods in various stages of digestion are detained for varying periods. Such contact makes possible the establishment of local sensitization in any part of the alimentary canal, even in the rectum, because of the presence of undigested foods especially when hypermotility occurs. Though this localized allergy may be similar to contact allergy in the skin, the atopic type of allergy resulting from specific antibodies in the blood and tissues of the gastrointestinal tract is the more probable explanation of the symptoms from food allergy. The frequency with which these antibodies are not demonstrated by positive skin tests can be explained by their presence in the gastrointestinal tissues and absence in the skin or because of sensitization to the starches and at times to pectins of foods as reported by Lietze. These latter reactions can be demonstrated only by immunological technique and not by skin testing.

The origin of clinical food allergy in the gastrointestinal tract may largely depend on an inherited predisposition and may result in the development of localized allergy in any part of the alimentary canal as in the mouth, duodenum, small or large bowel, or rectum. The predisposition to allergy, moreover, may be present in a localized area, so that epigastric or oral allergy or chronic ulcerative colitis or duodenal ulcer may occur in more than one member of the same or previous generations. And as stated on page 13, the inherited tendency to develop the same manifestations of allergy to the same food may occur.

Excessive eating of a food may result in localized allergy in various parts of the gastrointestinal tract, and as discussed on page 13, in manifestations of food allergy in other tissues of the body. It is possible that such sensitization might arise when a long-ingested food is temporarily eliminated for weeks at a time. We have never had clinical confirmation of this origin of food allergy, though we have seen the development of asthma to aspirin while it was discontinued for three weeks after its constant use for thirteen years and the development of severe dermatitis to phenobarbital after it had temporarily been stopped.

Food allergy produces its many clinical manifestations at any time of life contrary to the opinion of some students that it occurs with decreasing frequency in adult life and practically never in old age. Though food allergy develops frequently in infancy and childhood, its origin in adolescence, adult life, and not infrequently in old age has been increasingly evidenced in our practice for fifty years. In 1936 we reported a man, sixty-five years of age, who for the first time developed milk allergy causing bronchial asthma. Such origin of various manifestations of allergy to many other foods has repeatedly occurred in our patients. Many other patients have developed manifestations of food allergy after the age of sixty or seventy years. The failure of many physicians to realize this occurrence is due to the negative or fallible skin reactions to foods, the usual failure to study possible food allergy with trial diet especially in a strict and adequate manner with our elimination diets, and the usual

failure of test-negative diets to control food allergy.

Food allergy which develops in infancy or childhood may become inactive in two to ten years, with a disappearance of its manifestations, as reported in Chapter 1. In late life such potential food allergy may be activated again to the same or other foods causing the previous or other clinical disturbances.

DIFFERENTIAL DIAGNOSIS OF GASTROINTESTINAL ALLERGY

We have always emphasized the necessity of a detailed history of all previous and present symptoms; the importance of all indicated physical, laboratory, and x-ray examinations; and the necessary consideration of functional and psychic disturbances which might be responsible for the GI symptoms while a diagnosis of food allergy is made. It must be remembered, however, that the symptoms may be due to food or other types of allergy alone or that both allergy and the organic or psychic abnormalities conjointly may be responsible. Food allergy must receive adequate study usually with the initial use of our FFCFE diet in possible GI allergy, especially if previous medical investigations by other physicians have not given relief.

Abdominal distention, pain, cramping, belching, nausea, vomiting, diarrhea, or constipation in varying combinations and degrees often associated with headache and fatigue, body aching, confusion, dopiness, and other symptoms of allergic toxemia and fatigue (Chapt. 19) attributed by previous physicians to possible organic causes and especially to tensions and nervousness often have been markedly or completely relieved with our control of previously unrecognized food allergy.

Food allergy must not be ruled out because of the demonstration of organic disease. Thus a hiatal hernia must not rule out food allergy as a cause of epigastric distress. Food allergy should be ruled out by use of the FFCFE diet before an operation on moderate hiatal hernias. Diverticulosis revealed by x-ray must not rule out food allergy or other etiologies as a possible cause of diarrhea or left-sided abdominal distress. As discussed in this chapter, food allergy requires study as a logical cause of duodenal ulcer and a predisposing cause of acute or chronic appendicitis. And as emphasized in Chapters 6 and 7, food and less often pollen allergy requires study as the usual sole cause of CUC and regional enteritis.

TREATMENT OF GASTROINTESTINAL ALLERGY

Study of Food Allergy With the Fruit-Free, Cereal-Free Elimination Diet

Our FFCFE diet is advised in all cases of possible gastrointestinal allergy to foods. If there is a diet history of definite dislikes or probable allergy or large scratch reactions to individual foods in the diet, they should be omitted or substituted with similar relatively nonallergenic foods. Because of the possibility of allergy to tea when allergy to fruits and flavors is being studied, tea should not be added until symptoms are relieved for one or two months. Initially, water or possibly sparkling water, containing no citric acid, to which sugar is added is the only allowed drink. More detailed directions for the preparation of the diet are to be found in Chapter 3.

As advised in Chapter 3, the soy-potato or rice-potato bakery products, if rice is tolerated as discussed below, must be made in the patient's home by our recipes. Someone in the family of the physician or the physician's office assistant or a dietitian should use the recipes until satisfactory muffins can be made. Then, making of bread may be achieved. With the knowledge that satisfactory products can be made with the recipes, the physician can assure his patients that recipes are effective. Or the physician may find an honest baker who will make such products for sale, as does Bray in Oakland. That many bakery products sold in health food stores as being wheat-free in the western states contain wheat gluten or wheat flour has been determined.*

Our first elimination diets in 1931 excluded wheat, milk, eggs, fish, chocolate and coffee, condiments, and specific fruits and vegetables which we have found to be most frequent causes of gastrointestinal allergy. Increasingly in the next ten years the frequency of allergy to many or all fruits in the gastrointestinal tract justified the use of our FFCFE diet, which we have advised for nearly twenty years. If the patient knows that legumes and especially soy cause indigestion or definite allergy, soy-potato bakery products and other legumes are eliminated. To maintain weight and nutrition, it is necessary to include more white potato, fruit-free tapioca pudding, sugar, and the milk-free products with sesame or cottonseed oil when soy-potato bakery products are excluded from the diet. Important and more detailed advice about the use of elimination diets is found in Chapter 3.

As with all elimination diets, the diet must be maintained strictly for two to three weeks because of the delay of elimination of previously eaten foods from the body. And continued delay in the decrease in tissue pathology resulting from chronic food allergy often requires strict adherence

---

*Studies have been conducted by Arthur Lietze, Ph.D., in our Immunochemical Laboratory for the Study of Food Allergy, Samuel Merritt Hospital, Oakland, California.

to the prescribed diet for a longer period. The amelioration of food allergy in some patients in the summer and its exaggeration in the fall, winter, and early spring also must be remembered.

If symptoms are not relieved in three to four weeks with the FFCFE diet, then a minimal elimination diet should be ordered for three to four weeks. Emphasis must be placed on maintenance of nutrition and weight.

The challenge is to evolve a diet which relieves the gastrointestinal symptoms for at least two to three weeks or for a longer period if symptoms before dieting had recurred every two to four weeks. When such relief has been obtained, single foods can be added daily for three to five days, eliminating any which reproduce symptoms.

With these provocation tests, it may be found that allergy is not present to cereal grains, milk, eggs, and even to some or all fruits. It must be emphasized that possible allergy to added foods can be determined only when the patient is on a diet which keeps him symptom-free. Though allergic symptoms may arise in five to sixty minutes after ingestion of a food, they usually are not apparent to the patient until four, twelve, twenty-four hours, or only after the food has been eaten on two or more successive days. This delay in the development of symptoms after provocation tests in the usual cumulative or chronic type of food allergy makes the use of our elimination diets for diet trial superior to the Rinkel technique, in which evidence of food allergy is expected within a half-hour after provocation tests.

In the study of possible fruit allergy with our FFCFE diet, it is important that all flavors, spices, and condiments be excluded. It is also important that commercial foods containing citric acid such as minute tapi-

oca and sparkling water, as made by the Canada Dry Company, should not be used. When marked allergy to all fruits occurs, moreover, allergy to vitamin C in vitamins administered by mouth or parenterally must be kept in mind. Flavored candies, beverages, and gum must be avoided. It is important that no toothpastes, powders, or denture fixing pastes be used, since they all contain flavors. It is especially important that flavored mouthwashes and gargles be avoided. Even if the mouth is rinsed after their use, the minute amount remaining in the mouth or entering the blood through the oral mucosa before rinsing the mouth can prevent relief of symptoms in the stomach or intestines resulting from allergy to flavors or fruits. Flavors of fruits and condiments in medications of all types often produce symptoms in fruit-sensitive patients. Even sips of wine-flavored medicine caused severe cramping and diarrhea in a patient with allergic diarrhea resulting from fruit and condiment allergy.

Possible allergy to chlorine in water or to allergens of vegetation fish, as of mussels in the water pipes of London, or to other unusual ingredients justifies the substitution of distilled or pure spring or well water for city tap water. Possible allergens in filter pads or devices, as hair or even chemicals, must be remembered.

That such allergens can enter the blood through the oral mucosa is supported by activation of GI allergy to fruits through the entrance of grape allergens even through the vaginal mucosa after the use of vinegar douches by two patients. Moreover, gastrointestinal allergy to fruits has been activated in some of our patients by the inhalation of molecules of fruits in the air when the odor of the fruit is apparent. One patient allergic to citrus fruits sneezes repeatedly on entering a room where such fruit is present. Two of our patients with allergic colitis resulting in part from fruit allergens suffer exaggeration of their colitis when they inhale the air emanating from the ripened fruit on trees adjacent to their homes. One patient who develops asthma from tomato has symptoms when the odor of tomato is in the air from a cannery two blocks from her house.

And while food allergy is being studied with this diet, smoking tobacco, especially cigarettes, must be stopped not only because of tobacco allergens which enter the gastrointestinal tract but also because of possible fruit juices which flavor some brands. In place of flavored chewing gum, moreover, paraffin used to seal jellies is an excellent substitute.

The above discussion of the maintenance and manipulation of the FFCFE diet and of the necessary avoidance of fruit and other flavors and in some patients of vitamin C is important information for physicians who are challenged with the relief of the various manifestations of gastrointestinal allergy. When physicians only use lists of foods we advise in this diet without giving detailed menus to patients who are not aware of (a) the importance of avoiding traces of fruits, flavors, condiments, and of foods not included in the diets; (b) the time necessary for foods to leave the body; and (c) the usual delay in the development of allergic symptoms after provocation tests and other information in Chapter 3 and in this chapter, desired relief of allergic symptoms is not forthcoming. The challenge of relieving the acute, recurrent, chronic and often invaliding symptoms of gastrointestinal allergy will be aided by the study of our recorded long experience and the use of our trial diets in many cases for weeks or even months until successful use of the diets becomes possible.

Medications in GI Allergy

1. Since food allergens probably remain in the body for one to three weeks, severe GI symptoms therefrom may require such time to gradually decrease or disappear after elimination of allergenic foods. If soreness, pain, burning from edema, and inflammation resulting from allergic vasculitis in the gastrointestinal tissues as visualized in severe oral canker sores is severe, small doses of Prednisone or more concentrated commercial corticosteroids such as triamcinolone orally or even parenterally in reducing doses for five to seven days is justified for relief. Corticosteroids also decrease cramping and abdominal pain, diarrhea and tenesmus in allergic diarrhea, and regional enteritis and such symptoms with blood and mucus in CUC as discussed in Chapter 6. As the allergenic foods are revealed and deleted with elimination diets, the gastrointestinal symptoms usually are controlled without corticosteroid therapy. Occasionally small doses of corticosteroids are justified for more than a few days if pollen allergy is present until desensitization to allergenic pollens gradually relieves GI symptoms resulting from such allergy.

2. Healing of canker sores seems to be hastened by applying 70 to 90 percent ethyl alcohol in small phledgelets of cotton to the lesions for one to two minutes. Strict adherence to the FFCFE diet and possible use of corticosteroids are important for relief or prevention of recurrences.

3. The burning, belching, and distention in the stomach is benefited by bicarbonate of soda, milk of bismuth, and aluminum hydroxide. Because of the necessity of eliminating all flavors and condiments, such medications must be unflavored.

4. The pain from severe allergic gastritis may be such that codeine one-fourth to one-half grain by mouth and if necessary

hypodermically every three to eight hours may be indicated. And such codeine is justified for severe symptoms from food and if present pollen allergy in CUC and regional enteritis. The necessity of this drug decreases as allergenic foods leave the body.

5. If initial or continued constipation is present, drugs such as phenolphthalein, cascara, and others should be replaced by milk of magnesia, mineral oil, and if increased bulk in the colon is desirable, by ground psyllium seeds such as Konsyl® to which allergy has not been encountered.

6. Finally, all other medications should be stopped because of possible allergy to drugs. We have not found so-called anti-spasmodics necessary. As stated above, some fruit-sensitive patients are allergic to vitamin C and occasionally to B vitamins.

7. Since aspirin allergy may produce gastrointestinal symptoms as well as bronchial asthma and cutaneous allergy, such possible allergies must be remembered. The severe gastritis at times with bleeding and even hemorrhage from continued aspirin therapy, especially in large doses, must be remembered.

Because of the less frequent allergy to synthetic vitamins than to animal or vegetable preparations, the former should be prescribed.

SUMMARY

1. The frequency of gastrointestinal allergy in adults as in children (reported in Chapt. 25) must be recognized by all physicians including internists, gastroenterologists, abdominal surgeons, and allergists.

2. Though food allergy is the usual cause of perennial gastrointestinal symptoms, exaggerations during the spring, summer, and fall often arise from pollen allergy or at times seasonal foods.

3. Symptoms in the mouth, esophagus, stomach, small and large intestines, and rectum as a result of such allergies are in the statistics of 270 cases and also in an additional 150 cases in this chapter.

4. The role of food allergy (especially to fruits) in the mouth, particularly in canker sores and in epigastric allergy causing the upper abdominal distress and associated symptoms, are indicated in 270 cases in Table VIII.

5. Failure to recognize allergy, especially to foods, leads to many unnecessary abdominal operations and a diagnosis of psychoneurosis.

6. Duodenal and gastric ulcers are best explained by canker sore-like lesions especially because fruit, condiments, and other foods eliminated from our fruit-free cereal-free elimination diet.

7. Allergy to foods and at times to pollens causes inflammation of the small bowel, especially RE, discussed in Chapter 8.

8. Allergic diarrhea resulting from foods with no evidence of CUC must be recognized and studied for atopic allergy. Allergic peritonitis resulting from food allergy occurs.

9. In the colon, mucous colitis has been called asthma of the colon because of cramping spasms and mucus.

10. Pruritus and proctitis are usually due to allergy, as is allergic eczema (Chapt. 14).

11. Allergy in the cecum and appendix with or without secondary infection accounts for many unnecessary appendectomies.

12. Localized allergy, especially to foods,

causes dilatation and bleeding from the mucosa in the mouth, stomach, duodenum, and small and large bowel.

13. Pollen allergy as a cause of symptoms throughout the gastrointestinal tract receives special discussion.

14. Roentgen ray findings characteristic of allergy in the GI tract are reported. Finally, procedures for the diagnosis and treat-ment of gastrointestinal allergy are summarized.

15. The importance of control of food and less often inhalant allergy in the causation of CUC and RE is emphasized in Chapters 6 and 7.

16. Allergy especially to foods produces inflammation and muscle spasm and dilated blood vessels with resultant hemorrhoids.

Chapter 6

Chronic Ulcerative Colitis—Allergy in Its Etiology

S ince we supported in 1942 Andresen's report of food allergy as the major initial and continued cause of chronic ulcerative colitis (CUC) and recorded for the first time pollen allergy as a major cause with or without food allergy, this role of atopic allergy as the major cause of the eczematous inflammation and resultant ulceration has been increasingly confirmed in our practice.

CUC in adults will be the main challenge in the first part of this chapter. The importance of such allergy to foods and also to pollens in children and adolescents is extensively discussed in the second part.

In 1958 Andresen again wrote to us: "The only factor which I have found to be almost invariably the cause of this disease had been allergy, usually to foods." Added to this we have reported pollen, with or without food, and at times, drug allergy, since 1942. When allergy is the sole cause, the symptoms and tissue changes gradually reduce or disappear with the control of the allergies. When complicating secondary infection, anemia, hypoproteinemia, or avitaminosis is present, its treatment also is required.

The following evidence favors allergy as a primary cause:

1. Gastrointestinal allergy, usually to foods and at times to pollens and drugs, is frequent in any part of the GI tract from the mouth to the anus. This susceptibility to allergic reactivity is shown by the local passive transfer of antibodies to foods in colostomies. The many manifestations of GI allergy have been discussed in Chapter 5.

2. Allergy best explains the primary lesions of CUC. The erythema, granularity, friability, and serous mucous and bloody discharge are duplicated in the skin of acute allergic dermatitis, the characteristics of which should be observed and studied by physicians in order to understand the role of allergy in CUC. This continued serous exudation and bleeding may cause hypoproteinemia and anemia.

3. Small or large mucosal ulcers are explained by allergic vasculitis, thromboses, and necroses as are all canker sores, especially to foods, according to our experience (see p. 101). Tryptic digestion from enzymes flowing down from the pancreas into the colon and intestine may cause superficial or gross bleeding, denudation of the mucosa, perforation, and peritonitis.

4. Fever often occurs from allergy alone, as shown by relief of all symptoms of CUC including fever by the control of food and/or pollen allergy with no antibiotics, corticosteroids, or drugs. However, secondary infection as a moderate or serious complication may also be responsible for fever when present. It is always necessary, of course, to rule out *Salmonella* and viral infections including serum or viral hepatitis, pyrogenic bacterial infections in liver and lung, TB parasites, regional enteritis, Hodgkin's disease, and lymphomas.

5. Chronic allergy can produce fibrous

and scar tissue, as seen in the scarring of the corneas from ulcers as reported in Chapter 20 resulting from food allergy. Moreover, the scarring from duodenal inflammation and ulceration can arise from allergy to foods, as discussed in Chapter 5. Thus allergy, with or without secondary infection, may cause irreversible fibrosis resulting in a tubular ahaustric bowel or narrowing or stricture of the colon. Acute and chronic inflammation in the esophagus, duodenum, small bowel, and especially in the terminal ileum as a result of the allergy causing CUC also occurs.

6. Remission in CUC can be explained by the tendency of clinical food allergy to cease or decrease in degree. Such refractoriness after an allergic attack also occurs in bronchial asthma, allergic headaches, or migraine. It may be due to the exhaustion of the specific antibodies to the causative food or other allergen during the previous exaggeration of symptoms. The decrease of food allergy during the summer, reported by us for many years, and the seasonal influence of pollen allergy can also explain these remissions.

7. Localization of CUC in the rectum or other part of the colon is similar to localization of eczema in the skin. Spreading of CUC through the entire colon is also similar to the spreading of allergic dermatitis from the original site of involvement to other areas or over most of the skin.

8. Colitis may be the only manifestation of allergy, or clinical allergy may occur in other tissues. As occurs in other clinical food allergy, scratch tests usually are negative. This occurrence of negative skin reactions therefore requires diet trial with our elimination diets for the study of probable food allergy. Because skin reactions to pollens are negative in 10 to 15 percent of sensitive patients, a history of symptoms

activated from March to December justifies the consideration and treatment of such possible pollen allergy.

Statistics on 170 cases of CUC whose histories, studies, and treatment we personally conducted during a seventeen-year period up to 1959 follow. There were about twice as many females as males. The average onset was in the mid-twenties, ranging from 1½ to 40 years.

In addition to the statistics on the 170 cases reprinted in this chapter, those of the familial history of probable or definite clinical allergy, results of scratch reactions with food and inhalant allergens and the x-ray findings in the colons are printed in our articles in 1959 and 1960.

Supporting food and (less often) pollen allergy as the major cause of CUC are the results from our control of such allergy in these 170 patients reported in 1959 and 1960.

In spite of our continued confirmation of Andresen's recognition that CUC results from an eczematouslike inflammation because of food allergy and also because of pollen and drug allergy, there have been no reports of such allergy except to milk by Truelove and Taylor. Though milk is one of the most common allergenic foods, clinical allergy infrequently arises from one food in any single manifestation as proven

TABLE XII

CHRONIC ULCERATIVE COLITIS
(170 CASES)

Females:	111	Hospital cases:	103
Males:	59	Office cases:	67
Age of onset		25.6 years (1-71 years)	
Age at 1st visit		31.1 years (1½-78 years)	
Previous duration		3.9 years (1½-40 years)	
Degree of CUC:			
Grade 4 (most severe)			26.2%
Grade 3			41.0%
Grade 2			30.0%
Grade 1			3.8%
History of probable food allergy			56.0%
History of probable milk allergy			35.3%

in our many cases. Therefore, we are assured that the study of allergy to many foods with our strict elimination diets (as we have advised in the last 30 years and as summarized in this chapter and volume) with or without control of pollen, other inhalant, and possible drug allergies would reveal the frequency of several foods, including milk, as we have long reported.

Failure to advise this important study of atopic allergy in many separate medical articles on CUC and in textbooks on internal medicine and gastroenterology is most unfortunate for the many victims of CUC and could be remedied by the physician's study and control of atopic allergy as we advise. Ability to fulfill this responsibility requires time, effort, and successful utilization of advice in this volume and not casual reading of a brief discussion of the elimination diets in a manual or article.

Thus there was definite evidence of the role of food and/or pollen allergy in 88.6 percent of the relieved patients. Suggestive evidence in the additional 14.4 percent probably would have been more definite if excellent cooperation had occurred.

The role of the control of food and/or of pollen allergy alone or with corticosteroid and azulfidine therapy is shown below.

The good results that have been obtained in cooperating patients with our control of food and/or pollen allergy and when required, adjunctive therapy in additional patients since 1959 has decreased the reason

TABLE XIII

CAUSES OF CUC AS INDICATED BY RESULTS OF ANTIALLERGIC STUDY AND THERAPY

	%
Food allergy alone	41.0
Pollen allergy alone	2.9
Food and pollen allergy	10.6
Food and probable pollen allergy	15.0
Pollen and probable food allergy	8.0
Questionable food and pollen allergy	7.4
Undetermined probable causes	7.0

TABLE XIV

RECURRENCES AND EXACERBATIONS

Explained by breaks in the diet in	47 patients
Explained by inadequate pollen therapy in	23 patients
Depression, refusal to eat, and infection (in 1945) in	1 patient
Total	71 patients

for the 22.4 percent of poor results reported in 1959. This improvement is largely due to our insistence on strict adherence to the necessary elimination diet and/or on indicated continued pollen therapy. When patients have adhered to the diet, eliminating their allergenic foods, and have been treated for existent pollen allergy, symptoms have been controlled with little or no corticosteroids. Azulfidine® has been of questionable or no help when allergy has been controlled with or without minimal corticosteroids.

The occurrence of cancer in only two patients up to 1959, in one of whom it was present when we first saw him, and in one case since then can be explained by the decreased or absent irritation in the colon which persists when atopic allergy is uncontrolled. This absence of cancer is note-

TABLE XV

GOOD OR EXCELLENT RESULTS

	%
With antiallergic therapy alone and no antibiotics, sulfonamides, ACTH or corticosteroids	49.4
Patients receiving antiallergic therapy and only sulfonamides	8.2
Only azulfidine	2.9
Only antibiotics	4.7
Sulfonamides and antibiotics	8.2
Sulfonamides, antibiotics, and ACTH and/or corticoids	4.1

Thus the above 132 or 77.6% of our 170 patients received good results with the above antiallergic therapy with or without the above drugs and hormones. It must be emphasized that these results were obtained with little or no ACTH and corticosteroids except for a few patients up to the time of publication of these statistics in 1950.

worthy, since CUC has been controlled in many of our patients for ten to thirty years.

CHARACTERISTICS OF CUC

Diarrhea and rectal bleeding with lower abdominal distress and cramping require study of possible CUC. Viral and infective diarrhea, animal parasites, gram-positive flora in stools from antibiotics by mouth, and achylia must be excluded. Diarrhea without bleeding or other evidence of CUC or x-ray findings occurs from allergic diarrhea alone, as emphasized on page 114.

In chronic cases x-ray in our 170 cases showed usual involvement of the entire colon, less frequently being confined to the transverse and/or distal colon. X-rays may be negative, the diagnosis depending on proctoscopy alone, as in seven of our cases.

That the colon may be the only shock organ of allergy is shown by the history of other probable manifestations of allergy in only 30 percent of our cases. The degree of CUC in these 170 cases is shown in Table XII.

Initial symptoms may be mild with or without bleeding or fulminating, with fifteen to twenty-five bloody liquid stools, tenesmus, cramping, and fever. After establishment of the CUC four to ten daily soft or liquid stools with varying blood, mucus, abdominal and rectal discomfort, malaise, and fever continue. Remissions may occur, as discussed on page 139.

Unless CUC is controlled, complications present before our treatment occur, as in 45 of our 170 cases as listed in Table XVI. All of these complications were present when first seen or occurred in the first two months of our therapy before our treatment was effective. After our control of CUC complications were rare, readily controlled, or absent. The relief of arthritis, erythema nodosum, and fever (in 30%) controlled

TABLE XVI

COMPLICATIONS
(Other than Fever in 45 Patients Only)

	%
Arthritis	4.0
Cancer of colon	1.2
Chondritis of ear	0.6
Erythema nodosum	4.0
Fever*	56.0
Fistula (anorectal)	5.0
Hemorrhage from colon	3.0
Iritis	0.6
Strictures	3.5
Necrotic reaction to vaccine	2.0
Parotitis	0.6
Perforation of colon	4.0
Pyoderma gangrenosum	1.0
Recto-vaginal fistula	8.0
Schizophrenia	1.2
Thrombophlebitis	8.0
Pregnancy (2 in each of 4 patients) of women	18.0

*Controlled in 35 of the 96 patients with anti-allergic therapy and no antibiotics, sulfonamides, or corticosteroids.

with antiallergic therapy and no antibiotics including pyoderma gangrenosum needs emphasis. Normal pregnancies and deliveries occurred in twenty women.

Treatment
Food Allergy

Food allergy must be studied in all cases especially when symptoms are perennial and often recurrently exaggerated, at times during the menstrual periods. The decrease of symptoms resulting from food allergy in the summer with exaggeration in the fall to late spring, reported by us especially in bronchial asthma, occurs in CUC as in one case of twenty-five years' duration which was absent or inactive during the summer months. Skin testing with the scratch method usually is negative to all allergenic foods. If three to four plus reactions occur, they may be indicative of food allergy, especially with a diet history of definite dislikes or disagreements to the foods. To be certain that allergy exists to the reacting food, however, a provocation test with the food must be done but only after the patient is symptom-free (see Chapt. 2). The foods responsible for the allergic inflammation in CUC can be determined after the prescribed diet has controlled the symptoms. Then additional foods can be added, eliminating those which reproduce symptoms (see Chapt. 3).

The role of atopic allergy in CUC was temporarily supported by the finding of gamma globulin antibodies to milk by Wright and Trueblood in 1961. Though these antibodies seem to be increased in milk-sensitive patients, their presence in normal people reduced their diagnostic value. Since then, reports of immunological reactions to allergens in the tissues of the colon and in its secretion have been reported, especially by Kirsner and co-workers, none of which have proved of diagnostic or therapeutic importance. Thus the role of atopic allergy must be studied by trial diet and by results of desensitization when pollen allergy is indicated, as we stated in the *JAMA* in 1963.

A diet history of food disagreements or dislikes suggests possible allergy. Such a history especially to milk was obtained in about 50 percent of our 170 patients.

If milk allergy is suggested by diet history or scratch test, its complete elimination may gradually control CUC. That milk allergy is the sole cause in some cases was first reported by Andresen and by me in 1942. Usually, however, allergy to other foods has also been responsible. In our opinion, if allergy to other foods as well as to milk had been studied by Taylor and Truelove in 1961, who reported milk as the cause of CUC, the importance of this allergy in CUC would have been evidenced. To rule out allergy because of failure to control CUC with the elimination of milk alone without the study of allergy to other

foods and the study of less frequent pollen and drug allergies is not justified, as shown by our good results reported during the last thirty years.

That lactose intolerance resulting from deficiency in intestinal lactase causes diarrhea and other abdominal symptoms must be recorded. But such deficiency cannot cause the pathological lesions and resultant symptoms of CUC. The activation of CUC by minute amounts of milk, even a few drops, as reported by us and by Andresen, who reported that "ten drops caused bloody diarrhea for three days," is explained by resultant allergic edema and vasculitis and not by a deficiency in intestinal lactase which produces diarrhea and cramping when relatively large amounts of milk are ingested.

Unless milk allergy alone is very probable and especially if a milk-free diet has failed to relieve the symptoms of CUC, allergy to other foods which we have found to cause CUC, including wheat and other cereals, all fruits, spices and condiments, chocolate, coffee, and selected vegetables, as well as milk, must be studied. For this our FFCFE diet is advised (see page 48). If improvement is not evident in two to three weeks, then a minimal elimination diet (Chapt. 3) should be ordered before ruling out food allergy as a possible cause. Such a minimal elimination diet with extra strained or ground meat or chicken, white potato, fruit-free tapioca pudding, and extra sugar can yield over 2,000 calories and up to 100 gm of protein a day. This diet with multiple vitamins and initial large doses of corticosteroids gradually reduced as improvement occurs will control most severe cases of CUC, including the fulminating ones. If initial anorexia is present, our meat-base formula with extra cane sugar can be given by mouth or intubated through the nose into the stomach for several days.

The preparation of the menus and recipes, strict and adequate use of the diet, maintenance of nutrition, and addition of foods after relief is assured are all discussed on pages 48 and 50. Necessary prevention of inhalation of air-borne molecules of allergenic foods must also be remembered, as evidenced by a case of activation of CUC with rectal hemorrhage from the odor of tomato twenty-four hours after they were canned in the home. Activation of CUC also occurred when a fruit-sensitive patient inhaled the odors of ripe fruit from trees near her kitchen window.

Decrease in diarrhea, abdominal distress, and fever in two to three weeks favors food allergy. In our series of 170 cases this improvement arose in an average of ten days, varying from one to thirty days. With the strict diet improvement should continue and increase for at least two to three months. Then other foods, one every three to five days, are added, including rice, oats, beef, eggs, extra cooked vegetables, and later (in 3 to 4 months) fish and cooked fruits, eliminating any which reactivates colitis. Because of the frequency of milk allergy, we do not add it even in traces for one to two years, especially if a history suggesting milk allergy is present. If definite evidence of milk allergy occurs in the history or with feeding tests after initial relief, we are emphasizing its complete elimination during the patient's lifetime. Severe prolonged recurrences of CUC, especially after a trial of milk, have occurred, leading to unnecessary colectomies and even death, as in Case 61 reported in our discussion of CUC in children in Chapter 6. Such lifetime elimination of other foods, definite allergy to which caused the CUC, is fully warranted. Prevention of

colectomies and the many complications, including death, of uncontrolled CUC justify such eliminations throughout life. That health and nutrition can be maintained even with minimal elimination diets plus vitamins, as described in Chapter 3, must be realized. The unfortunate failure to recognize and control food and less frequent pollen allergy leads to resultant colectomies and is responsible in large part for the increasing number of ostomy clubs, which would be fewer and usually unnecessary if atopic allergy as the major cause of the eczematouslike allergic inflammation in the colon was studied and controlled, as advised in this chapter and in Chapter 5.

Patients with CUC resulting from food allergy require continued policing to prevent even slight breaks in the prescribed diet. No foods should be taken unless ordered by the physician. Routine physical examinations and laboratory tests, x-rays of the colon, and sigmoidoscopy should be done every one to two years.

If relief from the elimination diet and indicated corticosteroid and other possible drug therapy does not arise in three to four weeks or decreases in subsequent months, sole or concomitant inhalant allergy, especially to pollens, or errors in the diet or allergy to one or more foods in the diet may be present. Presence of parasites or the presence of a gram-positive flora in the stool from excessive antibiotics must be rechecked.

Pollen Allergy

Pollen allergy alone is suggested by the onset and recurrence of CUC or when food allergy is an associated cause by an increase of symptoms during pollen seasons. We had two cases of CUC begin immediately after intradermal testing with pollen done because of a history of hay fever. One case of severe CUC developed rectal hemorrhaging of 3,000 cc of blood (replaced by transfusions) which occurred during twelve hours after forty large positive scratch tests to pollens occurred.

In the last thirty years we have had patients whose CUC was controlled by pollen therapy alone for twelve, seventeen, twenty, and twenty-seven years up to the present writing. One patient with CUC in seven previous pollen seasons was controlled by our pollen therapy during her cooperation for two years. In addition, food and pollen allergies in 30 patients were associated and food with probable pollen allergy in 16 of the 170 patients reported in 1959. The first case of CUC as a result of pollen allergy recorded by us was in 1942. This case was reported again in 1950, 1954, and 1959 and is still well controlled. Continued desensitization has been necessary because of recurrences of colitis in the pollen season when therapy was stopped for a few months.

Skin tests to pollens may be large and numerous or slight or absent. Positive reactions, moreover, occurred in 13 of 170 cases of CUC without clinical allergy to pollens. If the history indicates pollen allergy, in spite of negative scratch reactions, desensitization with antigens containing all important pollens in the patient's living area is given, starting with a dilution which largely fails to react intradermally. Doses are increased up to a tolerated dose. Weak dilutions even of the 1:500 to 1:5 million may give good protection. Desensitization must be continued until relief of pollen allergy continues for two to three years. It may be necessary for many years. Desensitization has been unsatisfactory in some of our cases and has justified colectomy below the midtransverse colon in three cases and total colectomy in a fourth case. Better cooperation in adhering to the prescribed elimination diet and in desensitization to pollens along with indicated corticosteroid therapy might have made this surgery unnecessary. One patient whose CUC was not satisfactorily controlled in California with pollen therapy has been comfortable in Seattle where other pollens are in the air for only six months compared with ten months in California. After the second year in Seattle, slight colitis has occurred during the grass season in spite of pollen desensitization. Moderate bleeding from duodenal inflammation but no ulcer has occurred in the last two years, evidencing her marked gastrointestinal allergy to pollens. An irritable, moderately spastic duodenum was shown by x-ray.

Adjunctive Therapy in CUC Resulting From Allergy

Corticosteroids and formerly ACTH were given to only 26 of our 170 patients reported in 1959, usually in the first weeks in severe or fulminating cases or with subsequent exacerbations nearly always arising from breaks in the diet or inadequate pollen therapy. They have never been given without the study of food allergy with elimination diets and/or pollen therapy. Continued, large daily doses of 20 to 40 mg of Prednisone have not been used. No rectal injections and no long administration of corticosteroids have been given. Because of our many good results using no corticosteroids, our challenge has been that of obtaining similar results in all cases. Possible perforation of duodenal ulcer during corticoid therapy must be remembered. A quiescent ulcer perforated in one patient. Since then, antacid therapy has been given to patients with a history of past or active duodenal ulcer.

Antibiotics are given if secondary infection is possible. The mycin drugs are preferred, though (when indicated) penicillin is given. We must, however, keep possible resultant allergy in mind.

As discussed in Chapter 5, diarrhea (at times severe) from overgrowth of gram-positive bacteria resulting from prolonged antibiotic therapy, especially with the mycin drugs, occurs in otherwise normal people or in those with CUC or RE or other gastrointestinal disease. This cause must be recognized and controlled with cessation of antibiotics and oral administration of Mycostatin® 500,000 units three to four times a day until gram-negative bacteria predominate in stools.

When food allergy and less frequent pollen allergy are controlled, previous Azulfidine® therapy is discontinued. Azulfidine has not been given or required for the relief of CUC when cooperation in our control of food and pollen allergy is obtained. Allergy to Azulfidine also has occurred.

For initial anemia, bleeding, and hemorrhaging, iron, vitamin K, vitamin B_{12}, liver extract, and transfusions are available.

With increasing confirmation of atopic allergy as the sole cause of CUC and our realization of the necessity of the immediate use of our elimination diets in the moderate or chronic cases, of the minimal elimination diets in soft or liquid frequent feedings in the severe and fulminating cases, and the use of initial corticosteroids in moderate or large doses according to the severity of the CUC, partial or total colectomies or colostomies have steadily decreased in frequency. In the last ten years none have been done during the initial control of symptoms or in the many patients who have continued their cooperation in our antiallergic control for from ten to even twenty-eight years.

In 1959 our review of 170 cases showed that from 1940 to 1947 eight ileostomies with or without colectomy were done in patients who had not cooperated in our antiallergic therapy and in three who had not benefited from such treatment. In the next twelve years, ileostomy and colectomy were done in three patients who were not helped by our therapy probably because of poor cooperation. In one patient whose CUC had been benefited by our therapy, surgery was done because of perforation of the sigmoid, in one patient because of severe hemorrhage and infection of the colon, and in four patients surgery was done in other hospitals after they had stopped our previous beneficial therapy. Colectomy distal to a midtransverse colostomy possibly because of our failure to control pollen allergy in five cases was done.

Study and treatments are necessary to continue for one to two months or more before possible control by allergy is excluded. Colectomies done in two to three weeks because of failure of medical treatment is unjustified and condemns many patients to an ileostomy life because allergy had not been studied at all or not for the necessary number of months. Colectomy because of fulminating CUC is not justifiable, since it can be controlled with initial sufficient corticosteroid therapy, reducing the doses gradually in one to three weeks and with indicated study and control of allergy to foods and pollens or occasionally drugs.

With our increasing experience and better cooperation of patients, no deaths from CUC or its complications have occurred in the last ten years. From 1940 to 1947 there were five deaths resulting from peritonitis and five deaths after ileostomies before antibiotics or corticosteroids were available. In the next twelve years there was one death from metastatic cancer of the colon and one from perforated ulcer in a debilitated man seventy-eight years of age. In the last ten years one girl twelve years of age died not from CUC but intractable anorexia nervosa.

Results Since 1959

In the last eight years twenty-four new cases of CUC have been studied. Total colectomy was done in two months in a woman because of irreversible, severe diffuse CUC. Colectomies in other hospitals were also done in a man and in a boy twelve years of age who cooperated in our therapy for only two months. Perusal of bulletins and publications evidences the constant concern about irritation of the stoma, possible complications, and at times subsequent operation on the ileum. The odor, difficulty with application, social and marital relations, and psychological problems were very present.

In other patients who have cooperated in our antiallergic and indicated adjunctive therapy, the role of food and less frequent pollen allergy continues to be confirmed.

Every case of CUC is entitled to an early, open-minded, and adequate study of allergy, as advised in this chapter, before colostomy is done, resulting in an irreversible ileostomy life and the constant physical and psychological distress which has led to formation of many colostomy clubs in this and probably in other countries. This was reemphasized in the *JAMA* in 1963.

Case Summaries—
Food Allergy as the Sole Cause

Case 29: A woman fifty-four years of age had had CUC for 3½ months. Sulfathalidine® had caused dermatitis. Weight had fallen forty pounds. Constipation with mucus and blood for ten years suggested CUC as a cause. Nausea and diarrhea for years had resulted from certain foods. Milk had long been disliked. X-rays showed CUC in the entire colon confirmed by proctoscopy. Hemoglobin was 57 percent. With our FFCFE diet the bloody diarrhea, cramping, and slight fever were relieved in eight days. No corticosteroids or Azulfidine were required. Stools were solid in twenty days. Control of colitis continued since then with a milk-free, egg-free and fruit-free diet.

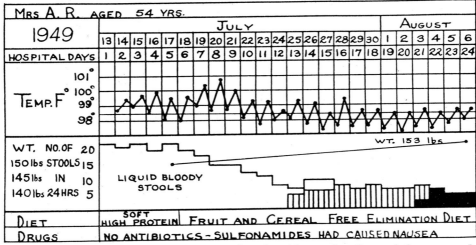

Figure 2. *Case 29:* Chronic ulcerative colitis for 3½ months. Loss of forty pounds. Sulfonamides caused dermatitis. Penicillin increased diarrhea. The patient had a life-long dislike for milk. Food allergy was indicated by relief of diarrhea with the elimination diet with no drugs or antibiotics and continued control for 4½ years with elimination of milk, eggs, and fruit. The increase in weight in the hospital continued up to 185 pounds in 1954.

Case 30: A woman thirty years of age was first seen in the county hospital in 1946 because of severe CUC for one year. A remission had occurred four months before from a milk-free bland diet and medications. Return to a general diet had reactivated severe CUC with high fever; bloody, liquid stools; anorexia; tenesmus; cramping; and loss of weight to eighty pounds (see Table XII, Case 5). X-ray showed a shaggy outline of the ascending colon with an ahaustral narrowed granular bleeding mucosa.

With our FFCFE diet with initial interval feedings and 2000 calories a day, bloody stools and fever reduced, and there were solid stools in two weeks. Corticosteroids and Azulfidine were not in use. Benefit from the sulfonamides was questionable. In twenty-five days all medications were stopped. In fifty days weight had increased twenty-two pounds in spite of no milk, wheat, and eggs in the diet.

In the twenty-two years since then, her CUC has been controlled with adherence to the FFCFE diet except when brief errors have occurred on three or four occasions. X-rays show an ahaustric narrow colon. Proctoscopy reveals a narrow rectum with a smooth nonerythematous nongranular mucosa. She passes two formed stools through a contracted anal canal. She is symptom-free, strong, active, and weighs 125 pounds.

The excellent control of severe CUC for twenty-two years with no development of cancer is due to her constant adherence to her elimination diet under our supervision. Corticosteroids and Azulfidine have never been given.

Fulminating CUC Resulting From Food Allergy

Case 31: A man thirty-eight years of age first developed CUC in May of 1939. It was fulminating in two months with pyoderma gangrenosum on the abdomen, an ischiorectal abscess, and fatal prognosis. After moderate relief three to five liquid at times bloody stools continued. Another fulminating attack with pyoderma gangrenosum on the neck and feet occurred in April of 1941. A postmortem permit was signed. In consultation, we ordered our FFCFE diet. Diarrhea and fever decreased, with recovery in 1½ months. No antibodies or corticosteroids were available in 1941.

In the last twenty-seven years his CUC has been absent except fulminating reactions in 1945 and 1950 when forbidden milk and fruit were eaten. He has worked every day in the automobile production line except during the war.

Since breaking his diet for three or four weeks in late 1967 he has adhered to our fruit and cereal-free elimination diet plus rice, additional cooked vegetables except onion and garlic, turkey, tea, and multiple vitamins, and in 1970 states: "I have enjoyed excellent health."

His physical examination, all routine laboratory tests, and x-ray of his lungs are normal. Roentgen rays of his colon six months ago revealed areas of scarring and some pseudopolyposis as a result of "chronic inactive CUC." No carcinoma or strictures were seen. No corticosteroids have been taken, except briefly two years ago after a break in his required diet. Tincture of opium, three to four drops one to three times a day, is taken for one to two days for slight diarrhea every one to three months, probably because of a slight break in the diet.

Comment: This was the first case of severe CUC we relieved with the FFCF elimination diet thirty years ago in 1939. Its fulminating character with recurrent high fever, excessive bloody diarrhea, loss of thirty pounds, the marked erythema nodosum on the abdomen and legs, preventing work in an automobile factory, and no health insurance in those days made treatment in the county hospital necessary. A fatal prognosis had been made, and an autopsy permit had been signed by the wife. Because of his fulminating disease (it being 10 years before cortisone and antibiotic drugs), an ileostomy fortunately had not been risked.

His remarkable gradual recovery with our fruit and cereal-free diet aided by three transfusions, vitamins and other medications, and probably by the sulfa drugs, with control of fever and diarrhea (see Fig. 3) heightened our conjecture that CUC causes an eczematouslike inflammation with resultant ulcerations from atopic allergy, especially to foods, associated with secondary infection and complications as discussed in this chapter and in our several medical articles during the last twenty-seven years.

When this patient was first seen, the exaggeration of symptoms in April and May suggested pollen allergy in spite of negative scratch reactions to pollens as a concomitant cause with food allergy. But the excellent gradual relief with adherence to our FFCF elimination diet and adjunctive therapy listed in Figure 3 in the hospital

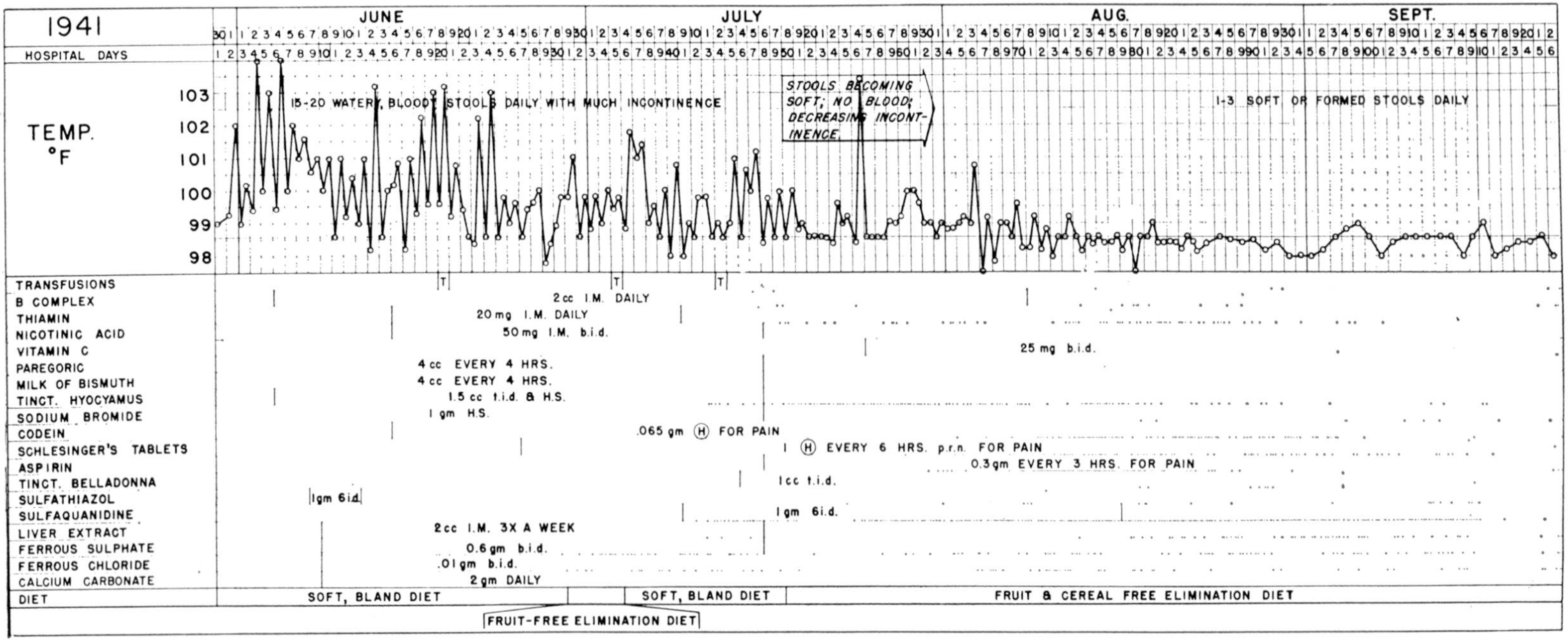

Figure 3.

dissuaded even empirical use of pollen desensitization.

In the twenty-seven years since then the excellent control of his CUC and his continued daily work as noted above has proved that food and not pollen allergy was always responsible for his CUC, which was life-threatening when we first saw him.

Pollen Allergy

Case 32: A man thirty-three years of age was seen in 1959 because of CUC, which had caused six to forty liquid at times bloody stools in the summer and fall with practically no winter symptoms for nineteen years. He had lived in Nevada, with the exception of two years in Germany where he was discharged from the army because of CUC in the summer of 1945. Incontinence during the summer necessitated wearing a towel between his legs. X-ray and proctoscopy confirmed CUC.

Scratch tests gave one and two plus reactions to summer and fall Nevada pollens. Even if skin tests had been negative, his history would have justified pollen therapy. Desensitization with an antigen containing pollens in the Nevada area prevented symptoms in the following summer. Perennial desensitization continued for fifteen years. Symptoms were controlled during the pollen season, except one year with pollen therapy was omitted. Initial doses of 1:50 million dilution were gradually increased to the 1:500 dilution. Symptoms were reactivated in the 1:50 strength.

His CUC was well controlled. He died of cardiac thrombosis in 1966.

Summary

1. Our study and treatment of CUC for thirty years indicates that erythema and edema from vasculitis and often resultant thromboses and necroses from allergic inflammation, especially to foods, less often to pollens, and occasionally to drugs is the major cause. Allergy to other inhalants needs study. Infectant allergy is not evident.

2. The colon may be the only shock organ of allergy. The family, personal, and diet histories may reveal no evident allergy.

3. Secondary infection, anemia, and avitaminosis must be considered.

4. Of 170 cases of CUC cooperating in our advised treatment published in 1960, 49.4 percent were controlled only with elimination of allergenic foods or at times with desensitization to pollens, with no sulfonamides, antibiotics, ACTH, or corticosteroids. There was confirmed food allergy in 113 (66.6 percent) of these patients.

5. Initial corticosteroids with their decrease and usual elimination with the gradual control of CUC in patients cooperating in our advised control of food allergy and, if indicated, pollen and occasional drug allergy are now advisable in most patients.

6. In the last twenty years no deaths have occurred, and no partial or total colectomies have been done in the last ten years in cooperating patients. Previous surgery in patients was due to inadequate control of pollen and food allergy and in part to irreversible pathology.

7. No deaths have occurred in thirty-two additional cases of CUC while they cooperated in our treatment since 1957.

8. Because of the importance of allergy to milk and wheat, we advise their lifelong, continued elimination. This advisability of lifelong control of food allergy, especially to milk and wheat and to a lesser degree eggs and other definite allergenic foods is emphasized in this chapter.

9. Though antibodies have been found to tissue antigens in the patient's colon tissues, their clinical significance is not established. If the effort and time being utilized in the determination of autoimmune or other serum antibodies were duplicated in studying and controlling atopic allergy to foods and less often to inhalants and drugs, our reported results from our advised treatment would receive

the definite confirmation which is so important for these patients.

10. Thus our results emphasize the importance of adequate, strict, and experienced study and treatment of atopic allergy in all cases of chronic ulcerative colitis rather than irreversible colectomies.

11. Though such study of allergy is mandatory in all cases of CUC, it is especially necessary and rewarding in CUC in infants and children, as advised in the next section of this chapter. We continue to affirm the following conclusions we published in the *JAMA* in 1963. It is our conviction that if atopic allergy were given the careful, accurate, and continued study we advise, its important role in the production of CUC would receive the confirmation it deserves, with resultant definite decrease in complications, in the need for ileostomies and colectomies, and in fatalities which are still common even with continued corticosteroid therapy.

ULCERATIVE COLITIS IN INFANTS AND CHILDREN

CUC in infants, children, and adolescents is due to atopic allergy, especially to foods and less often to inhalants, such as pollens, according to our experience reported by us for nearly thirty years. Evidence in the patient's history and from the tissue changes and pathology in the colon favor an allergic eczematouslike inflammation as the cause of the disease. This has received special discussion in the previous part of this chapter. Our good and excellent control of the allergy has decreased or eliminated the symptoms and the colonic inflammation in infants and older children as it has in the older patients, whose cases we have reported in various publications since 1942.

Because of our good or excellent relief of the symptoms and of the colonic allergic inflammation, we opine that our advised study and adequate strict control of atopic allergy to foods and less frequently to inhalants, especially pollens and at times drugs, are required in all cases of slight to severe and even fulminating CUC. Thereby ileostomies and colectomies increasingly have been prevented in practically all of our cooperating cases.

The necessary continued supervision by the patient and the unswerving cooperation of the child and parents for months, continuing at frequent intervals for years, are fully justified to prevent complications of uncontrolled CUC and a colectomy or ileostomy, resulting in a lifelong irreversible ileostomy.

Colectomy to prevent future cancer is not justifiable. With our control of allergy, cancer removed by surgery has only occurred in 1 percent of our cooperating patients and in one before our control was established.

After colectomy, moreover, possible extension of allergic inflammation of RE into the jejunum and duodenum, with stricture and fistula formation, and even into the stomach and terminal esophagus may occur if strict control of atopic allergies is not maintained. These results from uncontrolled food allergy and (less often) inhalant allergy would have been prevented by the control of initial causative allergy by our advice.

With control of allergy, membership in the increasing number of ostomy clubs of ostomy patients in most large cities is obviated. This includes parents whose children unfortunately have had colectomies or colostomies without adequate strict study and control of food and/or pollen and at times drug allergies which have prevented such surgery in children and has enabled surgeons to do ileocolostomies with a restoration of satisfactory colonic and recent function. Fortunately, total colectomy was not being advised when ileostomy was done in 1946, and 1941 (Cases 33 and 34).

We urge, therefore, that physicians who accept the responsibility of studying and relief of CUC in adults, especially in children, accurately follow our directions for the study and control of its allergic causes, which we have reported for thirty years. Without such dedication of the physician, surrendering to colectomy is comparable to cutting off the eczematous hand instead of determining and controlling existent causative food, inhalant, and drug allergy.

Case Histories

Case 33: A girl (C.D.) at the age of three years first developed in the summer of 1936 bloody mucus in the stools with increasing diarrhea up to twenty stools a day. In November, during an exploratory operation, the appendix and part of the ileum were removed. Moderate diarrhea and cramps continued thereafter in varying degrees for four to five years.

At the age of thirteen, in 1946, because of increased, bloody, mucoid, and loose stools and anemia, symptoms still being exaggerated in the summer, an ileostomy was done at a university hospital. X-rays had shown diffuse evidences of CUC throughout the colon. Bloody, liquid, ileal discharge continued after the operation. In 1947, twenty-two years ago, because of continued irritation of the stoma and bloody mucoid ileal discharge with marked depression, we were asked to study the patient for possible allergy. Scratch tests were negative to foods and pollens.

Because of her perennial symptoms continuing in the winter, food allergy was studied with a minimal elimination diet of lamb, potato, caramel tapioca, cooked carrots, squash, sugar, and Willow Run butter. No corticosteroids were given. In one month irritation of the stoma was reduced. The ileal discharge was thicker and only being passed four to five times in twenty-four hours.

Since the history indicated pollen allergy, even in the absence of skin reactions, desensitization with a 1:50 million dilution of a tree, grass,

and fall pollen antigen was given, the doses being increased as tolerated. Because of firmer, decreased ileal discharge and absent cramping and abdominal distress for over two years, the ileum was joined with the transverse colon in June of 1950. X-ray of the colon showed decreased but definite CUC. Though the terminal ileum was dilated, the colonic function was restored. Two to three formed stools were passed each day. In six months, however, severe pain and distention occurred in the abdomen, with indications of intestinal obstruction which was confirmed in the ileocolostomy union at emergency surgery. A new wider union was made.

Thereafter, her minimal diet was continued, with gradual addition of other foods, but wheat, cereal grains, chocolate, milk, eggs, and fruit have been entirely eliminated. One formed daily bowel movement has continued. Because of this marked relief, she worked as a secretary until her marriage at the age of twenty-six years. Pollen desensitization with a 1:5000 and later a 1:500 dilution continued. In 1953 she was well, working every day. She had a good appetite and weighed 121 pounds. There were two formed daily stools.

In 1954 because of a moderate anemia, oral iron, folic acid and B_{12} injections were given. Bowel movements continued to be increased to three to four a day each May and June. This justified continued desensitization to pollens. In 1958 she was still tolerating the 1:500 dilution.

In 1956 she was married. There have been three normal childbirths in 1958, 1960, and 1963. In the last ten years she has been on an entirely milk and wheat-free diet. No pollen desensitization has been administered for six years. No evidence of her former colitis or ileitis has occurred.

Case 34: With no previous illness, diarrhea with traces of blood started suddenly in 1941 in a boy (A.M.) eight years of age. Stools were negative for parasites. Proctoscopy and x-ray revealed CUC. With a bland diet and sulfaguanidine, varying relief occurred. In six months in November, however, a recurrence of severe bloody diarrhea and a liquid ileal discharge with fever and anorexia developed. An ileostomy was done. In four months there was retraction of the ileal stoma and in eight months a stricture of the terminal ileum, both of which required surgery. Thereafter, cramping and ileal liquid discharge increased, justifying the insertion of a small balloon in the terminal ileum which was inflated with air after its removal every three to four hours to release the accumulated ileal discharge and to relieve cramping. This required the mother's attention night and day. Weight reduced from sixty to forty-three pounds. He was bedridden most of the time. A soft bland diet containing milk, wheat, cereals, eggs, and other desired foods was allowed.

He was referred to us at the age of ten years in 1943 to study probable allergy as a cause of his ulcerative colitis and ileitus. He weighed forty pounds. His weakness was such that he could only stand by bending forward and supporting himself with his hands on his thighs.

His history revealed no personal or family history of allergy or possible food allergy. Scratch tests were negative to foods and inhalants. His blood count was normal except for a hemoglobin of 55 percent and RBC of 3,000,000. His serum proteins were 4.6 gm%. Urine was negative.

To study food allergy, rice, white potato, pearl tapioca cooked with sugar and flavored with burnt caramel, pureed carrots, peas, milk-free butter substitute, sugar, and salt were ordered. Sulfaguanidine 0.5 mg q.i.d., which had been previously given, was continued. B complex capsules b.i.d.; vitamin C, 100 mg b.i.d.; viosterol, 10 drops daily; and Caritrol® 5,000 units daily were given. For possible increase in bacterial immunity, respiratory bacterial vaccine 1:10 and vaccine containing colon bacillus 1:100 were administered hypodermically with a gradual increase twice a week for three months.

In one month he was stronger. Appetite was good. Necessary release of his ileal balloon because of cramps and pain had reduced from every two hours to every six to eight hours. In 1½ months the ileal discharge was solid ("hard to get out") instead of fluid. In two months he "felt wonderful" and "full of energy." Weight had increased ten pounds. An ileocolostomy was done by Dr. Dexter Richards, Sr., in spite of the opinion of two other surgeons that normal colonic function would fail because of the narrow ahaustric colon resulting from his CUC for 2½ years evidenced by our x-ray in October 1943.

In one month three to four formed bowel movements passed from his rectum daily. In February of 1944 hemoglobin was 80 percent. There were two to three formed daily stools. His father wrote: "His condition greatly exceeds my most optimistic expectations." Cooked squash, sweet potatoes, soy-potato bread and cookies, pears, peaches and apricot, and tea were gradually added to his original diet with no reactivation of his colitis. Back in his home in Seattle, his control continued. In April his hemoglobin was 78 percent.

In June of 1944 the family moved to the East Coast. We referred him to an internist who agreed to continue his diet. In July his serum protein was 6.1 gm%, hemoglobin 70 percent, and leukocytes 9,400.

In November of 1944 in response to the parents' question about the possible addition of milk, we emphasized its continued elimination. During the next three years his colitis did not recur. In 1945 his hemoglobin was 79 percent. In 1946 there was a slight recurrence of colitis resulting in our opinion, to deviations in his strict diet which are apt to occur unless strict supervision and policing of the patient's diet by the supervising physician occurs. Relief continued until November of 1947. Then there was a more definite reactivation of his colitis with a loss of eight pounds because of deviations in his diet and the activation of food allergy in the fall and winter, which we have long reported in Chapter 2.

Without our advice he consulted a prominent gastroenterologist who found "no definite evidence of reactivation of his colitis." "His general nutritional status is not too bad." He opined, however, that "eventually he will have to have a colectomy preceded perhaps with an ileosigmoidostomy." The probability of activation of his food allergy by deviations in his diet unfortunately was not considered by the gastroenterologist.

The importance of such food allergy in his case, in our opinion, should have been evident by the patient's history and the remarkable benefit from the control of his food allergy when I first saw him in 1943. Unfortunately, in our opinion, the elimination diet was replaced by a liberal bland diet containing milk up to a quart daily, milk having been excluded from his diet except for probable moderate deviations in the preceding five years.

After receiving this information about reinstatement of milk in his diet, I (Albert Rowe, Sr.) wrote the mother "that every trace of milk, wheat, and uncooked vegetables and fruits should be eliminated from his diet for many months to come. In fact, I would advise the elimination of milk for a much longer period." (Now we advise it throughout life.) "This elimination is not detrimental, as illustrated by the exclusion of milk in some people throughout life without any nutritional damage. My own sister, eighty-six years old, has never drunk milk or its products since infancy because of a lifelong dislike of milk and development of bronchial asthma when taken. There are only five small fillings in all her teeth. She is perfectly well except when she takes traces of milk which results in moderate asthma."

"I am afraid that the present diet will cause recurrences of ulcerative colitis and that gastroenterologists will increasingly favor total colectomy. Unfortunately this allergy in the colon tends to involve the small bowel, causing regional enteritis even after a colectomy is done if allergenic foods are not eliminated from the diet following colectomy. Recurrences of colitis in our patients have occurred when milk, wheat, and other forbidden foods have been added against our advice or when indicated control of inhalant allergy has been discontinued. The salvage of your son's colon is your important challenge. Do not fail to send me frequent reports about the maintenance of his diet, particularly if any symptoms develop." (This letter is still in our records of his case.)

The general diet was continued for ten years. He graduated from high school and college, married, and became associated with his father in business. His weight increased to 140 pounds; his height to 5'9".

In August of 1959 bloody diarrhea recurred, and ileostomy was reestablished without consulting us. We would have reestablished his elimination diet which had controlled his CUC in 1943. Liquid discharge from his ileum persisted after his operation. Fever and secondary infection developed, and finally jaundice occurred. After many transfusions while he remained in the hospital for two months with a reduction in weight to ninety pounds, he died.

Comment: The rapid relief of CUC and his gain in weight with our minimal elimination diet in 1943 without any medications after the first ten days indicates that this diet would have given relief when his CUC was reactivated at the age of twenty-eight years. Such relief is supported by the rapid relief of CUC during the first month in infancy, with the substitution of our meat-base formula for cow's milk at the age of one week.

Such control of food allergy, moreover, would have made the original ileostomy done at the age of eight years unnecessary. This in turn would have avoided the cramping, pain, constant liquid ileal discharge, and final use of the balloon in his ileum which had to be removed every two to three hours day and night by the mother for a period

of one year. The marked loss of strength and weight down to forty pounds when we first saw him at the age of ten years would not have occurred.

The excellent gain in weight and strength justifying the rejoining of his ileum in four months after our elimination diet was started showed that the foods in the diet plus vitamins and calcium assured adequate nutrition and increased weight without any animal milk, eggs, wheat, cereal grains, or other eliminated foods.

In this boy it was fortunate indeed that only an ileostomy without total colectomy was done before our study of possible atopic allergy was requested. In this boy food allergy proved to be the sole cause of his CUC as evidenced by the rapid relief of his symptoms, making an ileocolostomy possible in four months after our elimination diet was prescribed with resultant excellent reestablished function of his colon.

Case 35: A baby (F.G.) weighing 7½ pounds and 19½ inches in length at birth was given our meat-base formula on the third day because of diarrhea with traces of blood. Glucose and water had been taken during the first twenty-four hours. The meat-base formula was given instead of cow's milk because of its control in his sister of diarrhea resulting from cow's milk.

On the fifth day erythema and oozing developed on the genitals and buttocks, decreasing in the succeeding five weeks. Ten stools were passed after each feeding until the thirty-fifth day. No increase in weight had occurred. During this period only the meat-base formula was given. Banana flakes then caused crying, dilated pupils, aphonia, tachycardia, and drowsiness. About ten dark odorous stools were passed for two days. Hemoglobin was 3.5 gm at that time. Blood was given by vein, with an increase to 13 gm of hemoglobin in three days.

On the forty-second day an x-ray of the gastrointestinal tract revealed CUC in the descending colon and rectum. Moderate diarrhea and weakness continued because of which Paregoric, 20 drops daily, was prescribed, with a reduction in his stools. Our meat-base formula, 1200 cc a day, was his only nourishment.

Then Aristocort®, 6 to 8 mg daily, was ordered, and Fungizone® Ointment was applied to the eczematous areas with the administration of Mysteclin-F® by mouth because of a secondary fungus complicating the dermatitis of his genitals and buttocks.

In the eighth month weight was 10 lb, 8 ounces, and length 23¾ inches. His colitis was under good control. Pneumonia developed in both lungs, which was controlled with Chloromycetin® in five days.

At home he was receiving the meat-base formula, Aristocort, 8 mg daily, Mysteclin-F, and Vi-Penta drops daily.

Dr. Andrews of Louisville, Kentucky, who had prescribed the meat-base formula and cortisone since birth, then asked for our advice. In addition to his meat-base formula, we advised strained lamb, white potatoes, sugar, and in one week the addition of pureed peas and carrots.

He was then brought from Kentucky to the Children's Hospital in Oakland because of his failure to gain weight and possible adrenal insufficiency resulting from corticoids given for four months. A barium enema confirmed quiescent CUC in the descending colon and rectum. Blood count and electrolytes were normal. Sugar tolerance after sugar was fasting 78 mg%; in one-half hour 150 mg%, in one hour 102 mg%, in two hours 6.94 mg%, and in five hours 61 mg%. Plasma electrophoresis was normal.

Aristocort was then discontinued.

Diet in the hospital was our meat-base formula plus strained lamb, potatoes, rice, oatmeal, tapioca cooked with sugar and flavored with burnt sugar, Willow Run milk-free hydrogenated soy oil butter, salt and sugar, and sesame oil. Vi-Penta drops and 0.01 μg of B_{12} hypodermically were given twice weekly.

In two months at home he had gained five pounds and two inches in height. He passed two stools a day. No corticosteroids were given.

At the age of 17½ months, weight was 20 lb, height 31 inches, with a gain of 8 lb and 5½ inches in seven months. Soy-potato bread made by our recipes had been added. He was active and happy.

In the five years since 1964 he has been active and well. No reactivations of CUC have occurred. Milk, wheat, chocolate, and nuts are entirely eliminated from his diet.

Comment: The occurrence of bloody diarrhea in the first few days of life with the demonstration by x-ray of probable ulcerative colitis in the descending colon and rectum at the age of one month justifies the probability that this disease was present even at birth. The presence of these symptoms at birth supports the probability that the colon became sensitized *in utero* especially to milk allergens in the mother's diet during gesta-tion. The gradual initial control of this ulcerative colitis which has continued in the last five years justifies our report that this is the youngest reported patient in whom CUC has been controlled, particularly by the recognition and relief of food allergy without surgery. The relief after the third or fourth month until we saw him at the age of seven months depended in part on the use of costicosteroids. Our discontinuance of these corticosteroids at the age of seven months justified the conclusion that the control of his ulcerative colitis in the last three years has been entirely due to the elimination of allergenic foods.

The excellent gain in weight and maintenance of his nutrition, first with our meat-base formula and later with the other foods in our elimination diet together with calcium and vitamins, show that milk is not necessary for the maintenance of health, weight, and nutrition.

Summary

1. As in adults, CUC in infants and children is due to an eczematous inflammation with varying resultant ulcerations and complications because of food or inhalant, especially pollen, allergy alone or together, and less frequently to drug allergy.

2. With the control of such allergies and the indicated use of corticoids without which our good or excellent results in many of our adult patients and in Cases 33 and 34 were obtained before 1950. No colectomies have been done in infants and children when cooperation of the patient and parent has continued for more than two or four months. And former ileostomies have been replaced by ileocolostomies resulting from our control of allergy in Cases 33 and 34 with excellent control for over fifteen years. Then, in Case 34 a general diet was advised in Pennsylvania with fulminating recurrence of the CUC and death which would not have occurred if our advised control of food allergy had continued.

3. The history, laboratory findings, control of causative food and/or pollen allergies, our continued supervision and pa-

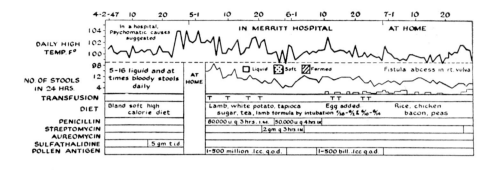

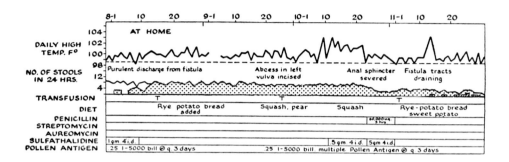

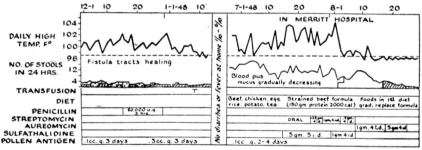

Figure 4. A girl twelve years of age. Allergy to pollens, especially grasses, as the major cause of CUC is indicated by its onset in July of 1946, relief in the winter, and return of fulminating colitis from March to mid-July of 1947; soft and decreasing stools with fever from infected fistulae in the fall; complete relief from January to June of 1948; and a lesser attack for 1½ months in June and July with continued insufficient pollen therapy. Since then, for 5½ years colitis has been entirely absent except for a slight increase in the formed stools in the summers of 1949 and 1951. Pollen desensitization has been continuous. Associated milk allergy has been considered but is in question.

tients' cooperation, and the excellent results from our antiallergic treatment with no corticoids before their availability in 1950 and since then with their minimal,

infrequent use to control symptoms after errors in diet are recorded.

4. Finally these case records emphasize atopic allergy as the cause of CUC and

the necessary cooperation of the patient and parents with the physician in maintaining and supervising antiallergic control by the informed and studious physician or specialist as we advise.

5. Since atopic allergy has received inadequate study and treatment by the profession, assiduous study of our discussion of diagnosis and control as summarized in this chapter and in our several articles in the last thirty years is the responsibility of the physician who accepts the responsibility and privilege of adequate study and control of CUC. He must not succumb to the temptation of surgical removal of the shock organ of allergy in the colon, placing the responsibility of control on the surgeons and condemning the patients, especially children and adolescents, to an irreversible ileostomy existence with its frequent complications and even death.

Chapter 7

Regional Enteritis—Allergy in Its Etiology

That regional enteritis (RE) is due to atopic allergy to foods, at times to pollens, and occasionally to drugs has been increasingly evidenced by our good or excellent results from the control of such allergies for over twenty years. This allergic etiology makes regional enteritis in the small bowel the equivalent of chronic ulcerative colitis in the colon. Though RE usually involves the jejunum and especially the ileum, it may involve the duodenum and lower esophagus, which requires study of possible allergy as we advise.

In 1953 in our article on "Regional Enteritis—Its Allergic Aspects," we reported that a possible role of allergy in the causation of regional enteritis had been suggested by Fenster, Kraemer, Bassler, Kullenkampf, Ravdin, and Johnston and Schepers from 1939 to 1945. Kaijser, in 1937, proposed the name "ileitis allergica" for regional enteritis arising from salvarsan. Tallroth, in 1943, and Blumstein and Johnson, in 1951, reported marked eosinophilic infiltration of involved tissues in regional enteritis.

Collins and Pritchett, in 1938, first reported ileocolitis resulting from possible food allergy. Diarrhea and fever for six years was rapidly controlled with our elimination diet. Then errors in the diet caused a marked relapse with a loss of fifty-five pounds. X-ray revealed regional enteritis and ulcerative colitis. After ileostomy improvement failed until the elimination diet was resumed. When relief was assured, the ileum was rejoined with the colon which functioned perfectly because of control of food allergy.

Of importance was the conclusion of Andresen in his book *Gastroenterology* in 1958 that RE is an allergic disease as is CUC as first reported by him in 1942. His further confirmation of this was prevented by his too early death.

In our article in 1953 we reported the following case of regional enteritis which had been controlled for five years by the complete elimination of milk. That deficiency in intestinal lactase cannot explain such relief or cause the pathology in the intestinal tissues in CUC and RE, best explained by atopic allergy especially to foods, is discussed in Chapter 25. This excellent control continued for another four years until the patient died of a cerebral glioma.

Case 36: A woman forty-one years of age had developed moderate nonbloody diarrhea with cramping and daily fever up to 101 F in 1941. This continued, and in 1945 roentgen rays revealed regional enteritis. Two feet of the terminal ileum were resected. Pathologic study showed markedly thickened intestinal wall. The serosa contained increased plasma cells, lymphocytes, and eosinophiles. Ulcerated areas were in the mucosa. Photographs showed 50 percent eosinophiles, tuberclelike lesions, and Langhans giant cells in the submucosa, as printed in our article.

Because of continued soft or watery stools, fever up to 101 F, fatigue, and a loss of fifteen pounds for two years after surgery, she was referred for our study of allergy. Roentgen rays showed disturbed mucosal patterns, edema of the mucosa, and narrowed areas in the lower jejunum and especially in the ileum, with hypermotility. There was no personal or family history of allergy. Scratch tests with foods and inhalants were negative.

With our fruit-free elimination diet of lamb, chicken, rice, white potato, sweet potato, carrots, squash, asparagus, tapioca caramel pudding, salt, sugar, water, and 50 mg vitamin C daily, all symptoms were controlled in three weeks. She then was passing formed stools daily. Gradually all foods were added in the next four months. Milk only reproduced diarrhea and slight fever.

X-rays of the small bowel each year showed steady decrease in former abnormal findings. In three years they were normal except for slight irregularity in the lower remaining ileum. Symptoms of regional enteritis were absent because of continued elimination of all milk.

In the last twenty years this control of regional enteritis has continued for one to seventeen years in twenty-six cases from the control of food allergy. In five patients concomitant pollen allergy has also required desensitization with multiple pollen antigens, as advised in Chapter 30. In one patient pollen allergy as the sole cause was indicated by excellent relief of former invaliding symptoms for seven years and a gain of 40 pounds during the last twenty years from pollen desensitization, injections of B_{12}, and without the elimination of any possible allergenic foods.

The following symptoms and complications had been present before our treatment in varying degrees: nausea, distention, abdominal pain, cramping, diarrhea, fever, mass in the right lower abdomen (in 4), canker sores, ileovesicular fistula (in 2), rectal fistula (in 1), weakness, depression, and loss of weight of five to twenty pounds in all except for fifty-five pounds in one patient. These symptoms had continued for one half to eighteen years (average of 5 years).

Our antiallergic therapy in fifteen patients began one half to nine years (average of 3½) after initial ileal surgery. Our

elimination diet was started immediately after ileal surgery in another nine cases. In two patients with regional enteritis of most of the small bowel as revealed by initial surgery, our elimination diet with initial large doses of corticosteroids which were gradually eliminated in two weeks relieved fulminating symptoms of regional enteritis, making massive intestinal resection unnecessary.

This control in these twenty-six patients has continued with no intestinal surgery for reactivated regional enteritis. Release of stricture of the ileum because of adhesions from initial surgery and enlargement of the ileocolonic union in a second patient because of obstructive symptoms from initial anastomosis only were required.

This absence of second intestinal surgery because of reactivation of regional enteritis is in marked contrast to second ileal surgery reported by Jackson in 40 percent of 104 operated cases, in 31 percent of 65 cases reported by Brown and Daffner, in 48.8 percent of such cases reported by Ferguson, and in 53 percent reported by Colp and Drulling, who stated recently (1969) that most resections for RE are followed by hospitalization one or two times and by additional operations.

We opine that the absence of second ileal surgery in our patients has been due to our control of atopic allergy.

The most recent report of results of surgical and adjunctive medical therapy in RE with no registered consideration of atopic allergy by Banks, Zetzel, and Richter in 145 cases of RE was published in 1969.

In 145 patients with RE having major abdominal surgery on the small bowel, 60 percent had two or more additional abdominal operations. Surgical mortality was

6.5 percent. Subsequent mortality in three decades because of RE was approximately 10 percent. Fistulae (not in rectum) developed in 37 percent, showing continued activity of RE. Abdominal abscess occurred in 23 percent. Thus an average of three operations indicated continued activity of the pathogenic process.

TABLE XVII

REGIONAL ENTERITIS IN 26 PATIENTS RELIEVED BY ANTIALLERGIC THERAPY

Case #	Sex	Age at Onset of RE (Yrs)	Yrs of Uncontrolled RD — When 1st Seen	Yrs of Uncontrolled RD — After Ileal Surgery	Yrs of Relief From Antiallergic Therapy	Additional Ileectomy After Initial Surgery	Cause — Food	Cause — Pollen
1	F	12	6	½	3	0	X	
2	M	30	9	9	4	0	X	X
3	M	22	18	8	13	0	X	X
4	M	12	6	*	2	0	X	
5	F	17	⅓	*	1½	0	X	
6	F	25	10	Exploratory; no ileal surgery (1)	5	0	X	
7	M	52	1	1½	6	0	X	
8	M	18	½	1⅓	4	Resection of stenosed anastomosis (1)	X	
9	F	43	3	1½	11	0	X	X
10	F	19	4	*	7	0	X	X
11	M	41	4½	¼	9	0	X	X
12	F	31	5	4	11	0	X	
13	F	43	9	3	17	Resection of stricture in upper ileum (1)		X
14	F	39	¼	Exploratory; no ileal surgery	5	0	X	
15	F	44	4	*	5	0	X	
16	F	33	15	5 (2 previous)	13	0	X	
17	M	31	4	4	9 (fair cooperation)	0	X	
18	M	15	14	*	7	0	X	
19	F	34	7	3	9	0	X	
20	F	33	6	4	6	0	X	
21	M	24	½	*	4½	0	X	
22	M	17	½	*	2	0	X	
23	M	17	8	*	1	0	X	
24	F	50	1½	1	2	0	X	
25	F	35	1	*	2½	0	X	
26	M	46	2	1	2½	0	X	

(1) Because of scar tissue and not recurrent ileitis.
*Placed on elimination diet immediately after surgery.

Compared with our results in twenty-six cases of RE cooperating in our study and control of food and less often inhalant allergy, additional surgery was done only in Case 5 in Table XVII because of failure to adhere to our prescribed elimination diet and in Cases 8 and 13 because of obstruction resulting from ileal strictures from initial disease and not because of its continued activity.

In our opinion the important study and control of atopic allergy especially to foods advised in this chapter would have controlled the RE after initial surgery or in nonobstructed cases without fistulae or secondary infection. The allergic enteritis, if diagnosed, might have been controlled without surgery if such strict control of atopic allergy had occurred.

We therefore advise study of atopic allergy to foods and less frequent inhalants, especially pollen, and allergy in all cases of RE first in the office or on entrance to hospitals for investigation or during or after emergency surgery.

In our opinion, with strict study of atopic allergy, complications will be decreased or prevented, subsequent surgery will be reduced and usually prevented, and the implacability of the pathogenic process will be reversed.

This failure to study and control atopic allergy, especially to foods, as advised in this chapter, we opine, explains in large part the fifty-six cutaneous complications of RE reported by Samitz, Dance, and Rosenberg, in 1970, especially anal, perianal, or vulvar fistulae or fissures or anal abscess, erythema nodosum, and the malabsorption syndrome occurring in their two hundred cases which did not occur in our twenty-six patients who long cooperated in our advised control of their atopic allergy, especially to foods, which

was not utilized by the writers or referred to in any of the fourteen articles in the references.

CONTROL OF ATOPIC ALLERGY

Possible food allergy requires its adequate study in all patients in whom seasonal occurrence of symptoms does not suggest pollen allergy as the sole cause.

If history with or without positive scratch reactions suggests allergy to milk, its entire elimination may give relief in one to three weeks. If this occurs, complete elimination of milk from the diet should continue for months or even for years if later provocation tests with milk reproduces symptoms.

Most regional enteritis, however, according to our reported experience is due to allergy to several foods, especially to milk, wheat, eggs, most or all fruits, condiments, chocolate, coffee, and other less allergenic foods. Thus for the initial study of possible food allergy our fruit-free elimination diet plus rice and minus beef and legumes is usually prescribed. Required protein, calories, additional vitamins, and calcium are necessary. The reader is referred to directions for the preparation and manipulation of the diet in previous publications and in Chapter 3 of this volume.

If scratch tests with common foods give large reactions to any foods in the prescribed diet, they are omitted. Intradermal tests are not advised, as discussed in Chapter 2. The clinical importance of large reactions to foods, however, must finally be determined by provocation tests after relief of symptoms of regional enteritis occurs.

If symptoms continue for two to four weeks in spite of strict adherence to the above diet, a minimal elimination diet such as rice, white potatoes, pearl tapioca, lamb, milk-free butter, salt, sugar, and water as advised in Chapter 3 should be followed before ruling out food allergy. If appetite for meat is impaired, strained meat or our meat-base formula made at home or by the Gerber Company may be ordered to increase necessary protein. Additional advice about the preparation and manipulation of these diets is in Chapter 3 and in our publications on chronic ulcerative colitis and regional enteritis.

Corticosteroids for the initial control of allergy, the dose varying according to the severity of the regional enteritis, may be indicated. The dose is reduced and eliminated with improvement. Triamcinolone 2 to 4 mg daily has been continued by only two of our twenty-six patients. Anemia must be controlled. Since absorption of B_{12} is often impaired in regional enteritis, especially after iliectomy and the blind loop syndrome, B_{12} injections every one to four weeks may be necessary for months or years.

Pollen therapy is indicated by the occurrence or activation of regional enteritis during the pollen seasons, by positive skin tests to pollens though they may be negative, and by other manifestations of pollen allergy. Control requires desensitization at times with initial, very weak dilutions of pollen antigens with a gradual increase as tolerated by the patient. At times it is advisable to move to an area in which causative pollens are absent.

Until symptoms are relieved by the control of atopic allergy especially to foods, cramps, abdominal soreness, and diarrhea

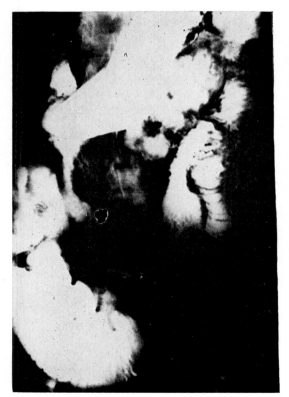 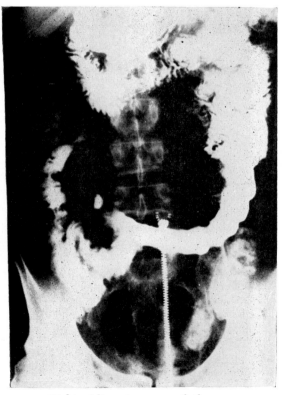

Figure 5. *Left:* Before our treatment eight years after ileal resection.   *Right:* After six years of therapy.

may require codeine, Lomotil®, or tincture of opium or an antispasmodic like Pro-Banthine® by mouth. Anemia may require iron or if severe, transfusions. Secondary infection may require antibiotics. Corticosteroids as advised above may be indicated until the causes of allergy are controlled.

In the challenge of relieving regional enteritis by control of allergy, indications for surgery must not be forgotten. Partial or nearly total stenosis from severe local allergic inflammation, fistulae, and later thick fibrotic granulomatous "hose pipe" bowel requires surgery. Postoperatively in the hospital and for years thereafter, our control of allergy with the cooperation of the patient should prevent reactivation of the regional enteritis in new areas which might necessitate second intestinal surgery, as it has in our twenty-six cases reported in this chapter.

CASE REPORTS

Case 37: A man thirty years of age developed six to ten bloody stools in 1953. Five feet of ileum was resected because of regional enteritis demonstrated by x-ray and later at operation. Watery stools up to twenty a day with cramping and abdominal soreness continued for nine years.

When referred to us to study possible allergy, he weighed 107 pounds, and weakness prevented walking or self-feeding. Serum potassium was 2.3 meq., and serum albumin was 3.3 gm.

The study of food allergy was carried out with our fruit and cereal-free elimination diet plus rice and minus soy. Potassium chloride and vitamins by mouth were also given. Weakness and diarrhea disappeared in three weeks. Nutrition, strength, and increased weight up to 145 pounds have been maintained for six years with complete elimination of milk, wheat, chocolate, coffee, and condiments.

Case 38: A man forty years of age had had abdominal cramping, soreness, and weakness for ten years when resection of sixteen inches of ileum was done because of regional enteritis. Two to five soft or liquid daily stools continued, and because of abdominal pain and severe nausea in five years, a second iliectomy was done.

During our study of possible allergy because of continued digestive symptoms, our cereal-free elimination diet gave relief in ten days. He felt "better than in fifteen years."

In one year diarrhea and cramping recurred attributed to inhalation of the odor of milk and fruit in a cannery. Against our advice a third ileal resection was done. With a general diet postoperatively, symptoms recurred in one month. Requesting our help again, his symptoms were controlled in two weeks by our fruit-free elimination diet with reducing doses of corticosteroids.

Excellent relief continued for four years. Then gradually he added wheat to his diet again without our advice. Resultant abdominal pain and nausea were controlled again by elimination of wheat with large and gradually reduced corticosteroids by mouth. With strict adherence to his diet for the last three years, no symptoms of regional enteritis have recurred.

Of note was the development of regional enteritis in his son and daughter in their early twenties confirmed by x-rays when their terminal ileum were resected. Strict adherence to their fruit and cereal-free elimination diet plus rice and oats and multiple vitamins has controlled symptoms except two moderate recurrences in the daughter because of breaks in her prescribed diet.

Comment: This is the only one of twenty-six patients who has had a resection of the small bowel after our initial control. Surgery was required because of the addition of wheat against our advice. The occurrence of regional enteritis in the patient's two children affirms familial occurrence first reported by Crohn and Yarmis.

That regional enteritis is due to atopic allergy to foods, at times to pollens, and probably to other inhalants or drugs as is chronic ulcerative colitis is evidenced by our good results given over twenty years.

Case 39: Regional enteritis for twelve years in a woman forty-six years of age in 1952 for which two feet of terminal ileum was removed was relieved of postoperative diarrhea and cramping, and our fruit and cereal-free diet alone was responsible. Gradual addition of foods proved milk alone responsible. Favoring atopic allergy was eosinophilia infiltrating mucosa, giant cells, and proliferative vasculitis.

Since then regional enteritis has been controlled in twenty-six cooperating cases for one to seventeen years (average 6.5 years) without second ileal surgery because of our control of food and less often pollen allergy. Initial ileostomy in twenty-two cases and ileotransverse colostomy with continuity in two cases were done.

Food allergy was controlled with our fruit and cereal-free elimination diet. Absent relief in two or three weeks or continuing severe symptoms indicated our minimal elimination diet.

Pollen allergy was the sole cause in Case 12 in Table XVII and was associated with food allergy in five cases.

Massive resections have been prevented with our control of food and indicated pollen therapy along with limited corticosteroid therapy in Cases 40 and 41.

Case 40: A woman fifty-two years of age had had invaliding regional enteritis, arthritis, and anemia for nine years unrelieved by ileotransverse colostomy with continuity three years before we saw her in 1949. Though scratch reactions to pollens were negative, exaggeration of perennial symptoms of regional enteritis during the pollen seasons for several years indicated pollen allergy as a major cause.

Her daughter had life-long diffuse eczema because of pollen allergy indicated by large scratch reactions to many pollens and good relief from desensitization.

Excellent control of the regional enteritis gradually developed in one year with desensitization at first with 1:10-12 dilution of a tree, grass, and fall pollen antigen which was gradually increased in strength as tolerated. Injections of B_{12} were given every two weeks. An elimination diet with no uncooked fruits or vegetables was ordered. With this pollen therapy and injections of B_{12}, weight increased forty pounds and active physical and social life became possible.

Comment: The excellent relief of this regional enteritis with normal physical and social activity resulting from pollen and B_{12} therapy alone indicates pollen allergy as the major cause. Since we first reported chronic ulcerative colitis resulting from pollen and to a lesser degree food allergy in 1942, we have relieved other cases of chronic ulcerative colitis with the control of pollen and associated food allergy.

REGIONAL ENTERITIS AND ILEO-BLADDER FISTULATA RESULTING FROM POLLEN AND FOOD ALLERGY

Case 41: A girl nineteen years of age was first seen in 1960 because of regional enteritis and a complicating bladder fistula with resultant cystitis. Abdominal distress was first noticed in May four years previously, increasing during the summer and early fall months, with a loss of ten pounds. Because of the continued abdominal distress, abdominal operation revealed regional enteritis in the terminal ileum. Her appendix was removed. At that time moderate cystitis was present because of which antibiotics were given at intervals during the next two years. Cystoscopy, in 1959, revealed polyps in the bladder with moderate cystitis. During the summer months of each year abdominal distress with rumbling and gurgling in the abdomen had been present and continued during the fall months. Slight fever developed, and in January feces in the urine were found. Because of this and the continued urinary tenesmus and cramping in her abdomen, transverse ileocolostomy and repair of a bladder fistula between jejunum and urinary bladder was accomplished. She was then referred to us in February, 1960, for the study of atopic allergy as a cause of her ileitus.

A history of flexural eczema at times since childhood and seasonal hay fever in the late spring and early summer months for several years was obtained.

Scratch tests revealed large reactions to practically all of the grass pollens, to many of the fall and tree pollens, and a one plus reaction to cat and dog which were in her house, which indicated their removal. She gave several questionable reactions to various foods which required study of possible food allergy as a cause of her cystitis. Allergy to milk was suggested by her lifelong lack of desire for milk.

Her drug history revealed edemas of the face on several occasions from aspirin. Allergy to other drugs was absent.

Blood and urine analyses when first seen were negative except for 6 percent eosinophilia.

Former cystitis from her ileobladder fistula had been controlled by antibacterial therapy after surgery.

Treatment and results: The start of this regional enteritis in the summer months with exaggeration in the following summer months together with her history of seasonal hay fever for several years and particularly because of her large reactions to grass and lesser reactions to tree and fall pollens indicated pollen allergy as a major or sole cause of her regional enteritis, the continuation of which led to the bladder fistula. Moreover, because of her aversion for milk and the persistence of her symptoms of regional enteritis to a moderate degree during the winter, food allergy was studied with our fruit-free, cereal-free elimination diet. Desensitization to a multiple pollen antigen which contained most of the spring pollens and lesser amounts of the fall pollens to which reactions had occurred was administered first in a 1:500 million dilution. The mother was instructed in the administration of this antigen biweekly for two months with a gradual increase from a 1:500 million into the 1:50,000 strength. During the rest of the year the strength of this antigen was gradually increased into the 1:5000 dilution given in increasing doses at weekly intervals. During the last eight years desensitization to this pollen antigen, at the present time in a 1:50 dilution, has been given at weekly intervals. In addition, milk, eggs, and uncooked fruits are still eliminated from the diet. She has taken rice and oatmeal and their bakery products in the last four years.

During this time there has been no activation of her former hay fever or of her regional enteritis during the pollen seasons. Blood count is normal and her physical examination done by her referring doctor is entirely satisfactory.

SUMMARY

1. That regional enteritis is due to atopic allergy to foods and at times to pollens and probably other inhalants and drugs is evidenced by our good results for over twenty years.

Favoring allergy are the following:

a) Eosinophilic infiltration of involved mucosa reported in many articles, as in Case 36.

b) Inflammation, edema, proliferative vasculitis, giant cell necroses, ulcerations, and fibrosis in the involved tissues are known results of chronic atopic allergy.

c) For many years students have suggested allergy as the possible cause of RE.

d) Evidence accumulated by Andresen and Rowe that allergy especially to foods and pollens is the primary cause of CUC requires study of allergy in the frequently associated or equivalent disease of RE.

e) The localization, spreading tendency, recurrences, fever, occasional inherited predisposition (as in one patient through father, daughter, and son), and the relief from corticosteroids in RE and CUC can be explained by allergy.

2. Excellent control of RE with our fruit-and cereal-free elimination diet with a final conclusion that milk allergy was the cause is reported in Case 39.

In the last eighteen years twenty-six cases of RE have been controlled for one to seventeen years (average 6.5 years) without second intestinal surgery because of their cooperation in elimination of allergenic foods found to be responsible with our fruit- and cereal-free diet and indicated pollen desensitization to pollen alone in Case 12, of Table XVII and pollen associated with food allergy in five cases.

Chapter 8

Bronchial Asthma Because of Food and Inhalant Allergy and Less Frequent Drug and Chemical Allergy

Food allergy, as emphasized in our book *Bronchial Asthma* (1963) and according to our experience for more than forty years, is of comparable or even greater importance than is inhalant allergy as a cause of bronchial asthma. We realize that this conclusion differs from that of most allergists. A recent guide for its treatment advises a well-balanced regular diet with no consideration of food allergy and no diet trial! To substantiate our opinion, observations and evidence accumulated during our long study of clinical allergy and especially of bronchial asthma supporting the importance of food and inhalant allergies will be presented in this chapter.

When food allergy especially is recognized and controlled and inhalant allergy is similarly dealt with as we advise, the infrequency or absence of infectant allergy as a rare primary and an infrequent secondary factor has become evident. Moreover, so-called vague, intrinsic causes have not been necessary to assume and psychosomatic causes of true bronchial asthma seem absent or of rare importance. Long sanitarium care and continued corticosteroid therapy except for small doses in some patients with obstructive emphysema have been unnecessary. Allergy to drugs as an occasional sole or associated cause, especially to aspirin and in one patient Orinase® has been recognized. Control of the cause resulting from allergy, especially to foods, as we advise in this volume justi-

fied by our published results for over three decades, and of equal or lesser frequency to inhalants rather than the temporary relief of symptoms by medications, especially by increasing use of corticosteroids, is the challenge of the medical profession. Atopic allergy especially to foods is the most logical explanation for bronchospasm and bronchorrhea. The too frequent use and expense of bronchodilator drugs by mouth, rectum, inhalation, and intermittent positive pressure have been greatly minimized and with strict cooperation of the patient, usually eliminated.

Our study and control of inhalant allergy and especially of food allergy as advised in this chapter and especially in Chapter 4 and in our books and medical articles for over thirty-five years greatly decrease and usually eliminate the severe, recurrent attacks of chronic bronchial asthma and its morbidity and mortality, which have been reported especially in England and Europe in the last two years. When control of asthma as advised in this volume has occurred, psychological and financial strains in the family have been prevented. In addition, such control, especially of food allergy, will decrease the use and the detrimental effects of too frequent adrenergic inhalant therapy, especially of intermittent positive pressure (IPP), which is not required by our cooperating patients with asthma and also obstructive emphysema, as we emphasize in Chapter 11.

Failure to control fool allergy is often responsible for uncontrolled asthma, unnecessary invalidism, and at times mortality not only in bronchial asthma but also in obstructive emphysema, as stressed in Chapter 11.

Failure of chronic asthmatics to respond to therapy, especially "prolonged desensitization to inhalants," in spite of sincere effort too often is due, we are convinced, to failure to study and control food allergy as advised, especially with our CFE diet in this chapter and in Chapter 3. With such study and control, especially of food allergy, I opine that the statement "Asthma offers medicine a challenge with its many complicated problems" by Sugahara in Japan would be largely answered as corroborative by Kaplan in South Africa in his article "Food Allergy—the Missing Link in Perennial Bronchial Asthma," in 1967.

This failure to recognize the importance of food allergy, we opine, is a "world-wide medical tragedy." With the important consideration, recognition, and control of food allergy, as advised in this volume, "a great step forward for mankind" will occur. Its importance in perennial nasal and pharyngeal allergy, bronchiectasis, and as a major cause of obstructive emphysema (Chapt. 11) as well as chronic bronchitis is emphasized in the next four chapters and especially in Chapter 30.

Failure to realize the importance of food allergy is due, in our opinion, largely to three causes: a) Food allergy too often is ruled out because of negative skin reactions to foods or of failure to relieve asthma with test-negative diets, which exclude only skin reacting foods. This is unfortunate for patients, since it is increasingly and generally recognized, as we have emphasized since the 1920's and

especially in 1933, that much chronic food allergy is not associated with positive skin tests and that many positive reactions, especially by the intradermal method, are nonspecific or are due to past or possibly potential allergy. b) This lack of recognition of food allergy arises largely from failure to use trial diets, especially our cereal-free elimination diet, adequately for sufficiently long periods of time. Skepticism about our conviction of the important role of food allergy in bronchial asthma is not justified by any physician who has not used our cereal-free elimination diet strictly as we advise in a large number of patients for a period of several months rather than a few days or several weeks. The great importance of this CFE diet for the study of food allergy has been emphasized in Chapter 3 as it is in this chapter. c) Finally, the failure to realize that most "colds" preceding or associated with recurrent attacks of bronchial asthma, especially in children (Chapt. 25), are due to initial activation of food allergy in the nose and sinuses before its major activity develops in the lungs, with resultant asthma, are usually responsible for the erroneous conclusion that bacterial infection or allergy is responsible for such attacks. That infectant allergy is not the cause of asthma is supported by the relief we have obtained in a large number of patients suffering with such regularly recurrent asthma when the underlying food allergy, at times associated with inhalant allergy, has been recognized and controlled. Our pathognomonic history of bronchial asthma, especially in children (Fig. 8) must be remembered in all countries by all physicians.

It is our urgent advice that all perennial bronchial asthma, chronic bronchitis, and obstructive emphysema with or without evident bronchial asthma in which inhalant allergy is not the assured cause must be studied for probable food allergy, especially with the accurate, adequate use of our CFE diet as advised in this volume and especially in this chapter.

CHARACTERISTICS OF BRONCHIAL ASTHMA RESULTING FROM FOOD ALLERGY

1. Bronchial asthma resulting from food allergy may develop at any time of life, as shown in the statistics in Table XVIII in this chapter. The relief of such asthma in all ages from the strict, adequate use of our CFE diet during four decades has established this conclusion. Thus patients, regardless of age, may develop bronchial asthma resulting from food allergy, alone or associated with inhalant allergy or resulting from inhalant allergy alone, occasionally because of drug allergy, and rarely if ever to infectant allergy. That bronchial asthma after the age of fifty-five years is due to the same causes as in youth and midlife will be emphasized.

2. Food allergy often produces regularly recurrent attacks of bronchial asthma, as emphasized in Chapter 2, followed by partial or incomplete refractoriness to the causative foods, as noted in Chapter 1. This refractoriness was first discussed by Schloss in 1920. It has been confirmed by us and other investigators since then and recently by Gerrard in four children of a family. The asthma may be preceded for a few hours or rarely for one or more days by nasal allergy, often with fever (Chapt. 24) because of foods (Fig. 13), suggesting an infectious cold as the cause. During the attack the reacting bodies in the nasal or bronchial tissues theoretically are gradually exhausted after which no symptoms recur until these antibodies reaccumulate above the reacting threshold. As these recurrent attacks continue, the interim refractoriness may decrease and result in slight-to-moderate persistent chronic asthma. However, regularly recurring activation of such perennial symptoms may continue as an equivalent of the former recurrent severe attacks. Such increased symptoms or attacks often are associated with or preceded by "head colds" and fever, making patients and their physicians erroneously conclude that infection rather than the causative food allergy is responsible.

This cyclic activation of bronchial asthma resulting from food allergy does not occur in all patients.

Case 42: Thus a girl nineteen years of age had had bronchial asthma at irregular intervals with no seasonal variations in childhood. At times no asthma occurred for two to four months. During the two months before we saw her, it had persisted constantly, keeping her in bed one or two days every week. She gave no skin reactions to foods, but three plus reactions to house dust and cat hair by the scratch method were obtained. Strict environmental control of dust and entire avoidance of cats for several weeks had given no relief. Food allergy was studied with our CFE diet. In two weeks her symptoms were less and absent in the following three months. Since then, eggs, milk, and cereal grains (including wheat) have reproduced symptoms on several occasions. Such persistent, irregular asthma may occur at any time of life. It always requires consideration of inhalant as well as food allergy. In this young girl the reactions to dust and cat hair were of questionable importance. In many patients, of course, inhalant allergy with or without food allergy is the cause of such chronic irregularly activated asthma.

3. Food allergy, especially when it causes bronchial asthma, is inactivated in certain patients during the summer months (Chapt. 1), so that allergenic foods cause little or no difficulty from early June to late or mid-August, September, October, or even into December.

The increased available solar radiant energy correlates with this beneficial effect. This benefit disappears in the fall, or as late as January, with a recurrence of asthma at that time and through the winter and early spring months when tolerance to foods is low. Relief occurs in the summer with recurrence of attacks in the fall. When such tolerance is higher, attacks may not start until November or even early January, recurring quite regularly thereafter until May or June. This seasonal effect on food allergy is emphasized in Chapter 2.

4. Food allergy in certain patients decreases or is absent away from the ocean (Chapt. 2). Floyer, Salter, Wyman, and Jimenez-Diaz and others previously have noted an increase of asthma in damp, low, and marine areas. This explains relief of some asthma resulting from food allergy in inland areas. In northern California we have studied many asthmatics who are relieved ten or more miles away from the ocean, over our coastal hills, with no attention to diet, and who have no asthma near the ocean when their food sensitization is controlled. This effect on food allergy probably is responsible for much relief of bronchial asthma in the desert and mountain areas of the United States, especially in the western states. It may account for relief of some patients in inland areas of Switzerland, Germany, Austria, Italy, and Spain. In the United States increase of asthma resulting from food allergy seems to occur in the inland areas of the Great Lakes and large river basins. Of interest is a patient with asthma living on the coast of Florida who was not only relieved in the summer months but also in the mountains of Georgia in other months of the year. The adequate relief of this asthma with the CFE diet at all times of the year in Florida on the coast showed that food allergy was the entire cause. Kantor *et al.* have shown that this

relief away from the coast is in no way a function of absence of inhalants.

5. Fever may arise from food (Chapt. 24), as from drug and serum allergy. Thus it often causes the fever for one to three days with recurrent attacks of asthma resulting from food allergy, especially in young children whose fever may rise to 103 to 105 F for one or at times two days. It may also cause more persistent fever, varying in degree and necessitating the consideration of all possible infections and other causes. Such fever may lead unfortunately to unnecessary bed rest in the home, hospital, or sanitarium, and at times to unnecessary operations, as discussed more fully in Chapter 24. When such fever occurs in asthmatics suffering with demonstrated or assumed food allergy, secondary bronchial infection or infection in other body tissues of course must be recognized and treated with indicated antibiotic drugs.

6. When bronchial allergy is due to food allergy, the lungs may be the only shock organ. As shown in Table XLIII, other tissues also may be affected by such allergies. Nasal and sinal allergies especially occur, and gastrointestinal allergy and allergic headaches are not infrequent. As already noted, eczema resulting from food allergy often occurs in infancy before asthma develops and may continue with bronchial asthma for varying periods thereafter. Other manifestations of food allergy also may occur.

7. The dietary history may or may not reveal dislikes or idiosyncrasies to foods responsible for bronchial asthma and for other allergic manifestations. The way to obtain such histories and the evaluation of such information are discussed in Chapter 2, as outlined below.

METHOD OF RECORDING HISTORY OF ASTHMATIC PATIENT

The systematic recording of the history expedites the diagnosis. Additional information will be obtained from the patient's answers to a questionnaire in our book *Bronchial Asthma* (1963). It may be recorded under the following headings:

Bronchial Manifestations: Onset, frequency, periodicity, and chronicity of the attacks or of persistent symptoms; the amount and character of the sputum; frequency and degree of cough; fever; complications; former history of bronchial symptoms; and geographic and seasonal influences, if any.

Nasal and Sinusal Symptoms: Duration, amount, and degree of seasonal or perennial nasal congestion, blocking, sneezing, itching, nasal or postnasal discharge, sinusal congestion or pain, and former history of head colds or sinusitis.

Dermatoses: Onset, duration, and distribution of allergic dermatitis (eczema), contact dermatitis, urticaria, or angioneurotic edema during life, with possible etiologic comment.

Gastrointestinal Symptoms: Occurrence of canker sores and other oral, gastrointestinal, and abdominal symptoms, with their duration, degree, characteristics, and possible relation to allergy.

Recurrent Headaches: Migraine, biliousness, fatigue, or "toxic states."

Genitourinary, cardiovascular, glandular, nervous, or *psychoneurotic disturbances* with data for or against allergy as a primary or complicating cause.

Dietary History: Dislikes or disagreements for foods of all types and habits of eating. Questions such as "Do you drink milk, eat eggs, or eat spinach?" may suggest allergy, digestive inefficiency, whims or fancies, or psychoneuroses as causes. Potential or active nutritional deficiencies

must be recognized, as emphasized by Minot.

Drug History: Possible allergy to medicaments used even infrequently.

Environmental History: The kinds of carpets, curtains, furnishings, mattresses, pillows, bedding, furs, clothing, animals, plants, flowers, cosmetics, toilet accessories, and other similar information concerning the living, sleeping, working, and recreational environments. Likewise, the names of trees, shrubs, and flowers; the character of the surrounding region, whether built up or in the country; its proximity to barns, animals, fields, orchards, forests, or marshes; the amount and character of dusts; and similar information.

Family History: Bronchial, nasal, cutaneous, gastrointestinal, or other symptoms, especially migraine, recurrent headache, toxic or bilious states in several generations, and progeny, with a record of possible familial ingestant, inhalant, or contactant sensitizations; other unusual information concerning familial diseases, longevity, and dietary habits.

Residences: Their possible relation to allergy.

Past History: Past or present infections or illnesses not noted above.

Menstrual history and the possible influence of allergy.

Operations: Years and results of operations, especially on the nose and throat.

Habits: Amount of tobacco and alcohol and their influences on allergy.

ALLERGIC CAUSES OF BRONCHIAL ASTHMA

Our studies for forty years increasingly have indicated the approximately equal or greater importance of food than inhalant allergy as the sole or a concomitant cause of bronchial asthma. They have also shown occasional asthma from various drugs, especially to aspirin, and in one patient whose extremely severe asthma was due to Orinase and its questionable origin from infectant causes. This is shown in the statistics in Table XVIII.

BRONCHIAL ASTHMA IN CHILDHOOD

Our opinion that food allergy is of great importance in the causation of bronchial asthma in childhood depends on our analysis of the causes in 411 infants and children whose bronchial asthma was treated and controlled during six years up to and including 1946 (see Table XVIII) and on good results in formerly published articles before corticosteroids were available. This importance of food allergy has been increasingly confirmed in the last twenty years, as reported in our book *Bronchial Asthma—Its Diagnosis and Treatment* in 1963 and especially in two articles on asthma in infants and children because of food allergy in 1959 and 1968.

The typical and in our opinion pathognomonic history of bronchial asthma resulting from food allergy in childhood has been increasingly recognized by us for over thirty years, as reported in our books in 1944 and 1963 and in articles on bronchial asthma, especially in 1959 in the *JAMA* and in *Asthma Research* in 1967. It is characterized by cyclic attacks in the fall and winter and up to early May, being less frequent or absent in the summer. They are often preceded by nasal symptoms resulting from food allergy and not infection.

The characteristics of this history are graphically shown in Figure 6. Since it occurs most often in children, it is also printed in our extended discussion and advice on the causes and treatment of bronchial asthma in children in Chapter 25. Since it also continues into adolescence and less often into adult life, it is printed in this chapter in which the causes and results of treatment which we have advised for over forty years in bronchial asthma in adolescents and adults are reported.

Bronchial asthma resulting from food allergy alone usually begins in the first three years, especially from the sixteenth to twenty-sixth months. At times it is preceded by infantile eczema which disappears or decreases before or when the asthma develops. Such asthma, however, can continue through childhood and into adult life. The attacks usually recur every two to eight weeks. Coryza, nasal congestion, and sneezing resulting from nasal allergy rather than from an infectious cold may precede the asthma by four to twenty-four hours or may arise with and continue throughout the attack.

TABLE XVIII

CAUSES OF BRONCHIAL ASTHMA IN 1491 CASES AS DETERMINED BY
GOOD RESULTS FROM ANTIALLERGIC CONTROL AND MEDICATION

	0-5 Yrs 156 Cases %	5-15 Yrs 255 Cases %	15-55 Yrs 907 Cases %	55 Up 173 Cases %	Total 1491 %
Food with or without other allergies	88	78	72	82	76
Food allergy alone	40	25	20	40	26
Inhalant and other allergies	57	70	80	66	73
Pollen and other allergies	50	64	70	57	66
Pollen allergy alone	3	8	25	9	18
Animal emanations and other allergies	6	6	7	11	8
Miscellaneous inhalant and other allergies	5	5	4	16	7
House dust and other allergies	9	10	19	20	18
Bacterial and other allergies	1	1	1.5	3	1.7

Note: Data covers the 7 years before 1948 before corticosteroids were used.

RECURRENT ATTACKS OF BRONCHIAL ASTHMA DUE TO FOOD ALLERGY ESPECIALLY IN CHILDREN

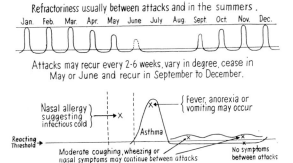

Figure 6. Pathognomic history of bronchial asthma resulting from food allergy, especially in childhood, which continues into adult life as such or with interim symptoms resulting from incomplete refractoriness to food allergy between attacks. This history is emphasized in Chapter 25 and referred to throughout this volume.

Complete relief between these frequent attacks may continue during a one-year or three-year period. Then moderate symptoms between attacks may develop if food allergy is not controlled, or they may occur from the onset of the asthma. This is best explained by the failure of the assumed antibodies to fall below the reacting threshold. Then patients have daily coughing in varying degrees with or without wheezing and dyspnea with exercise and especially on retiring and at intervals through the night. These moderate continued symptoms are often recurrently exaggerated, being an equivalent of the former or usual cyclic attacks of asthma resulting from food allergy.

This usual regularity of attacks or exaggeration of symptoms resulting from food allergy may be changed by various influences. These include temporary delay in the increase of the specific reacting bodies sufficient to produce the severe attacks of asthma or a temporary decrease in the allergic reactivity or even a partial anergy, all of which are hypothetical and are only supported by clinical observations. These attacks and symptoms in certain patients are also favorably influenced in inland dry areas and also in the late spring and summer months, as already discussed. Further extended discussion of bronchial asthma in childhood and early adolescence appears in Chapter 25.

When this typical history resulting from food allergy occurs, as emphasized in Chapter 25, its control alone relieves asthma with no desensitization, vaccine therapy, or corticosteroid therapy.

BRONCHIAL ASTHMA IN ADULTS BETWEEN THE AGES OF FIFTEEN AND FIFTY-FIVE YEARS

As indicated in Table XVIII food and inhalant allergies have been found of approximately equal importance in adults from the age of fifteen to fifty-five years based on our analysis of apparent causes in 907 such asthmatics treated with good or excellent results during 1940 to 1947 and in former published series. This frequency of food allergy has been increasingly confirmed in our practice for over thirty years. To recognize this frequency of food allergy, the aforementioned characteristics of food allergy in Chapter 1 have to be remembered. It is necessary to study food allergy with the experienced and proper use of our CFE diet and at times with its modifications when perennial asthma exaggerated in the fall to late spring, recurrently exaggerated, or occurring in attacks every three to six weeks with varying degree of interim symptoms occurs. As noted already, the frequency of food allergy alone was 20 percent in these adult patients compared with its greater frequency of 40 percent in children and in old age (Table XVIII). Our analysis indicated that food allergy with or without other allergies occurred in 72 percent, compared with inhalant allergy and other sensitizations in 8 percent. Infectant asthma occurred in no patients and was only a rare complicating or secondary factor. Moreover, in no patient was nasal surgery or tonsillectomy responsible for the good results. Removal of infection in gums and around teeth seemed of possible importance in only two patients. If this persistent study of food allergy with similar study of inhalant allergy had not occurred, infectant asthma might have been assumed as an exclusion diagnosis in many patients. This great infrequency of bacterial allergy does not minimize the necessity of recognizing secondary or acute infection in the lungs and of course in other tissues of the body and of institution of proper treatment, as discussed in this chapter and in Chapter 2.

As in the younger group, allergy to house dust and fungi in our area is probably less than in damper or colder areas. If more of our patients had lived in rural areas and had slept on hair or feather mattresses and had been more exposed to animals of various types, the frequency of allergy to animal emanations, feed dusts, and other environmental allergens would have been increased.

BRONCHIAL ASTHMA RESULTING FROM FOOD ALLERGY IN ADULTS

In contrast to children and especially infants, the regularly recurring attacks of bronchial asthma resulting from food allergy were less frequent in adults. Perennial symptoms of varying degrees of asthma and expectoration usually resulted from food allergy. Moreover, the frequent regularly recurring intensification of symptoms every two to eight weeks with preceding or associated increased nasal allergy suggesting infectious "colds" especially from early or late fall to late spring usually re-

sulted from food allergy at times associated with inhalant allergy. Then from mid-June to late August the asthma often was absent or definitely diminished when food allergy was the sole or major cause. The recurrence of exaggeration of nasal and bronchial allergy in the fall months because of activation of food allergy must be emphasized. Many patients must remain on their required elimination diet and especially our CFE diet during the fall, winter, and at times the early spring months for many years in order to control their bronchonasal allergy resulting from foods. A moderate number of these food-sensitive asthmatics, moreover, were greatly or entirely relieved in dry, inland areas (Chapt. 2).

It is necessary to emphasize, as shown in Table XVIII, that inhalant allergy always has to be considered. The perennial asthma, especially when persistent through the fall and winter months, requires thorough consideration of house dust, animal emanations, and miscellaneous inhalant allergies along with food allergy as possible causes, especially if strict, adequate use and manipulation of our CFE diet as advised in Chapter 3 do not yield the desired results. When asthma is not controlled by evironmental control and desensitization to indicated inhalants and if indicated with stock and especially autogenous dust antigens, failure to study and control food allergy as we advise often is responsible for failure to obtain satisfactory relief.

The importance of inhalant allergy is emphasized later in this chapter.

CASE HISTORIES

Case 43: A woman thirty-eight years of age had had bronchial asthma for twelve years, recurring from September to May for six years after "head colds" and constantly for six years except in July and August.

Perennial nasal allergy and polyps had occurred for years. Scratch tests were negative except for a few pollens. Examination showed diffuse bronchial asthma. Chest x-rays showed hyperinflation and depressed diaphragms. With treatment with our CFE diet, asthma was relieved in three weeks with no medications. Weight increased from 90 to 106 pounds in six months. Rice and corn caused asthma.

Objecting to the diet, she consulted another doctor for two years. All foods were eaten, and asthma continued. Weight fell to 82 pounds. Then she asked that we reorder her CFE diet. In two months she was doing all her housework and gained twenty-two pounds in six months.

Comment: The pathognomonic history of asthma resulting from food allergy was confirmed by excellent relief with our first treatment and again three years later. The relief depended on control of food allergy and on no desensitization or vaccine therapy.

BRONCHIAL ASTHMA IN PATIENTS OVER THE AGE OF FIFTY-FIVE

Our experience especially justifies the conclusion that food and inhalant allergies are the causes of practically all bronchial asthma in patients over the age of fifty-five years (Table XVIII) as they are in the younger groups. With this opinion Tuft, Kern, and others agree. This shows that patients over the age of forty or fifty, as we have emphasized since 1931 and especially in 1946, can develop or maintain sensitizations to foods and inhalants as in previous years. And why should they not so react, except when in a cachectic or debilitated state when anergy might occur? A contrary opinion is not justified because reacting bodies to inhalants and especially to foods are not demonstrated with skin tests or because test-negative diets fail to relieve asthma. Matsumura and co-workers have also shown decrease in serum antibodies but persisting allergy with aging. In older children over twice as many asthma patients failed to react to any allergens as in younger groups. Many of these patients proved to be food-sensitive. Food allergy, determined by

results of treatment, as a sole cause in 40 percent of this series and associated with inhalant, drug, and rarely if ever with bacterial allergies in 42 percent (Table XVIII) cannot rationally be doubted by any physician who has not used our CFE diet in the accurate and adequate manner for more than a few weeks in many patients as advised in this book and our other publications.

Likewise, inhalant allergies must receive open-minded study in this older group. The history often will suggest such allergy. The clinical significance of positive skin reactions and a history of possible inhalant allergy which occur less often in patients over the age of fifty-five years than in younger adults must be studied with strict environmental control and if necessary with desensitization therapy discussed below.

With this recognition and control of food and inhalant allergies, moreover, the present trend to attribute chronic bronchial asthma over the age of forty years to bacterial allergy or to vague intrinsic causes including emotional and psychosomatic influences as major causes will be reversed. Then these latter factors will assume their true role as activators of underlying atopic allergic causes, the control of which allows psychosomatic disturbances to occur without recurrence or definite exaggeration of bronchial asthma. With our advised control of bronchial asthma, true infectious colds can occur as in other ages without recurrence of asthma.

This control also accounts for our use of no long-term corticosteroid therapy to relieve bronchial asthma in children, in adults, and in the elderly, as reported later in this chapter. And it is responsible for the excellent or good relief of the symptoms of obstructive emphysema without continued use of intermittent positive pressure therapy, of bronchodilator drugs, and with little or no corticosteroids, as reported in Chapter 11.

Case Records

The following record illustrates food allergy as the cause of longstanding bronchial and nasal allergy in a patient sixty-one years of age treated for fifteen years unsuccessfully with vaccine, dust extracts, repeated antral washings, nasal surgery, and intranasal therapy. Two other records of asthma resulting from food allergy are summarized.

Case 44: A woman sixty-one years of age had had "colds" with wheezing, coughing, and expectoration lasting two to four weeks every one to three months from early fall to late spring for twenty-five years. Nasal congestion and postnasal mucus had been frequent.

Relief had failed from injections of dust, pollen, and vaccines every week for twenty years. Antral surgery and washings and removal of polyps had not helped.

Diet history revealed no idiosyncrasies to foods.

Skin tests were slightly positive to pollens, eggs, milk, and fish.

Treatment: Because of the recurrent asthma, decreased in the summer and failure of injectant therapy, food allergy was studied with our CFE diet. Relief occurred in three weeks and has continued. Symptoms recurred with cereal grains and milk in the fall to late spring.

Pollen and vaccine therapy was not given. Nasal polyps did not reform with strict adherence to the CFE diet to which other fruits and vegetables gradually were added.

Case 45: A man sixty-six years of age had had increasing tightness in the chest, coughing and some wheezing, nasal congestion, and postnasal mucus for five years with no previous nasobronchial symptoms. For one year asthma had continued daily from "sunset to sunrise" except in the summer. Hospitalization was necessary in February, March, and May.

His mother and two maternal uncles had asthma.

X-rays of lungs had indicated moderate emphysema.

Scratch tests with foods and inhalants were negative. Intradermal tests gave one to two plus reactions to pollen, dog, horse, and house-dust allergens.

Treatment: With our CFE diet and inhalation of 1:100 epinephrine, asthma was absent in three weeks, and light farm work was resumed. Relief has continued but requires the strict CFE diet in the fall, winter, and spring. Cereal grains and milk cause no asthma in the summer.

Comment: Onset of asthma in old age and inactivation of food allergy in the summer are illustrated in this case. No injections of inhalants or vaccines were given. Continued asthma rather than recurrent attacks with interim relief in the fall to late spring characterized his history.

Case 46: A woman sixty-six years of age had had "winter asthma" for four years in Ohio attributed to coal smoke. Desensitization to molds had failed. Moving to Berkeley, California, to avoid coal smoke also failed to relieve asthma. Milk exaggerated her asthma. Aspirin caused itching of hands and feet. Her uncle had asthma.

Skin testing revealed positive reactions to fall pollens and feathers and negative reactions to foods.

Treatment: With our CFE diet and potassium iodide, asthma was absent in two weeks. This relief continued for two weeks during a visit in Ohio in spite of coal smoke inhalation. Since then our CFE diet has been necessary to control asthma. Other foods were tolerated in the summer but not in the fall and winter. Desensitization to pollens has not been given.

DIAGNOSIS OF FOOD ALLERGY IN BRONCHIAL ASTHMA
History

The typical, in our opinion, pathognomonic history of bronchial asthma resulting from food allergy in children summarized in this chapter and especially in Chapters 2 and 25 indicates food allergy as the sole cause. The recurrent attacks every two to four weeks often with initial nasal allergy and fever suggesting an infectious cold but really resulting from food allergy and the relief between attacks and in the summer which history occurs in children especially after eighteen to twenty-four months may be less typical in infancy up to six to ten months. Then, as previously noted, croup or modified asthma and nasal symptoms often occur from food allergy for a few days every one to two weeks as discussed in Chapter 25.

This typical history may continue into adolescence and occasionally from twenty to 40 years, as already discussed.

In adult life and old age bronchial asthma resulting from food allergy produces more perennial symptoms with wheezing, coughing and shortness of breath nearly every day. Careful questioning, however, often reveals exaggeration of symptoms for a few days every two to four weeks, being the equivalent of the recurrent attacks in childhood resulting from food allergy. Any symptoms may decrease or be absent during the summer.

Thus all bronchial asthma which occurs in the fall, winter, and spring with or without a decrease in the summer requires study of food allergy. The exception is when asthma is definitely a result of animal emanations or environmental allergens, the removal of which definitely relieves the asthma. Such inhalant allergy of course may be associated with food allergy, as indicated in Table XVIII. Asthma resulting from food allergy in the fall and winter also may be associated with allergy to pollens as to mountain cedar and acacia in the winter and those which produce asthma in the late spring and summer. This prevents relief in the summer which would occur if food allergy were the only cause. Our routine plan of recording the history of bronchial asthma from the viewpoint of allergy is advised in later pages of this chapter and in Chapter 2.

Skin Testing for Food Allergy

As discussed in Chapter 2, scratch tests with food allergens along with those with inhalants are routine in our practice, although scratch tests often fail to reveal any or all foods causing clinical allergy. This is justified by large reactions which occur at times to foods which may cause immediate symptoms. Provocation tests to determine actual clinical allergy to such reacting foods, however, are necessary, as discussed in Chapter 2. Smaller reactions often are of no clinical value, being nonspecific or a result of past or potential allergy. Much chronic cumulative food allergy is not indicated by positive scratch tests. Since intradermal reactions to foods which have not occurred with the scratch method often are nonspecific, such tests are not done in our practice. Moreover, death has been reported from such intradermal tests (Chapt. 2).

If skin testing is not available or is of questionable value particularly when done in a commercial laboratory, indicated study of food allergy without skin testing with our CFE diet as advised in this chapter and Chapter 3 is important.

Other Tests for Food Allergy

Serum γ-globulin antibodies to milk, eggs and wheat have been reported in the last decade. Their diagnostic value, however, has become increasingly questionable in part because of their occurrence in the sera of nonallergic people. Moreover, γE globulin, not γG, γA, or γM globulins, seems to be the major form of the reagin responsible for the positive skin test and clinical allergy, according to Ishizaka.

The leukopenic index first reported by Vaughan and the pulse test of Coca are of questionable value in diagnosing cumulative or chronic food allergy (see Chapt. 2).

TEST-NEGATIVE DIET

In some patients total elimination of foods giving large scratch reactions and of those foods to which definite dislikes, known clinical allergy, or disagreements exist may gradually control some bronchial asthma and other manifestations of food allergy. Because of the fallibility of skin tests in determining clinical food allergy, however, such test-negative diets usually fail to control the allergic symptoms.

Though cow's milk is the most common allergenic food during life, allergy to other foods also usually occurs, except in early infancy before even traces of other foods are eaten. However, as suggested in Chapter 3, the complete elimination of milk and its products for three to four weeks, especially if there is a history of distaste, aversion, or disagreement to it, may initiate diet trial. In infants its entire substitution with soy milk or our meat-base formula as advised in Chapter 3 and especially in Chapter 25 is recommended.

ANTIBODIES TO STARCH (LIETZE)

About half of our food allergy patients' sera react strongly with starch in a radial immunodiffusion test. Starch allergy accounts for nasal and bronchial symptoms in some of our patients. A still larger portion of our emphysema patients' sera react in the starch test. These patients are relieved of bronchorrhea and bronchospasm by our CFE diet. On the basis of these findings we removed potato starch from the diet of one patient with asthma unrelieved by the CFE diet. Removal of starch from the elimination diet successfully relieved her asthma.

An extended discussion of serum anti-bodies to protein and starch by Arthur Lietze, Ph.D., is in Chapter 28.

STUDY AND CONTROL OF FOOD ALLERGY BY TRIAL DIETS

Because of the fallibility of the skin tests in determining clinical food allergy, diet trial with the exclusion of foods commonly productive of allergy must be used for the diagnosis of such allergy.

Though cow's milk is the most common allergenic food, allergy to other foods also usually occurs. However, as advised in Chapter 3, the complete elimination of milk and all of its products, especially if there is a history of dislike or disagreement to it, for at least three to four weeks may initiate diet trial.

Usually in practically all of our patients suspected of suffering from food allergy, allergy to other foods, especially cereal grains, eggs, chocolate, and other foods which less frequently cause food allergy, is studied with our CFE diet. This necessity of limiting the foods to those in the prescribed diet, of using our published menus and recipes, of maintaining nutrition and a desired weight, and of modifying the initial diet of allergy to foods in the diet is suspected by patient or physician is published in detail in Chapter 3. This chapter requires careful reading together with the accurate strict use of the CFE diet in several patients for more than two to three months to acquire success and efficiency in its use. Good results require strict adherence to these directions based on our successful use of this diet for forty years.

After relief is assured for two to three times as long as former relief, foods one by one can be added as advised in Chapter 3, eliminating any foods which reproduce symptoms. The method of adding such foods and the realization that resultant asthma may not occur in the summer or between attacks when refractoriness to food allergy may be present are discussed in Chapter 1.

The strict cooperation of the patient must be policed by the physician. The slightest deviations will prevent desired relief when food allergy is causative. Bakery products must be made by our recipes at home or by a trusted and regularly inspected baker, as emphasized in Chapter 3.

DIAGNOSIS AND CONTROL OF INHALANT ALLERGY

Inhalant allergy is indicated by the history of bronchial asthma, nasal or other manifestations of allergy arising during pollen seasons, or from inhalation of animal emanations, dusts, spores of fungi, or other airborne allergens. At times asthma from inhalants is not apparent in the initial history, especially if perennial or persistent asthma is present and skin reactions to inhalant allergens are slight or absent. It may become evident because of later evidence of inhalant allergy supported by the good results from specific desensitization to suspected inhalants and strict environmental control as advised in Chapter 3.

Though inhalant allergy has been the sole cause of bronchial asthma in our practice in from 3 to 75 percent, it has been associated with food allergy in approximately 42 to 53 percent of our cases except in young children and especially infants, as indicated in Table XVIII. In our patients pollen allergy as the sole cause occurred in only 3 percent of our children up to the age of five. It increased to 8 percent in children and to 25 percent in adults. Animal emanations including silk and other allergens in fabrics as the sole cause were infrequent in our patients, since few of them were on farms or in contact with many animals. Silk allergens from silk filters in vaccine occur, as reported by Coleman (1957) and Friedman *et al.* (1957). Associated with food and other inhalants, animal emanation allergy is more frequent.

It must be emphasized that asthma does occur at times to dogs, cats, horses, cattle, pigeons, parakeets, and other birds as the sole cause. This is indicated usually by skin reactions to the allergens and especially by the history. We have a few patients with asthma from deer dander or pigeon or other bird emanations alone. Also, asthma at times is attributed wrongly to animal emanation allergies, as in a veterinarian whose asthma had been attributed to such allergy rather than to unrecognized food allergy, the control of which with our CFE diet entirely relieved his asthma.

The frequency of pollen allergy as a sole cause would have increased if all moderate or brief asthma associated with severe hay fever had been included and especially if our practice had been in areas where ragweed is abundant. And if many more of our patients had lived where animals are frequent, as on farms or in various other occupations, asthma from their emanations as a sole cause would have been more common.

The role of house dust as a sole or associated cause of asthma in our opinion has been overemphasized because of the frequency of nonspecific reactions to house dust.

This opinion harmonizes with that of the Research Committee of the British Tubercular Association in 1968 that relief of asthma was no better with injections of aqueous extracts of house dust than with control solutions with or without environmental control of house dust. Assurance that allergy exists to pure house dust rather than to other inhaled allergens in the environment was difficult to establish. The as yet unconfirmed role of allergy to mites is discussed below.

When other inhalant and especially food allergies have been recognized and controlled, house dust alone as a cause of bronchial asthma rather than its other allergenic ingredients has decreased in the last twenty years since the statistics in Table XVIII were evaluated.

ALLERGY TO MITES

That allergies from mites in the house, especially in mattress or furniture dust, cause some clinical allergy attributed to house dust was first suggested by Voorhorst, Spieksma, *et al.* in Holland in 1967; confirmed by Maunsell *et al.* and Pepys *et al.* and Brown and Fler in England in 1968; confirmed by Miyamoto in 1967 in Japan; and confirmed by Mitchell, Woharton, *et al.* in 1969 in the United States. *Dermatophogoides, Deulinea,* and especially *D. pteringssimus* especially in mattresses and furniture dust are most common in Europe. Related *D. fascinae* was reported most common in Ohio. Though definite skin reactions to extracts of mites occur in patients reacting to house dust, clinical allergy especially in nasobronchial tissues to house dust by desensitization with allergens of mites awaits further confirmation. A comprehensive review article by van Bronswijk and Sinha has recently appeared (1971).

If such allergy exists, strict environmental control, as advised in Chapter 4, in a hospital room or with plastic covers on mattress, pillows, and furniture with desensitization to autogenous house dusts and to allergens of such mites should be remedial. Since the diet of these mites is reported to be human dander, strict per-

sonal cleanliness is also indicated.

That symptoms attributed to house dust in spite of strict environmental control may be relieved with study and control of definite or marked food allergy must be remembered.

TREATMENT OF FUNGUS ALLERGY

In our practice in Northern California and in a considerable number of other patients from other western states and fewer from other areas of the United States, asthma and other manifestations of clinical allergy from airborne fungi are less evident than is reported by some allergists in other areas. We have evidence of allergy to *Alternaria* especially in patients from our agricultural Central Valleys. Occasional asthma from fungi grown from dusts and molds in homes and especially basements has been supported by relief of asthma resulting from environmental reduction of molds and by desensitization with autogenous fungus extracts. Good results from treatment of bronchial asthma, however, have depended according to our analysis on desensitization with stock or autogenous antigens of fungi only in a few patients. It is our opinion that with the adequate study and control of inhalant allergy, especially to pollens and animal emanations and especially with our advised study of food allergy, indications of fungus allergy will be minimized. We agree with Vanselow (1968) that the value of desensitization to fungus allergens needs further evaluation. Desensitization to fungi along with that to pollens, dusts, and other inhalants in so-called "conventional antigens" too often is given for months or years with no relief of bronchial asthma or other manifestations of allergy in patients suffering with unrecognized food allergy alone.

Inhalant allergy resulting from miscellaneous inhalants including orris root, karaya, and other vegetable gums in hair-setting solutions; pyrethrum; glue dust; cottonseed; kapok; hay, grain and feed dusts; tobacco; and also allergic reactions to fly and insect venoms is discussed in Chapter 4 on nasal allergy.

SKIN TESTS WITH INHALANT ALLERGENS

When inhalant allergy is suspected, initial scratch tests with all important inhalant allergens in the patient's environment (Chapt. 2) which are possible causes of the patient's asthma should be done. In our practice we nearly always depend on scratch tests, realizing the fallibility and possible danger of intradermal tests. If intradermal tests are done, they should only be performed with inhalants that have given negative or slight reactions by the scratch tests. Too often intradermal reactions are nonspecific or not indicative of clinical allergy. They should never be done, moreover, with cottonseed, flaxseed, or glue or with dilutions of other inhalants stronger than 1:500 because of possible severe general reactions therefrom.

As with foods, all positive inhalant reactions do not indicate clinical allergy. An unquestioned history of clinical allergy or positive provocation inhalant tests with the reacting inhalants must determine their allergenicity. Thus reactions to tree, grass, and fall pollens may occur in a patient allergic only to fall pollens.

TREATMENT OF INHALANT ALLERGIES

Environmental control in the home or working environments as advised in Chapter 18 often relieves allergy to animal emanations, dust, silk, or miscellaneous inhalants. Efficient control of pollen, dust, and other inhalant allergens, according to detailed advice in Chapter 30, and if necessary air filtrating mechanisms may reduce or control resultant allergic symptoms.

When elimination of inhalant allergens is impossible, desensitization with antigens containing the responsible inhalants is indicated. The success of such therapy depends on the amount of the allergenic inhalant that is in the air. Thus desensitization to black walnut, olive, or cedar pollens in patients who live under or in groves of such trees which produce clouds of pollens may only give partial relief. Continued perennial desensitization with maximum tolerated dilutions for two to three years may produce desired protection. Moving away during the pollination of such trees may be required, especially during the first year of desensitization.

Though desensitization to emanations of animals in patients who constantly care for them often is successful with large tolerated doses repeated weekly for two to three years, it may be unsatisfactory. We have desensitized milkers allergic to cow emanations and veterinarians and those in constant contact with animals in occupations and home who are allergic to horse, cat, dog, or other animal dander.

Initial onset of asthma or other manifestations of allergy after moving into a house requires study of allergy to emanations of animal pets or other environmental allergens in the house even though skin reactions are absent. This was recently emphasized by the relief of severe asthma in a new residence by the removal of all dusts containing emanations of cats formerly in the house, as advised on page 87, and by continued desensitization to a cat dander as advised to control pollen allergy on page 82.

The preparation of antigens containing inhalants and the method of their administration to produce desensitization, advised in Chapter 30, are amplified in our book *Bronchial Asthma—Its Diagnosis and Treatment*, 1963, and in our current textbooks.

The importance of the control of inhalant allergy is discussed in Chapter 4 of this volume.

INFECTANT ASTHMA

Evidence of infectant asthma in our practice and in our clinic has steadily decreased to a minimum in the last thirty-five years. As we have reported in our texts and medical journal articles, especially in the *JAMA* in 1959, the nasal symptoms and fever even up to 104 F which often occur before and during recurrent attacks of bronchial asthma in children and less often in young and older adults are due to activation of food allergy rather than to infectious colds, as we have emphasized previously. The fever which occurs in these first one to two days of the attacks in about 50 percent of the cases, as shown in Table XLIII, is nearly always due to sudden activation of allergy to foods, as is fever which arises from allergy to drugs and sera as confirmed by us for thirty-five years. When inhalant and especially food allergy is adequately studied and controlled in patients with perennial bronchial asthma, chronic bronchitis, and in obstructive emphysema (Chapt. 11) at times along with temporary corticosteroid therapy, the symptoms often are controlled without any evidence that infectant or intrinsic causes are major factors. We have used no stock or autogenous vaccines to control chronic bronchial asthma or nasal allergy for over forty years. Vaccines are only used to raise immunity to adenoviruses or respiratory bacteria,

hoping to prevent actual infectious colds.

Though infection superimposed on bronchial asthma may require antibiotics, failure of such medication alone to control recurrent bronchial asthma or chronic bronchitis helps to rule out infection as the sole cause.

The reported association of infection in most asthma either as a complication or a cause will be less apparent and usually absent if atopic allergy to inhalants and especially to foods is studied and controlled as advised in this volume as it has been by us for many years in our office and hospital, necessarily in cooperating patients.

The conclusion of other allergists, most recently in 1969 and 1970, that infectant asthma resulting from assumed increased susceptibility to infection is the cause of recurrent attacks of asthma, especially in childhood, because of gradual reduction of such attacks while stock vaccine is given every one to two weeks for two to even five to six years with the reported disappearance of attacks in only 25 to 60 percent of cases is unjustified unless the study and control of food allergy as we advise has been done in a strict and adequate manner and has failed to relieve the asthma. Excellent relief of attacks reported by us in 50 infants and children in 1959 and in 130 cases in 1967 with the control of food allergy as we advise with no desensitization or vaccine therapy is evidence against infectant allergy as the cause of the asthma. We have many children whose attacks have continued every two to six weeks for one to six years. Their attacks have necessitated frequent previous hospitalization often with the incorrect diagnosis of bronchopneumonia despite the continued administration of stock vaccines with or without attempted desensitization to inhalants, whose attacks have been controlled in one or two months with strict adherence to our CFE diet with no desensitization to inhalants, vaccine therapy, or continued medication. This control has also eliminated worry of parents, frequent hospitalizations, expense of medical and drug therapy, change of climate, parentectomy, prolonged sanitarium care and treatment, and of great importance, long-term corticosteroid therapy. Study and control of food as well as inhalant allergy with our CFE diet advised in Chapter 3 should be routine in all adults and children with perennial asthma especially when recurrent and activated in the fall to late spring. Such study is mandatory in children, as more fully discussed in Chapter 25.

Perennial asthma or chronic bronchitis in adults including those in old age moreover cannot be attributed to infection, intrinsic or psychosomatic causes because of negative skin reactions to inhalants and foods, or failure of empiric desensitization with "conventional inhalant antigens" without adequate study and control of inhalant allergy. In some of these patients pollen allergy in the pollen seasons also must be recognized and treated, and environmental allergy in the home or working environments must be controlled, especially in the fall to late spring. But many cases of asthma formerly attributed to infectant causes, especially when asthma is decreased or absent in the summer, in our opinion are due to unrecognized and uncontrolled food allergy alone.

PSYCHOLOGICAL INFLUENCES IN BRONCHIAL ASTHMA

Uncontrolled recurrent or perennial bronchial asthma in spite of continued manipulation of the diet, environmental control, desensitization, vaccine therapy, and the gamut of drugs, even corticosteroids, at times with changes of climate and recurrent or prolonged hospital or sanitarium residence results in discouragement, depression, and at times frustration in parents and relatives. This occurs especially from the resultant interference in home, occupational, educational, and recreational activities and when semiinvalidism results. The resultant concern and increased frustration of parents and their constant effort to understand and relieve the causes of recurrent and often invaliding bronchial asthma in their children are interpreted by some psychologists to overprotection or even parental rejection which increases the child's symptoms.

Though these psychological problems and disturbances in personality have existed in some of our adults and their families and in some children and their parents when we have first seen them, the relief of the asthma in the very large majority with our study and control of inhalant and especially of food allergy which too often has received inadequate or unfortunately no previous attention gradually eliminates the mental disturbances in patients and relatives. As the parents realize that the severe recurrent attacks, with or without interim symptoms, are controlled with strict elimination of allergenic foods and/or with the control of inhalant allergy, they no longer feel that their "child is different." Parents and children are relieved of their apprehension and anxiety which had resulted from the uncontrolled asthma. Parentectomy and separation of the child from the family for one or two years therefore should not be done unless adequate study of food allergy, especially with the CFE diet and/or proper control of inhalant allergy, has been carried out as advised in this volume and in our book *Bronchial Asthma—Its Diagnosis and Treatment*, 1963. Beneficial effects ascribed to parentectomy may often be due to change of climate only. With our control, especially of food allergy, sanitarium care has not been necessary in any of our children when their cooperation and that of the parents have been adequate.

We agree with Dubo, McLean, and Sheldon from their evaluation of eighty-one unselected children with chronic asthma that there is no stereotyped "asthmatic personality" and that overprotectiveness by the mother is not a general finding. Other conclusions from this study minimize the psychological aspects of bronchial asthma which have steadily decreased in our patients with the antiallergic control and minimal adjunctive drug therapy when necessary, as discussed in this volume. In our opinion, moreover, asthmatic children rarely if ever intentionally wheeze to relieve emotions or to gain affection or concern of parents, relatives, or nurses.

Irritability, restlessness, nightmares, incorrigibility, tantrums, listlessness, fatigue, difficulty in concentration and in school work, and other symptoms in the syndrome of allergic toxemia and fatigue (this is discussed extensively in Chapt. 19) which we have reported in the literature for thirty years may be associated with bronchial asthma and are relieved with the control of inhalant and especially of food allergy. Occasionally an epileptic equivalent has to be recognized and controlled with Dilantin or a similar drug. The relief of character and personality changes by the control of causative food allergies, as we have reported since 1932, received important support by Clarke in 1939, as summarized in Chapter 16.

INTRINSIC ASTHMA

This diagnosis has been made by some allergists, especially by Rackemann, when an evident family history of clinical allergy and definite skin reactions to inhalant or food allergens are absent or when attempted control of possible food or inhalant allergy and even of assumed bacterial sensitization has not relieved the asthma. Some unrecognized allergy possibly from hidden infection or the results of metabolic, endocrine, or some obscure inherent factor or chronic disease also has been fruitlessly considered. The diagnosis therefore is indicative of uncertainty and is a preferred explanation based on pure assumption.

In our practice these unrelieved cases have gradually decreased in the last three decades as our control of inhalant and especially of food allergies has improved. In these patients previous or associated "recurrent or chronic bronchitis or sinusitis" has frequently been relieved with the control of the causative allergies, especially to foods.

Thus asthma of this type, especially in adults and old people, must not be relegated to intrinsic or unknown causes but must challenge the physician and especially the allergists with continued investigation and study, hoping to relieve the antigen-antibody reaction which it must be assumed is responsible.

SECONDARY FACTORS

It has long been apparent that bronchial asthma in particular, nasal allergy, and to a lesser extent other manifestations of allergy are exaggerated by but not primarily due to so-called nonspecific factors. Dusts of all types, especially in inhalant-sensitive patients, may exaggerate symptoms, even when specific allergy to them is absent. Odors, smokes, and chemical fumes, especially from burning sulphur, formaldehyde, paints, lacquers, varnishes, and refrigerating chemicals, exaggerate uncontrolled or activated subclinical allergy. This is in addition to the actual petrochemical allergies which may exist. Changes in temperature, weather, humidity, and wind may be such causes. The detrimental effect of the fall, winter, and early spring; proximity to the ocean; or in some patients residence in low inland areas in river basins or near large bodies of fresh water on food allergy has long been reported by us.

At times the inhalation of fumes, dirt, and smoke has been the assumed cause of bronchial asthma which is entirely relieved with control of allergy, especially to foods.

The exaggeration of asthma by acute or chronic nasal and bronchial infections is generally reported. That such infectant allergy, however, is a rare allergic cause of bronchial asthma and that "colds" and infective diseases will not cause its symptoms when the usually overlooked food and less often inhalant allergies are controlled has been emphasized above and throughout this volume. Moreover, the mistake must not be made of attributing "colds" preceding recurrent attacks of bronchial asthma, especially in children, to infection rather than to the activation of food allergy which is responsible for such attacks.

Bronchial asthma recurring before or during menstrual periods is usually due in our opinion to activation of food and possibly inhalant allergy which causes no interim symptoms. Such asthma before or during periods is often controlled when atopic allergy, especially to foods, is recognized and relieved. Bronchial asthma and other manifestations of allergy may disappear after the first weeks of pregnancy, probably because of increased corticoids from pituitary stimulation. Anergy especially to food allergy arising during pregnancy also is a possible explanation. Asthma or another allergic manifestation reappears with the culmination of pregnancy. It may occur during pregnancy from some food

eaten only then or in excess. Thus asthma during pregnancy in one woman was due to milk taken only during gestation.

UNRELIEVED BRONCHIAL ASTHMA

Valuable information about today's available beneficial therapy of bronchial asthma resides in the statistics of our 325 patients unrelieved during the seven-year period before 1948 when 1491 cooperating patients received good or excellent results from our treatment in those years before corticosteroids and ACTH were generally available. That such results can be obtained without these hormones needs recognition and emphasis because of their unfortunate and increasing present use in bronchial asthma. As emphasized in this volume, they should never be used except in intractable or severe asthma unless persistent, experienced, and adequate study and attempted control of inhalant and especially of the usually unrecognized food allergy, as we advise, and the infrequent drug and very rare bacterial allergies are steadfastly continued in order to eliminate their use entirely. In those few patients whose asthma is not satisfactorily controlled with such persistent control of the probable allergic causes, relief of symptoms with ephedrine, aminophylline, and epinephrine hypodermically and by inhalation and other similar drugs should be accepted rather than surrendering to the relief of the continued use of corticosteroids.

Thus during this seven-year period 1491 cases of bronchial asthma were well controlled with our therapy and without hormones except briefly in a limited number. Of the 325 additional cases only 7 percent gave good cooperation and only 7 percent cooperated for more than six months. Though treatment based on complete history, physical examination, x-ray, laboratory tests, and skin tests was immediately advised, 40 percent of the patients failed to report after the initial visit though there was evidence that some of them did follow the diet with benefit. Brief cooperation for only four weeks occurred in 27 percent of the 325 patients and for only one to three months in 15 percent, a minimum of six months being required before reporting good results.

It is obvious that excellent cooperation during the four seasons for even one year would have greatly reduced this number of unrelieved patients. Today many of them undoubtedly have received and are probably conditioned, unfortunately, to corticoids given by other physicians with their potential harmful effects and future bodily impairments which will be increasingly apparent with continued use.

Because of the increasing realization of the many complications and dangers of continued use of corticoids and ACTH, even in small doses, they should never be used except briefly in status asthmaticus, very severe asthma, and in small doses in some patients with obstructive emphysema, as noted in Chapter 11, or other chronic allergy. Realization of these dangers is important because of the increased use of these hormones by physicians, especially in the control of bronchial asthma, as advised unfortunately by many medical contributions and particularly by unwarranted claims in advertisements of the many commercial pharmaceutical companies with little or no warning about possible complications and no emphasis on the adequate and strict study and control of inhalant, occasional drug, and especially of food allergy as we advise. This long use of corticoids is rarely preceded or accompanied by any experienced study and indicated control of the allergies, as we advise, which would make the hormones unnecessary.

It must be emphasized that the recurrent noninvaliding symptoms of bronchial asthma during exercise, in the early morning, or on arising should be controlled with ephedrine, aminophylline, epinephrine by inhalation or hypodermically, or other therapy and by the continued study and control of the causative as yet unrecognized inhalant and especially food allergies and not with continued corticoids or ACTH therapy.

The conditioning of the asthmatic to corticoids is illustrated in the following case:

Case 47: A woman fifty-three years of age was relieved of perennial bronchial asthma of ten years' duration with our CFE diet and the decreasing use of aminophylline, ephedrine, and potassium iodide. This relief continued for three months with strict adherence to her diet. Being free of asthma, she journeyed to Denmark to visit relatives, where her diet was stopped and severe asthma recurred. In the hospital she was given ACTH and corticoids. During the last three years severe asthma has recurred when 4 to 8 mg of triamcinolone have not been taken in spite of her strict adherence to the diet which had given her the initial excellent relief.

TABLE XIX

UNRELIEVED BRONCHIAL ASTHMA IN 325 PATIENTS STUDIED
DURING THE 7-YEAR PERIOD BEFORE 1948 WHEN THE
1491 RELIEVED PATIENTS WERE TREATED

	0-15 Yrs	15-55 Yrs	55 Yrs Up	Total Pts
Number of patients	61	202	173	325
Good cooperation	7	15	7	29 (9%)
Poor cooperation	54	187	55	296 (91%)
Time of treatment				
None	31	73	25	129 (40%)
1 to 4 weeks	17	54	17	88 (27%)
1 to 3 months	1	37	13	51 (16%)
3 to 6 months	2	28	4	34 (10%)
6 to 12 months	10	20	3	23 (7%)

DRUG ALLERGY

Drug allergy produces bronchial asthma infrequently compared to the many cutaneous, joint, hepatic, and gastrointestinal manifestations and fever arising therefrom. This clinical allergy is explained by the union of the drug or chemical with a body protein or hapten to the combination of which a specific antibody forms and persists in the body. Thereafter the entrance of the drug into the body results in an allergic reaction, occurring often to a minute amount and at times immediately to a severe degree. It is a much less frequent cause of bronchial asthma than foods and inhalants. Every history therefore must record any suggestion of asthma or other allergic manifestations and any drugs, hormones, or antibiotics recently administered or given in former years to which sensitization may have developed.

Of all drugs acetylsalicylic acid or aspirin most frequently causes bronchial asthma, as reported by Prickman and Buckstein, by Friedlaender and Feinberg, and others. This has been reported in approximately 3 to 5 percent of young and especially older asthmatics. Allergy to aspirin, it must be remembered, also causes urticaria, localized edema, gastrointestinal symptoms including gastric bleeding, and less frequently other allergic symptoms. Though such asthma usually is moderate, it may be severe and even fatal. Therefore it is good to suspect aspirin sensitivity in allergic patients, especially in asthmatics, and to prescribe 1 grain followed by 2 to 3 grains in an hour or so to determine whether any possible sensitization occurs from such small doses before giving large consecutive amounts. If it exists, the patient must never take any medication containing aspirin, remembering its inclusion in practically all remedies for pain, headache, and arthritis.

Other pain-relieving drugs including sodium salicylate, para-aminosalicylic acid, antipyrine, phenylbutazone, acetophenetidin and acetanilid, and especially amidophyrine produce varying manifestations of allergy but rarely bronchial asthma. Severe asthma developed in one hour after oral Orinase three different times in a man sixty-eight years of age who had bronchial asthma and bronchitis relieved by our control of food allergy.

Increasing realization of the frequency of clinical allergy from penicillin must restrict its administration to the control of infections resulting from pneumococci, streptococci, syphilis, gonorrhea, and other pathogens requiring its use. When its use is advisable, it should be given with great caution, especially if there is a previous history of definite clinical allergy.

Sudden unpredictable fatalities from anaphylactic shock, including bronchial spasm from the parenteral and also the oral administration of penicillin, even of the new penicillins wrongly heralded as nonallergic, are the chief deterrents to its use. Moreover, the development of clinical allergy seven to twenty days after its administration during which time sensitization and other symptoms and fever occur, as in the serum sickness of Von Pirquet and Schick, is frequent. When the common urticaria and angioneurotic edema with severe pruritus are the main results, they often persist for weeks or even months until all traces of the penicillin disappear from the body and all traces of it are eliminated from the patient's foods, such as nearly all commercial milk and its products.

Thus the administration of any penicillin is open to criticism unless other antibiotics or even sulfonamides have failed to control infections. This is especially true in the treatment of respiratory infections which occasionally complicate bronchial asthma except when penicillin is indicated in pneumococcal or streptococcal infections as demonstrated by sensitivity tests or cultured bacteria. Since infectant asthma in our experience is rare, antibiotics and especially penicillin should not be given routinely when attacks of asthma occur. The allergic causes should be controlled as we advise. If a complicating or associated infection is definitely demonstrated, antibiotics other than penicillin are advisable for a limited time.

The intramuscular injection of penicillin even in the first months of life because of moderate nasal or bronchial symptoms and fever and often with slight or no fever is especially unjustifiable because of the possible resultant sensitization or development of severe or even fatal clinical allergy. For definite infection it should not replace a broad-based antibiotic by mouth.

Opinions vary about the value of skin testing in determining allergy to penicillin. Collins-Williams and Vincent and Berger and Eisen obtained little help. Matheson, according to Glaser, found positive reactions when the immediate serious allergy was present and negative tests in the delayed type. Harris and Vaughan also reported such negative reactions, indicating that the skin sensitizing antibody was not responsible for the allergy to penicillin and also the limitations of skin testing in the diagnosis of clinical allergy.

Kern and Wimberly advised testing with a fresh dilution of 10,000 units in 1 cc first by the scratch method and then conjunctively. If both are negative, 0.02 cc of this sterile dilution can be injected intradermally. If these tests are positive, oral or parenteral penicillin is inadvisable. If an infection such as streptococcal, pneumococcal, or luetic requires penicillin, its careful and

gradual increase with preliminary and concomitant corticoid therapy may be justified.

Asthma and other clinical allergy also arising from streptomycin would be more apparent if it were in greater use. Fortunately such allergy to other mycin drugs is rare and apparently is never serious. Clinical allergy to animal serum and biologics is discussed in our book on asthma in 1963.

Alexander has listed reports of rare and usually moderate asthma from acacia, karaya, and tragacanth gums; fish oils; chlorotetracycline (Aureomycin®); diphenhydramine hydrochloride (Benadryl®); cocaine; dehydrochloric acid (Decholin®); meperidine hydrochloride (Demerol®); digitalis; fennel; heparin; ipecac; liver extract; mercurials; chymotrypsin; pancreatin; papaine; para-aminosalicylic acid; penicillin; propophyllin; pyromen quinine; sesame seeds; stramonium; sulfacyanates; sulfonamides; malt extract (Taka-Diastase®); tannic acid; thiamine; tragacanth, viomycin sulphate, and frequently from castor bean gums and its oils. Fatal anaphylactic and more frequent severe reactions have been reported to sulfobromophthalein sodium by Venger.

We have observed severe bronchial asthma from Orinase when taken after it had been discontinued for two months.

The claim that refining vegetable oils removes all allergens is not proven and is exemplified by asthma and other allergic symptoms which resulted in patients we have studied who have developed asthma and other allergic symptoms after the ingestion of cottonseed oil. Recent biochemical research is demonstrating the existence of many different lipids, all of which are oil-soluble.

Allergic shock with asthma was reported to cocaine by Waldbott and to procaine

0.3 to 0.5 percent of patients to whom it is given. Death may occur, as reported by Unger and Unger. Because of this and its more rapid action and also because of the absence of reports of asthma and shock especially with intramuscular and intravenous administration of corticoids, they are used in our practice instead of ACTH. Fatal asthma was reported by Maunsell, Pearson *et al.* after parenteral ACTH. Further justification for the use of corticoids is the evidence that ACTH is not necessary to activate adrenal function when it is decreased by previous corticoid therapy.

Severe allergic reactions to trypsin and its questionable mucolytic effect contraindicate its use in bronchial asthma.

Asthma From Animal Sera

Asthma with or without anaphylactic shock and even death occurs with the first injection of animal serum, especially of the horse, when there is an inherited or natural "sensitivity." For this and other reasons, intradermal testing is never done on a patient who gives a positive reaction to horse serum by the scratch method. Deaths after the intradermal testing with horse serum were recently emphasized by a death from a 1:10 dilution reported in the *Journal of the American Medical Association*. Previous scratch and ocular tests would have contraindicated such intradermal injection. The outstanding discussion by Ratner of the anaphylactic and serum sickness type of reaction and the serious involvement of the nervous tissues from serum allergy must be remembered.

Therefore, immunization of everyone to tetanus toxoid every three to four years is imperative so that a booster injection of tetanus toxoid rather than tetanus antitoxin will suffice to stimulate immunity when penetrating wounds occur. This is especially important in allergic patients and par-

ticularly in those who have any suggestion of allergy to animal emanations. Serum allergy also develops when horse or other animal sera are given for the rare diphtheria of today where immunity has not been established by previous injections of diphtheria toxoid. It also occurs when animal serum is given to control botulism. Antipneumonic sera used over twenty years ago has been replaced by antibiotics. Sensitization to horse serum may arise from ingestion of horse meat or mare's milk.

Asthma and clinical allergy from tetanus and diphtheria toxoid, clinical allergy from transfusions, and tetanus prophylaxis are discussed in this chapter.

DEATH IN BRONCHIAL ASTHMA

Death in bronchial asthma has usually occurred in intractable cases, though it has resulted during anaphylaxis from injections of antigens, sera, drugs (especially aspirin), and as recently noted by Pearson in England from an anaphylactic reaction to ACTH. Messer, Peters, and Bennett discussed 304 deaths in asthmatics at the Mayo Clinic in a forty-year period. Of these 11.3 percent died in status asthmaticus and 10.4 percent from complications of asthma. The remaining 78 percent died of causes other than asthma. Williams and Leopold recently reported 101 patients who died during status asthmaticus. Two thirds were females. Ninety percent had asthma for over ten years. Necropsies were done in fifty-four cases.

Death in bronchial asthma in recent years is less frequent than in previous decades because of the increasing recognition of its allergic causes, the realization of the danger of sedation (especially with opiates and even with moderate amounts of barbitals), the use of antibiotics and corticoids when indicated, and the better treatment of intractable asthma as advised in this volume.

During the seven-year period when our 1491 well-controlled asthmatics were treated from 1940 to 1948, death occurred in eight patients, three of whom were seen in consultation. Since 1948 only one death resulting from intractable asthma has occurred in our cooperating patients.

Death also occurred in the following patients who were seen in consultation and had not been studied and controlled especially for probable food allergy as we advise.

Sedation with opiates, barbitals, and in one case with paraldehyde by mouth and rectum had been given in seven patients without our advice. Two of these patients seen in consultation expired in two days from cerebral paralysis occurring in coma because of anoxia from intractable asthma for relief of which morphine had been administered. One patient with severe asthma was seen in consultation because of pneumothorax which resulted a few hours later in sudden death. Death occurred in another patient addicted to opiates who refused to cooperate in any antiallergic treatment. Another patient died of cardiac failure in a prolonged attack of asthma. Death occurred in four of these patients after discontinuance of our CFE diet which had previously controlled their asthma. Three of these were being treated by other physicians and received sedatives before death. One developed asthma on a vacation after a break in her diet. Barbitals given by another physician had produced anoxia and cerebral paralysis before she returned to our care in the hospital. This irreversible cerebral paralysis which results in three to four minutes of anoxia with cyanosis was also operative in three of the other

deaths when sedation had been administered.

It is probable in our opinion that treatment advised in this chapter for intractable asthma would have prevented the moribund state in several of Leonhardt's patients reported in 1961. Adequate hydration with 5 percent invert sugar and not 5 percent glucose (see page 468) and the disuse of all sedation and adequate doses of corticoids and antibiotics which were not reported in his records along with other therapy advised in this chapter which have relieved intractable asthma and prevented death except in one patient in the last fourteen years in our practice might have been beneficial. We disagree particularly with sedation in the treatment of bronchial asthma as with phenothiazine derivatives, chloral hydrate, barbitures, and paraldehyde, which had been given in his first case.

This infrequency of fatalities in our practice has largely depended moreover on our strict control of existent inhalant and especially of food allergy as advised in this volume, on the elimination of all sedation, and on the necessary cooperation of patients.

The increase of fatal asthma reported by Speizer *et al.* in 1968, by Barach and Segal in 1968, by Shannon *et al.* in 1968, by Pearson in 1968, and by Palm *et al.* in 1969 has not occurred in our practice in the last fifteen years.

The 100 percent increase in deaths in asthma in England and Wales reported in 1969 was attributed largely to overuse of bronchodilator drugs and insufficient corticosteroids and by Inman and Adelsyein in 1969 to overuse of pressurized aerosols. Since deaths from bronchial asthma have markedly decreased in our patients and since no long-term corticosteroid therapy, no IPP, and little or no hand-operated adrenergic aerosol therapy has been given, we opine that our strict study and control of food allergy in all cases of severe and especially perennial bronchial asthma best explains our excellent results. Contraindications and dangers of long-term IPP therapy receive emphasis in Chapter 30. Evidence of such study with our CFE diet or its modifications as advised in this volume is not found in any of these reports of increasing morbidity and deaths.

We emphasize again the great importance of study and control of food allergy as advised in this volume, in our book on bronchial asthma in 1963, and in our several articles on bronchial asthma in the last thirty years along with control of inhalant (especially pollen and drug) allergies which has been responsible for our decreased morbidity and minimal mortality. Along with such control of food allergy, the use of little or no corticosteroid therapy, the use of no aerosol intermittent positive pressure therapy and minimal inhalation adrenergic drugs only by the hand atomizer, the use of no sedation therapy in asthma (especially in severe asthma or status asthmaticus) are added reasons that are responsible for no increase in occasional fatalities which we have long reported in our books and published articles. Of all these reasons our strict study of possible food allergy in all perennial asthma as well as in chronic bronchitis and obstructive lung disease must be emphasized, especially because of the absence of acceptable evidence in publications of other students of its adequate study and control as we have long advised.

COMPLICATIONS, SEQUELAE, AND ASSOCIATED MANIFESTATIONS OF BRONCHIAL ASTHMA WHICH REQUIRE CONTROL OF ALLERGY AND OTHER THERAPY

1. Obstructive emphysema arises most frequently from perennial allergy—all-year-round inhalant and especially from uncontrolled food allergy—continuing for many years. That such atopic allergy to foods with or without inhalant allergy is the best explanation for shortness of breath arising from bronchospasm as well as of resultant destructive changes in the capillaries and other tissues in the alveoli and adjoining areas is discussed in Chapter 11.

When the bronchial airways including the terminal bronchioles are obstructed by mucosal edema and especially by bronchospasm and by mucus from allergy in the mucosa during severe recurrent attacks of asthma, especially those resulting from food allergy, with subsequent interim relief between the attacks, the emphysema is temporarily relieved with no resultant irreversible destruction. But when asthma persists because of failure to recognize and control the atopic allergy, particularly to foods, and in spite of bronchodilating medications including adrenergic intermittent positive pressure therapy, the destructive changes from the progressive and increasingly invaliding obstructive emphysema occur.

As emphasized in Chapter 11, progression of these destructive changes and the resultant morbidity and too often mortality have been prevented by our control of atopic allergy, especially to foods, with little or no adjunctive therapy, always in necessarily cooperative patients, as advised in Chapter 3.

2. With control of atopic allergy as advised above, the bony deformities of the chest from longstanding bronchial asthma

and resultant emphysema, especially in children and adolescents, will not occur, or if established, will be prevented from their usual progression, providing the control of atopic and possible secondary infection is maintained in the cooperating patient.

3. With unrecognized, progressive emphysema destructive changes in the alveoli and adjacent tissues cause bullae formation in the lungs as well as air-containing blebs under the pleura, rupture of which causes pneumothorax or even massive collapse.

4. Subcutaneous emphysema is infrequent in severe asthma, as reported by Sheldon and others. Rupture of the superficial air blebs permits air to pass into the tissues of the mediastinum and even into the tissues of the face and upper back. Crepitations are revealed by palpation and evidenced by auscultation. Atelectasis occurs in small or larger areas or an entire lobe from blocking of its airway by edema and occluding mucus, resulting from uncontrolled food allergy with or without inhalant or drug allergy. Friedman and Molony reported six cases requiring bronchoscopic aspiration plus antibiotics for relief.

5. Prickman and others have reported bronchostenosis resulting from localized narrowing from allergic inflammation with or without infection in a bronchus and not because of plugging of mucus alone. Suppressed breath sounds, fremitus, and increased x-ray translucency are diagnostic.

Mucoid impaction of the bronchi with a V-shaped x-ray shadow, its vertex pointed to the hilum, or with a cluster of grapes reported by Greer may require surgery to remove the obstruction and diseased tissues. Our control of allergy, especially to foods, as advised in this chapter and in Chapter 3, would be important to establish or continue.

6. Massive collapse because of complete blocking of a bronchus is serious but uncommon. Death may occur, as reported by Clarke, Maxwell, and others. This requires advice of a chest surgeon along with continued control of allergies as advised in this volume.

7. Spontaneous pneumothorax is uncommon but dangerous, occurring in patients with perennial asthma associated with emphysema. Large ruptures of vesicles extending through the pleura cause sudden severe pain, dyspnea, and even death. Small openings cause increasing pneumothorax. Favorable results as reported by Clarke and by Faulkner and Wagner and hoped for recovery by Elliot occur.

8. Bronchiectasis usually develops from uncontrolled bronchial asthma in children as a result of food allergy and at times inhalant allergy. This has been emphasized in Chapter 10, in which the important control of allergy, particularly to foods, and other advised therapeutic procedures are summarized.

Pulmonary fibrosis may occur with bronchiectasis or with chronic bronchitis as reported in Chapter 9.

When continued fever, purulent sputum, and bronchial cough persist, antibiotics selected by tests of cultured sputum are important. Bronchopneumonia must be recognized and correctly controlled.

9. Chronic bronchitis causing cough and expectoration with or without wheezing is usually due to atopic allergy. When the symptoms are perennial or exaggerated during the fall, winter, and early spring months, food allergy and to a lesser extent environmental inhalant allergy are responsible. When fever is present, secondary infection must be recognized and controlled.

10. Nasal allergy, as discussed in Chapter 12, is usually due to the same atopic

causes as is the concomitant bronchial asthma. When perennial and especially when exaggerated in the fall and winter months, food allergy with or without environmental allergens must be studied and controlled. When fever and purulent sputum or discharge from the sinuses occur, antibiotics are required.

Haziness or opacity in x-rays of the nasal sinuses is practically always due to allergies that are responsible for the asthma. In 1491 of our asthmatics relieved by antiallergic control, nasal allergy occurred in 78 *percent.* This caused the boggy, pale nasal mucosa at times with enlarged turbinates and nasal polyps as discussed below.

Our realization that these findings are due to allergy and not infection has prevented the Luc-Caldwell operations on the antra with their radical exenteration, as advised especially by Grove, for the control of bronchial asthma. If relief of asthma occurs from such surgery, it is temporary and disappointing, as reported by many allergists, especially by Rackemann and Wille, Schenck and Kern, Piness and Miller, Agar and Cazort, Unger, and others. There is a general agreement with the opinion of Lewis, written in 1934 as follows: "In my opinion of all the affections in the human organism where surgery has been not only the least beneficial but in addition largely harmful, allergic vasomotor and hyperplastic affections of the nose have been the most outstanding. Especially and positively is this so where radical operations upon the sinuses in addition have been done." There is no justified evidence, moreover, that infection in the sinuses is a frequent complication and especially a cause of bronchial asthma in children. The failure of relief of bronchial asthma from operations on the sinuses and in the nose itself adds support to our con-

clusion and that of many other allergists that infectant asthma is rare.

Surgery on any sinus in which chronic purulent infection is present, as indicated by associated pain, fever, leukocytosis, and increased polymorphonuclear leukocytes, may be required if conservative irrigations of the sinuses and antibacterial therapy are not effective. Unless such infection is very probable, however, washing of the antra because of hazy or opaque findings revealed by x-ray or transillumination is not justifiable. Possible introduction of pathogenic bacteria into the sinuses may have resulted in purulent sinusitis.

11. Mucous polyps may develop in the nose and maxillary sinuses when nasal allergy with or without bronchial asthma occurs. They may be single or multiple, varying in size, at times obstructing one or both nasal passages. They usually contain eosinophiles. They arise in the nasal mucosa, especially under the turbinates. Originating in the antra, they may be confined therein or may project through the foramen, resulting at times in pedunculated polyps obstructing the nasal cavity. They may also develop in the ethmoids, projecting into the nasal passages. Kern and Schenck especially emphasized their occurrence only in allergic patients. Hansel expressed the opinion of allergists that antiallergic study and control should precede or at least be concomitant with their surgical removal. Without such allergic therapy, these polyps nearly always recur in a few weeks to months according to the degree of the persistent allergy.

Our study and treatment of patients with nasal polyps, as stated in Chapter 12, have long indicated that food allergy in contrast to inhalant allergy is the usual cause. The perennial activity of allergy from the common foods eliminated from our CFE diet producing its allergenic effect minute after minute for months and years explains the gradual development of polyps and their recurrence after removal better than does seasonal pollen allergy or intermittent allergy to other inhalants. In those patients with nasal allergy to animal emanations and environmental or occupational inhalants, which are inhaled minute after minute without respite for months on end, such continuous allergic reactivity could also be responsible for such polyps. However, in our experience food allergy is the challenge in practically all cases. Long-continued control of it is required to prevent recurrence of polyps after surgical removal. We have witnessed reduction of small, multiple polyps but not the subsidence of large and especially pedunculated polyps by antiallergic treatment.

12. Vascular allergy in the lungs, especially when generalized and usually fatal periarteritis nodosa occurs, may be present in bronchial asthma. Eosinophilia of 30 to 40 percent and even up to 84 percent in the asthmatic should suggest this complication. Generalized vasculitis is indicated by symptoms from involvement in the gastrointestinal, renal, or nervous tissues; fever; eosinophilia (which may be absent); leukocytosis; anemia; enlarged spleen; and severe malaise. Contributions of Rackemann and Greene and especially of Harkavy and subsequent writers, have emphasized the importance of recognition of the occasional periarteritis nodosa or of such vascular allergy in patients with severe bronchial asthma.

13. Finally, any of the diseased states which may produce dyspnea, wheezing, or coughing may occur in patients with true bronchial asthma. Though such occurrences are rare, they must be remembered, emphasizing the necessity of a carefully recorded history, a complete physical examination, and all indicated laboratory and roentgen ray studies to discover all pathological conditions as well as probable bronchial asthma.

14. The challenge of food and less so of other atopic allergy in Goodpasture's syndrome is discussed in Chapter 22.

CONTROL OF MODERATE, SEVERE, AND INTRACTABLE BRONCHIAL ASTHMA IN ADULTS

Recognition of the causes and initial relief of symptoms of moderate, severe, and intractable bronchial asthma immediately requires the steps outlined below. Treatment of bronchial asthma in infants and children is discussed in Chapter 25.

1. Possible or evident food allergy requires immediate study with the strict use of our CFE diet or its modification as we advised in this chapter and in Chapter 3 in all office patients and those requiring hospitalization. The diet is ordered by the physician in office or hospital as follows: Cereal-Free Elimination Diet (Rowe) modified if indicated by history or large scratch reactions, minus foods in the diet, or plus similar foods as advised in Chapter 3. Dietitians know this diet and its modifications and its necessary strict preparation. Office assistants rapidly learn how to instruct patients in its accurate use, especially with our *Elimination Diet* Booklet.

2. Possible or evident inhalant allergy in the home, working, or recreational environments justifies strict control of environmental airborne allergens as advised in this chapter and in Chapter 30.

3. When pollen or possible fungus allergy causes seasonal symptoms, reduction of such airborne allergens by air filtration mechanisms, changes in location, and gradual desensitization to demonstrated

causative pollens as advised in this and other chapters is important.

4. Recognition and elimination of possible allergenic drugs, medications, and other chemicals are required.

Control of symptoms by medications and therapeutic measures until recognition and control of food, inhalant, and less frequent drug and chemical allergies reduces or eliminates such therapy as required in the following degrees of bronchial asthma.

Medications Indicated for the Relief of Bronchial Asthma Until the Allergic Causes Are Recognized and Controlled

Before enumerating and discussing the medications available for the control of the shortness of breath, wheezing, coughing, expectoration and symptoms of its varying complications including infection, and of moderate severe and intractable bronchial asthma, the following objectives in its control need emphasis.

1. Such medications are only justified to relieve the symptoms of asthma until the necessary adequate study and control of the causes of atopic allergy to inhalants, drugs, and especially foods have relieved the symptoms.

2. As long as medications are required, the physician must continue to discover and control remaining allergenic causes, remembering that sensitization to various inhalants and other ingestants which are infrequent causes of bronchial and nasal allergy must be suspect. As emphasized in this chapter, intrinsic unrecognizable causes are not supported by our long experience.

3. Relief of bronchial asthma must be maintained with the elimination and control of inhalant, drug, and especially of too often unrecognized food allergens and not by drugs and other medicaments alone,

especially by long-term corticosteroid and/or adrenergic inhalant therapy and especially with intermittent positive pressure (IPP).

4. A serious criticism of the commercial advertisements of bronchodilating drugs or adrenergic aerosols and especially of corticosteroids for the control of asthma is the absent emphasis of the physician's responsibility to study and control the atopic allergy to inhalants and drugs and especially to foods necessarily according to our long experience with trial diet by our CFE diet as advised in this volume. It is only with adequate accurate study and control of the causes of atopic allergy that bronchial asthma was relieved in our cooperating patients with little or no drug therapy before 1950 and since then with no long-term corticosteroid or IPP adrenergic aerosol therapy as emphasized in the rest of this chapter.

MODERATE BRONCHIAL ASTHMA

Moderate bronchial asthma present at the initial conference with the physician or continuing after control of severe asthma requires the following procedures.

Study of possible food allergy especially with our CFE diet as advised in Chapter 3 and also of possible inhalant allergy with skin testing and environmental control is imperative, as advised in this chapter. Along with this the temporary use of corticosteroids may be indicated, as advised below.

1. Epinephrine hypodermically 0.2 to 0.5 cc of the 1:1000 dilution every one-half to six hours according to age and severity of the asthma is especially effective. Intramuscular injections are contraindicated. Doses for infants and children are advised in Chapter 25.

Parents or patients must be instructed

in its administration. If slower acting epinephrine in oil is given intramuscularly, sesame oil is advised rather than peanut oil, which causes allergy in some patients. Sus-Phrine® may also produce longer relief.

2. Ephedrine with or without aminophylline and a sedative in tablets or in suspension relieve moderate symptoms. Isuprel® sublingually produces less nervousness. Oral Racephedrine alone or with aminophylline (Amodrine®) or aminophylline alone may be effective.

3. Inhalation of epinephrine 1:100, of racemic epinephrine hydrochloride 1:1000, or isoproterenol (Isuprel) hydrochloride 1:200 relieves mild asthma.

Since Graeser and us, in 1935, first advised limited inhalation therapy with epinephrine 1:100 for relief of bronchial asthma, no detrimental effects from its moderate use have occurred in our practice. Isuprel 1:200 may be more effective.

When two to three drops of 1:200 Isuprel or of epinephrine 1:100 in 2 cc of salt solution are inhaled from a hand-activated atomizer or with compressed oxygen or washed air, expectoration of thick mucus may be increased.

Positive pressure breathing with the Bennett, Bird, or other apparatus is not used or necessary in our practice because of relief of bronchospasm and bronchorrhea from our control of atopic allergy to foods and when indicated, to inhalants with decreasing use of corticosteroids and bronchodilator drugs as advised in this chapter.

The use of epinephrine 1:200 by a hand atomizer first advised by Graeser and us in 1935 rather than by IPP itself is favored in the recent study of Morris *et al.* Improvement depends on inhalation of "nebulized bronchoactive or mucolytic medications and not on the use of positive pressure

itself." Disuse of pressure, moreover, avoids the danger of high inspiration pressure as discussed by Morris *et al.*

Our good results in the relief of shortness of breath in bronchial asthma, chronic bronchitis, and especially obstructive emphysema as reported in Chapters 8, 9, and 11 has depended on our study and control of atopic allergy to inhalants and the too often overlooked and uncontrolled food allergy and the limited use of bronchodilating drugs and limited and no long-term corticoid therapy, adrenergic inhalation therapy being utilized by hand atomizers as Graeser and us first advised in 1935, and the disuse of IPP.

With our control of allergy, especially to foods, and the limited or no drug therapy, the gloomy forecast of the burgeoning and increasing chronic obstructive pulmonary disease (COPD) is usually reversed.

Additional reasons for the disuse of or very limited use of adrenergic aerosol therapy especially with intermittent positive pressure mechanisms are presented in the Appendix of this volume especially because of its detrimental effects and unnecessary expenditure for apparatus and operating personnel.

4. Limited value of disodium cromoglycate by inhalation compared with epinephrine or Isuprel is reported by Williams, Jr., and Kane, Herxheimer, and others since 1967 and recently by Chen *et al.*

5. Rectal suppositories containing aminophylline or theophylline from 3¾ to 7½ grains according to age benefit bronchial asthma. They are not advised in children under the age of five years. It may be absorbed better in the rectum when suspended in water. More rapid relief in adults occurs when given intravenously during a three- to five-minute period.

6. If dehydration is present, increased

fluids by mouth may suffice. Intravenous fluids with invert sugar rather than corn glucose solution advised below in the treatment of severe and intractable bronchial asthma infrequently are necessary in moderate asthma.

7. Sedatives, including Demerol, and barbiturates (except small doses of phenobarbital) or of a tranquilizer are contraindicated as discussed below in severe and intractable asthma. Dermatitis from phenobarbital given alone or with ephedrine or other drugs occurs.

8. Since corticosteroids hasten the relief of bronchospasm and bronchorrhea, their use for three to seven days to control moderate symptoms is justifiable. An initial daily dose of 15 to 30 mg of prednisone or 10 to 25 mg of triamcinolone or comparable doses of other corticosteroids as tabulated in Table XX with gradual reduction during five to twenty days to one tablet or none daily is advised.

With the control of food and inhalant allergy, no long-term corticosteroid therapy has been required in any child or adult except for 2 to 8 mg of triamcinolone or comparable doses of other corticosteroids in a few patients with perennial asthma who have received such previous long-term therapy and in about 60 to 70 percent of patients with obstructive emphysema, as discussed in Chapter 11.

Increasing articles advising long-term corticosteroid therapy with oral therapy even every other day as by Briggs, in 1968, has not been necessary for the control of perennial asthma in any of our cooperating children or adults because in our opinion of our adequate sufficient study of food allergy and indicated inhalant allergy as we advise.

Realization and recognition of the various complications of corticosteroid and corticotropin therapy as reported in all advertisements of manufacturing companies are summarized as follows:

Corticoids are justified during the treatment of severe intractable bronchial asthma. As antiallergic therapy controls the symptoms, corticoids must gradually be stopped. Corticoids are preferable to ACTH. Corticoids may be justified, moreover, if invaliding asthma fails to respond to adequate continued antiallergic therapy as advised in this volume. Their continued use, however, is only allowable with continued effort to control the causative allergies without their use and with the approval of another physician in consultation. Segal *et al.* found that prolonged and even intermittent steroid therapy in children suppresses the pituitary-adrenocortical function, causing a poor response to the administration of ACTH even for 4½ months. The physician who allows continued use of corticoid too often is committing the patient to prolonged therapy which may be impossible to stop and which does not effect a cure of asthma or other clinical allergy. Side effects may not occur for weeks or months, but complications must always be anticipated. The onset of complications such as infections, peptic ulcers, or pancreatitis by corticoids must be realized.

Possible complications as noted by Segal, Attinger, and Goldstein listed below must be explained to the patient so that he can report any which may arise. Hemograms, urinalysis, and blood pressure determinations must be done every three to four months if these hormones are continued even in small doses. Hypokalemia must be counteracted with potassium by mouth.

Less serious complications:
Facial mooning, acne, edema, hirsutism and skin pigmentation

Headaches, bodily aches, pains, weakness, lassitude

Mild euphorea to mild depression, mental and physical hyperactivity

Hypertension, tachycardia

Hyperglycemia, glycosuria, aggravation of existing diabetes

Myopathy, muscle cramps (especially in the quadriceps from dexamethasone)

Depressed thyroid function

Impaired tissue repair and healing

Increased gastric acidity and pepsin

Thrombophlebitis

Sensitivity reactions to ACTH (intramuscularly)—skin rashes, pruritus, urticaria, occasionally wheezing and angioneurotic edema

Hemorrhagic skin manifestations

More serious complications:

Potassium deficiency, muscular weakness

Negative nitrogen balance

Osteoporosis, fractures (especially in women after menopause and in immobilized patients)

Masked infections, spread of existing infection, serious spread of nonpathogenic inhabitants of the gastrointestinal and respiratory tracts

Mental confusion to severe psychosis and convulsions

Exacerbation of quiescent ulcers, development of peptic ulcers, hemorrhage and perforation of the gastrointestinal tract

Pancreatitis (Nelp, Siegel, and Levin)

Activation and spread of unsuspected or inactive tuberculosis

Sensitivity reactions of anaphylactic shock, especially from ACTH

Growth suppression when the dose of prednisone (or other corticoids) is greater than 5.1 mg per square meter of body surface per day (Van Metre and Pinterton)

Fever from etiocholanalone and other steroid metabolites (Kappas *et al.*)

Most serious complications:

Withdrawal syndrome—"adrenocortical storm"

Poor tolerance to trauma, shock, and infections

Active atrophy of adrenal cortices, making continued corticoids necessary

Deaths from adrenal insufficiency from stress in patients who have received continued corticoids

Repetitive or continued corticosteroid or ACTH therapy for a period in excess of seven days is unjustifiable without concomitant, adequate study and indicated control of probable or existing food, inhalant, drug, and chemical allergy. With the gradual control of these allergies, the hormones can be discontinued. Failure on the part of manufacturers to stress this responsibility of all physicians in their advertisements and brochures is to be seriously condemned. It is the responsibility of editors of medical journals, our allergy and other medical societies, and also of the Food and Drug Administration to emphasize this necessity in such publications.

When corticoids or ACTH have been administered for several weeks or months without due consideration of attempted control of inhalant and especially food allergy, their discontinuance should be attempted in two to four weeks after indicated antiallergic therapy is established. Reduction in dosage, however, must be gradual and extend at times over a period of from one to five months to permit the adrenals suppressed by previous therapy to regain normal function. During the period of withdrawal and within the ensuing six to twelve months, resumption of corticoid or ACTH therapy may become necessary on an emergency basis during stress periods associated with injury, severe illness, and surgery.

When these hormones have been administered for several months for the control of bronchial asthma and other allergic manifestations, their discontinuance may not be possible without a reactivation of severe symptoms in spite of continued antiallergic therapy without recurrence of moderate or even severe symptoms. In such situations, antiallergic control and other therapeutic measures including the oral administration of potassium should be continued as long as hormonal therapy is employed in the attempt to eliminate its use.

All persons receiving these hormones should have results of a recent chest x-ray and a tuberculin reaction recorded. Such individuals should be given wallet or purse cards indicating that corticosteroid or ACTH are or have been administered.

CORTICOSTEROID THERAPY

No long term corticosteroid therapy to control perennial bronchial asthma has been required in our adult patients including those in old age when strict cooperation in our study and control of inhalant and especially food allergy have been obtained. However, in spite of their apparent cooperation in our antiallergic therapy, small continued doses of corticosteroids of 2½ and at times 10 mg of prednisone or lesser doses of triamcinolone have been required in about one-half of our older patients with obstructive emphysema or occasionally in adult asthmatics who have previously received long-term corticosteroid therapy. That such good results without continued corticosteroids can occur is shown by the excellent results we reported in 1946 to 1947 from our control of food and inhalant allergy three years before corticosteroids were available. That such study and control of atopic allergy as well as emotional factors usually make long-term corticosteroid therapy unnecessary has been stressed by Ford and others, including Fontana, as stated in our discussion of such therapy of asthma in children in Chapter 25. When small doses are required, mild unrecognized allergy to foods in the diet or slight deviations therefrom or varying degrees of uncontrolled inhalant allergy must be suspected and if suspected or discovered, controlled. The increase of allergy to foods and the more frequent inhalation of indoor airborne allergens in winter, as emphasized in Chapter 1, must be remembered.

This minimal or no long-term corticosteroid therapy is in marked contrast to its common use in chronic bronchial asthma reported in this and other countries. Our scrutiny of such articles yields no acceptable evidence that inhalant and especially food allergy has been studied and controlled as we advise. Thus Maunsell, Pearson, and Livingstone, in England (1968), reported its use in 170 patients to control perennial bronchial asthma. Their long-term use of corticosteroids for one-half to nine years (av. 4.3 years) with good results in only from 53 to 62 percent, moderate relief in 22 to 33 percent, failure in 7 to 10 percent, and death in 5 to 7 percent is not comparable to our published results during a seven-year period before corticosteroids were available (p. 183). That the results were approximately the same in their seventy cases with allergic factors, in seventy-five cases with only infective factors, and seventeen cases with "neither factor" can also be explained by failure to control atopic allergy to inhalants and especially to foods which has been our adamant responsibility in all cases of perennial asthma or asthma in the fall and winter for over thirty-five years.

Reasons for failure to recognize food allergy explained in Chapter 1 are reiterated throughout this volume. In the last 500 of our hospital cases in the last fifteen years, only 3 deaths have occurred in comparison to 8 in their 170 cases in a ten-year period in spite of long-term corticosteroid therapy in each one. This again can be explained by our immediate study and efforts to control food and inhalant allergies.

The side effects of corticosteroids they also report including facial edema, glycosuria, and status asthmaticus from continued corticosteroid therapy reported by other physicians resulting from the withdrawal of corticosteroids are very infrequent in our patients because of our use of no long-term corticosteroid therapy except with intermittent minimal doses in a few patients noted above.

Speizer, Doll, and Heaf report increased mortality since long-term corticosteroid therapy and pressurized aerosol broncho-dilators have been used. Moreover, in a report by Joseph in 1968 in Australia on long term corticosteroid therapy in perennial asthma, there is no evidence of adequate, strict study and control of atopic allergy to inhalants and especially to foods, the importance of which has long been emphasized in our practice. The important complete withdrawal of corticosteroid therapy in only 4 percent and his statement that such steroids may have to be continued throughout life are not justified unless atopic allergy especially to foods has been studied and hopefully controlled as advised in this chapter and in our other publications.

We opine, moreover, that the increase of deaths from bronchial asthma reported by Gandevia in 1967 in Australia up to fifty-two per one million in females would be definitely less if the control of atopic allergy, especially to foods, with adjunctive therapy we advise in this chapter and in our book *Bronchial Asthma—Its Diagnosis and Treatment,* 1963, were assured. Deaths in bronchial asthma have already been discussed in this chapter.

The many side effects of long-term corticosteroid therapy reported by the drug committee of the American Academy of Allergy in 1967 including edema of the face, glycosuria, hirsutism, and others, at times even death, resulting from stopping long-term corticosteroid therapy do not occur in our cooperating patients because of our disuse of such therapy except for minimal doses in a few patients noted in the first part of this discussion. It must be remembered that if glycosuria occurs in a patient as a result of possible corticosteroid therapy, a decrease in steroids usually controls it. If the asthma is controlled before possible allergy to corn has been determined, corn glucose by mouth should not be given because of possible reactivation of the asthma from corn allergy. Invert sugar instead of corn glucose by vein is equally important, as advised on page 468.

Case 48: A patient sixty years of age. Bronchial asthma had caused coughing, wheezing, and shortness of breath every day, especially on awakening, exaggerated every three to four weeks, increasing in the fall, winter, and early spring months with improvement during July and August for four years since the age of twelve years. In spite of desensitization to pollens, dust, and fungi every week for four years, relief had increasingly required prednisone recently from 35 to 75 mg daily for three years to maintain relief and prevent serious asthma. In spite of inhalation of epinephrine with a hand atomizer one to four times a day and intermittent positive pressure inhalation of epinephrine two to three times a day, no decrease in daily steroids had occurred. Even though her history was indicative of our pathognomonic history of bronchial asthma resulting from allergy, such allergy had never been recognized.

Colic and constant crying for seven to eight months in infancy followed by recurrent colds and coughs with no fever particularly in the fall and winter months in childhood, as emphasized in this chapter and in Chapter 25, indicated food allergy as the major cause. Much postnasal mucus best explained by food allergy had continued throughout her life. In February one year previously she had been hospitalized for two weeks because of pneumonia associated with continued asthma. A general diet at that time was prescribed!

Continued asthma had caused nervousness, tension, and at times definite depression.

Her diet history revealed a lifelong dislike for

milk and a moderate dislike for eggs without any other suspicions of possible food allergy.

Her environmental history revealed no evidence of inhalant allergy even though desensitization to inhalants had been continued weekly for four years with no benefit.

Family history revealed perennial nasal allergy in the mother.

She lived in Maine except for the previous four weeks in our San Francisco Bay Area.

Pneumonia with exaggerated asthma had occurred in the fall several times in the last six years.

Tonsillectomy at the age of six had not benefited the nasal allergy.

Physical examination was negative except for moderate diffuse rhonchi and wheezing throughout both lungs. X-ray of the lungs revealed hyperlucency in an enlarged chest. Pulmonary function tests were normal after adrenalin hypodermically, as were her blood, urine, and sedimentation rates.

Skin tests gave one to two plus reactions to several animal emanations, grass, fall and several tree pollens, and a two plus reaction to eggs. Scratch tests to other foods, including milk, were negative.

Treatment and Results: Because of her likely allergy to milk in infancy and her dislike for milk and eggs, study of food allergy to these foods and other common allergenic foods with strict adherence to our CFE diet was advised. Such study was also indicated by the pathognomonic history of bronchial asthama resulting from food allergy. Corticosteroids were reduced from 75 mg to 16 mg in three days and to 2 mg a day in twelve days. Ephedrine was eliminated in two weeks. Intermittent positive pressure was immediately discontinued. In two months the asthma had been entirely absent for four weeks. Because of long-term corticosteroid therapy, the triamcinolone was continued with 2 mg a day.

Control continued with strict adherence to her CFE diet until Thanksgiving, when wheat, milk, and eggs, were taken without our advice for two days, resulting in rapid return of her severe asthma, necessitating hospitalization and temporary increase in her corticosteroids to obtain relief. Since then, with strict adherence to the elimination diet and 2 mg of corticosteroid daily, her asthma has been entirely controlled without any other medications for the last five months.

CONTROL OF ASTHMA WITH LITTLE OR NO MEDICATIONS

Discontinuance of all medications through the control of atopic allergy is the physician's challenge not only in moderate but severe (including perennial chronic asthma) and often intractable asthma.

This can only occur with adequate relief of existent inhalant, drug, and especially food allergies as has resulted with our CFE diet and at times its modifications (Chapt. 3).

Food allergy, as emphasized, unfortunately is too frequently ignored or inadequately controlled for reasons we have reiterated in this volume. Without its recognition, patients with perennial bronchial asthma with or without emphysema and chronic bronchitis too often are given detrimental long-term corticosteroids, antispasmodic medications, and unnecessary desensitization to conventional multiple antigens containing pollens, dust, fungi, and miscellaneous antigens, along with injections of vaccines often one to two times a week for months or even years, as for twenty years in a previously-summarized case, when the recognition and control of food allergy alone would control the asthma with no injectant therapy and little or no medications. This has been emphasized in our publications on asthma for many years, as in *Progress in Allergy* in 1952, *JAMA* in 1960, and especially in our book on bronchial asthma in 1963.

Retarded growth and underweight from chronic asthma and rehabilitation for relief of asthmatics are discussed in the above book on pages 139 to 144. Nostrums and other empiric therapy advised in bronchial asthma and therapies formerly used in bronchial asthma are also discussed in the above book.

STUDY, TREATMENT, AND CONTROL OF SEVERE BRONCHIAL ASTHMA

Severe bronchial asthma characterized by shortness of breath, wheezing, coughing, bronchospasm, and mucoid expectoration continuing through the day and night especially with exercise and at 1 to 5 AM often requires hospitalization. If it is not incapacitating, treatment in the office and home can be effective.

Our advised study and control follow:

1. Immediate study and control of possible food allergy with our CFE diet, inhalant including pollen, and less frequent drug, chemical, and rare infectant allergies is mandatory.

2. Immediate important relief of symptoms until control of food, inhalant, less frequent drug, and rare infectant allergies occurs requires the following medications:

a) Epinephrine 1:1000 hypodermically (not intramuscularly) 0.15 to 0.5 cc according to degree of asthma and age, one to six times in twenty-four hours, usually gives temporary or partial relief. Local necrotic skin lesions (Arthus phenomenon) from allergy to epinephrine given for relief of asthma for many years as reported by us in 1948 is shown in Figure 7.

b) Epinephrine 1:100 or Isuprel 1:200 by inhalation is available. Aminophylline 3¾ to 7½ grains by rectum and (to relieve severe asthma) by vein every eight to twelve hours is also advised for relief.

c) Corticosteroid therapy is indicated immediately for the control of severe asthma in patients treated in the office and at home. Intramuscular injections of 20 to 40 mg of Solu-Medrol® or triamcinolone together with 8 mg two to four times daily for two to three days orally are advised. As relief occurs, the dose is gradually reduced to 4 mg two times a day in five to seven days and is further reduced or stopped in ten to twelve days providing study and control of food, inhalant, and existent drug allergies are continued.

In patients treated in the hospital, corticosteroids can be given 20 to 40 mg of Solu-Medrol or triamcinolone or comparable doses of other corticosteroids intramuscularly one to three times a day, the amount varying with the degree of asthma. Oral doses, as above, are gradually reduced and eliminated in one to two weeks. Since an important complication of such therapy is peptic ulcer with the activation, bleeding, or even perforation of a duodenal ulcer and

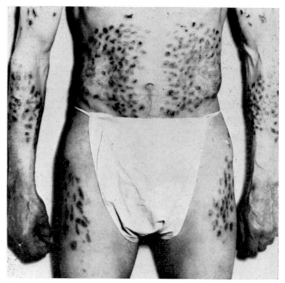

Figure 7. Cutaneous necrotic changes of the Arthus phenomenon from long-repeated subcutaneous epinephrine reported by us in 1948.

since our experience indicates the frequency of allergy, especially to fruits, as a major cause of duodenal ulcer (Chapt. 5), fruits should be eliminated from the diet with our FFCFE diet when a healed or active ulcer is suspected. An x-ray of the stomach or duodenum in the second or third day of corticosteroid therapy is advisable. As the asthma improves, the above diet must be continued, and unflavored aluminum hydroxide by mouth is advised five to six times daily. With this diet and an unflavored antacid medication, cortico-steroids can be continued and gradually reduced and eliminated.

If an old or present ulcer is not a problem, the corticosteroid can be continued and reduced as advised above, using the CFE diet with no antacid therapy.

d) Patients treated in the office must drink more water than desired to relieve possible dehydration, especially if an elevated hematocrit is found.

If dehydration is present in the hospital-treated patients, in addition to extra water by mouth, intravenous 5 percent invert sugar in water is given up to 1 to 3000 cc daily for one or two days. In one 1000 cc each day 4.5 percent sodium chloride may be included. Invert sugar made from sucrose is advised instead of corn glucose because of the exclusion of corn and its products in our CFE diet and to prevent severe prolonged allergic symptoms in a corn-sensitive patient from intravenous glucose which has occurred in corn-cereal sensitive patients who have received 5 percent glucose by vein before our control of cereal grain allergy and before our realization of the importance of using invert sugar. Chemical analysis in our research laboratory has revealed 1 mg of antigenic residue per bottle of dextrose. What allergist would knowingly inject 1 mg of allergen intravenously into a patient suffering from asthma?

e) If serum determinations of K, Na, Cl, and Mg reveal a deficiency, this must be relieved intravenously or by mouth. Until the gradual control of food and inhalant allergies relieves asthma, many different medications are available for relief of bronchospasm, bronchorrhea, and shortness of breath as already advised for the control of moderate asthma in this chapter.

f) Ephedrine with or without amino-phylline and mild sedative by mouth.

As severe asthma is relieved, continued treatment as advised above for relief of moderate asthma is continued until strict control of food and/or inhalant allergy with cooperation of the patient allows the reduction of medications to a minimum or their entire elimination as discussed above.

TREATMENT OF INTRACTABLE BRONCHIAL ASTHMA (STATUS ASTHMATICUS)

Immediate study of allergy to foods, inhalants including pollens, less frequently to drugs and chemicals, and rare infectants as advised on page 202 is imperative.

This should be considered a serious medical emergency and is best treated in the hospital. Dyspnea is usually extreme; shallow abdominal breathing may predominate. Orthopnea is usual, with arms or hands often resting on thighs or on a table or chair. Wheezing, rales, and rhonchi are suppressed by severe generalized bronchospasm and by varying degrees of mucosal edema and obstructing mucus in the pulmonary airways.

Immediate limitation of foods to those in our CFE diet is imperative even when pollen or other inhalant allergy seems the undoubted cause. If nausea is present, foods in the diet should be liquid, minced, or pureed until abatement of the asthma creates a desire for regularly cooked foods in the diet.

Study and control of definite or possible inhalant and less frequent drug allergy with environmental control are especially important. Immediate study of allergy to foods, inhalants including pollens, and drugs and chemicals advised on page 202 is mandatory.

Relief of initial intractable and less severe continued symptoms with medications, intravenous fluids, limited or no sedatives, indicated antibiotics, and no intermittent positive pressure therapy and the following medications is necessary:

1. Epinephrine 1:1000, 0.2 to 0.5 cc, according to age and weight should be given hypodermically and repeated in ten to fifteen minutes if necessary. If after four injections there is little or no relief, the patient probably is temporarily epinephrine-fast. After relief occurs with the proper medications, epinephrine usually is again beneficial, given every two to six hours according to the resultant relief.

2. Aminophylline 3¾ to 7½ grains in adults and 1½ to 3 grains in children according to age and weight given slowly intravenously during a three-to six-minute period or intramuscularly is often beneficial. It is contraindicated under the age of five years. The dose may be repeated every six to twelve hours. It may be incorporated in necessary intravenous fluids or injected directly into tubing, given intramuscularly, or given by rectum. Overdosage may produce peripheral vascular collapse and even death. The most frequent toxic symptom is vomiting. Administration should be stopped at once if toxic symptoms appear.

As improvement occurs, aminophylline can be continued by rectal suppositories or fluid rectal instillations, 3½ to 7½ grains according to age, every six to twelve hours. As symptoms decrease with the control of food and/or inhalant allergy or of infrequent drug allergies, aminophylline usually with ephedrine by mouth and epinephrine 1:1000 hypodermically are indicated.

3. Corticosteroids administered intramuscularly must be given immediately as advised in the above treatment of severe asthma in doses depending on the severity of the asthma. In our practice Solu-Medrol or triamcinolone have been used with excellent results. Adequate doses, 20 to 40 mg intramuscularly, should be repeated every three to six hours until definite relief

of the shortness of breath, wheezing, and bronchospasm occurs. Concomitant oral administration of one to two tablets of the chosen corticosteroid every four to six hours also is advisable. As relief occurs, the oral can supplant the parenteral administration. If the corticosteroid is only given by mouth, dosage should begin with six to eight tablets with a gradual reduction in one to two weeks to two and later to one tablet daily. These doses are indicated in all patients with status asthmaticus or severe bronchial asthma except in infants and young children, as discussed in Chapter 25. Our experience indicates that therapeutic initial failure from corticosteroids most frequently results from inadequate dosage in the first two to four days. Corticosteroid therapy in infants and young children is advised in Chapter 25.

The physician's responsibility is to gradually reduce and discontinue corticosteroids as the increasing control of atopic allergy occurs because of the detrimental effects of such corticosteroids.

Corticotropin (ACTH) intramuscularly or intravenously given every four to six hours is less effective. It is not used in our practice because relief is delayed in comparison to that obtained from corticosteroids. Moreover, there is no evidence that its intermittent administration prevents adrenocortical depression when steroids are given. Maximum adrenocortical response to it, moreover, occurs only after four to five days. Specific sensitivity to it also may develop. True organ sensitivity to the pituitary also may occur, requiring complete cessation of corticotropin therapy. Many allergic reactions and several deaths from ACTH given intramuscularly and by vein have been reported according to Hill and Swinburn, Unger and Unger, and others. In addition, Zucker and Bendo, in 1961, reported cyanosis, apnea, and shock in an asthmatic in ten minutes after an intravenous infusion containing aminophylline and forty units of ACTH. With epinephrine 1:1000 by vein, artificial respiration, oxygen by intermittent positive pressure, and 10 mg of hydrocortisone by vein, recovery occurred. Such allergy therefore favors the use of corticosteroids instead of ACTH when necessary in bronchial asthma. Rapid allergic or anaphylactic reactions have not been reported from their use.

Recommendation of prednisone administration on alternate days in steroid-dependent asthmas tends to justify its continued long-term therapy which is not required in any child or adult who is cooperative in our study and control of inhalant (especially food) and less frequently drug allergy as advised in this chapter and throughout this volume. In our opinion the ignorance of inadequate control of food allergy, which our continued adequate study and control has proved to be negligence, is responsible for most long-term corticoid therapy. Physicians are controlling allergy with steroids and drugs rather than accepting the challenge of determining and controlling a patient's allergies, of which the food sensitivities are especially responsible for the bronchospasm and shortness of breath.

Since long-term corticosteroid therapy, even in doses of 10 to 20 mg, has not been required to control perennial bronchial asthma or other manifestations of atopic allergy in patients cooperating in the control of inhalant, drug, and especially of food allergy as advised in this volume, we have not tried or evaluated the effect of large oral doses of corticosteroids of 20 mg, 50 mg, or larger doses every other day. The challenge of all physicians to relieve clinical atopic allergy by the study and control of its causes especially those re-

sulting from foods must be accepted. Reports of relief from large doses of corticosteroids every other day tend to justify such long-term therapy, relieving the physician, including allergists, of their responsibility to obtain relief by adequate study and control of the allergy, especially to foods, as advised in this volume.

TABLE XX
ORALLY ADMINISTERED CORTICOSTEROIDS*

Drug	Dosage (mg)
Cortisone acetate	25
Hydrocortisone	20
Prednisone (Delta®, Deltrasone®, Sterane®, Meticortin®)	5
Prednisolone (Co-Hydeltra®, Meticortelone®)	5
Triamcinolone (Aristocort®, Kanacort®)	4
Methylprednisolone (Medrol®)	4
Dexamethasone (Decadron®, Deronil®, Gammacorten®)	0.75
Paramethasone (Haldrone®)	2
Celestone	0.6

Parenterally Administered Corticosteroids†

Cortisone acetate—aqueous suspension	100
Hydrocortisone sodium succinate (Solu-Cortef®) (IV or IM)	100
Prednisolone sodium succinate (Meticortelone, soluble, Hydeltra—T.B.A.®)	50
Prednisolone butylacetate (Hydeltra—T.B.A.)	40
Methylprednisolone (Solu-Medrol) (IM or IV)	40
Triamcinolone (Aristocort)	40

*Maximum single table size.
†Maximum single dose.

4. Fluid and electrolyte therapy also is most important to correct dehydration and electrolyte deficiency in the blood and tissues. Decreased potassium occurs with continued corticosteroid or from indicated digitalis therapy. Fluid deficits are frequently large, 2000 to 4000 cc in adults and less in children according to the degree and duration of the status asthmaticus.

Since allergy to cereal grains, including corn, in our experience requires immediate study with our CFE diet, 5 percent invert sugar made from sucrose rather than corn glucose in water is given intravenously. Clinical allergy from corn glucose sold for intravenous use, at times severe, has occurred in some of our corn-sensitive patients. The possible continued bronchial edema, mucus, and spasm from 50 to 200 gm of corn glucose in 5 percent glucose solutions intravenously for one to several days must be realized. Death in a woman with intractable asthma given 2000 to 3000 cc of 5 percent glucose by vein for three days was best explained by continued bronchospasm and resultant heart failure from allergy to corn allergens in glucose. Another corn-sensitive patient developed severe bronchospasm decreasing in four days after 2000 cc 5 percent glucose was given by another physician because of a general temporary reaction from a pollen injection. The disuse of glucose by vein also has been emphasized by Rinkel and Randolph when corn allergy is possible.

Continuous intravenous therapy during the first twenty-four to seventy-two hours may be advisable if dehydration is severe, especially if the veins are small. Water or dilute juice of fruits in our CFE diet and sugar, if tolerated by mouth, must be encouraged. Serum sodium, chloride, carbon dioxide, and potassium determinations, along with sound clinical judgment and experience, must guide such therapy. Hematocrit determinations will indicate the initial degree and gradual relief of dehydration. Sodium chloride should be limited to 1000 cc of one-half normal solution in 5 percent invert sugar solution one time daily with additional 2000 to 3000 cc of 5 percent invert sugar in water through the rest of the twenty-four hours, the amount depending on dehydration and blood chloride and hematocrit determinations. Increased renal excretion of sodium and potassium occurs in severe asthma.

Potassium and magnesium can be added to the intravenous fluid the first day and as indicated thereafter. Potassium salts (20-60 mEq) intravenously or 4 to 8 gm orally should be given each day when large doses of corticosteroids are used. It must be remembered that cellular potassium deficiency may exist in status asthmaticus even though the serum potassium is 5 to 6 mEq because of concentration of the blood before dehydration is relieved. Fluid and electrolyte therapy in infants and children is discussed in Chapter 25. Reduced potassium therapy is necessary as corticosteroids are gradually reduced and stopped. To aid expectoration of bronchial mucus, water and fluids by mouth must be increased as intravenous fluids are decreased and discontinued. Requiring the patient to drink 200 to 300 cc of water every one to two hours until recovery may be advisable.

5. Antibiotic therapy is advisable with large doses of corticosteroids in intractable asthma. This is necessary to counteract frequent secondary infection which may be masked by these hormones. In contrast, antibiotics are not indicated for an initial "cold" with or without fever, which as we have emphasized throughout this volume are due to food allergy and not infection, though secondary infection may at times be present.

The choice of antibiotics with this corticosteroid therapy must be governed by the resistance to local hospital staphylococci and other possible or cultured bacteria in the sputum. One antibiotic for possible gram-negative and a second for gram-positive organisms at first parenterally may be advisable. These should be given before culture and sensitization studies on the sputum are available if pneumonitis is probable. After such tests are done, a change of antibiotics may be indicated. Unless a bacterium is cultured that only responds to penicillin, other antibiotics are preferable because of the frequency of allergy to penicillin. This is especially true if there is a previous history of possible or definite allergy to penicillin.

Oral as well as parenteral administration of penicillin has caused rapid fatality. If such a reaction occurs, epinephrine 1:1000 must be given hypodermically and if relief is not apparent, 0.3 cc can be given slowly by vein along with artificial respiration. Epinephrine 1:1000 can be repeated hypodermically in five to ten minutes if the emergency continues. The occurrence of marked cutaneous or other tissue allergy seven to twenty days after penicillin therapy also must be anticipated. All of this favors the use of another antibiotic rather than penicillin in most cases. Allergy to penicillinase to control such reactions also discourages its use, as reported by Weiss and others.

6. Sedation of any type is initially contraindicated because it tends to suppress conscious respiratory effort which is absolutely necessary until symptoms of intractable asthma are relieved. It also increases CO_2 saturation in the blood. Death may result from such sedation. This contraindication applies especially to morphine, other derivatives of opium, and even to large doses of codeine. We agree with Ratner and others that meperidine hydrochloride (Demerol) should not be given because of its suppression of the coughing reflex and of the activity of the respiratory center, both of which are important to maintain the coughing reflex. Moreover, narcotizing doses of codeine, barbiturates, and other sedatives by suppressing the respiratory center and respiration lead to anoxia and even death in status asthmaticus. Sleep induced by such medication may also cause definite cyanosis, shock, hypotension, and even death in spite of restoration of normal amounts of oxygen, CO_2, and electrolytes in the blood and body tissues. A cerebral death occurs because of irreversible damage in the brain from anoxia which lasts for more than three minutes. A postmortem demonstrated such decortication with softening in the cerebral cortex, corpus striatum, and globus pallidus as reported in one unconscious patient kept alive, unfortunately, for one year. Finally, habit formation from any of the drugs is a constant danger.

7. Humidified oxygen should be administered only by nasal catheter or a plastic mask for hypoxia and cyanosis, utilizing an oxygen flow of 6 liters a minute. Such hypoxia is determined by cyanosis of the tongue and mucous membranes instead of the fingers. This cyanosis is primarily due to obstruction of the airway from edema and bronchospasm. Oxygen is of little benefit, however, until such obstruction is decreased by medication. It infrequently is required except in severe unrelieved intractable asthma. Positive pressure breathing in these patients is contraindicated. Helium-oxygen with such apparatus is not necessary with the therapy which we are recommending.

It must be remembered that continued oxygen therapy in bronchial asthma may produce confusion, stupor, coma, and even death when a continued increase in CO_2 in the blood has occurred in chronic or intractable asthma, especially when complicated with emphysema. The stimulating action of CO_2 on the respiratory center decreases, being partially supplanted by hypoxia. When this is relieved with arterial saturation with inhaled oxygen, ventilation is diminished and CO_2 in the blood rises with serious or fatal results. Thus oxygen inhalation must be properly supervised and interrupted at regular intervals, especially if the respirations fall below twelve per minute. Occasional rupture of the stomach or distal esophagus because of entrance of the catheter into the esophagus (reported by Walstad and Conklin and also by Longobardie *et al.*) must be remembered.

GLOMECTOMY

The moderate to marked relief of bronchial asthma from glomectomy reported by Nakayama and later by Overholt has not been confirmed. Indications of its possible use have steadily decreased in our practice with our adequate study and control of food allergy with the CFE diet and if necessary with its modifications which are indicated. As cooperation of the patient continues, indicated adequate desensitization with environmental control when inhalant allergy is an evident challenge is required.

We agree with Prigal and practically all allergists that various surgical procedures by thoracic and neurosurgeons for relief of bronchial asthma are to be definitely avoided.

Comment

With immediate consideration of food and inhalant allergy, medications, and control of fluid and electrolyte deficits advised above, bronchospasm is usually diminished in a few hours. If it persists, the inhalation of bronchodilators including epinephrine 1:100, 2.25 percent racemic epinephrine (Vaponefrin®), or isopropylarterenol (Isuprel or Aladrine®), together with a wetting agent such as water or Alevaire®, by nebulization may decrease the spasm and aid expectoration of mucus. If our advised diet, environmental control, and adequate parenteral corticosteroids are utilized, however, the routine use of inhalation therapy, especially in intractable or recurrent bronchial asthma, is unnecessary. No routine intermittent positive pressure therapy

with adrenergic drugs is used in our hospital, office, or home therapy of asthma or obstructive emphysema, especially because of detrimental effects which occur as reported in Chapter 11.

In longstanding, severe, and finally intractable bronchial asthma, retained mucus in the bronchial tract not only occludes the bronchioles but at times the larger and main bronchi. The bronchospasm and increasing mucoid obstruction of the airways at times intensify anoxia, resulting in death especially if sedation has been prescribed.

It must be emphasized that in our practice deaths have not occurred except in a few patients as a result of our immediate study of inhalant and especially food allergy along with adequate initial parenteral doses of corticosteroids, relief of deficiencies of fluids with invert sugar instead of corn glucose solutions, the use of no sedation, and the use of other medications as advised in this chapter.

In intractable bronchial asthma, cardiac decompensation must be recognized. Right ventricular failure with cor pulmonale occurs most often. A large tender liver is the most reliable sign rather than cyanosis alone, venous distention in the neck, or edema. Continued intractable asthma also causes tachycardia and varying degrees of hypertension. It is possible that vasculitis and other tissue changes from atopic allergy occur in the pericardium and also in other vascular tissues, as reported by Harkavy and others (Chapt. 26). Thus changes in the ECG extrasystoles, exaggerated if they have previously occurred, may arise. Digitalization and later quinidine therapy may be required. Diuretics including diazides and aldactizide with maintenance of potassium requirements with the advice of a cardiologist are important if edema especially in the feet and legs and other evidence of cardiac decompensation occur.

Vasopressor therapy is indicated if severe shock develops in spite of the above treatment.

In the rare patient where intractable asthma does not respond to the above recommendations and where a near moribund condition indicates possible death, the mechanical therapy by an anesthesiologist in cooperation with the allergist as summarized in this chapter may be advisable.

SUMMARY OF INFORMATION ABOUT THE CHARACTERISTICS, STUDY, AND CONTROL OF BRONCHIAL ASTHMA

1. Allergy to foods is a more frequent cause of bronchial asthma than inhalant allergy, especially in the fall to late spring and particularly in childhood and old age.

2. With good control, possible infectant, intrinsic, and emotional causes decrease to a minimum or disappear.

3. There is a pathognomonic history of bronchial asthma resulting from food allergy characterized by cyclic attacks for two to five days every two to five weeks, especially in the fall to late spring, absent or less severe in summer.

4. Other manifestations of clinical allergy and occurrence of other disease states must be recognized and controlled.

5. Information from positive scratch tests with ingested foods and inhaled allergens must be correlated with the patient's history. Their importance must be evaluated with provocation ingestant and inhalant tests.

6. A complete physical examination with indicated laboratory and x-ray studies to recognize other diseases and complications of bronchial asthma including emphysema, bronchiectasis, and cardiovascular disease is mandatory.

7. Food allergy rarely may be controlled by a diet eliminating specific foods suspected by the patient or physician as causes of the allergy or giving large scratch tests.

8. Because of the frequency of negative scratch reactions and the clinical fallibility of positive reactions, diet trial with our CFE diet or a modification usually must be used in a strict and adequate manner not for three weeks but for a minimum of six months as advised for thirty years and emphasized in this volume.

9. Negative scratch reactions occur in 10 to 15 percent of pollen-sensitive patients. Desensitization to inhalants is important in such patients as well as in those whose scratch reactions indicate allergy to inhalants. Desensitization with initial tolerated doses of such inhalants, increasing to a maximum tolerated dose, and repeating it for more than two years is advised.

10. Indicated environmental control is important.

11. Medications for control of moderate, severe, and intractable bronchial asthma, decreasing the doses as control of atopic allergies occurs, is advised in this chapter.

12. Limited initial use of corticosteroids with their decrease and discontinuance as control of the atopic allergy occurs is advised.

13. No long-term corticosteroid therapy is required with our treatment except for small doses in some chronic asthmatics previously treated with long-term corticosteroid therapy or in some patients with severe obstructive emphysema (see Chapt. 11).

14. Limited adrenergic aerosol inhalant therapy with the hand atomizer Graeser and I (Albert Rowe, Sr.) first advised in 1937 is reduced to a minimum when inhalant and especially food allergy is controlled as we advise. With control of atopic allergy in obstructive emphysema, such therapy by intermittent positive pressure

is not required, as reported in Chapters 11 and 30.

15. In addition to the discussion of causes and their recognition with the method of control of moderate, severe, and intractable bronchial asthma in this chapter and in children's asthma (Chapt. 25), discussion of additional aspects of asthma can be found in our work *Bronchial Asthma— Its Diagnosis and Treatment*, 1963. Summaries of forty-seven cases in infants, children, adults and the elderly who were relieved of their perennial symptoms, usually a result of food allergy, with or without inhalant allergy especially to pollens are presented, and the book is recommended reading.

16. The physician's challenge to determine the allergic causes of the patient's bronchial asthma, recognize the complications, and extend maximum relief justifies his thorough study and expertised use of information in this chapter, in Chapter 25, and also in our book on bronchial asthma in 1963 in order to obtain the maximum results with his patients available as a result of our study and treatment of this disease during the last fifty-four years.

Chapter 9

Food Allergy in Chronic Bronchitis

CHRONIC BRONCHITIS

Our good results in the control of chronic bronchitis from the study and control of food allergy emphasize such allergy as its major cause. This is true not only in the nonobstructive type but also in chronic bronchitis present in varying degrees in obstructive emphysema as reported in the previous chapter. Food allergy requires study especially in chronic bronchitis occurring only or exaggerated in the winter months, remembering the definition of Fletcher that chronic bronchitis is present when a chronic cough with expectoration lasts for at least three months in at least two consecutive years. As we reiterate through this volume, one of the major characteristics of food allergy is the recurrence or the activation of its manifestations during the late fall, winter, and into the early spring months, with a decrease or inactivation during the summer (Chapt. 1).

Allergy as a factor in chronic bronchitis was supported by several participants in the International Bronchitis Symposium in the Netherlands in 1960. One stated that many authors opine that the cough, dyspnea, and production of sputum "can only be understood when both asthma and bronchitis are considered the expression of a common 'asthmatic' constitution." Herxheimer also stated that "asthma and bronchitis are likely to be one and the same disorder. This becomes more probable by the presence of a high percentage of eosinophiles in the sputum of asthmatics as well as of bronchitics."

Favoring allergy are the eosinophiles in the sputum and bronchial walls in chronic bronchitis. Orie reported sputum eosinophilia (greater than 60%) in twenty-seven of thirty-five cases. Brille reported such eosinophiles in 57.1 percent in the blood in 34.9 percent of 123 bronchial biopsies and 41 percent of the sputa in patients with chronic bronchitis. He stated "that allergy is very probably an important factor in many cases of chronic bronchitis, but its appreciation is unfortunately not yet assured." Hers noted "eosinophilic leukocytes, histiocytes, and eosinophilic granules in the bronchial wall in chronic bronchitis," which cells are "accepted" as an expression of "an allergic constitution." Goslings made a similar conclusion. Orie, Sluiter, *et al.* emphasized the asthmatic constitution in asthmatic bronchitis, obstructive emphysema, and bronchiectasis and the development of right heart failure from poor control of the symptoms in his very informative chart.

In spite of this evidence of allergy in chronic bronchitis, the study and control of allergy have not been rewarding. Studies of inhalant allergy with desensitization to suspected inhalants and environmental control with or without vaccine therapy have only yielded partial, questionable, or no relief.

Except for our increasing study and control of food allergy in chronic bronchitis in the last thirty years, moreover, such allergy has received little or no consideration. This is due a) to the usual exclusion of food allergy by negative skin tests to foods which, as we have emphasized for years, often occur in cumulative chronic food allergy or b) to failure of test-negative diets (if skin reactions occur to foods) to relieve the symptoms of chronic bronchitis. This is due to the recognized fallibility of positive skin reactions to foods which cause clinical food allergy, as emphasized in Chapter 2.

Our conviction that food allergy is a major cause of chronic bronchitis has resulted from our good or excellent control of the moderate to severe cough and varying degrees of expectoration (bronchorrhea) with the strict and adequate use of the CFE diet as advised in Chapters 3 and 8. This relief of chronic bronchitis with moderate to abundant mucoid expectoration associated with obstructive emphysema with the strict use of our CFE diet as reported in the preceding chapter emphasizes the important role of food allergy in these pulmonary diseases. The control of chronic bronchitis with this diet, and when necessary with initial corticoids and antibiotics, is discussed below in the control of chronic bronchitis.

As emphasized in this volume, good results with our elimination diets have depended on the patient's strict cooperation in excluding all traces of foods other than those listed in the initial diet. Bakery products must be made as advised a) by our recipes by a trusted baker supervised and inspected by the physician or b) at home by these recipes. The butter substitute must be entirely milk-free. Slight deviations from the diet especially away from home and inhalation of odors of food excluded from the diet must be avoided. That previously ingested foods remain in

the body for one to two weeks or more and that pathological changes in the shock tissues of allergy as in the lungs gradually decrease in one to two or more months emphasize the necessity of adhering to the diet until relief of symptoms is assured. Residual irreversible pathology from long-standing food allergy often persists in spite of the long elimination of allergenic foods. The necessity of strict cooperation of the patient and adequate supervision and policing of the diet and of the patient's adherence thereto is the physician's responsibility, as is his precise execution of directions for required medications or surgical procedures in other medical service to his patient.

UNCERTAIN ORIGIN OF CHRONIC BRONCHITIS FROM OTHER CAUSES THAN ALLERGY

The importance of this recognition of food allergy as the major cause of chronic bronchitis with or without obstructive emphysema (OE) is emphasized by the failure of previous investigations to establish infection from viruses or bacteria as the cause of the malady. None of the various antibiotics nor the use of viral, stock, or autogenous vaccines of respiratory bacteria has given relief at all comparable to that from our antiallergic control. Though daily penicillin or tetracycline reduced morbidity, Francis and Spicer reported little resultant decrease in recurrent attacks of bronchitis. Though the noncapsulated hemolytic influenzae bacteria are commonly grown from the sputum of patients with chronic bronchitis, injections of this bacteria in a vaccine failed to give desired relief. This evidence against infection as the major cause of chronic bronchitis does not rule it out as a secondary factor which occurs in varying degrees in some cases. And this is especially true when complicating saccular bronchiectasis is present, wherein the elimination of purulent sputum continues even though allergy especially to foods may be an initial or major cause of the chronic bronchitis with or without bronchospasm as discussed in the second part of this chapter.

If cough and especially purulent expectoration continue, the sputum must be cultured, and concomitant antibiotics may be indicated. In occasional cases variant forms of pulmonary *Cryptococcus*, as discussed by Tynes, Mason *et al.* in 1968, may need consideration.

It is generally accepted, moreover, that inhalation of air pollutants from coal, petroleum, and other mineral and organic combustibles and from the dusts of agricultural, mineral, and other industrial products increases the morbidity and less frequently the mortality in chronic bronchitis, bronchial asthma, and obstructive emphysema. Since there is no definite evidence that such irritation can cause these chronic respiratory diseases, a predisposition to their development must be assumed. Such predisposition can be explained as allergic or asthmatic in nature, as favored in the Symposium on Chronic Bronchitis in 1960 and as indicated in our practice. It is possible that nearly all of the morbidity and less frequent mortality resulting from marked increase in smog in London and various industrial areas in England, Europe, and in various large cities in our country occur in patients who already have these chronic respiratory diseases. It is also probable that if the allergic causes of these diseases, especially food allergy, were controlled that the serious detrimental effects of smog would be greatly decreased. That the absence of the predisposition to pulmonary allergy helps to explain why the serious effects of smog are limited to a small percentage of the total population is important to emphasize.

That food allergy should be studied as advised in this chapter as a possible cause of longstanding pneumonitis or chronic bronchitis of "unknown origin" is important to remember. When allergy is a possibility, our cereal free elimination diet instead of a general or even soft diet should be routine.

MORBIDITY AND MORTALITY FROM CHRONIC BRONCHITIS

Because of the evidence favoring allergy, especially to foods, as a major cause of chronic bronchitis (CB), study of such allergy should be routine as it is in perennial bronchial asthma and obstructive emphysema. This is especially so because of the prolonged morbidity with increased mortality from chronic bronchitis reported by many students. Orie reported mortality equal to that of pneumonia and pulmonary tuberculosis combined. Many absences from work from CB occur in England and Europe, as evidenced in the report of Francis and Spicer of the loss of 22 million working days because of CB in England and Wales in 1955 and 1956, this being one-fourth of all absences of males from work. In spite of this morbidity, our careful scrutiny of many articles on CB in England as well as in other countries including the United States reveals no adequate study of allergy, particularly to foods, in any considerable number of patients.

PATHOLOGY IN ALLERGIC PULMONARY DISEASES

Atopic allergy in the lungs produces different manifestations depending on the different allergic reactions in varying pulmonary tissues. This is comparable to the different manifestations of atopic allergy which occur in the skin, including a) erythema resulting from allergy in the superficial cutaneous capillaries; b) hives, with or without erythema, resulting from allergy occurring in scattered areas of superficial skin capillaries; c) localized swellings arising from allergy in the deeper cutaneous blood vessels; d) allergic dermatitis characterized by erythema and diffuse permeability of the cutaneous capillaries with exudation of serum and often with oozing, crusting, thickening, and scaling of the skin; e) chronic lesions arising from vascular allergy causing resultant thromboses; or f) parenchymal inflammation in localized areas of the lungs occurring in Loefflers Syndrome.

In like manner different manifestations of pulmonary allergy, especially to foods, have been increasingly recognized in our practice because of major or minor allergic reactions in different pulmonary tissues. Thus in CB there is mucosal inflammation and edema with enlargement of the goblet mucus-producing glands with hypersecretion of mucus, infiltration of eosinophiles, and of other cells arising from allergic inflammation in the bronchial walls. In bronchial asthma there is widening and hyalization of the basement membrane and hypertrophy of the smooth muscle layer; hypertrophy of the mucus-producing glands with resultant excessive bronchial mucus; cellular infiltration especially with eosinophiles; and varying degrees of vasculitis in the parenchyma. In obstructive emphysema there are varying degrees of destruction of alveoli which may result from vascular allergy, especially from foods. This can result from minute thromboses and occlusion in the small blood vessels, including the capillaries; in the walls of the alveoli, with resultant necroses and destruction of the alveoli; and varying degrees of inactivation of the tissues in the parenchyma of the lungs because of

allergic vasculitis. This vasculitis can also arise from tobacco, varying allergic vascular susceptibility to which can explain why some people smoke excessively for twenty to forty years with no resultant CB or obstructive emphysema as shown by our pulmonary function tests and also by our lung scans after intravenous injection of ^{131}I.

Since our good or excellent control of the symptoms of OE reported later in Chapter 11 depends in our opinion on our antiallergic control of bronchospasm and to a lesser extent of bronchorrhea, evidence of such allergy and resultant bronchospasm requires more study in autopsy specimens of the lungs than has been published in the literature.

DIAGNOSIS OF CHRONIC BRONCHITIS

Uncomplicated chronic bronchitis in which allergy to foods is the major cause is characterized by persisting cough at times in paroxysms, along with varying amounts of mucoid expectoration exaggerated or only occurring during the fall to late spring. The sputum usually contains eosinophiles. If it also contains excessive pus cells with or without fever, probable or actual secondary infection requires antibiotics. The sputum is distinctly different from the purulent sputum of bronchiectasis. The frequency of negative scratch tests and the fallibility of positive reactions to foods which occurs emphasizes the failure of test-negative diets in practically all cases to reveal food allergy. Tests with inhalants, especially with pollens, at times reveal potential or active inhalant allergy which may be of secondary or at times major importance.

After the cough and expectoration in CB are controlled by antiallergic therapy advised below, pulmonary function tests and x-rays of the lungs may be normal. If the CB, however, has been perennial, with exaggeration in the fall to spring for several years, secondary infection superimposed on the allergically involved bronchial tissues with varying degrees of resultant pulmonary fibrosis may develop. Such pulmonary fibrosis and increasing bronchiolar markings through the lungs are seen in x-rays. Moderate decrease in pulmonary function tests may occur in spite of the absence of bronchospasm when severe Hammond-Rich syndrome may result.

If chronic cough and expectoration occur in patients with a history indicative of bronchial asthma, the study and control of the allergic causes of such asthma and associated bronchitis must be done according to our advice in Chapter 8. If pulmonary function tests, x-rays of the lungs, lung scans if available, and the clinical history indicate obstructive emphysema, the study of allergy and control of symptoms is the challenge, as advised in Chapter 11.

TREATMENT OF CHRONIC BRONCHITIS

Because of the evidence of allergy as a major cause of CB and the relief we have obtained with the study and control of food allergy, our CFE diet should be immediately prescribed instead of a general diet. Ruling out food allergy in the causation of chronic bronchitis is not justified by a physician unless adequate study of such allergy with this CFE diet has been done for several months, especially in the fall, winter, and spring, when food allergy is activated (Chapt. 1). The initial use of corticosteroids, with their reduction and usual elimination in two to four weeks, is recommended as advised in our chapter on bronchial asthma and OE in Chapters 8 and 11. As emphasized in Chapter 3 the excuse for not ordering this diet that it is not possible to prepare in Europe or even in this country is refuted by the ease of its use in many

hospitals in California and throughout the United States and its accurate use by a host of our patients and parents during the last forty years.

Ordering of this diet in hospitals and home is described in Chapter 3. The list of foods, menus, and recipes with emphasis on the strict adherence to the diet for adequate periods to study food allergy are also detailed in Chapter 3. After relief is assured, provocation tests as advised will gradually determine allergic foods necessary to continue to eliminate from the diet. The decrease of allergy to foods in the summer may allow addition of other foods in July or August. If symptoms recur, especially in September to December, our strict CFE diet must be resumed.

Until the initial symptoms are controlled, corticosteroids are usually advisable, reducing them from large to minimal doses with their usual elimination in two to four weeks. With evidence of secondary infection, indicated antibiotics for limited periods are required.

Our study and control of atopic allergy, especially to foods, and initial corticosteroids have given relief which has continued with little or no steroid therapy. Similar results from steroids require strict control of indicated allergy, especially to foods, with strict maintenance of the elimination diet, as in our Case 49.

If asthma is associated with chronic bronchitis, its treatment as advised in Chapter 8 is required.

As allergenic foods leave the body and allergic reactivity in the pulmonary tissues decreases, the symptoms of CB decrease and usually disappear without continued corticosteroids or other medications. If inhalant allergy is or becomes evident, its control as advised in Chapters 3 and 8 is necessary. Though pollen allergy may be the sole cause of bronchitis in the pollen seasons, it is of questionable or of no importance in the winter, when pollens are out of the air.

CASE RECORDS OF CHRONIC BRONCHITIS

Case 49: A man eighty years of age had coughed through the night and less during the day for three years. The exaggeration of coughing, even to the point of gagging, for one to two weeks every month during the winters favored food allergy as the cause. Dyspnea even with exertion was absent. Previous colds and coughs had been absent. He fortunately had stopped smoking for twenty-five years.

FEV_1 was 65 percent and the third second was 87 percent. Maximum breathing capacity was 123 percent of normal. Scratch tests with inhalants and food allergens were negative.

Study of food allergy with our CFE diet relieved cough and expectoration in one month. Provocation feeding tests with milk, wheat, corn, rice, and coffee reactivated the bronchitis.

Case 50: A man sixty-seven years of age had been awakened with abdominal distention and coughing at 3 AM for eight months. Coughing also occurred with stairclimbing, rapid walking, or lifting. Life-long nasal congestion and postnasal mucus had been present. Epigastric distention had been present forty years.

X-rays of his gastrointestinal tract and gallbladder were negative. Scratch tests with foods and inhalants and routine laboratory tests were negative.

Food allergy was studied with our FFCFE diet, fruits being eliminated because of indigestion. After relief, feeding tests revealed reactivation of the cough and nasal allergy from milk, cereal grains, chocolate, and coffee. Continued elimination of fruits was required to prevent former distention.

DIFFUSE INTERSTITIAL PULMONARY FIBROSIS

Diffuse interstitial pulmonary fibrosis is characterized by progressive dyspnea and a chronic, hacking, dry or slightly productive cough. Its report in four acute cases by Hamman and Rich (1944) explains its continued designation as the *Hamman-Rich syndrome*. Its usual chronicity, however, favors the name *chronic, diffuse, interstitial fibrosis,* as emphasized by Gross (1962). Dr. Scadding (1960) suggests the name *sclerosing alveolitis.* Rare blood mucus suggests secondary malignancy.

In advanced cases shortness of breath (SOB) occurs with slight exertion. Slight cyanosis may increase with exercise. Decreased expansion of the chest and movement of the diaphragms with diffuse hoarse rales and scattered rhonchi, often constant coughing with little or no wheezing, or prolonged expiration differentiates it from obstructive emphysema (OE). Heart sounds are easily heard in contrast to OE. Clubbing of the ends of fingers occurs even before onset of respiratory distress. In chronic severe cases cor pulmonale occurs.

X-ray reveals a diffuse micronodular or microfibrotic picture, especially in the lower lungs. This often appears before cough or SOB.

Progressive contraction of interstitial connective tissue often causes small radiotranslucencies of a "honeycomb lung." Pleural involvement seen in lupus erythematosis, rheumatoid arthritis, and esophageal thickening and immobility seen in scleroderma separate it from these maladies. Complicating malignancy producing larger nodules is rare.

The common physiological abnormalities—impaired diffusion of oxygen across the air-blood interface causing "the alveolar capillary block" syndrome described by Scadding resulting in hypoxemia and a normal or slightly increased pH and low oxygen tension—are present. Frequent hyperventilation causes an elevated alveolar oxygen tension. Respiratory alkalosis is rare.

Explanation of usual hyperventilation was discussed by Marks, in 1967, in his excellent article from which most of the above information, containing forty-eight references, has been summarized and to which the reader is referred.

As Marks states, in spite of increasing recognition and study of this malady by clinicians, radiologists, physiologists, and pathologists, when a final diagnosis of diffuse idiopathic insterstitial pulmonary fibrosis is made "specialty interest fades and the practitioner is left with a most difficult therapeutic problem with little help from his consultants." Atopic allergy, especially to foods, has received no consideration before our present study.

As Stack, in 1965, stated, the unrestricted disease invariably follows a progressive course, leading to gradual deterioration and death in a few months to several years.

Scadding (1960) concluded that the rate of progression varied inversely with age.

These serious and progressive results we opine require the study and control of definite or probable allergy, especially to foods, which has yielded the good nonprogressive benefit in the next case.

Along with bacterial and viral infections causing pneumonitis, collagen vascular diseases, and the autoimmune reactions to lung tissue, allergy to foods, inhalants, and bacteria have been considered causes. Evidence of an assured etiology, however, has never been published. We opine that this may be changed by study of atopic allergy, to foods particularly, as we advise below.

Though hypersensitivity has been indicated by varying degrees of improvement in some patients with corticosteroid therapy, as reported by Scadding in twelve patients in 1960, he stated that improvement usually was stopped with his discontinuance of the hormone because of possible danger of continued corticosteroid therapy.

Because of this improvement in some patients with corticosteroids, study of possible atopic allergy to foods and to possible inhalants as advised in this volume would have been justified.

The excellent control of coughing and increasing SOB resulting from our study and control of food allergy with decreasing and later elimination of corticoids in the following case of diffuse interstitial fibrosis of the lungs justifies such study in other cooperating patients as we advise in this volume, especially in Chapters 2, 3, and 8.

Bilateral Interstitial Fibrosis

Case 51: A man fifty-seven years of age had had nearly constant coughing with moderate clear expectoration but no fever since "pneumonia" five months before in February. Bilateral interstitial pulmonary fibrosis had been diagnosed by x-ray. Shortness of breath had increased for two years; "Can only walk one block" and moderate cardiac decompensation was found. Treatment with antibiotics and steroids gave questionable benefit.

He had recurrent bronchitis and coughing in the fall to late spring for over twenty years, with "pneumonia" five times in his youth and again at twenty-seven, twenty-eight, and fifty-five years of age.

Nasal congestion and sneezing had occurred from hay and grain dust with no seasonal hay fever in the spring or summer.

Diet history indicated no dislikes or disagreements for foods.

Drug history of allergy was absent.

Environmental history indicated sneezing from hay and grain dusts as noted above.

Familial history of respiratory disease or allergy was negative.

Physical examination revealed a moderately cyanotic man, with shortness of breath, exaggerated with constant unproductive coughing and exertion. Crackling rales in the lower lungs; marked clubbing of the fingers; an enlarged chest, especially anterior-posteriorly; and a three plus enlarged prostate were found. Blood pressure was 140/90.

X-rays of the lungs taken on 8/7/67 and 9/17/69 showed evidence of diffuse, chronic, and progressive parenchymal lung disease which appeared to be a chronic progressive fibrosis. There was an increase in the disease process between the dates when the films were taken. Several rib fractures had also appeared in the interval.

Pulmonary function tests showed total vital capacity of 1900 cc (77% of normal). FEV_1 was 1600 cc, 63 percent of normal; FEV_2 was 2450 cc, 96 percent of normal; FEV_3 was 2500 cc, 100 percent of normal; and MBC was 64 percent of predicted.

Lung scan after injection of ^{131}I was normal.

Arterial blood studies on 8/7/67 showed pH 7.46, pCO_2 36 mm, O_2 saturation 95 percent, and pO_2 78 mm.

Blood count showed hemoglobin 77 percent, white blood count 21,350, 39 percent neutrophiles, 53 percent lymphocytes, and 2 percent eosinophiles.

Three months later blood count showed hemoglobin 74 percent, white blood count 14,950, 70 percent neutrophiles, and 30 percent lymphocytes. Sedimentation rate was 49 mm per hour (Wintrobe, corrected). The hematocrit was 37 vol%.

Skin testing revealed one plus reactions to several grass pollens, and one plus to wheat, milk, eggs, tomatoes, and mustard.

Treatment and results: Food allergy was studied with our CFE diet. Aristocort 4 mg three times a day for four days was given, and pertussis and respiratory vaccine 1:10 hypodermically at four-day intervals was administered. The undiluted strength was reached gradually and continued.

Because of cough and shortness of breath in July, desensitization to tree, spring, and fall pollens was given up to 0.7 cc of the 1:50 dilution for the last two years.

With the continuation of the diet and the Aristocort 4 to 8 mg daily, coughing has been absent, and shortness of breath definitely was reduced. He could walk six blocks without increase in shortness of breath, compared with the one block with severe shortness of breath when first seen.

With deviations in diet shortness of breath and some coughing recurred, helped by Tedral® tablets, one to three daily, and inhalation of epinephrine 1:1000 every one or two hours but only for one to three days. No corticosteroids were taken.

9/10/69. *Pulmonary function tests:* Vital capacity 1750 cc FEV_1 was 1300 cc, 74 percent; FEV_2 170 cc, 100 percent; and MBC was 38 percent. Lung scan after injection of ^{131}I was normal.

3/1/70. The above relief continued until SOB and coughing increased in late October because of eating commercial soy-potato bread containing gluten from wheat. With resumption of triamcinolone 12 mg t.i.d. for three days and resumption of a soy-potato bread minus wheat made by the wife, coughing stopped and SOB disappeared in one month. In the last two months cough has been absent and SOB has disappeared, allowing him to walk four to five blocks. He continues to take 2 to 4 mg of the corticoid daily.

Thus the control of food allergy with control of the less important pollen allergy has controlled these symptoms from pulmonary fibrosis and prevented the usual progressive deterioration in this disease.

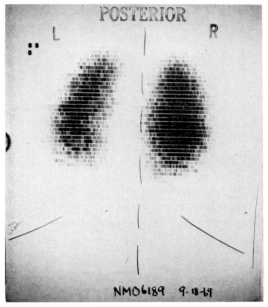

Figure 8. Uniform labelling of both lung fields with radioactivity. No change since the study of 6/6/67 (2 years). *Interpretation:* Normal lung perfusion by scan.

SUMMARY

1. Food allergy as a major cause of chronic bronchitis is supported by the following:

(a) Its exaggeration from early fall to late spring, especially in the winter, which is a characteristic of food allergy (Chapt. 1).

(b) Recognition of an asthmatic constitution and wheezing by European allergists.

(c) Failure to establish infection as the cause.

(d) Frequent eosinophiles in the sputum.

(e) Our excellent results from the study and control of food allergy for many years.

2. Though inhalant allergy may be present, it is infrequently a sole or major cause.

3. If symptoms continue in the late spring and summer, pollen allergy requires study and control.

4. Study of probable food allergy and its control require strict, adequate use of our CFE diet or its modifications as advised in Chapters 3 and 8.

5. Initial and adjunctive use of corticosteroids and of indicated antibiotics for secondary infection are advised in this chapter.

6. With this important recognition and control of allergy (predominantly to foods) morbidity, absenteeism, complications, and mortality from chronic bronchitis usually will be reduced to a minimum.

7. The challenge of study and treating progressive pulmonary fibrosis (Hamman-Rich syndrome) for probable causative atopic allergy, especially to foods, is discussed and illustrated by my results in Case 49.

Chapter 10

Role of Food Allergy in Bronchiectasis

The following information justifies the study of atopic allergy, to foods in particular, in the partial causation of symptoms and the possible origin of bronchiectasis.

Israels, Warringa, and Lowenberg in their article on bronchiectasis in *Bronchitis Symposium* published by Charles C Thomas in 1961 stated that an "asthmatic constitution with allergic alterations in bronchi is a (major) factor in the origin of bronchiectasis." They stated that some of its symptoms may be "residual signs of preexisting bronchial asthma." This does not develop "behind a tuberculous stenosis, foreign body or caseous apical tuberculus." Such "patients may have allergic antecedents" and symptoms "like those of asthmatic allergic patients." They pointed out that bronchiectasis often develops in early life when bronchial asthma is frequent and that some of the symptoms in patients with bronchiectasis may not be due to it but rather to residual effects of preexisting bronchial asthma. Hers stated that "bronchiectasis may result from a viral plus a bacterial infection which destroys the walls of some bronchi in patients with bronchial asthma" or "asthmatic constitution." He also commented on the occurrence of longstanding chronic bronchitis in which the asthmatic constitution so often is evident, as discussed in the last chapter. Brille opined, moreover, that bronchiectasis may arise from obliteration of bronchioli, especially in children who have recurrent bronchio-litis, which always requires the study of food allergy according to our experience (Chapt. 25).

Additional information about the important consideration of atopic allergy, especially to foods, in the initiation of bronchiectasis in Chapter 25 on clinical allergy in childhood is important because of its usual origin in childhood and the frequency of bronchial asthma and of other manifestations of nasobronchial allergy, especially to foods in these young patients.

In addition to the above evidence of probable allergy as a cause of symptoms and as a possible predisposing cause of the bronchiectasis itself, as summarized above, the relief of symptoms arising from the control of food allergy in the following cases of bronchiectasis justifies the study and control of such allergy by physicians.

CASE REPORTS

Case 52: A man forty-five years of age living in Idaho had had bronchiectasis for over thirty years with increasing shortness of breath, coughing, daily expectoration of 6 to 12 oz of purulent sputum, discouragement, and especially weakness for eight to ten years.

Repeated colds and coughs, which always suggest allergy, especially to foods, had occurred in childhood, with increasing cough and purulent expectoration in his teens. At twenty-two years of age, marked bronchiectasis was diagnosed with bronchograms. Cough and expectoration continued, and bronchograms confirmed bronchiectasis again in ten years. Daily expectoration of purulent sputum up to 8 oz a day with severe coughing, shortness of breath, and weakness increased. IPP therapy with micronephrine and 40 percent oxygen three times a day for three years with penicillin by mouth daily for three weeks every two months had been ineffectual. He could walk slowly and drive an oil truck but could not run oil into tanks and could not climb stairs. Medical advice from six physicians and two university clinics gave no help.

He gave no history of allergy except for its probable role in recurrent colds and bronchitis in childhood and as a cause of bronchospasm and cough causing increasing shortness of breath. Scratch tests gave two to four plus reactions to most grass, fall, and tree pollens in Idaho. Slight reactions occurred to several fungi and two plus reactions to eggs and milk. Blood and urine analysis were negative. Pulmonary function tests were not done because of possible contamination of the apparatus from his purulent sputum. Peak flow volume, however, was 240. Sputum examination showed gram-negative and gram-positive cocci. Culture gave many alpha streptococci and *Neisseria*. Diffuse cylindrical and saccular bronchiectasis was confirmed by bronchograms done by David Dugan, M.D., who opined that surgical resection was contraindicated.

Treatment and results: To study food allergy our CFE diet was ordered in the hospital. Aristocort 8 mg q.i.d. was given. No IPP therapy was ordered.

When he left the hospital in seven days, Aristocort was reduced to 4 mg daily. Shortness of breath and cough had decreased, as had his purulent expectoration from 8 to 3 oz a day. Strict adherence to our CFE diet was stressed. Desensitization to all season Idaho pollen antigens was discontinued during the late fall months. Aristocort was stopped.

In the last 2½ years his shortness of breath has disappeared. Strength has increased, so that he delivers oil products by truck. He has bought three oil stations operated with the help of three men. "His wife cannot believe his energy and vigor." He walks and works with no shortness of breath and "is leading the dance." "Formerly he had to sit around and feel sorry for himself." In spite of large skin reactions to pollens, his relief

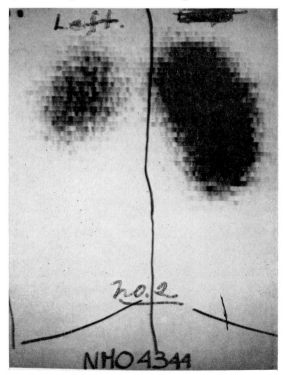

Figure 9. *Left:* 12/12/66. Reduced pulmonary arterial perfusion to the right lung base. Absent perfusion to the lower two-thirds of the left lung. *Right:* 12/23/68. Reduced perfusion of the upper half of the left lung and absent in the lower half. *Conclusion:* The right lung base is better filled with radioactivity, with a moderate increase in the left lung. (Oscar Powell, M.D.)

has occurred with no desensitization therapy and with control of food allergy only.

Two times he has broken his diet, with resultant shortness of breath and increased cough and expectoration for five days. Therefore, he adheres to our CFE diet plus tea and any desired vegetable or fruit except onion. He uses no IPP therapy, no corticoids, and no bronchodilator drugs. Though he continues to expectorate 2 to 3 oz of purulent sputum a day, his strength, vigor, and feeling of well-being enable him to work from 7 AM to 6 PM and to enjoy home life and sleep well. In the last two years he has operated his three oil stations, and he and an assistant are delivering oil products in his entire county in Idaho. Because of the marked reduction in expectoration of purulent mucus, absence of fever and toxicity, and his increased strength and well-being, resection of his involved lung is no longer considered.

Indicative of improvement is the increased filling of his right lung with radioactivity on lung scans during the two years of decreased symptoms of bronchiectasis from control of his food allergy and no intermittent aerosol inhalation therapy, corticoids, or bronchodilator drugs, as shown in Figure 9.

Comment: Because a possible role of atopic allergy in bronchiectasis has not been considered by the medical profession, only a few cases have been referred to us as allergists. The possibility of allergy, especially in saccular bronchiectasis, moreover, seemed unlikely to us until the article by Israels *et al.* was published in 1961. Thus, when the above patient was referred three years ago, we accepted the challenge of studying atopic allergy, especially to foods.

During the last forty years as we have studied and controlled large numbers of patients with perennial bronchial asthma, as we reported especially in 1946 and 1963, other asthmatic patients with cylindrical bronchiectasis and abundant nonpurulent sputum have been benefited by our antiallergic therapy and especially by our control of food allergy. The presence of bronchiectasis in some patients probably was not

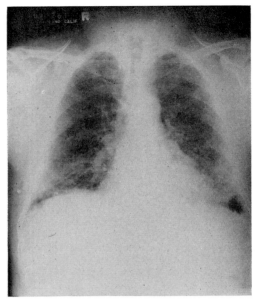

Figure 10. 12/20/66. Lungs moderately hyperlucent, with increased hilar markings. Diffuse fibrous and degenerative tissues in bases, especially on the left. Diaphragms are flattened.

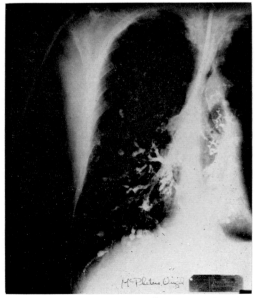

Figure 11. 12/23/66. Marked saccular bronchiectasis first diagnosed twenty-four years ago originating in childhood when asthma resulting (we opine) from food allergy was present.

realized because bronchiograms were not ordered. And as stated above, possible allergy in saccular bronchiectasis had not been considered.

The following case of cylindrical bronchiectasis with incapacitating cough and bronchorrhea has also been relieved with our CFE diet.

Case 53: A man fifty-eight years of age with cylindrical, nonsaccular bronchiectasis, diagnosed by Chevalier Jackson in Philadelphia in 1950, with a history of constant bronchial coughing and bronchorrhea up to 1 pint of nonpurulent sputum daily for over two years was referred because of possible allergy twenty-five years previously.

His history revealed perennial nasal allergy and probable bronchial asthma for twenty years before onset of symptoms when first seen. Though scratch tests to inhalants and foods were negative, they did not rule out clinical allergy, especially to foods.

To study food allergy, our CFE diet was ordered. During his ten-day stay in the hospital, his cough and bronchorrhea rapidly decreased in spite of no antibiotics or corticosteroids, the latter not being available. In the following year entire relief continued with an entirely milk-free and cereal-free elimination diet. This patient had been unable to work for two years and was referred by a physician in New Mexico where climatic change had given no relief.

Apparent shortness of breath and coughing in two additional patients with moderate saccular and cylindrical bronchiectasis of many years' duration have been definitely relieved with adherence to our CFE diet with initial corticosteroids, which now have been eliminated. All foods other than milk, cereal grains, eggs, and coffee are gradually being added.

Because of the possible and in our opinion definite role of atopic allergy in causing the symptoms and the pathogenesis of bronchiectasis, it is most important to recognize and control the allergic causes of bronchial asthma, recurrent bronchitis, bronchiolitis, and perennial nasal allergy in childhood and in young adult life so that bronchiectasis will not develop. It is especially necessary to prevent the establishment of the saccular type, with its resultant purulent expectoration which cannot be eliminated without resection of the involved lobes of the lung. And since such probable allergy is perennial, often exaggerated in the fall and winter and early spring, food allergy especially requires adequate and experienced study as advised in this volume.

SUMMARY

1. That atopic allergy requires recognition and control in bronchiectasis was advised by Israels *et al.* and Hers and Brille in 1961, as is necessary in bronchial asthma.

2. Its usual onset in children often after attacks of recurrent bronchiolitis or asthma, which in our experience is usually due to food allergy, favors it as the initial major cause and as a continuing, exaggerating factor with or without inhalant allergy in childhood and continuing into adult life.

3. The control of atopic allergy usually to foods has reduced the expectoration and cough from cylindrical bronchiectasis to a minimum or entirely, as in Case 52.

4. Therefore, such allergy, especially to foods and when indicated to inhalants, needs strict and adequate study both in cylindrical and saccular bronchiectasis.

5. Adjunctive benefit from antibiotics and vaccine therapy is important in saccular bronchiectasis, as discussed in this chapter.

Chapter 11

Food and Inhalant Allergy in Obstructive Emphysema

Excellent or marked relief of symptoms of obstructive emphysema with varying degrees of chronic bronchitis by the control of food allergy and less often of inhalant allergy with no IPP adrenergic aerosol therapy and with minimal or no corticosteroids or bronchodilator drugs was reported by us in twenty cases at the meeting of the AMA in 1964 and confirmed in an additional sixty cases as reported in *The Journal of Asthma Research* in 1967 and increasingly in subsequent cases in the last three years.

Diagnosis was based on pulmonary function tests, lung scans, x-rays, clinical history, and physical examination.

That perennial bronchospasm and less frequent bronchorrhea in OE require the accurate and adequate study and control of atopic allergy to foods, especially, that we advise, is emphasized by the good or excellent relief of such symptoms with our control of such allergy. No adjunctive intermittent positive pressure therapy and minimal or no corticosteroids or bronchodilator drugs are required. Less frequent inhalant allergy, especially to pollens and less often to animal emanations, dusts, and to other miscellaneous airborne allergens, if indicated by the history and by positive scratch tests, also requires environmental control and if necessary, desensitization therapy, as advised in Chapter 8. These results justify our opinion that the study and control of such possible or evident atopic allergy is mandatory in all cases of OE.

Our recognition and control, especially of food allergy, we opine, will reduce invalidism, morbidity, absenteeism, disability insurance, cost of IPP machines, drugs of many types, psychiatric investigations, inhalation technicians' efforts, sanitarium care, and mortality.

Our results stress the importance of control of allergy which we advise in the treatment of all cases of OE in which bronchospasm and varying degrees of bronchorrhea are present. Atopic allergy, primarily to foods, offers the best explanation. Definite evidence of such allergy may not be present, but its consideration is justifiable in all cases, particularly with bronchospasm. This control is especially necessary when a former history of bronchial asthma has preceded the shortness of breath (SOB) of OE or when a previous allergic predisposition is evident in a carefully recorded history. In some patients histories of perennial nasal allergy with or without postnasal mucus and former nasal and bronchial colds, especially in the fall, winter, and spring months are revealed, indicating possible food allergy (Chapt. 2). Aversions or dislikes for foods, often of long standing, indicate possible food allergy. This is especially true of milk, which justifies study of allergy to it as well as other common allergenic foods excluded from our CFE diet as a cause of increasing bronchospasm and unrecognized bronchial asthma. Chronic bronchitis, which is often associated with or may precede OE, also requires the study of allergy, especially to foods, as emphasized in Chapter 9 instead of infection as its major cause.

The history of former or associated bronchial asthma in a large majority of our patients supports our opinion and that of Banyai and Herxheimer that bronchial asthma plays a major role in the symptoms of OE. Sluiter and Orie made the important statement, "The vast majority of patients with emphysema represent the final stage of a basic asthmatic disorder." Hers and other investigators reported by Orie and Sluiter in 1961 recorded eosinophiles in bronchial tissues and bronchorrhea, emphasizing a common "asthmatic constitution." Orie, in 1961, expressed the common opinion that chronic bronchitis with or without obstruction is due to an unknown underlying cause which our successful results indicate is atopic allergy usually to foods. This has been emphasized by Kaplan (1967) in South Africa with his use of our CFE diet in his article "The Elusive Link in Incurable Bronchial Asthma—Food Allergy."

The great importance of the study and control of food allergy in chronic nonspecific bronchopulmonary disease (CNSBPD) justifies its further discussion and emphasis in Chapter 30.

The recognition of bronchial asthma and its equivalent, the asthmatic predisposition emphasized by Orie and Sluiter in their reports of conferences in Europe, and the evidence of such allergy in our own cases, as confirmed by our good and excellent results from our control of atopic allergy especially to foods, necessitates our disagreement with investigators who conclude that asthma and OE are entirely different diseases. Discussion of this continues in Chapter 30.

We opine that if these patients are studied with an open mind about atopic allergy as we advise, this difference would not be supported. If atopic allergy, especially to foods, had been so studied, more evidence

of allergy with the use of corticosteroids as reported by Klein, Salvaggio, and Kundur in 1969 would have occurred but only in cooperating patients.

The failure of OE to develop in all patients with longstanding seasonal and especially perennial asthma can be explained by localization of the causative allergy in the bronchi and bronchioles without involvement of the capillaries of the alveoli.

Because of our reports since 1947 that food allergy is the sole cause of bronchial asthma in 25 to 40 percent of all cases, even in old age, and is associated with inhalant allergy in an additional 40 to 25 percent, food allergy has been studied in OE importantly with our CFE diet, continuing its use for an adequate period as advised in this chapter and in Chapters 3 and 8. Our emphasis on food allergy as justified by our results without any IPP therapy with little or no corticosteroids is important because of failure of its recognition and control in the literature by other investigators. Thus in pages of the reports of the two European conferences in 1961 and 1964 and in their literature since then, searching of the texts reveals no adequate consideration, study, or control of atopic allergy, especially to foods.

PERSONAL CASES

Summaries of four cases of OE in which food allergy plays a major role follow:

Case 54: A man sixty-two years of age entered the Merritt Hospital in June, 1966, because of invaliding coughing and shortness of breath with exertion, moderate wheezing, and expectoration up to two cups of mucus daily. These symptoms had increased for six years and had been definitely exaggerated in the preceding five months. He had coughed steadily after 5 AM each day associated with wheezing and shortness of breath for three to four hours. Lesser symptoms continued during the day.

Since childhood nocturnal coughing and nasal congestion with discharge had persisted without

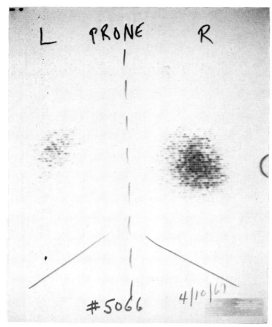

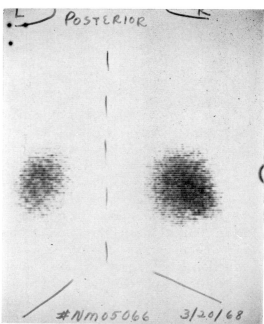

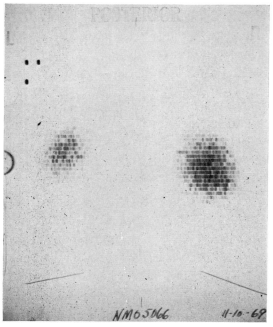

Figure 12. *Left:* 4/10/67. Lung scan: nearly complete obliteration of arterial blood flow in the left lung and reduced flow in the upper half of the right lung. *Right:* 3/20/68. Lung scan chest roentgenogram: hyperinflation and flat low diaphragm. *Bottom:* 11/10/69. No significant change in perfused areas in scans taken 8/19/66, 4/10/67, 3/20/68, and 11/10/69.

Symptoms had not decreased in the preceding three years before which one package of cigarettes had been smoked daily for thirty years.

Physical examination revealed diffuse rhonchi, wheezing, and suppressed breath sounds in his moderately enlarged chest. Blood pressure was 150/96. X-ray of the lungs showed increased translucency and flattened smooth diaphragms. Routine laboratory tests were negative except for 13,200 leukocytes. Scratch testing gave two plus reactions to wheat, milk, and eggs; three plus to tobacco; one plus to several grass pollens; and two plus to tree pollens.

Vital capacity was 3,600 cc, FEV$_1$ 31%, FEV$_3$ 71%, and MBC 69%.

Lung scan revealed limitation of pulmonary blood flow to the mid lungs (see Fig. 12).

An ECG was normal with no evidence of cor pulmonale.

Opinion and treatment: OE with asthmatic bronchitis, increasing cough, and shortness of breath for one year and life long nasal congestion

fever, especially in the winter, indicating probable food allergy.

His symptoms had increased tension, nervousness, and depression for which a tranquilizer had been taken for three years.

Corticosteroids and antibiotics especially in the fall and winter had yielded no continued benefit.

and discharge with no fever, exaggerated in the fall and winter, justified the study of atopic allergy, especially to foods, with our CFE diet.

Adrenalin, 1:1,000, 0.5 cc every one to four hours hypodermically, and Aristocort, 40 mg t.i.d. intramuscularly for three days continuing in decreasing oral doses was ordered. 1000 cc of 5 percent invert sugar, rather than 5 percent glucose, with 7½ grains of aminophylline intravenously were given slowly the first day. Aminophylline 7½ grains by rectum was given at 9 PM for three nights. To control possible secondary infection, though no fever was present, Achromycin® 250 mg t.i.d. was given for three days. Dacron pillows were ordered.

He left the hospital with good relief in eight days. Strict adherence to our CFE diet together with Aristocort 4 mg t.i.d. for two days, b.i.d. for two days, and one time daily thereafter was ordered.

The importance of food allergy is evidenced by excellent control in the last 3¾ years and no evidence of increase of OE.

Steady improvement continued for three months until recurrence of coughing, wheezing, and shortness of breath occurred when he ate wheat and milk against orders.

With the reestablishment of relief effected with adrenalin and brief moderate doses of Aristocort, his cough, nasal allergy, former nervousness, and shortness of breath resulting from limited exertion have been very well controlled. Therapeutic measures include strict adherence to our CFE diet and 2 mg of Aristocort one to two times a day only at intervals. He has traveled by auto three times to Missouri. He has lived in the San Joaquin Valley with no activation of the OE or chronic asthmatic bronchitis. Respiratory infections on three occasions have been controlled with Achromycin, but there has been no activation of his OE or chronic bronchitis. He is working part-time as a custodian in his church, does light work at home, and is able to walk several blocks without stopping because of shortness of breath.

This marked relief of symptoms of OE and chronic bronchitis has depended on the strict elimination of allergenic foods utilizing our CFE diet to which other vegetables and fruits have been added. Relief has also depended on soy-potato bakery products made at home or obtained from a cooperating baker whose products are free of wheat, milk, and other grains excluded from the CFE diet as determined by Arthur Lietze, Ph.D.,

in the Merrill Food Allergy Research Laboratory at the Merritt Hospital (see Chapter 26).

That this relief of bronchospasm, SOB, and nasal discharge resulted from our control of food allergy and not from a decrease in the destructive changes in the lungs is indicated by no change in his four lung scans done in the Nuclear Medical Laboratory of the Merritt Hospital in Oakland on 8/19/66, 4/10/67, 3/20/68, and 11/10/69 and in his pulmonary function tests during the last 3½ years* of his strict adherence to our CFE diet with minimum or no Aristocort and with no adrenergic aerosol therapy by hand atomizer or intermittent positive pressure.

Case 55: A woman sixty-seven years of age had had perennial bronchial asthma for forty-nine years with increasing shortness of breath and bronchospasm for eight years. Study of allergy with our CFE diet was ordered. Aristocort 8 mg t.i.d. for three days was gradually stopped in two weeks.

For two years symptoms have been absent except for shortness of breath on fast walking. The diet has been maintained. Wheezing and shortness of breath from provocation tests with cereal grains, milk, eggs, chocolate, and coffee justified their continued elimination. She uses no corticosteroids or drugs. She sleeps well. Weight of 86 lbs is maintained. She walks three blocks to an office building. She has never smoked. IPPB therapy has never been used. In the last six months all foods except milk as such has been tolerated with no reactivation of symptoms. Whether this tolerance continues especially during the winter remains a question.

Present VC is 1600 cc, FEV₁ 50%, FEV₃ 75%, MBC 61%, and pO₂ 84 mm. Hg, pCO₂ 38.5 mm, Hg, pH 7.41.

The continued excellent relief is best explained by the control of food allergy without drugs, corticosteroids, or IPPB and not by a decrease in the destructive lung disease.

PATIENTS' TESTS AND X-RAYS

Statistics on the first fifteen of forty-six patients published in 1967 in whom pulmonary function tests, especially the FEV₁, lung scans, x-ray findings, clinical history

---

*Report of O.M. Powell, M.D., Director of the Nuclear Medical Laboratory, Merritt Hospital, Oakland.

and physical examination, and indicated OE are in Table XXI.

Pulmonary function tests were done for our office or by A.C. McCuistion, M.D., in the Pulmonary Function Laboratory at the Merritt Hospital. Residual volumes in forty patients varying from 0.75 to 7 liters above normal values supported the diagnosis of obstructive emphysema.

Initial tests were done two to eight weeks after initial control of severe and often incapacitating bronchospasm and less severe bronchorrhea by our medications as advised in this chapter and by the immediate study of and control of food allergy with our CFE diet and indicated environmental control. Desensitization was used to control indicated inhalant allergy, especially to pollens and to those inhalants that are not eliminated from the inspired air by environmental control. Pulmonary function tests on the first one to two days before initial control of assumed bronchial asthma in these patients showed greater airway obstruction, as shown in Table XXI.

The average results of tests for vital capacity, FEV_1, FEV_3, and MBC were the same or only slightly increased after one-half to four years of good or excellent control of symptoms, as summarized in Table XXI.

Thus it appears that the marked clinical improvement was not due to a decrease in the destructive lung disease but to control of bronchospasm and varying mucosal edema resulting from the control of allergy, especially to foods.

LUNG SCANS

As advised by Lopez-Majano, Tow, and Wagner, lung scans have been done in thirty-four of the forty-six patients and in seven other patients in whom initial peak expiratory flow rates were determined rather than pulmonary function tests. The reduced arterial blood flow indicates probable obstructive lung disease of a moderate to severe degree in varying parts of one or both lungs with obliteration of even two-

TABLE XXI

PULMONARY FUNCTION TESTS, LUNG SCANS AND X-RAY FINDINGS
INDICATING OBSTRUCTIVE EMPHYSEMA IN 15 RELIEVED PATIENTS

			Tests 2-8 Weeks After Initial Control of Bronchospasm					Tests After Relief of Obstructive Symptoms for 1½ to 4 Years						
Case	Age	Sex	VC %	FEV 1 sec %	FEV 3 sec %	MBC %	Years of Control	VC %	FEV 1 sec %	FEV 3 sec %	MBC %	Lung Scan	X-Ray	Amount of Relief
1	59	F	73	40	70	35	2	57	38	65	35	3+	4	3
2	53	F	88	45	69	61	1	92	44	77	62	3+	2	4
3	65	M	70	28	48	25	1½	65	26	52	28	3+	4	3
4	59	M	53	30	55	20	½	59	27	52	25	3+	3	4
5	51	M	100	34	57	39	1	105	34	62	40	3+	4	4
6	62	M	54	56	90	51	1	70	51	70	60	4+	4	4
7	54	M	51	50	74	33	1	62	50	72	36	2+	4	3
8	59	F	110	44	72	50	½	94	40	76	55	1+	4	3
9	59	M	80	43	70	47	4	90	43	69	49	2+	4	4
10	71	M	98	52	65	80	1½	64	57	86	56	3+	3	4
11	66	F	63	53	86	37	½	56	56	78	53	2+	4	4
12	61	M	85	47	85	56	½	88	57	82	60	2+	3	4
13	53	M	90	57	76	80	1	94	56	80	78	2+	2	4
14	65	M	53	55	74	35	3	55	53	82	47	2+	4	4
15	68	M	80	46	75	40	3	81	44	76	43	2+	4	4

Note: The results in the first 15 of the 46 patients published in 1967 are reprinted.

TABLE XXII

PEAK FLOW RATES, PULMONARY FUNCTION TESTS, LUNG SCANS AND
X-RAY FINDINGS INDICATING OBSTRUCTIVE EMPHYSEMA IN 7 RELIEVED CASES

Case	Age	Sex	Initial Peak Flow Rate	Years of Control	VC %	FEV 1 sec %	FEV 3 sec %	MBC %	Lung Scan	X-Ray	Amount of Relief
1	67	M	140	½	52	37	84	27	4+	4	4
2	73	M	160	¾	27	52	96	27	2+	3	4
3	73	M	120	½	112	52	88	40	2+	4	4
4	72	M	240	½	90	42	77	41	2+	3	4
5	68	F	180	1	102	62	87	56	3+	1	4
6	60	M	120	4	85	61	93	62	2+	1	4
7	49	F	220	1½	116	56	87	60	2+	1	4

Note: The results in 7 of the 14 patients published in 1967 are reprinted.

thirds of both lungs as indicated by 1 to 4 (maximum) in Tables XXI and XXII.

X-RAYS OF LUNGS

Indications of obstructive emphysema in the x-ray of the lungs are graded 1 to 4 in Tables XXI, XXII, and XXIV: (1) hyperinflation, (2) hyperinflation and depressed diaphragm, (3) hypertranslucence and flat diaphragm, and (4) the former with widened intercostal spaces and increased A-P diameter of the chest.

PATHOLOGY IN THE PULMONARY TISSUES IN OBSTRUCTIVE EMPHYSEMA INDICATIVE OF ALLERGY

In view of the importance of atopic allergy, especially to foods, indicated in our practice in OE, pathological evidence of

such pulmonary allergy needs additional study. As in intractable bronchial asthma, eosinophiles are numerous in the bronchial mucus in OE, as emphasized in the Symposium on Bronchitis edited by Orie and Sluiter in 1961. There occurs an increase in the activity of goblet cells in the bronchial mucosa which is responsible for the bronchial mucus. The bronchial walls are often infiltrated by eosinophiles, histiocytes, and eosinophilic "granules."

Because of the marked bronchospasm in OE, which we are relieving in varying degrees with the control of allergy to foods particularly and less often to inhalants and with initial large doses of corticosteroids which can be decreased to a minimum or eliminated in seven to twenty days, more microscopic studies in the walls of the small

TABLE XXIII

VARIATIONS AND AVERAGES OF PULMONARY FUNCTION TESTS
IN 46 CASES OF INDICATED OBSTRUCTIVE EMPHYSEMA

	Tests Done 1-2 Weeks After Initial Control of Bronchospasm	Tests Done After Control of Bronchospasm for ½-4 Yrs	Averages %	Normal Values
Vital capacity (% of predicted value)	30-136		82	Over 85%
		32-138		
FEV 1st sec. (% of predicted value)	28-60		46	75-80%
		26-64	47	
FEV 3rd sec. (% of predicted value)	48-100		76	90-97%
		52-94	78	
M.B.C. (% of predicted value)	20-80		48	75-80%
		32-81	51	

TABLE XXIV

RESULTS OF PULMONARY FUNCTION TESTS DONE IN 1967

FOR VC, FEV₁, FEV₃, AND MBC

			Tests in 1-2 Days Before Control of Bronchospasm					Tests After Relief of Obstructive Emphysema for 1-2 Months						
Case	Age	Sex	VC %	FEV 1 Sec %	FEV 3 Sec %	MBC %	Inc. in FEV 1st Second	VC %	FEV 1 Sec %	FEV 3 Sec %	MBC %	Lung Scan	X-Ray	Amount of Relief
1	65	M	84	19	47	27	9	70	28	49	25	3+	4	3
2	59	M	53	20	50	16	10	53	30	55	20	3+	4	4
3	51	M	104	22	53	35	12	112	34	57	39	3+	4	4
4	52	F	103	50	83	40	13	128	73	92	78	1+	1	4
5	51	M	102	50	70	51	15	116	65	93	58	3+	3	4
6	59	M	60	25	63	40	18	80	43	73	47	3+	4	3
7	44	F	70	45	77	55	27	82	72	97	67		3	4
8	51	F	72	42	80	30	23	73	65	84	36		1	4
9	48	F	94	35	84	66	23	101	58	80	59	2+	1	4

Note: On the first 1 or 2 days of our initial study the results were definitely lower than those done in 2-8 weeks resulting from our control of initial bronchospasm and bronchorrhea. These statistics were published in 1967.

bronchi and bronchioles in OE should be done. Possible presence of metaplasia of the mucosa, hypertrophied basement membrane and smooth muscle as well as an increase in eosinophiles in the submucosa which occur in severe bronchial asthma needs to be investigated. Moreover, evidence of allergic vasculitis in the pulmonary tissues which could produce thromboses and necroses and disintegration in the alveolar walls and interstitial tissues requires investigation.

ANTITRYPSIN DEFICIENCY AND EMPHYSEMA

It has been found that patients with antitrypsin deficiency in their serum are very likely to develop emphysema. Nevertheless, the great majority of emphysema patients do not have this deficiency. Fagerhol and Hauge (1969) found that in many types of chronic pulmonary disease 8 out of 503 patients (1 out of 14 emphysema) had an antitrypsin deficiency, whereas 0.8 patients would statistically be expected to have this deficiency. This means that a patient who has chronic pulmonary disease has only about two chances out of a hun-

dred of having the deficiency. Those patients who do have the deficiency, however, have an extremely high chance of developing chronic pulmonary disease, but they characteristically develop it at an early age (under 40) and not in later years.

STARCH AND EMPHYSEMA

Because of the demonstration of IgA globulin antibodies to starch, particularly in sera of emphysema patients by Lietze, Volkheimer's report of presence of starch particles in the small blood vessels of the lungs is of interest.

INCORRECT OR OVERLOOKED DIAGNOSES OF OE

An incorrect diagnosis of OE is not infrequent, causing unfortunate concern in the patient and family because of the increasing morbidity and mortality which are being reported from OE in medical and lay publications. Emphysema is being misdiagnosed at times because of questionable or slight shortness of breath or coughing, a slightly flattened or low diaphragm in the x-ray, or symptoms of bronchial asthma without abnormal pulmonary function tests or abnormal lung scans.

Some of these maladies, moreover, may produce moderate changes in pulmonary function tests, x-rays of the lungs, and lung scans which also result from OE. Careful diagnostic study therefore must be made. However, if the FEV$_1$ is over 70 to 75%, the FEV$_3$ is over 90%, the MBC is over 75%, and the lung scan reveals no decrease in the arterial blood flow in the lungs, OE can be excluded. If these tests approach normal in one to two months with the control of atopic allergy, bronchial asthma rather than OE also is indicated.

The shortness of breath, coughing, and wheezing, moreover, may be wrongly attributed to some of the maladies listed in the differential diagnosis of bronchial asthma instead of to OE. Cardiac disease especially may be blamed. Thus the decision that shortness of breath and wheezing are due to OE requires accurate pulmonary function tests and lung scans if available.

When the common complication—cor pulmonale—arises from OE, the shortness of breath, cough, and wheezing may be due to right heart failure as well as to symptoms of OE caused by pulmonary allergy. Edema of the legs may result from pressure of the depressed diaphragms.

HISTORY AND SKIN TESTS

In our sixty patients a history of bronchial asthma or of an asthmatic predisposition occurred in 85 percent of them. Where this was not evident, there usually was a history of perennial nasal allergy or of chronic bronchitis, indicating probable allergy especially to foods. That bronchial asthma was probable in 70 percent of the family histories was evidenced in a well-taken history of the immediate family and relatives.

The ages varied from twenty-nine to seventy-three years (av. 57 years). Obstructive symptoms had occurred for one to fifteen years (av. 3.6 years).

Positive scratch tests to foods were present in only twenty-six cases. Such tests usually did not correlate with subsequently incriminated allergenic foods. Because of the fallibility of positive and negative scratch reactions in determining clinical allergy to foods, our CFE diet rather than a test-negative diet was used adequately and strictly to study food allergy.

Slight to definite reactions occurred to pollens in eighteen cases and to animal emanations, fungi, and dusts in a small number. Though environmental control was advised in most patients, its necessity in all cases was questionable. When history indicated exaggeration of symptoms to inhalants, especially pollens, desensitization to them is done.

EVIDENCE FAVORING ALLERGY TO FOODS AND PROBABLY TO TOBACCO AS A CAUSE OF OBSTRUCTIVE EMPHYSEMA

Destruction in the walls of the alveoli and adjacent tissues characterizing obstructive emphysema is best explained in our opinion by vasculitis with resultant thrombosis and necrosis in the capillaries of the alveolar walls resulting from allergy to foods as well as to tobacco. Bronchospasm causing most of the shortness of breath is best explained by contraction, especially in the bronchioles; varying degrees of cough and bronchial mucus by mucosal edema; and secretion in the small bronchioles. The latter also explains coughing and mucoid expectoration varying according to the degree of localized mucosal allergy.

Without bronchospasm resulting from allergy, shortness of breath would be minimal from the destruction of the alveoli alone, as evidenced by no increased shortness of breath at rest after unilateral lobotomy, providing bronchial asthma or obstructive emphysema is absent. Similarly, atrophy in the alveoli without bronchospasm usually occurs in most senile emphysema.

Favoring food allergy as the cause of shortness of breath in obstructive emphysema is our confirmation for seven years of the marked relief of shortness of breath in two to eight weeks from the total and continued elimination of allergenic foods with the use of our CFE diet or its modifications, aided with little or no adrenergic inhalation therapy and especially with no intermittent positive pressure. Little or no oral corticosteroids or bronchodilator drugs are required except for initial relief in the first two or three weeks until allergenic food residues leave the body.

Allergy is also indicated by the marked relief from large initial doses of corticosteroids and of moderate doses of bronchodilator drugs, both of which can be reduced to a minimum or discontinued entirely, as allergens in the causative foods or tobacco, if allergy to it is a cause, leave the body in one to four weeks.

Moderate relief of symptoms of shortness of breath from limited use of corticosteroids has also been reported by Scadding and others.

That allergic vasculitis to allergens in foods, tobacco, and probably at times to other inhalants best explains the destructive changes in the lungs diagnosed by pulmonary function tests and particularly by lung scans is supported by the absence of shortness of breath, abnormal pulmonary function tests, and lung scans in those people who have developed no allergy to lifelong daily ingested foods or to daily inspired inhalants. This is especially true of tobacco, even after continued smoking of

two to three packages of cigarettes daily for thirty to forty years. Demonstrating the unimportance of tobacco smoke is the second reported failure to induce pulmonary emphysema in rats by inhaled tobacco smoke by Aviado *et al.* in 1970.

Cigarettes were smoked in quantities of one to three packs a day for fifteen to forty-five years by 76 percent of our patients who were relieved by our therapy. Though severe symptoms of OE usually occurred in heavy cigarette smokers who were relieved by our antiallergic control, they also occurred in 24 percent of patients who had never smoked, indicating that atopic pulmonary allergy, especially to foods, was the common cause of obstructive lung disease in these nonsmokers.

The marked infrequency of tissue changes of OE in lungs removed for cancer resulting from long-inhaled tobacco smoke also does not favor allergy to tobacco as a cause.

That allergy to foods is of greater probable importance than to tobacco is evidenced by failure of lasting relief of symptoms of obstructive emphysema even with limited corticoid therapy in our patients who have never smoked or have discontinued smoking for months or even years until our advised control of food allergy has been established for more than a few weeks. Statements that the etiology of centrilobar emphysema is accurately known to be due to cigarette smoking are premature when cessation of smoking does not ameliorate the SOB and food allergy therapy does.

That obstructive emphysema and chronic bronchitis can result from atopic allergy to foods or tobacco without definite clinical evidence of bronchial asthma, except bronchospasm, and that chronic asthma often occurs without emphysema is explained by the long-recognized localization of allergic reactivity in only one area of a tissue or vital organ. Thus localization of allergy in the alveoli in perennial bronchial asthma is comparable to localization of eczema only on the hands or fingers and not in other cutaneous areas or in the conjunctiva or cornea and not in the sclera, retina, or lens of the eye (Chapt. 20). Thus localized allergy, especially in the alveoli and small bronchioles, to foods and probably to tobacco and less often to other inhalants best explains obstructive emphysema. Therefore, the recognition and control of food allergy as we advise supported by our good and excellent results reported in this chapter and in our articles in the literature for the last seven years are important challenges and responsibilities of the medical profession.

CONTROL OF FOOD ALLERGY

The relief of invaliding symptoms of emphysema and chronic bronchitis in the group of sixty patients we reported in 1967 and as we reported in twenty cases in 1965 justifies the immediate study of food allergy with our CFE diet and the control of less frequent pollen or other inhalant allergies. Hospital dietitians are glad to cooperate in the preparation of the CFE diet, and office patients are easily instructed in its use. Since food residues remain in the body for two or more weeks and because a longer time is needed for chronic tissue changes in the lungs from atopic allergy to decrease, strict adherence to the diet is imperative.

After relief for six weeks other vegetables and fruits, one by one, may be added as we have advised in Chapter 3. After relief is assured for three to four months, wheat, milk, other cereal grains, eggs, chocolate, coffee, and fish may be tried. If symptoms recur, recently added foods must be eliminated. Bakery products must be made by a baker supervised by the patient or made in the patient's home. Unlisted wheat products in commercial bakery products have been determined in our Immunochemical Laboratory by Dr. Lietze, as reported in 1967. Since food allergy often decreases in the summer, provocation feeding tests are best done in the fall, winter, and spring. Less frequent inhalant allergy must be controlled.

CONTROL OF INHALANT ALLERGY

Though environmental control to reduce possible allergy to animal emanations and house dust was encouraged in most patients, allergens in the home were of minor importance to food allergens. Desensitization to dog and horse dander was given in only one patient, who was also allergic to foods. Pollen desensitization was given to twelve patients because of former hay fever in the spring or fall and positive reactions to pollens. Food rather than pollen allergy explained the perennial symptoms usually exaggerated in the winter.

CONTROL OF SYMPTOMS IN OUR SIXTY PATIENTS

Hospitalization was necessary because of severe invaliding symptoms in 30 percent of patients. To study allergy to foods, our CFE diet was ordered. In very sick patients it was first given with soft, minced, easily eaten prescribed foods. To control allergy, large doses of corticosteroids intramuscularly or by mouth were given for three to four days until bronchospasm, rales, and shortness of breath became minimal. Then oral corticosteroids were reduced to a minimum or eliminated in two to four weeks. This benefit from corticosteroids also reported by Lowell supports the major role of allergy in OE. Klein *et al.*, in 1969, reported improvement in spirometric values from brief use of corticosteroids in six of eighteen cases of obstructive lung disease. Better results similar to ours would have resulted with control of food and possible inhalant allergy as we advise. Questionable or poor results from former use of corticosteroids are explained by failure to study and control allergy especially to foods as we advise. Relief with no continued corticosteroid therapy has occurred in 30 percent of our patients as noted below. Possible activation of a duodenal ulcer requires antacid therapy and the elimination of fruit and condiments from the CFE diet as advised in Chapter 5. Fluid and electrolyte deficiencies were corrected. Because of possible corn allergy, 5 percent invert sugar instead of 5 percent dextrose was given by vein (see Chapt. 8). Water was encouraged. Epinephrine by injection or inhalation and aminophylline were given as required. Complicating cardiac impairment or pulmonary infection necessitated control. IPPB therapy in hospital and later in office or home was not required when study and control of allergy, especially to foods, as we advise were strictly maintained. In three to ten days ability to walk about the hospital with minimal or no shortness of breath occurred in all patients.

Moderate symptoms justified study and control of symptoms only in the office in 65 percent of patients. The CFE diet was ordered immediately. Initial large oral doses of corticosteroids gradually were reduced or stopped in two to three weeks, as emphasized in Chapter 30. Epinephrine given hypodermically by the patient or by inhalation was advised. Aminophylline rectally helped initial bronchospasm.

Continued relief at home is maintained by strict unquestioned adherence to the CFE diet as discussed above. In 70 percent of the patients, triamcinolone 2 to 6 and rarely 8 mg a day by mouth is justified, especially for one to three days after slight

breaks in the diet to give maximum relief to the shortness of breath. Epinephrine or Isuprel by inhalation and Ephedrine-Aminophylline tablets, one or two a day, at times are given for moderate or intermittent bronchospasm. No medications or corticoids were required for continued relief in twenty patients. Relief has continued without breathing exercises or any IPPB therapy in all cooperating patients.

CONTROL OF ATOPIC ALLERGY MAKES THE USUALLY ADVISED THERAPY UNNECESSARY

With the control of allergy, especially to foods, as advised in this chapter with or without minimal corticosteroid and bronchodilating therapy, good or excellent relief of symptoms in practically all cases of OE and chronic bronchitis occurs without use of adjunctive therapeutic measures as advised in medical articles, manuals and textbooks, and in rehabilitation programs for relief of OE and other obstructive lung disease. Our treatment has included or required:

1. No IPPB therapy with adrenergic aerosols.
2. No breathing exercises in classes or clinics.
3. No postural drainage except in definite bronchiectasis.
4. No oxygen therapy except as indicated in cardiac decompensation.
5. No "tapping of the chest" or breathing through pursed lips.
6. No tracheostomies except in rare emergencies.
7. No emphysema belts.
8. No or rare psychological therapy as encouragement from relief of symptoms occurs.

These conclusions about present-day forms of therapy based on our good and excellent results in the control of shortness of breath and other symptoms of obstructive emphysema harmonize with the recent conclusions of Emirgil, Sobol, *et al.* that the three forms of usual therapy, namely (a) antibiotics and nebulized bronchodilator, (b) IPP adrenergic therapy, and (c) breathing exercises, do not influence the course of chronic bronchitis and OE. It emphasizes atopic allergy, especially to foods, which with our advised decreasing and finally little or no drug therapy has been responsible for the good and excellent control of chronic bronchitis and OE we report in this chapter and in Chapters 8, 9, and 10.

The necessity of considering vascular allergy to tobacco in the walls of the alveoli and adjacent tissues as an additional cause of obstructive emphysema along with the danger of cancer from the inhalation of tar and other irritating substances emphasizes the necessity of its entire disuse in obstructive lung disease, even though 20 percent of our proved patients with OE have been nonsmokers.

The importance of the control of probable allergy to foods and to a lesser degree to inhalants and the cessation of inhaled tobacco smoke is emphasized by the increased morbidity and mortality from obstructive lung disease, especially of OE, as reported by the Public Health Service. Its statistics state deaths from chronic bronchitis and obstructive emphysema have doubled every five years. Even in 1965, according to Hepper *et al.*, 23,700 deaths were reported from obstructive emphysema and chronic bronchitis by the Public Health Service. In 1964, moreover, chronic respiratory disease contributed to fifty thousand deaths. OE was second to heart disease as a cause of social security disability in males and yearly pensions were up to ninety million dollars. It was estimated that at least 10 percent of the males

over the age of forty had evidence of obstructive lung disease in the Mayo Clinic.

Recognition of atopic allergy as the main cause of obstructive lung disease, especially of OE, as supported by our results from its recognition and control by our cooperating patients in our opinion will greatly reduce morbidity, mortality, the necessity of disability payments, and the over ninety million dollars paid for social disability each year, as recorded in 1965.

With relief and control of atopic allergy many of our patients have continued or resumed a gainful occupation. Since we have not used intermittent positive pressure, the cost of these apparati, estimated through our questionnaires to hospitals and clinics throughout the country to be over ninety million dollars, and the expense of technician-therapists in hospital and emphysema clinics, plus the expense of additional personnel and housing in operating of such clinics would, we are assured, be markedly reduced if atopic allergy were controlled with minimal or no adjunctive corticoid and drug therapy that we have used to obtain published results. These have been obtained without instruction in and the use of breathing exercises in emphysema clinics and with no intermittent adrenergic inhalation therapy as stated above.

Patients advised in the Mayo Emphysema Clinic according to Hepper *et al.* reported in 1968 that "some help in understanding the disease" and its problems was obtained in 67 percent, improvement occurred in 37 percent, no change occurred in 38 percent, and that the symptoms had increased in 19 percent during the ensuing year. Six percent did not answer the questionnaire.

In these clinics technician-therapists occupy a major role in the operation of the clinic under the supervision of a physician. Such clinics and technician-therapists in emphysema clinics in our hospital cases have not been necessary to obtain our good results.

With relief of symptoms with minimal or no dependence on the above adjunctive procedures, frustration and discouragement in patients because of failure of relief from previous medical therapy and the publicized serious prognoses and increasing mortality from OE, nervousness and tension are greatly reduced, which has made psychological therapy and counsel unnecessary.

With this recognition and control of bronchial allergy, especially to foods, "the dilemma in therapy" and the "R factor" are largely answered, the increasing morbidity and mortality in this country can be reversed, the relief of cor pulmonale and right-sided heart failure are expedited, and the need of emphysema classes and inhalation therapists and emphasis on the grave prognosis will be decreased. Increased physical activity and a return to gainful occupation are possible.

Skepticism of a physician about the great importance of atopic allergy, especially to foods, as the major cause of the symptoms of obstructive emphysema with varying chronic bronchitis will gradually disappear after study and control of such allergy, with resulting decrease in our initially advised bronchodilator drugs, and corticosteroids has been maintained in more than a few cooperating patients for more than two to three months.

SUMMARY

1. With control of atopic allergy, especially to foods, marked or good relief was reported in sixty private patients in 1967 and in an additional thirty-five patients in the last two years, with indicated obstructive emphysema and chronic bronchitis, confirming our report in our first twenty patients in 1964. The crippling, progressive course of this disease in cooperating patients has been prevented.

2. Formerly used bronchodilator drugs, inhalant therapy, and corticosteroids which had given little or no lasting relief have been greatly reduced or eliminated.

3. No IPPB therapy has been used or required.

4. Relief has allowed increased activity and in some patients a return to gainful occupations.

5. The good or excellent relief of symptoms of obstructive emphysema depends primarily on the control of bronchospasm and bronchorrhea resulting from our control of food and less frequently of inhalant allergy and not on the reduction of the destructive parenchymal changes in the lung, the cause of which, in our opinion, is also best explained by vasculitis and resultant necroses from such allergy.

6. Though cigarettes were smoked for years by forty-six patients, emphysema developed in fourteen nonsmoking patients with asthmatic predispositions.

7. Since relief has not been accompanied with definite improvement in pulmonary function tests, it is best explained by relief of bronchospasm, mucous membrane edema, and bronchorrhea resulting from control of atopic allergy, especially to foods.

8. This importance of allergy, especially to foods, in obstructive emphysema and chronic bronchitis is similar to that in bronchial asthma in all ages which we have long reported as determined with our CFE diet and emphasized in Chapters 3 and 8 of this book. With the study of food allergy as advised, its major role in the causation of OE will receive important confirmation by other physicians.

9. Initial strict elimination of all cereals as well as of milk, eggs, chocolate, and less

allergenic foods in the study of food allergy must be emphasized.

10. This study of atopic allergy, especially to foods, as we advise therefore is a primary major challenge in all patients with these chronic respiratory diseases. The allergic cause of bronchospasm, especially to food, must be found and eliminated. Reliance on bronchodilating drugs by inhalation or orally and corticosteroid therapy is unjustified.

11. As evidenced in repeated lung scans, there is no decrease or increase in the destructive changes in the lungs even though SOB and other symptoms of OE have been uniformly decreased in patients cooperating in our control of allergy, especially to foods, with minimal or no adjunctive drug therapy.

12. Skepticism about this importance of food allergy and to a lesser extent inhalant and especially pollen allergy is not justified unless its adequate study and control as we advise with limited or no adjunctive inhalant or oral bronchodilating drugs in more than a few patients for several months and not for three weeks has been continued.

Chapter 12

Perennial Nasal and Laryngeal Allergy Resulting From Food and Inhalant Allergy

Food allergy, alone or with inhalant allergy, is in our experience of forty years the common cause of perennial nasal allergy. With its recognition, possible chronic or recurrent infection in the nose and sinuses becomes a minimal cause. As discussed below, recurrent fever with attacks of nasal allergy is often due to food allergy rather than to infection. Failure to recognize food allergy is due to the fallibility of the skin test, failure of most "test-negative diets," to reveal such allergy, and failure to use a trial diet, especially our CFE diet, for its study.

A typical history suggesting food allergy follows: Congestion and intermittent or constant nasal blocking with varying watery or mucoid discharge occur. Increase of symptoms from food allergy in ocean areas, with decrease in inland and especially dry areas, may occur. Exaggeration in the winter half of the year is usual. Sneezing and itching resulting from food allergy are less than in inhalant allergy. Some tickling, upward or lateral pushing and picking of the nose, loss of smell and taste, sniffling, mouth-breathing, noisy breathing, and snoring are frequent. Soreness of the throat, hoarseness, and postnasal mucus causing hacking, gagging, and throat-clearing arise. Disturbed, restless sleep and in childhood sleeping on knees or pounding of the head may occur.

The nasal mucosa is edematous and pale. Eosinophiles usually are in the mucus.

Edema and vacuolization of the cytoplasm in the ciliated columnar epithelial cells which are wiped from the nasal mucosa may indicate food allergy, according to Byron, in contrast to nuclear and cytoplasmic degeneration resulting from the common cold.

Nasal polyps in our experience are usually due to food allergy. Regrowth has been retarded or prevented in our patients when food allergy is continually and strictly controlled.

DENTAL DEFORMITIES IN CHILDREN RESULTING FROM PERENNIAL NASAL ALLERGY, ESPECIALLY TO FOOD

Perennial nasal allergy causes mouth breathing and resultant occlusion and V-shaped dental arches, as discussed by Marks in 1965 in which references to many other articles in which allergy received little and usually no consideration are listed.

Since food allergy requires special study together with less frequent inhalant allergy, it is important to study and control it in the strict and adequate manner advised in this chapter and in Chapters 2 and 3. Less frequent and less important inhalant allergies must be controlled.

FOOD AND INHALANT ALLERGY IN TWO-HUNDRED PRIVATE CASES OF PERENNIAL NASAL ALLERGY

The frequency of food and inhalant allergy singly and of food in association with inhalant allergies in two hundred private cases controlled by us in five or more years is shown in Table XXV. In comparison to the sole role of food allergy in 42 percent, its role in association with inhalant allergy varied from a dominant to a minor role.

FOOD ALLERGY AS THE SOLE CAUSE OF PERENNIAL NASAL ALLERGY

Because of the frequency of food allergy as the sole cause, histories on fifty such cases relieved with the use of our CFE diet with no injections of inhalant antigen or vaccine are shown in Table XXVI. Because of the fallibility of and frequent absence of scratch reactions to allergenic foods, test-negative diets usually fail to reveal food allergy and are not used in our practice.

Many patients had used nose drops, non-allergenic pillows and bedding, environmental control—all with no benefit. Previous desensitization with such inhalants for months and in two cases for seven years had been of no help. Partial or marked relief occurred, however, in two to three weeks with the control of food allergy with my CFE diet alone.

That infection itself or infectant allergy rarely if ever causes perennial nasal allergy is increasingly evident to rhinologists and allergists. Previously assumed infection has led to unrelieving operations on the turbinates and sinuses. Antral washings, windows in the nasal antral walls, and Luc Caldwell operations have been done for assumed infection. Thereafter, secondary infection often resulted. This complication, with the unrelieved nasal allergy resulting from unrecognized food and/or inhalant allergy, has produced increased distress and even semiinvalidism.

COMMENTS ON STATISTICS IN TABLE XXV

The nasal allergy resulting from food allergy in these patients occurred in all ages from one-half to sixty-one years. This finding refutes the claim that food allergy rarely or never occurs after forty years. The frequency of congested and blocked noses and of so-called repeated head colds in young children resulting from food allergy is not shown because of the limited number of children in this group. Thus the adenoid facies and malocclusion of teeth from long-continued mouth-breathing and the common upward pushing of the nose from chronic food allergy are not emphasized. Recurrent serous otitis media and fever resulting not from infection but to food allergy are exemplified in two case histories.

This perennial nasal allergy continued on an average of fourteen years, varying from one to fifty-nine years. Lasting relief from local therapy, decongestants, vaccines and desensitization to inhalants, and from operations of the septa, sinuses, and polyps when utilized had failed. The relief from our control of their food allergies alone emphasizes the importance of their recognition.

Intermittent or constant blocking of the nose with congestion occurred in 72 percent. Moderate watery and at times mucoid

TABLE XXV

FREQUENCY OF FOOD AND INHALANT ALLERGY IN 200 PRIVATE PATIENTS CONTROLLED FOR 5 YEARS

		Age First Seen	
		Average: 27.8 years	
Food allergy alone	42%	0-10 years	15%
Food and pollen allergy alone	21%	10-20 years	16%
Food, pollen, other inhalants	20%	20-50 years	48%
Inhalant allergy alone	10%	50-77 years	21%
Duration of symptoms: 1-55 years (Average: 8.1 years)			

Note: No cases of seasonal hay fever as a result of pollens, with or without fungus allergy, are included.

discharge was usual. Sneezing in 22 percent and itching in only 18 percent were less frequently due to food than to inhalant allergy especially to pollens. Blocking of the ears and reduced hearing occurred in 16 percent. Earache and serous otitis media would have been more frequent if more infants and children with perennial nasal allergy had been studied.

The perennial symptoms usually varied in degree. As in bronchial asthma resulting from food allergy, there were intermittently exaggerated symptoms, at times every two to eight weeks in 28 percent. The increase in symptoms in 40 percent of these patients from the fall to late spring, especially in the winter, is explained by the exaggeration of food allergy during these seasons, which we have long reported in bronchial asthma resulting from food allergy. Improvement in symptoms in the summer in 14 percent was less frequent than that which occurs in bronchial asthma resulting from food allergy.

In our experience head and bronchial colds every two to eight weeks in the fall to late spring with relief during the summer, especially in children and young adults, always require the study of recurrently activated food allergy rather than infection as the major or sole cause. Fever up to 103 F is usually due to food allergy rather than infection (read Chapt. 24).

This perennial nasal allergy was the only manifestation of clinical allergy in 33 percent. Headaches, usually with nasal blocking, occurred in 42 percent. There was previous bronchial asthma in 24 percent. Many of the gastrointestinal symptoms in our opinion were due to food allergy. Continued and especially severe nasal allergy, particularly blocking, caused distressing fullness, pressure, and even pain in the nose in 22 percent and in the antra in 14 percent. These symptoms were at times associated with headaches, restlessness, and varying insomnia, fatigue, dopiness, depression, confusion, generalized aching especially in the neck and shoulders, and other symptoms of allergic toxemia and fatigue which occurred in 26 percent of these patients. Such symptoms often impaired ability to work and to enjoy friends, entertainment, reading, radio, or television.

Family history was negative for evident allergy in 28 percent. Probable nasal allergy in 48 percent and bronchial asthma in 20 percent show the tendency to inherit similar manifestations of allergy.

DIAGNOSIS OF FOOD ALLERGY

Though the history, as already summarized, is very indicative of food allergy, inhalant allergy may be the sole or an associated cause. Perennial symptoms, especially in winter, and the nonexaggeration or absence of symptoms during pollen seasons excluded pollen allergy. Moreover, history suggesting allergy to animal emanations, miscellaneous inhalants, or house dust was absent.

Though recurrent attacks of exaggerated nasal blocking, postnasal mucus, and pressure in the nose often with fever of 100 to 103 F for one to three days every three to six weeks with interim blocking and postnasal discharge occur, such attacks and fever (not resulting from infection) are much less frequent than the typical recurrent attacks characteristic of bronchial asthma resulting from food allergy emphasized in Chapters 8 and 25.

The diagnosis of food allergy was confirmed by the relief of the nasal symptoms by the elimination of allergenic foods determined by our diet.

Skin testing was done by the scratch or puncture method with all important foods and inhalants including fungi. As in most chronic food allergy, negative scratch

TABLE XXVI

STATISTICS IN 50 CASES OF PERENNIAL
NASAL ALLERGY RESULTING
FROM FOOD ALLERGY

*(No desensitization to inhalants or vaccine
utilized to obtain our relief)*

Age (average)	38.5 years (5½-70)
Males	52%
Females	48%
Age of onset (average)	21.5 years (½-61)
Duration (average)	14 years
Blocking and congestion	72%
Congestion (nasal) alone	70%
Pain in nose	22%
Pain in antra	14%
Worse in winter	22%
Better in summer (1 better in Arizona)	14%
Sneezing	22%
Itching	8%
Otitis media	6%
Attacks of increased symptoms	28%
Fever with recurrent attacks	4%
Blocking of ears and reduced hearing	16%
Polyps	8%
Septum operations	14%

Other manifestations:

Bronchial allergy	24%
Coughing	18%
Eczema	8%
Urticaria	12%
GI symptoms	26%
Toxemia and fatigue	26%
Headaches	42%

Family history:

Bronchial asthma	26%
Nasal symptoms	48%

History suggesting:

Food allergy (milk 22%)	36%
Drug allergy (especially penicillin)	12%
Inhalant allergy	6%

Skin reactions:

Foods	24%
Pollens	44%
Animal emanations and miscellaneous inhalants	28%
House dust	24%

X-ray of sinuses:

Hazy antra	24%
Opaque	6%

Eosinophilia (Blood):

3%-10% (1 case 20%)	24%

Previous unsuccessful desensitization to
inhalants 18%

reactions to foods usually occurred. The one and two plus reactions in 24 percent infrequently harmonized with the foods which caused the nasal allergy. Since relief

occurred with the diet alone and with no desensitization or strict environmental control, the skin reactions to various pollens in 44 percent, animal emanations and miscellaneous inhalants in 28 percent, and to house dust in 24 percent were either nonspecific or indicative of past or potential allergy.

When any evidence of relief from diet trial fails in two to three weeks, foods in the diet are suspected or inhalant allergy as suggested by skin tests and at times by history alone is reconsidered.

Though this chapter emphasizes food allergy as the sole cause of perennial nasal symptoms, the frequent occurrence of inhalant allergy, alone or associated with food allergy, must be remembered.

STUDY AND CONTROL OF FOOD ALLERGY WITH TRIAL DIET, ESPECIALLY WITH THE CEREAL-FREE ELIMINATION DIET

Because of the fallibility of skin testing in determining food allergy, it is studied with trial diet utilizing our CFE diet. If milk allergy is indicated by diet history, beef also is excluded or given only one to three times a week. Though milk allergy is the sole cause in an occasional case, other foods along with milk, especially those excluded from our CFE diet, are the usual causes. If allergy to other foods in the diet is suggested, they also may be omitted.

Our experience, as discussed in Chapter 3, emphasizes the importance of eliminating all cereal grains as well as milk, eggs, wheat, and other less common allergenic foods in the initial diet. Without this initial elimination of all cereals, the number of good results is reduced. Strict adherence to the diet for two to three weeks, maintenance of protein intake by eating enough meat and fowl, and sufficient calories and vitamins to maintain nutrition and a desired weight must be emphasized. Our published menus, recipes, and directions for the use of the diet, as detailed in Chapter 3 of this book, are given to every patient.

The directions advised in Chapter 3 for prescribing, manipulating, and maintaining the CFE diet are essential for its successful use. The manipulation of the diet is summarized as follows:

If some relief occurs in two to three weeks, the diet must be maintained for another one or two months until relief is assured. That it takes weeks for tissue changes from chronic food allergy to gradually decrease is shown in the figures in Chapter 14. During this period additional fruits and vegetables can be tried every three or four days. We have found fruits and vegetables to be less frequent causes of allergy than milk, cereal grains, eggs, chocolate, coffee, and fish. When relief is assured for two to three months, rice, oatmeal, rye, and wheat may be added, one every four or five days, and later eggs, milk, and gradually other foods can be tested, eliminating any which reproduce symptoms. Soy- or lima-potato bakery products made by our recipes and the advised milk-free butter substitute are necessary until rice, rye, and later wheat and their bakery products are tolerated.

If some improvement does not occur in two to three weeks, beef and (rarely) soy, suspected vegetables or fruits, or at times white potatoes can be eliminated. Moreover, if a distaste or possible allergy exists to soy beans or lima beans, bakery products thereof can be omitted, providing weight is maintained with plenty of white or sweet potatoes and tapioca cooked according to our recipes, extra sugar, and the prescribed butter substitute and oil. White potatoes at times also cause allergy.

If such accurate diet trial fails to relieve symptoms, the following must be considered:

1. Definite nasal polyps prevent relief even though the diet is correct. After excision, especially if previous removals have occurred, our elimination diet should be maintained. In our experience food allergy is the usual cause of polyps as discussed later in this chapter. This is emphasized especially in Chapter 8.

2. If polyps are absent, inhalant allergy may be the cause, either alone or with food allergy, as illustrated in a subsequent case.

Because of the necessity of desensitization to inhalants for one or more years, the initial recognition of food allergy when it is a sole cause is most important. With control of unrecognized food allergy, some patients were relieved in two to four weeks who had obtained no help from desensitization with conventional antigens containing pollen, animal emanations, fungi, and house dust allergens even for three, five, or seven years. Thus with an open-minded attitude toward food allergy, we are assured that much injectant desensitization therapy can be prevented.

Food allergy must be studied in every case of perennial nasal allergy in young and older children and subsequent years, even in old age, as the sole cause or associated with inhalant allergy.

MEDICATIONS FOR TEMPORARY RELIEF

Until control of causative allergy relieves nasal congestion and especially blocking, antiallergic medications are justifiable. There are a few patients, especially children, who tolerate long nasal blocking, especially if pain and nasal and postnasal discharge are minimal. Usually the symptoms listed in Table XXVI, however, are so disturbing not only to the patient but to parents, relatives, and associates that temporary respite with drugs is important until allergy is controlled.

1. Antihistamines, preferably the long-acting ones, may relieve moderate distress. The choice depends on resultant relief, degree of resultant drowsiness, and other effects.

2. Decongestant drops or sprays in the nostrils also give varying relief. For relief of severe nasal allergy, Privine® and especially Afrin® by drops or spray are more efficient than other antihistamines lasting for six to twelve hours. Such use is justifiable for comfort, control of emotions, nervousness, and tension. With the control of the allergy, especially to foods, the patients themselves discontinue such intranasal medication showing no habit formation. Privine and especially Afrin every eight to twelve hours have been most effective in our patients.

3. Prednisone is also justifiable in daily oral doses of 10 to 25 mg until relief from the elimination diet with or without control of inhalant allergy arises. Triamcinolone 2 to 4 mg two to three times a day is preferred in our cases. Thereafter, its gradual omission in one to four weeks as relief from control of the allergies increases is the physician's definite responsibility. Its longer use is rarely justified.

These medications, therefore, are only justifiable with adequate and experienced study of causative allergy, especially to foods, so that drugs can be discontinued. Relief from the control of food allergy moreover occurs in some patients whose nasal allergy has not responded to empiric desensitization to inhalants such as pollen, animal emanations, miscellaneous inhalants, house dust, and even fungi for months or years.

CLINICAL EXPERIENCE

1. Perennial nasal allergy resulting from food sensitization usually causes varying combinations and degrees of nasal congestion, intermittent or continuous nasal blocking with moderate or absent sneezing. Itching from food in contrast to inhalant allergy usually is absent.

Case 56: A boy (T.E.) seven years of age had had nasal congestion and blocking with sniffling, mouth breathing, nose pushing, snorting, and snoring with no itching perennially for four years. For his first three years he had had a deep bronchial cough for two to three weeks intermittently from fall to late spring. He also had recurrent sore throats with "head colds." He was irritable and dopey. He was not fond of milk. A Dacron pillow and blanket had not helped. Removal of tonsils and adenoids had failed. The grandfather had asthma.

A hemogram, urinalysis, x-ray of the lungs and sinuses, and scratch tests with important inhalants and foods were negative except for a hazy antra and a three plus reaction to house dust.

Treatment: With our CFE diet, nasal symptoms and cough decreased in ten days. In one month all symptoms were absent. Corticosteroids were not available. He was not irritable or dopey. His personality was "entirely different" (read Chapt. 25) and energy increased. Symptoms recurred with wheat, milk, and eggs. A long-used decongestant was discontinued after ten days.

Comment: This history was typical of perennial nasal allergy from foods. During the first three years he had had recurrent bronchial asthma during the fall to late spring, pathognomonic of food allergy. It is probable that his recurrent sore throats and so-called "head colds" were due to recurrently activated food allergy rather than to infection.

His diet history suggested allergy to milk. Food allergy being the likely cause, the dog, carpets, and pads on the floors were not removed. It is probable that the Dacron pillow and blankets were unnecessary. His reaction to house dust was probably nonspecific.

Case 57: A woman (D.R.) thirty-five years of age had had sneezing, nasal congestion, and coryza on arising and during the days increasingly for several years. Itching had been absent. Dopiness and confusion had occurred. There had been no other clinical allergy. She disliked milk. Inhalant allergy was not apparent. There was nasal allergy in her father and hay fever in a sister. Tonsils and adenoids had been removed.

Physical examination, urinalysis, hemogram, sedimentation rate, and Kline test were negative except for a pale, edematous nasal mucosa and a blood eosinophilia of 11 percent. Scratch tests showed one plus reactions to dog, goat, and wool emanations and to house dust. One to three plus reactions occurred to several grass, fall, and tree pollens and 1 plus to milk, carrots, almonds, and cocoa.

Treatment: In two weeks our CFE diet produced a "clear head and nose for the first time in several years." Gradual addition of other foods showed that milk and egg were causative.

Comment: This typical uncomplicated history of perennial nasal allergy was due to eggs and especially to milk allergy which she always disliked. Confusion and dopiness evidenced mild allergic toxemia resulting from food allergy. The absence of itching and of exaggeration of symptoms in the spring to fall was against allergy to the skin-reacting inhalants, especially pollens. No desensitization to inhalants was given.

2. Nasal allergy resulting from food allergy may be recurrently exaggerated at times with fever in the fall to late spring especially in children.

Case 58: A girl (K.S.) thirteen years of age had nasal congestion and blocking with postnasal mucus and occasional sneezing but no itching all of her life. Symptoms had been exaggerated, with fever up to 104 F every month since infancy associated with sweating and weakness. Penicillin had been given with no help. The attacks were less frequent in summers. Bronchial asthma occurred twice in the first two years. Bronchitis had accompanied some attacks since then.

Diet, drug, and environmental histories were negative for allergy. Her mother had hay fever. Tonsillectomy eight years ago had been of no help.

Physical examination was negative except for an edematous, pale nasal mucosa with mucus and congested pharynx. X-rays of lungs and sinuses, urinalysis, and hemogram were negative. Scratch tests gave 1 plus reactions to cow's and goat's milk and to a few spring pollens and fall pollens.

Treatment: With our CFE diet, nasal symptoms improved in two weeks. Some nausea and fever of 99 F were present in four weeks but with no severe attack. Thereafter, attacks were absent.

In the last two years only milk, wheat, rice, and corn have reproduced symptoms. No injectant, corticosteroid, or antibiotic therapy had been given.

Comment: This perennial nasal allergy exaggerated in definite attacks with temperature up to 103 to 104 F, particularly during the fall to the late spring months, is an equivalent of the pathognomonic history of bronchial asthma resulting from food allergy which we have been long reporting.

3. Perennial nasal allergy may be accompanied with recurrent aural pain or discharge (serous otitis media). Relief from our CFE diet indicates food allergy. Such allergy occurs in the eustachian tube and/ or in the middle ear, with or without a secondary infection. This nasal allergy with monthly serous otitis and fever up to 104 F simultaneously in identical twins for eight years was relieved with our diet (Cases 65 and 66).

4. Perennial nasal allergy may be associated with pain in the nose and antra with dull or sick headaches.

As indicated in Table XXVI, pain in the nose in 22 percent and in the antra in 14 percent of our patients was relieved with the elimination diets. Headaches, often persistent with nasal blocking and pressure or in both sides of the head or nuchal area, occurred in 42 percent, at times with nausea or vomiting. With the proper elimination diet, relief usually occurred.

5. Perennial nasal allergy resulting from foods rather than from apparent pollen allergies is illustrated in the following case:

Case 59: A woman forty years of age had had since aet ten in November and recently every two weeks attacks beginning with soreness of the throat and irritation of the nose, coryza, and fever up to 101 F the next day. Soreness of the throat, loss of voice, and decreased hearing often occurred. These symptoms had handicapped her teaching for thirteen years. Pain and blocking of the ears usually occurred on the second day. Attacks were more frequent in the fall to late spring and less severe and often absent in the summer.

Eczema in the flexures and backs of ears had been present in the teens, being rarer in occurrence since then.

During attacks there had been marked fatigue and impaired ability to teach. Attacks, especially the fever, had been blamed on "colds" by several physicians. Penicillin was given during attacks until allergy to it developed twenty years ago.

Diet history revealed slight aversion to milk and dislike for fruits.

Her father had perennial hay fever always suggestive of food allergy.

Scratch tests were negative except a four plus reaction to English plantain and slight ones to several grasses. Laboratory tests were negative except eight percent eosinophilia and haziness in the antra by x-ray.

All symptoms were relieved in one month with our CFE diet with no uncooked fruits or vegetables. After relief, provocation tests with individual fruits and corn reproduced symptoms.

Comment: Food allergy was indicated by the regular, recurrent attacks, better in the summer (Chapt. 1). Fever was also relieved, as is fever in recurrent attacks of bronchial asthma resulting from food allergy in children. Her recurrent sore throats, most perennial nasal discharge, hoarseness, loss of voice, and fatigue because of food allergy have been relieved by adequate, experienced use of our CFE diet as we advise.

6. Unrecognized food allergy prevents good results from desensitization therapy for evident or probable inhalant allergy.

Case 60: A woman (Mrs. S. W.) thirty-eight years of age had coryza with varying nasal blocking and sneezing without itching for three years, exaggerated in the spring but continuing in the fall and winter.

Epigastric distress, cramping, and diarrhea had occurred from milk and fruits. She disliked eggs, crab, and the cabbage group of vegetables.

Sinus x-rays were negative. Scratch testing revealed reactions to grasses and a few summer and fall pollens. Desensitization to many pollens and animal emanations for two years had failed.

Treatment: Food allergy was studied with our FFCFE diet. Desensitization to a multiple grass and pollen antigen was given. Cortisone, 25 mg t.i.d., was given only for three days, gradually eliminating it in two weeks. In three weeks blocking had disappeared for the first time in three

years and other nasal and gastrointestinal symptoms and fatigue were absent.

For five years elimination of milk, eggs, chocolate, and tomato have been necessary to control nasal allergy and fatigue. Tomato and milk also cause epigastric distress and nausea. Lamb causes headache, swelling of the eyes, and nausea. Desensitization to pollens is still necessary in the spring, summer, and early fall.

Comment: This perennial nasal allergy was not controlled by desensitization to inhalants and corticosteroids for two years. Symptoms were rapidly controlled, however, with our FFCFE diet. Desensitization has also been necessary to control nasal allergy during the pollen seasons. Relief of epigastric symptoms has depended on the elimination diet, in part a result of the elimination of all fruit.

7. Perennial nasal allergy resulting from foods had prevented relief from nasal operations on the sinuses, septa, and turbinates and removal of recurrent polyps.

Case 61: A woman thirty-five years of age had had recurrent nasal symptoms with antral pain, nasal discharge, buzzing, and blocking of the ears with no itching for twenty-seven years. Symptoms had been exaggerated during three to four head colds in the fall and winter. Tonsillectomy and eight nasal operations had given no benefit. For 1½ years coughing and wheezing spells, lasting for several days, had occurred. Diet history revealed apparent nasal blocking from corn, milk, eggs, and wheat. Spices, condiments, and rich foods caused epigastric burning. Asthma had occurred in a paternal uncle and "sinus problems" in the father.

Physical examination, hemogram, urinalysis, and Kline test were negative. Scratch tests with inhalants and foods gave many slight reactions. X-ray of the sinuses revealed thickened membranes in the antra and residual evidence of windows in both antra.

Treatment: Because of perennial nasal symptoms unrelieved by 8 operations and her suggestive history of food allergy, this was studied with my CFE diet. Nasal symptoms were relieved in 4 weeks. For 12 years it has been necessary to eliminate cereals including wheat, eggs, milk and dried beans to control her nasal and bronchial allergy. Former recurrent head colds and epigastric distress have been absent.

8. Perennial nasal allergy is often as-

sociated with allergic toxemia and fatigue, as we have long reported.

Case 62: A man (M.Z.) forty-eight years of age had had nasal congestion and marked post-nasal mucus for many years increased in the fall and winter. For four years constant blocking was so great he could not "even sneeze." With these symptoms, generalized headaches had increased. Severe fatigue was unrelieved by sleep. Loginess, inability to concentrate or remember, depression, and pain in the head with thinking had prevented work as a food checker for eight months. Sometimes he felt "as if I would lose my mind." Epigastric burning and distention had continued for three years. He had long disliked milk. Fruits increased epigastric distress. Physical and laboratory examinations and scratch tests with inhalants and foods were negative except for edema of the nasal mucosa, postnasal mucus and a one plus reaction to house dust.

Treatment: With our FFCFE diet, all symptoms decreased in a week and were absent in seven weeks. He resumed work, being free of his nasal allergy and "able to think and face the day's work."

During the last four years milk, wheat, and other cereals have reproduced nasal and cerebral symptoms and fatigue. Epigastric burning and distention have been controlled by elimination of cooked and uncooked fruits. Vitamin C is being given.

Comment: Food allergy in the nasal and adjoining meningeal and probably cerebral tissues explains the severe nasal blocking, postnasal mucus, severe headaches, and allergic fatigue and toxemia. Relief of epigastric symptoms depended on elimination of fruits.

HOARSENESS AND APHONIA RESULTING FROM FOOD ALLERGY

Laryngeal allergy causing hoarseness and aphonia requires accurate study of food allergy with or without less important allergy to inhalants. Perennial nasal and bronchial allergy including bronchial asthma and other manifestations of bronchial allergy reported in this volume may be present and continue unless such allergy, especially to foods, is recognized and controlled as we advise. Treatment for as-

sumed infection with antibiotics and other treatment by physicians including specialists usually fail to give relief, as evidenced in the following patient.

Case 63: A woman fifty-two years of age had had hoarseness with "loss of voice to a whisper" for two months in December seven years ago, again for three months starting in December three years ago, another for six months a year ago, and again since November for the last four weeks. An irritative cough producing slight, greenish mucus was present. Antibiotics and other therapy from six physicians including two otolaryngologists had been ineffectual.

Frequent "colds with hacking coughs" with postnasal mucus and snoring had been present all of her life. Other possible manifestations of allergy, including headaches, had been absent.

Diet history of possible disagreements or allergies to foods was absent. Drug history likewise was negative. Environmental history suggesting inhalant allergy was absent. Hay fever was present in two sons.

Skin tests with food and inhalant allergens were negative. X-ray of lungs and sinuses and other laboratory tests were also negative.

Treatment and Results: The recurrent attacks of laryngeal congestion, especially in the winters, required study of possible food allergy with the CFE diet. To help reduce probable allergy, Aristocort 20 mg intramuscularly and 4 mg by mouth t.i.d. was given. "Unbelievable" relief was present in one week. Then the corticosteroid was gradually eliminated in one week. Voice was normal and cough absent in two weeks. In two months voice was normal, and she felt better than she had in many years.

In the last 2½ years hoarseness and aphonia have been absent except for a week after slight breaks in the diet occurred. Milk, eggs, and cereal grains must be eliminated to prevent laryngeal allergy and aphonia.

ROLE OF FOOD ALLERGY IN NASAL POLYPS

It is generally agreed that allergy is the probable cause of recurrent nasal polyps.

Kern and Schenck receive the credit for stressing the importance of allergy in the etiology and treatment of nasal mucous polyps in 1933 and 1934. Their analyses of 232 cases, their emphasis on the frequency of nasal polyps in bronchial asthma, their photographs of microscopic sections and occurrence of varying tissue eosinophilia, and their discussion of the English and German literature are worthy of the reader's review. In 1957 Blumstein and Tuft discussed their results of antiallergic treatment of recurrent nasal polyposis in an important contribution of 160 cases. Seventy-two percent had bronchial asthma, 47 percent had none, and 53 percent had multiple polypectomies while they cooperated in treatment. Less frequent operations occurred in 21 percent of the latter cases. No relief occurred in 31 percent, which we opine would have been reduced if food allergy had been treated as we advise. Aspirin allergy occurred in 12.5 percent.

Favoring food allergy is the occurrence of polyps in patients who have varying degrees of perennial nasal allergy which always requires consideration of allergy to foods. The recurrence after surgical removal and the perennial increasing degree of nasal polyps are best explained by persisting allergy to continually eaten foods. Moreover, failure of recurrence resulting from strict use of our CFE diet in cooperating patients who had had from two to eight and more, as in one patient, recurrences after thirty-one polypectomies emphasizes the importance of food allergy.

Against pollen allergy as a sole cause is the persistence and increase in the polyps when pollens are absent from the air in winter and the failure of continued pollen desensitization when such allergy is indicated by skin tests or history to prevent recurrences after surgical removal. The absence of itching in the nose and eyes, of sneezing, and of other manifestations of pollen allergy, especially in the winter, is against a pollen etiology.

Against allergy to animal emanations, house dust, and miscellaneous inhalants is the usual failure to prevent recurrences of polyps with strict environmental control in the home and working environments and from continued desensitization even with conventional antigens often used empirically containing pollens, dusts, spores of fungi, animal emanations, and miscellaneous inhalant allergens.

Against infection as a cause is the failure of alleviation of polyps after attempts to control infection by intranasal or sinal surgery, after administration of stock and autogenous vaccines, and from antibiotic therapy. The cloudiness or even opacity especially in the maxillary sinus is explained by allergic edema with or without polypoid regeneration of the antral mucosa. Rare infection, however, must be recognized by pain, fever, abnormal blood counts and presence of pus in the sinuses themselves. This infection of course requires antibiotics and advice of a surgeon. The removal of mucosa and polyps from the maxillary antra by a Luc Caldwell operation, however, without definite evidence of infection does not eliminate perennial nasal allergy in the regenerated tissues. Prevention or recurrence of nasal polyps also may not result from such surgery. And similar failure of relief usually occurs after antral windows are established by surgery followed by repeated irrigations of the antra which are affected by allergy rather than infection. Secondary infection unfortunately may result from such irrigations through the nonsterile nasal passages. These surgical procedures have not been done in our practice for over thirty-five years in patients with nasal polyps and varying degrees of perennial nasal allergy.

Perennial nasal allergy so frequently a result of food allergy alone is always present in varying degrees when recurrent nasal polyps occur. When removal of large nasal polyps, which usually originate in the maxillary antral mucosa, rapidly relieves nasal blocking continuing for weeks or several months, perennial allergy in the nasal mucosa may be slight. However, if perennial nasal allergy is marked, causing nasal congestion and blocking by itself, polypectomies may not relieve the blocking for more than one to two weeks while the effect of local anesthesia continues. When multiple small polyps originate in the ethmoidal sinuses, the degree of relief from nasal blocking depends on the degree of allergy in the nasal mucosa. When such mucosal allergy is present, its relief as well as prevention of polyp formation depends on the control of allergy, especially to foods, as advised below.

As stated above, the control of food allergy with strict, continued adherence to our CFE diet has prevented recurrence of nasal polyps in the large majority of our cooperating patients. Such study is not necessary after removal of initial nasal polyps, providing blocking of the nose is rapidly relieved and longstanding nasal allergy, as discussed in this chapter, is absent. Study of food allergy is justified, however, if such polyps have been removed two or more times during a period of six to twelve months, indicating a predisposition to their formation best explained by food allergy. And such control of food allergy is also important if in addition to recurrent polyps, perennial nasal allergy persists.

Since it requires weeks or several months for nasal polyps to recur after surgical removal, control of food allergy with adherence to our CFE diet must be vigorously maintained for long periods before prevention of their recurrence is assured.

Case 64: A man (W.N.) forty years of age had had nasal congestion and discharge all of his life with no itching and moderate sneezing with recurrent blocking briefly helped by four polypectomies. Openings into antra for five years had not helped. No asthma or typical hay fever had occurred. One son had nasal congestion.

Physical examination, urinalysis, hemogram, and Kline test were negative except for an edematous nasal mucosa. Small polyps had recurred since last removal three months before. Scratch tests were negative to foods and inhalants.

Treatment: With our CFE diet, nasal congestion and coryza were controlled. In eight years polyps have not recurred with a milk-free and egg-free diet.

SUMMARY

1. Food allergy is the common cause of perennial nasal allergy.

2. The typical history resulting from food allergy includes varying nasal congestion, blocking, and nasal and postnasal discharge with moderate paroxysmal sneezing and little or no itching compared with that resulting from inhalant allergy throughout the year.

3. Common failure to recognize food allergy is due to absent or fallible skin reactions to allergenic foods, failure of a test-negative diet to relieve symptoms, and failure to use a trial diet for which our CFE diet has been important.

4. Symptoms may be exaggerated in the fall, winter, and early spring in recurrent attacks, at times associated with fever resulting from food allergy rather than infection.

5. Marked nervousness, emotional instability, mental dullness, impaired concentration, and other symptoms of allergic fatigue and toxemia may occur.

6. Statistics on fifty cases of perennial nasal allergy resulting from food sensitization alone, relieved with the CFE diet alone with no injections of vaccines or desensitization to inhalants, are presented. Many

more cases are not listed because of unnecessary, often brief, injectant therapy.

7. These results emphasize the responsibility of controlling such cases with diet alone without the routine and often empiric unfortunate desensitization to one or several assumed causative inhalants given too often to most cases of perennial nasal allergy. In spite of absence of relief resulting from uncontrolled food allergy, such desensitization may be continued for one to even seven years.

8. Though food allergy often is the sole cause, concomitant inhalant allergy and its control may be important. Occasional inhalant allergy as the sole cause of perennial nasal allergy also must be recognized.

9. Though pollen may be associated with other inhalant allergy in causing symptoms during the spring, summer, and fall, it is not a factor in the winter.

10. The cases described in this section of this chapter, however, were due to food allergy alone. Recurrent head and bronchial colds resulting from allergy, especially to foods, are also discussed in Chapter 7.

PERENNIAL NASAL, PHARYNGEAL, AND LARYNGEAL ALLERGY RESULTING FROM INHALANTS

Though perennial symptoms continuing into the fall and winter as well as in the spring and summer always require the study and indicated control of the most frequent cause, namely food allergy, as emphasized in the first part of this chapter, allergy to the emanations of animals in the home or area of employment or recreation, dusts from kapok and cotton mattresses, wool and insecticides in carpets, allergens in agriculture or industry, in working areas, allergens in hay and grain dusts together with allergens of fly and insect emanations, tobacco smoke, cosmetics and perfumes,

and various other miscellaneous airborne allergens in addition to airborne pollens requires study and (if present) advised control.

For the study and control of these airborne inhalants, the reader is referred to their discussion in the second section of Chapter 4.

Consideration of such inhalant allergens is emphasized by a possible history of exaggeration of symptoms from such environmental allergens. In these patients varying degrees of environmental control, as advised in Chapter 4, are advisable. Pillows containing Dacron are advised until allergy to feathers is entirely excluded. This consideration of inhalants other than pollen must be routine even though the usual cause of perennial nasal and sinal allergy, namely food allergy, as emphasized in the first section of this chapter, is the most important and too often unrecognized and uncontrolled cause.

Pollen allergy always has to be considered and evaluated in these patients with perennial nasal symptoms. Though other inhalant and food allergens individually or together may in varying degrees cause the perennial symptoms, pollen allergy may be a minor or definite concomitant cause during the pollen seasons evidenced by exaggeration of symptoms in those periods especially if reactions to pollens occur. If such exaggeration is not evidenced in the history or by seasonal activation of symptoms, positive reactions do not necessarily prove clinical allergy to such pollens.

Thus:

1. Food allergy as discussed in the first section is the major and often the sole cause of perennial nasal, sinal, pharyngeal, and laryngeal allergy.

2. Allergy to inhalants other than pollen,

usually indicated by history and skin tests, is a less frequent cause.

3. Though allergy to pollen is rarely a cause in the winter, except from mountain cedar in the western states and acacia in California, it may be a combined cause with other inhalants and also food allergy during the pollen seasons.

Ear Allergy

Otologists, allergists, and other physicians must recognize atopic allergy as a cause of tissue changes and resultant symptoms in the outer, middle, and inner ear especially a) when other manifestations of clinical allergy, particularly in the nasal, sinal, and bronchial tissues are or have been present; b) when the history indicates possible food or inhalant allergy; or c) when the diet and environmental histories and scratch tests indicate such possible allergies. Though associated manifestations of allergy in the nasobronchial, ocular, cutaneous, gastrointestinal, central and peripheral nervous, genitourinary, and musculoskeletal tissues may occur in various frequencies, the ears may be the only shock organ, as is true of the frequency with which eczema of the hands may be the only manifestation of cutaneous allergy.

This recognition of and control of otological as well as of nasal allergy often makes the following surgical procedures unnecessary: a) removal of tonsils and adenoids, b) resection of the nasal septum and swollen turbinates, c) washing of sinuses for assumed infection, or the d) Luc Caldwell operation. With the control of food allergy e) nasal polyps after their initial surgical removal may not recur, providing food allergy and the less frequent causative inhalant allergy are properly controlled. Since symptoms of otological allergy often occur in patients with nasosinal allergy, the reader is referred to Chapter 12 on nasal allergy.

If allergy to inhalants and especially to foods continues in the middle ear, thickening of membranes and possibly scar tissue impair the function of the hammer, stirrup, anvil, and also the tympanum, so that permanent decrease in hearing results, at times requiring relief from expertised surgery.

Relief of indicated food and/or inhalant allergy requires study and treatment, as advised in Chapter 8.

CHRONIC EXUDATIVE SEROUS OTITIS MEDIA

Recurring attacks of inflammation, edema, and exudation of serous fluid in the middle ear with resultant pain and bulging of the drum in infants and children and less often in adolescents and adults always require study and control of food allergy as a major probable cause. The usual regular recurrence of these attacks every two to six weeks and their decrease or absence in the summer especially favor food allergy, as emphasized in Chapters 1 and 8. The history of these attacks is similar to or equivalent to the history of recurrent bronchial asthma resulting from food allergy confirmed by us for over thirty years, as emphasized in Chapter 8.

As in such bronchial asthma, fever associated with this serous otitis media is practically always a result of food allergy rather than infection, especially when the discharge from the middle ear is not purulent and the fever subsides with or without temporary corticoid therapy and with the immediate use of our CFE diet (see Chapt.

3). Such regular recurrent serous otitis media resulting from food allergy (eggs and milk) was reported by Noun in 1942.

If secondary infection is suspected, especially if pus is present in the aural discharge, antibiotics for a few days are justified. That the fever is often due to food allergy as it is in recurrent attacks of asthma resulting from food allergy is stressed in Chapter 8. If fever is slight or absent, antibiotics are not required. If infected tonsils and/or an infectious head or bronchial cold are present, antibiotics are justified even though allergy is the sole cause of the serous otitis media.

Along with this recurrent serous otitis media, varying degrees of nasal and sinal allergy with or without allergic bronchitis or bronchial asthma are present. When food allergy is controlled as we advise, all sino-bronchial symptoms are gradually relieved. These manifestations of food allergy often have caused sickness, invalidism, much medical attention, absence from school, and parents' concern for months or years, as evidenced in Case 65 for nine years.

Removal of tonsils and of adenoids, even "two or three times," fails to terminate these attacks of serous otitis media which result from food allergy. With adequate control of allergy, especially to foods, the insertion of plastic tubes through the drum into the middle ear to allow discharge of fluid and to relieve pressure becomes unnecessary. Many of these children are underweight even though they are encouraged or at times forced to drink up to a quart of milk to which they have an aversion and are allergic.

If the causes of serous otitis media are not found, otorrhea may continue for more than a few days, and in some cases varying degrees of chronicity associated usually with other manifestations of allergy occur.

The refractoriness which develops after three to five days during a regular attack decreases in degree, and a persisting allergic reaction in the middle ear and eardrum develops, especially in the fall and winter when exaggeration of food allergy occurs.

LITERATURE

Allergy has been suspected as a cause of recurrent serous otitis media by otologists, other physicians, and allergists for many years. Lewis suspected it in 1929, reporting recurrent serous otitis in six children, with spontaneous rupture of the ear drums. He commented on the futility of myringotomy without lasting relief.

Proetz, in 1931, reported allergy to eggs, potato, chicken feathers, and horse dander as a cause of serous otitis media. Another author reported recurrent otitis media in a boy eight years of age who was chronically ill. He also had nasal and bronchial allergies and was restless, nervous, and irritable. He was being forced to drink one quart of milk a day, which he definitely disliked. The removal of tonsils and adenoids had been of no benefit. Plastic tubes had been inserted through his eardrums for several weeks. Relief gradually occurred with the elimination of wheat, milk, and eggs. Noun, in 1942, reported chronic otorrhea resulting from food allergy. This was associated with tinnitus or vertigo and at times nystagmus, indicating allergy in the inner ear, as noted in our following discussion of vertigo. He reported two cases of recurrent otorrhea, one attributed to allergy to eggs and meat and the second attributed to tomato and eggs, to which a four plus skin reaction occurred, and one other in a boy of eight years of age in whom recurrent attacks associated with fatigue and impaired health were relieved by the elimination of tomato and eggs. After relief a doughnut caused immediate vomiting and cramps and in three days an attack of serous otitis media. Gradual relief occurred during the next two to three weeks.

Food allergy as the sole cause of this recurrent serous otitis media was indicated by the regular attacks approximately at monthly intervals preceded by nasal allergy incorrectly suggestive of a "head cold," which history is identical with that of recurrent attacks of bronchial asthma in children long emphasized by us as being a result of food allergy alone, as we have recorded in Chapters 8 and especially in 25.

In these cases reported by Noun, irritability, restlessness, fatigue, and bad health characteristic of the allergic fatigue and toxemia syndrome we first reported in 1931, as reported in Chapter 19 of this volume, also were relieved when food allergy was controlled (see Chapt. 25).

Watson (1969) in England reported hearing loss from chronic exudative serous otitis media (glue ears) in 4.4 percent of 1,777 children five years of age and in 4.1 percent of 1605 thirteen-year-olds.

Cases 65 and 66: Identical twins, first seen at the age of nine, had had attacks of nasal congestion and blocking of the nose with a bronchial cough associated with a fever up to 102 F always associated with serous otitis media in each boy, recurring at the start of the attacks which recurred at approximately monthly intervals. Pain in the ears with bulging of the eardrums always occurred. Two or three times a year lancing of drums was necessary. In other attacks spontaneous discharge of a serous nonpustular fluid relieved the pain.

Indicating food allergy as a probable cause was the usual absence of these attacks during June and July up to mid-August. Antibiotics had always been given for three or four days during the attacks. Removal of tonsils in each boy at the age of four and of adenoids at the age of eight had not decreased the frequency, severity, fever, or aural discharge. During the first two years a croupy cough occurred with each attack, and in

those years steam inhalation was given under tents over the bed in the nighttime during the attacks and for a week or so afterwards from the early fall to late spring. For the preceding three years both boys had had much postnasal mucoid discharge along with nasal congestion. Hacking cough had occurred, moreover, nearly every night between the attacks, decreasing or being absent in the summer.

Dermatitis on the legs and arms of each twin with itching of the nose and eyes occurred during the spring months, indicating pollen allergy.

Diet history revealed a lifelong dislike for milk in both boys. With urging, however, milk had been drunk, and ice cream, butter or cheese had also been taken nearly every day in their lives. Eggs had been definitely disliked up to three years before.

Drug history revealed no evident idiosyncrasies. Chlor-Trimeton® 8 mg twice a day had been taken every day except in the summer, with no relief of the serous otitis media.

Environmental history revealed no evident allergy to airborne allergens except from pollens during the spring. The first boy gave two plus scratch reactions to several tree, grass, and fall pollens. The second boy gave lesser reactions to similar pollens. Scratch tests with foods were negative in both boys.

Urinalysis was negative, and the blood counts were negative except for 10 percent eosinophiles.

X-rays of the sinuses and chest were negative.

Family history revealed seasonal hay fever in the maternal aunt. The maternal grandmother had chronic congestion of the nose and sinuses. The father had chronic sinusitis.

Treatment and results: Food allergy was definitely indicated because of the regular recurring attacks of serous otitis media accompanying the activation of nasal and bronchial symptoms at monthly intervals for nine years and also because of the relief of these symptoms during the summer months.

To study such food allergy, our cereal-free elimination diet was prescribed, along with a multiple synthetic vitamin and calcium carbonate one-half teaspoonful daily. In one month aural, nasal, and bronchial symptoms had not recurred except for slight pain in the ears for a few hours but with no fever or discharge. The diet was maintained. Environmental control including a foam rubber pillow had been previously ordered for several years without benefit.

After the first month there was no return of the attacks of serous otitis media, nasal and bronchial symptoms, and fever, the cereal-free diet being strictly maintained. In three months the mother stated that "they had never been so well." They had increased energy. Former restlessness, irritability, and disturbed sleep had disappeared. To the diet additional fruits and vegetables, turkey, and fish were gradually added in the next six months. In the winter when rice had been added for four days, there was a moderate reactivation of nasal and bronchial symptoms including sniffling and coughing and slight pain in the ears in both boys. This disappeared gradually one week after the rice was eliminated. In one month corn produced similar symptoms. In eight months milk for three days caused greater reactivation of the nasal and aural symptoms.

With the strict diet no attacks of otitis media associated with nasal and bronchial symptoms and fever occurred for two years. Then after a moderate break in the diet, one boy developed pain and fluid in the ears which disappeared in ten days with the return to the strict diet.

During the last nine years of the control of food allergies, two or three mild respiratory infections have occurred each fall or winter without any evidence of nasal or bronchial allergy and no recurrence of the otitis media or fever. To increase resistance to such respiratory infections, mixed respiratory and viral vaccines have been given in moderate doses every two to four weeks.

During the last four or five years rice and corn, fish, and as stated before, all vegetables and fruits have been added to the diet without return of their initial symptoms. Weight in both of the boys has increased from 57 pounds to 140 pounds at the present time.

Tunnel Vision From Wheat Allergy

No complications have occurred except for the development of tunnel vision in January, 1966, after one of the boys had eaten wheat in moderate amounts for a two-week period. An ophthalmologist had been consulted. Because of suspected intracranial pathology, studies were made by the ophthalmologist, who ordered an EEG and an encephalogram. When the mother reported the findings to us, I suspected edema from reactivated food allergy, probably in the occipital lobes. With corticoids by mouth in decreasing doses over a period of a week and the elimination of wheat, this tunnel vision disappeared. It recurred a year and a half later after eating wheat in June and July at his grandfather's home. Tunnel vision recurred around the first of September when, as we have long emphasized, food allergy becomes activated. Rapid relief with the elimination of wheat and the brief use of corticoids by mouth is recorded in Chapter 20.

Criep, 1942, in his study of seven pairs of identical twins reported similar symptoms especially from food allergies and often identical skin reactions to allergens but no cases with such identical symptoms as in these patients.

COMMENT

Though food allergy best explains the regular attacks of perennial serous otitis media with interim refractoriness and absence of symptoms, inhalant allergy requires consideration, as illustrated by the occurrence of five recurrent attacks of such otorrhea in six months in a girl six years of age who was relieved when she stopped feeding pigeons, which she had been doing previously for eight months. This indicates that other inhalants also need consideration, as reported by Derlachi of relief of recurrent serous otitis media by desensitization to house dust. Solow and Updegraff also reported similar inhalant allergy as a cause. This relief from continued desensitization may be due to nonspecific rather than specific relief of allergy.

That continued attacks of serous otitis media along with perennial nasal and spinal allergy, even after adenotonsilectomy, can produce bilateral impairment in hearing with tympanic retraction and fluid in the middle ear is shown by 95 percent relief of nasal symptoms and impaired hearing when Derlachi eliminated wheat, beets, and beet sugar from the diet of one patient. The elimination of oatmeal relieved "severe conductive hearing loss" in the right ear which had resulted from recurrent attacks of nasal allergy and bronchitis associated with weakness and fatigue with fever up to 103 F which had not been controlled by desensitization to house dust and with antibiotics and histamines. This therefore justifies the study of food allergy in practically all cases of recurrent serous otitis media even though inhalant allergy seems to be a definite possibility. Derlachi also reported otorrhea associated with nasal allergy in a woman fifty-nine years of age because of milk allergy rather than house dust, to which desensitization had been given for many months with no benefit. Thus such control of atopic allergy often to foods alone may relieve symptoms, preventing middle ear surgery and controlling ringing noises and other symptoms continuing after such surgery.

ALLERGIC DIZZINESS, VERTIGO, AND MENIERE'S SYNDROME

Dizziness, vertigo, and Meniere's syndrome are discussed as a conjoint entity, Meniere's syndrome associated with nausea, vomiting, tinnitus, and some deafness being its maximum manifestation. When any degree of this syndrome occurs, allergy, especially to foods, as stated by Urbach and Wilder, requires definite consideration.

Along with or before the study of allergy as a cause of this syndrome, the following possible causes must be studied and eliminated: generalized viral or bacterial infections, infection and abscesses in the sinuses, cerebral arteriosclerosis, strokes, new growths, hemorrhages in the labyrinth, toxemia from chronic diseases, anemia, toxic or allergic reactions to drugs, allergic migraine, and headaches.

LITERATURE ON DIZZINESS AND MENIERE'S SYNDROME

Quincke, in 1893 and especially in 1921, suggested that Meniere's syndrome might be due to an angioneurotic edemalike involvement of the labyrinth of the internal ear or its nerve supply. Kobrak (1928) agreed to such a possibility. Dederding (1930) also reported three cases associated with angioneurotic edema and suggested transient edema of the vestibular apparatus as a cause.

Duke (1923) first suggested that this syndrome might be due in certain patients to foods and included two case records of food sensitization in his original article. He personally reaffirmed this opinion to us on several occasions in 1923 to 1934 and told of another patient whose dizziness because of food allergy was such that he would fall on the street. Balyeat (1933) reported tinnitus, vertigo, nausea, and migraine in a man thirty-five years of age from milk allergy. The former diagnosis had been neurosis.

Malonge, according to Bray (1934), reported two cases of Meniere's syndrome resulting from allergy to orris root and house dust. A case of dizziness, vertigo, and nausea immediately on entering a barn, as noted by Yandell (1933), was possibly due to localized edema in the brain from allergy to inhalants. In line with this case was the intense vertigo, tinnitus, nausea, and vomiting in periodic attacks for fourteen years from allergy to orris powder. Reactions to house dust and orris allergens were present, and he reported successful control of such vertigo with specific desensitization to such allergens. Levy (1934) encountered a case of tinnitus aurium resulting from inhalant allergy to dog hair.

Proetz (1931) studied one patient who had the syndrome for five years. Milk in minute amounts even in traces of butter reproduced the attacks. Allergy to iodides also caused attacks. Urbach and Wilder (1934) recorded Meniere's syndrome, with frequent lapses of consciousness, urticaria, angioneurotic edema, vomiting, and mucous colitis relieved by a milk-free diet. It is possible that the good results from a diet low in sodium combined with ammonium chloride therapy, as advised by Fustenberg, Lashmet, and Lathrop (1934) in patients with Meniere's disease, were due to relief of allergic edema. It is possible that such edemas may produce mild tinnitus, dizziness, or deafness. Transient deafness with or without tinnitus, gastrointestinal symptoms, and at times headaches or other allergic symptoms probably may arise from allergy. Two such cases of intermittent deafness relieved by the elimination of specific foods have come under my observation. It is possible that other tissue disturbances than edema, such as allergic vasculitis, also are responsible.

DIZZINESS FROM HYDROPS OF LABYRINTH BECAUSE OF EXCESSIVE INTAKE OF SODIUM CHLORIDE

Since these symptoms, especially dizziness, may result from hydrops in the labyrinth because of increased sodium in the blood, relief from a salt-free diet may occur. When study of food allergy is indicated, moreover, a low salt diet and diminution of other sodium such as that in sodium carbonate and in baking powders are important. Tolerance for sodium chloride can be determined by its careful addition to an elimination diet, moreover, if food allergy is a major cause.

Case 67: We reported attacks of vertigo in a woman sixty years of age who had mucous colitis for twenty years. The control of food allergy with our elimination diet eradicated dizziness as well as the colitis. Henoch's purpura associated with the usual abdominal and joint symptoms also had occurred as a result of food allergy (Chapt. 22) at the age of forty-five for several months.

Case 68: Another patient became so dizzy after eating eggs or apples that she had to lie down immediately for two or three hours. We studied three other patients with severe sudden dizziness relieved by the elimination of specific foods. Two

additional patients had intermittent deafness with moderate dizziness resulting from food allergy, one with severe gastrointestinal allergy and possibly bacterial allergy.

Our experience points to the advisability of replacing skin tests as used by Duke in 1923 with diet trial using our elimination diets because of the frequency of negative skin reactions in food allergy. He stated that Meniere's syndrome results from lesions involving "either the labyrinth or peripheral end organ, the primary neuron or vestibular nerve proper, its tract or the central nuclei in the medulla or mid-brain of the vestibular nerve apparatus." He emphasized that acute infectious diseases, syphilis, hemorrhage into the labyrinth, tumors, abscesses, and traumatic injuries must be ruled out.

One of his cases resulting from food allergy follows. The symptoms were relieved by epinephrine hypodermically and by the elimination of the causative foods; they were reproduced by the ingestion of the foods and by the intracutaneous injection of the extracts of these foods.

Case history reported by Duke: An unmarried woman thirty-five years of age complained of attacks of dizziness, nausea, and fainting. The family history was negative for allergy. She had had hives every summer for fifteen years and had a urinary bladder allergy (read Chapt. 21) controlled by the elimination of certain fruits and vegetables one year before. Her present symptoms had been present slightly for several years, being exaggerated for the past several weeks. The severe attacks caused her to fall to the floor and lasted from one-half to three hours, recurring every day or two. Many examinations, including careful otological and roentgen ray studies of sinuses were negative. Adrenalin relieved the attacks as did a vegetable and fruit-free diet.

Richet and Rowe, in 1930, reported vertigo in a patient with ophthalmic migraine associated with a "falling" sensation. Examination of the central nervous system and spinal fluid revealed no abnormality. Symptoms were controlled with the elimination of fruits, vegetables, and nuts.

Atkinson, in 1941, reported Meniere's syndrome relieved with the elimination of milk, eggs, and beef. He gave niacin 50 mg one to three times a day with benefit.

Dohlman incriminated milk and wheat.

Dean reported Crisco and cottonseed oil as such and in Crisco as a cause.

Urbach reported a case of cerebellar disturbance with dizziness and tinnitus because of eggs, pork, and tomatoes.

Yandell, in 1931, reported labyrinthine storms with vertigo from allergy to orris root in a boy fourteen years of age.

Jones, in 1938, reported dizziness and vertigo from edema in the Eustachian tubes and fluid in the internal ear in a boy seven years of age resulting from chocolate, nuts, and wheat. He also reported allergic labyrinthitis with recurrent dizziness one to two times a week relieved by the elimination of milk.

Criep reported eight cases of vertigo with associated symptoms which he attributed to allergy to foods with or without associated inhalant allergy. Summaries of these cases are included in this chapter because of the indicated role of inhalant and especially of food allergy as reported by this experienced allergist of national repute. These typical cases with paroxysmal dizziness alone and also complicated with varying degrees of nausea and vomiting, ringing in the ears and tinnitus characteristic of Meniere's syndrome were relieved by Dr. Criep by the control of food with or without concomitant control of inhalant allergy.

Case 69: A man forty-two years of age had sudden recurrent attacks of dizziness with moderate deafness associated with cold sweats, nausea, and vomiting for fourteen years. A family history of allergy and positive skin tests to several foods were obtained. Elimination of specific allergenic foods gave lasting relief.

Case 70: A man twenty-four years of age had paroxysmal dizziness, pain in the occiput, nausea and some vomiting, buzzing and ringing in the ears, and disturbed equilibrium for several years. The severity and persistence of the symptoms kept him in bed for three to four weeks at a time and at one time for several months. Familial hay fever and perennial asthma were present. Skin tests were positive to many foods. Licking stamps produced an attack attributed to the sweet potato in the glue on the stamps. Control of food allergy gave relief for five years except for three slight attacks because of deviations in the diet.

Allergy to drugs and sera may cause this endolymphatic edema or recurring edema in the labyrinth. Toxic involvement of the eighth nerve from streptomycin also must be remembered.

Study and control of food allergy according to our experience is best done as we advise in this volume, especially in Chapters 2 and 3. When relief fails or before study as outlined above is begun, other causes of dizziness must be investigated by specialists as advised by rhinologists and otologists and discussed by Elia in 1968.

IMPAIRED HEARING BECAUSE OF ALLERGY FROM EDEMA IN THE EUSTACHIAN TUBES

Decreased hearing may occur from a) closure of the nasal opening into the Eustachian tubes or b) edema in the Eustachian tubes arising from edema of the nasal mucosa resulting from perennial food allergy and less often inhalant allergy. It also occurs from edema in the tubes themselves, usually with edema in the middle ear without definite nasal blocking from allergy, especially to foods. Nasal allergy from pollen or environmental house, occupational, or recreational airborne inhalants or dusts can also cause edema in the Eustachian tubes, middle ear, or possibly in the cochlea, resulting in impaired hearing. Perennial involvement however is usually due to food allergy.

When blocking in the nose occurs from mucosal edema and nasal polyps, food allergy in our experience also is the probable cause (see Chapt. 11). This requires the accurate and adequate use of our CFE diet for two to three weeks before in preparation for removal of the polyps and afterward to prevent their return.

Probable inhalant allergy requires indicated environmental control and desensitization to airborne pollens, especially pollens which cannot be eliminated from the air inspired by the patient.

Case 71: Edema of Eustachian tubes because of food allergy:

A man fifty-five years of age had had blocking of the Eustachian tubes much of the time for eight years and constantly for the last six years. Increased deafness and ringing in the ears had occurred. Frequent blowing out of the tubes, over 150 times, had given brief relief. With colds, inflations had been requested every one to two days. Frequent antibiotics had been ineffective. Corticoids were not available in 1949 when I first saw him. There was no blocking or polyps or itching of the nose.

Bronchial asthma or bronchitis had never occurred.

For several years fatigue, "not being rested on awakening," dopiness, and lack of energy indicating allergic toxemia described in Chapter 19 were present.

Diet history revealed a lifelong distaste for milk (always indicating milk allergy).

His drug and environmental and familial histories were negative for possible allergy.

Physical examination was negative except for moderate retraction of ear drums and postnasal mucoid discharge.

Routine laboratory tests including a sedimentation blood test and x-rays of sinuses were negative.

Scratch tests were negative to ingested foods and inhaled allergens in his environment.

Opinion, treatment and results: The edema in the Eustachian tubes for eight years, especially in the fall, winter, and early spring, and the lifelong distaste for milk justified the study of food allergy with our CFE diet. Food allergy best explained the perennial full feeling in the Eustachian tubes.

The diet was ordered in 1949 before corticoids were available.

In two weeks closure of ears, ringing, and deafness had decreased and in one month had disappeared. Relief continued for two months. In four months symptoms remained under control even with the addition of rice, oats, corn, coffee, fish, all vegetables, and fruits gradually to the diet. Symptoms recurred when milk, wheat, and eggs had been eaten. In five years relief from the blocking of the Eustachian tubes, ringing in the ears, impaired hearing, and fatigue and dopiness had continued from the continued elimination of the above foods.

ADVISABILITY OF CONTROLLING FOOD ALLERGY BEFORE AND AFTER OPERATIONS FOR OTOSCLEROSIS

Case 72: A woman fifty-seven years of age had had postnasal mucus with nasal congestion localizing especially in her ears for twenty years. Roaring in her ears started two years previously in the spring. Otosclerosis was diagnosed, and the anvil, hammer, and part of the stapes which "were frozen" were removed. Since then a fullness in and around the ear with constant noises had persisted with moderate impairment of hearing in the left ear. The distress in the ears, roaring, and noises had been worse since the operation, especially in the spring and early summer.

Food allergy was not suggested by the history.

Codeine caused nausea. Phenobarbital had caused hives.

A canary was in the house. Walnut trees were near the home.

Her father had hay fever.

Scratch tests were negative to foods and inhalants. X-ray showed haziness in each antrum.

Treatment: Because of perennial nasal symptoms, our CFE diet was ordered to study possible food allergy in spite of negative skin reactions. Desensitization to a multiple pollen antigen was given because of exaggeration of symptoms in the spring and summer.

Noises and fullness in the ears and discomfort in the right ear decreased, especially in the last eight months of her antiallergic control. Hearing in the left ear improved. An advised operation on the left ear similar to that on the right has not been necessary.

Hence, control of allergy before operation on bones of ears and after operation is important.

Though control of her food and pollen allergies before surgery probably would not have obviated the surgery, mild allergy would be relieved and make surgery unnecessary.

ALLERGIC DERMATITIS OR ECZEMA OF THE EARS

Longstanding eczema of the ears in thirty cases seen by us in the last twenty-five years occurred on all or most of the outer surface of the ears in 80 percent, on the back of the ears in 23 percent, in the ear canals alone in 17 percent, and in the canals associated with eczema on the outer ear surfaces in 27 percent, as reported in our statistics in Table XXVII compiled from our records of these relieved patients. In the other 83 percent moderate eczema also occurred in other areas of the skin, varying in each area from 10 to 30 percent in frequency. Eczema of the ears was the major manifestation of cutaneous allergy in all thirty patients. No cases of brief duration of eczema of the ears were tabulated.

Interesting is the average age of forty-seven years with no patients of ten years or less, the average being increased by the inclusion of one case of eighty years. The average duration of unrelieved eczema of the ears of fifteen years is also increased by the inclusion of the six cases of eczema of the ears of varying severity for four to twenty years. The predominance of females, if confirmed by other allergists, may be due to the greater irritation of the ears by soap, cosmetics, and hair and scalp sprays by women which activates potential eczema resulting from food allergy.

Exaggeration of the aural eczema in the fall, winter, and early spring months in 23 percent occurs less often than in bronchial asthma in children and in allergic bronchitis resulting from food allergy alone (see Chapt. 9 and 25). Food allergy was

TABLE XXVII

ECZEMA OF THE EARS IN 30 CASES

Males	5
Females	25
Age (11-80 years)	av. 47 yrs
Duration (1-61 years)	av. 15 yrs
Areas Involved:	
Outer surfaces of ears	24 (80%)
Ears and canals	8 (27%)
Back of ears	7 (23%)
Eczema only in ear canals	5 (17%)
In other skin areas	25 (83%)
Scalp	9
Neck	10
Hands	7
Genitals	8
Eyes	3
Torso	4
Arms	5
Legs	3
Winter Exaggeration	7
Personal History of Allergy:	
Asthma	6
Urticaria	2
Indigestion	6
Former eczema	1
Fatigue	4
Depression	1
Nasal allergy	1
Family History:	
Hay fever	4
Asthma	3
Headaches	2
Eczema	7
Skin Tests (scratch):	
Food	0
Pollen	5
Diet History:	
Suggesting food allergy	14 (47%)
Milk	10 (30%)
Causes:	
Food alone	21
Food and pollen	9

adjudged the sole cause by us in approximately 84 percent of our thirty cases. Exaggeration in the summer in 16 percent correlates with our conclusion that pollen allergy was the sole cause in 6 percent and was associated with food allergy in ten percent. The occurrence of other probable manifestations of allergy in the personal and family histories varying from 6 to 24 percent indicates the frequency of allergic predisposition in these patients.

Eczema only in the ear canals causing

itching, scaling, crusting, serous discharge, and varying degrees of aching and pain is more frequent than indicated in our statistics. One woman forty-five years of age with eczema only of the ear canals for twenty years had lasting relief from food allergy with our cereal-free elimination diet. Many patients with eczema of the ear canals, moreover, have used antibiotics and corticoid ointments as advised by physicians or purchased at drugstores with resultant temporary or partial relief. Lasting relief at times has occurred after a slight infection is controlled with an antibiotic ointment or when irritation from a plastic plug in the ear canal has been discontinued.

Study of the allergenic causes including drugs or contact allergy as from nail polish, earphones, or ear wax removers always needs consideration in cases of this type. Eczema from allergy to alloys of nickel in earrings and bows of eye glasses as well as to the plastic in the bows of eye glasses is always necessary to remember. The itching and at times aching and pain in the ear canals with involvement of the tympanum often is distressing, causing nervousness, irritability, and restless sleep.

Our statistics do not indicate allergy to environmental inhalants other than pollens. Such inhalants need consideration, however, if experienced adequate control of food and pollen allergy fails to relieve the symptoms. Moreover, it is always necessary to take into consideration contact allergy until relief occurs. A Dacron pillow rather than a feather, foam, hair, or kapok pillow should be used. Also, possible allergy to wool blankets or other fabrics in bedding must be considered. The reader is referred in this regard to our discussion of allergy to contactants of many types and to drugs, medicaments, chemicals, and dyes in Chapter 20 on ocular allergy and in Chapter 14 on allergic eczema.

Possible seborrhea as a major or complicating factor in eczema of the ears, especially on the backs of the ears, must be remembered.

The relief of seborrhea occurs with the application of Mycostatin, Achromycin, or other "mycin" ointments or the long-utilized tars and salicylic acid ointments and at times mercury ointment and lotions. Dermatitis with characteristic seborrhea, however, may clear when antiallergic control with initial corticosteroids, the use of our elimination diets, and when indicated control of environmental allergens and desensitization therapy occurs.

PERSONAL CASES

Case 73: A woman twenty-eight years of age had eczema in the ears and vulva perennially with exaggeration during the fall and winter months for ten years. Scratch tests with food and pollen allergens were negative. There was no other eczema on any other part of her skin. Food allergy was indicated by its perennial occurrence and its exaggeration during winter months. With our cereal-free elimination diet, the eczema was controlled. Definite conclusions about the specific foods excluded from the elimination diet were not possible because of failure of the patient to cooperate satisfactorily with provocation tests.

Case 74: A woman fifty-five years of age had eczema confined to the ears alone for eight years. Of interest was the absence of other definite manifestations of allergy in her personal and family history. Scratch tests with food and inhalant allergens were negative. Her diet history indicated probable increase of the dermatitis from the eating of fruit. With the use of our fruit-free and cereal-free elimination diet maintained strictly for two months in the last six weeks without any corticosteroids, the eczema was relieved. Provocation tests thereafter showed that fruits, milk, wheat, corn, and rice reactivated the eczema.

ECZEMA OF THE EARS FOR SIXTY-ONE YEARS AND OF THE VULVA AND PERINEUM FOR FOUR YEARS BECAUSE OF FOOD ALLERGY

Case 75: A woman sixty-five years of age had had dry and at times oozing and crusting eczema on the outer surface and backs of the ears, with exaggeration of the rims for sixty-one years except for moderate decrease during medical therapy for five years at the age of fifty. For the last four years an itching eruption had also been present on the inguinal, vulval, perineal, and perianal areas. She had been treated without benefit "by forty physicians." "Every ointment she heard of" had failed to give relief. All her life she had worn pads in the back of the ears and covered her pillows with a towel at night to absorb the oozing.

Perennial nasal allergy had continued for thirty years. Loss of smell had been present for six years. Her diet history revealed increasing oozing of the ears from chicken, turkey, and "candy." She had disliked milk all of her life. Eggs caused bloating and a "shivering sensation." There was no familial allergy except hay fever in a brother. Scratch tests with food and inhalant allergens were negative.

Physical examination and routine laboratory tests were negative except dermatitis, as described above.

Treatment: Because of the perennial, lifelong eczema and because of the diet history suggesting food allergy, it was studied with our CFE diet. Because of possible complicating seborrhea, 5 percent ammoniated mercury was applied to the erupted areas after they had been soaked with saline solution. This treatment was discontinued in about two weeks.

In one month the itching and dermatitis had subsided. In two months the eczema had disappeared for the first time in sixty years, and the eruption on the inguinal, vulval, and perianal areas had greatly decreased. Foods were gradually added to the diet during the next six months, and it was found that wheat, milk, chocolate, and eggs individually reactivated the dermatitis. In another year the eczema had been absent except when the above foods were ingested, even in small amounts.

Case 76: A woman eighty years of age had dermatitis of the outer ears and canals for thirty-four years. There was no seasonal variation. The marked exaggeration of her eczema, which had spread around the neck onto the anterior chest and over the breasts, had occurred during the last two years. Much dermatological treatment through many years and maximum x-ray therapy had been ineffectual.

There was no history of other manifestations of allergy, of food dislikes or disagreements, or of drug or environmental allergy. Scratch tests for food and inhalant allergens were negative.

Treatment: Because of the perennial eczema in spite of negative reactions to foods, food allergy was studied with our CFE diet. In one month all eczema had decreased except for a slight eruption on the earlobes. Hydrocortisone ointment used for three weeks relieved this residual eczema. To the strict CFE diet, vegetables, fruits, cereals, and fish were gradually added. The addition of milk, wheat, and eggs reproduced the dermatitis on the ear and neck. After relief occurred from the elimination of these foods, their allergenic effect was again confirmed by their addition to the diet.

DECREASED HEARING IN CHILDREN

Decreased hearing occurs especially in children from allergic edema in the mucosa of the nose and especially in the Eustachian tubes and membranes of the middle ear.

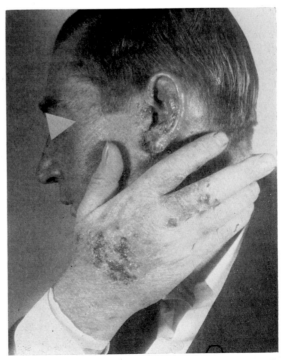

Figure 13. Eczema of ears and hands as a result of food allergy.

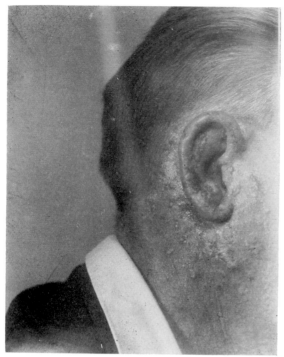

Figure 14. Eczema of ears resulting from food allergy determined with our CFE diet.

In ten children in our practice decreased hearing had been perennial, being exaggerated during the winter months, especially in eight of them, indicating food allergy. The nasal allergy and deafness had caused absences from school one-half or even three-fourths of the time in four children and less absence in four other children. Definite improvement had occurred in the summers in seven children. Rubbing of the nose, snoring, and noisy breathing with little sneezing and no itching were frequent. Nasal congestion, blocking of the nose, varying degrees of nasal discharge, and postnasal mucus causing a hacking cough had occurred especially in the fall and winter months. Serous otitis media had occurred in six children because of food allergy.

Bronchial asthma in three of the ten children, eczema in one, and hives in one

had occurred. Inefficiency in school work, inattentiveness, irritability, and fatigue in several children were present.

The family histories revealed nasal allergy in five and asthma in four of the ten children.

Skin tests were positive to milk in one child and to pollens in one.

Good to excellent results, depending largely on cooperation of the children and parents, resulted from our study and control of food allergy with our CFE diet and at times with its modifications.

DECREASED HEARING IN ADULTS BECAUSE OF FOOD AND INHALANT ALLERGIES

In adult life varying degrees of deafness occur when perennial nasal allergy is present, especially when blocking of the nose, mucosal edema, fluid in the maxillary antra, and postnasal mucoid discharge are present. Hearing is decreased when the nasal apertures of the Eustachian tubes are obstructed and especially when edema in these tubes is present. As stated in Chapter 11 on Perennial Nasal Allergy, sensitization to foods is the usual cause. Recurrent nasal polyps, which in our experience are nearly always due to longstanding food allergy, increase the blocking of the nose and resultant deafness. When this nasal allergy has started in childhood, continuing into adult life with or without nasal polyps, decreased hearing may be definitely exaggerated.

Along with the nasal blocking and edema in the Eustachian tubes, allergic inflammation and edema in the middle ear often occur in infancy and childhood and at times in young adults. Recurrent serous otitis media resulting from food allergy is also a frequent occurrence and may continue for months or even years.

Allergy in the middle ear may also produce continued inflammation without development of serous or mucoid secretion. In many of these people ringing, singing, or other noise in the ear is disturbing. Chronic allergy in the middle ear, moreover, may produce adhesions involving the bones in the tympanum, reducing their function, at times with involvement of the cochlea, causing varying degrees of loss of hearing.

When reduced hearing in children and adults occurs from edema of the Eustachian tubes and allergy in the middle ear, probable food allergy must be studied and controlled as advised in this volume. Allergy to environmental animal emanations and dusts may also be responsible, as previously discussed in this chapter and in Chapter 4. Deafness from edema in the mucosa of the nose, Eustachian tubes, and at times in the middle ear during the spring, summer, and fall from allergy to airborne pollens must also be remembered. Such deafness and associated symptoms, in our experience, from allergy to pollens are infrequent as compared to their origin from food allergy. Seasonal deafness controlled by desensitization to pollens in the air during the pollen seasons is illustrated in the following case. Food allergy also was exaggerated, especially in the winter.

Case 77: A woman forty years of age had had a "plugged up" right ear with fullness through the entire head with decreased hearing from April until late October for three years. In the last year moderate symptoms had persisted during the winter. Increasing loss of hearing had occurred, especially during the pollen seasons. Usual itching of the eyes because of pollen allergy was absent. Granulation of the eyelids on arising had been present for two years during pollen seasons.

Head colds and coughs had been occurring every month or so in the fall, winter, and early spring for several years. Severe wheezing and heaviness in the chest in the fall and winter months had been present, indicating bronchospasm resulting from probable food allergy. Post-nasal mucus also had been present for many years, especially in the winter months, since childhood, again suggesting food allergy.

There was no sneezing or itching in the eyes or nose.

Headaches often with nausea and vomiting had occurred with her periods for three years. Intermittent constipation had occurred. Vaginal mucus had been passed for many years.

All of these symptoms, especially the blocking of the ears with decreased hearing and headaches, had made her irritable, tense, and nervous. During the pollen seasons she felt fatigued and dopey, particularly during the menstrual periods.

Diet history revealed increased postnasal mucus from milk and cheese exaggerated during the fall and winter months.

Her drug history revealed the taking of four to six aspirins a day with no definite relief of symptoms.

Her environmental history revealed no indication of allergy to recreational or household inhalants.

X-rays of the chest and maxillary sinuses were negative, as were the blood count, VDRL, and sedimentation rate.

Scratch tests gave one plus reactions to several grass, tree, and fall pollens.

Treatment: Pollen allergy was indicated by history and slight positive skin tests in the spring to late fall as a cause of the edema in the Eustachian tubes and nasal passages. An antigen containing the airborne pollens in her environment during the spring, summer and fall months was started with a 1:500,000 dilution. It was gradually increased. In four months 0.60 cc of a 1:100 dilution was tolerated. With the repetition of this dose at weekly intervals during the last 2½ years, there has been no blocking of the ears and no reduction in hearing during the pollen seasons.

In order to study food allergy as a cause of her headaches and her vaginal mucoid discharge, our CFE diet was prescribed during the fall, winter, and spring months when these symptoms were definitely exaggerated. After relief of these symptoms, additional foods one by one were added and rice, oats, and eggs were tolerated. Canned corn and corn starch reproduced her headache and moderate blocking of the ears during the winter months. Omission of beef and egg, moreover, before and during her period eliminated her menstrual headaches.

With this treatment "wonderful, unbelievable"

freedom from symptoms occurred. She "feels like a new person." Repeated head colds and coughs during the winter were absent, and this for the first time in her life.

Comment: This record reports relief of blocking of the ears with decreased hearing and a full feeling throughout the entire head from April to late October by pollen desensitization. Skin reactions to pollens were slight or absent.

Her headaches (especially during her menstrual periods), vaginal mucus, and postnasal mucus present throughout the year, as reported in Chapter 12, were relieved by the elimination of allergenic foods. Canned corn and corn starch were found to reproduce headaches and moderate blocking of the ears. Beef and eggs especially reproduced her headaches.

COMMENT

Therefore, when deafness, with or without blocking of the nose or Eustachian tubes, is associated with perennial nasal blocking, especially when minimal or absent sneezing or itching is present, food allergy must be studied as we advise. Corticosteroids in reducing doses during a one to two week period will hasten relief.

When deafness occurs in the pollen seasons, desensitization is important. Possible allergy to animal emanations and miscellaneous inhalants is frequently relieved with adequate and strict environmental control. If it is impossible to eliminate all of the causative airborne allergens, desensitization to such allergens is indicated.

FOOD ALLERGY AND SURGERY

When operation of the bones of the middle ear is advisable, the control of definite or possible food allergy and less often control of inhalant and especially pollen allergy are important. With such control before and after surgery, postoperative symptoms from uncontrolled allergy will be diminished or prevented. The following case report illustrates such postoperative benefit.

Case 78: A man fifty-three years of age had had blocking of the Eustachian tubes, congestion in the pharynx, hoarseness, and tightness in the anterior neck most of the time for ten years. Recurrent "nasal colds" without fever had been frequent, especially in the late fall and winter. Advice from several physicians and specialists was ineffectual. Antihistamines two to three times daily gave limited relief.

Depression, drowsiness, fatigue, and frustration, increased in part from failure of medical treatment, continued.

Diet, drug, and environmental histories suggested no allergic cause except probable pollen allergy because of exaggerated perennial symptoms in the pollen seasons.

Physical examination and routine laboratory tests were negative. X-rays showed haziness in the maxillary antra. Scratch tests were moderately positive to tree, grass, and fall pollens in his area with negative reactions to other inhalants and foods.

Treatment: For four years continued elimination of wheat, milk, and eggs has been required to control perennial blocking of the Eustachian tubes, pharyngeal congestion, fatigue, and depression. Desensitization to the tree, grass, and fall pollens has relieved exaggeration of symptoms during the pollen seasons. Therefore, perennial food and seasonal pollen allergies are the established causes.

SUMMARY

1. Atopic allergy to foods and inhalants often involves the outer, middle, and inner ear and the Eustachian tubes with or without nasobronchial allergy or other clinical manifestations of such allergy.

2. Food allergy may be the sole cause when the manifestation is recurrent, especially in the fall to late spring, decreased or absent in the summer, as emphasized in Chapter 2.

3. Thus recurrent serous otitis media often with fever in spite of absent infection is usually due to food allergy alone, as it was for eight years in identical twins (Case 65) and other children reported in this chapter.

4. Food allergy as an important cause of dizziness, vertigo, and of Meniere's syndrome, as emphasized by Duke in 1923 and later by Criep in 1941, who determined such food allergy with our elimination diets, is emphasized. Such allergy has been long confirmed in our practice.

5. Impaired hearing from allergic edema in the Eustachian tubes from atopic allergy especially to foods is frequently encountered in our practice. Illustrative case reports are summarized.

6. Finally, eczema of the ears resulting from food allergy and when exaggerated in the spring into late fall to pollen allergy must be recognized and controlled as we advise.

Chapter 14

Atopic Dermatitis (Eczema) Resulting From
Food and Other Allergies

Atopic dermatitis (eczema) can arise from practically all food, inhalant, and drug allergens, as cited in Chapter 2, which cause the nasobronchial and other manifestations of allergy discussed in this volume. As in bronchial asthma, one or more food, inhalant, drug, or other miscellaneous allergens may individually or in multiples be responsible for this type of eczema. Rarely atopic eczema co-exists with contact dermatitis. Sensitization to various allergens may vary in degree. Mild sensitizations frequently exist, difficult to recognize, often without skin reactions, and the summation effects of several slight allergies may also be responsible for persistent eczema. As in bronchial asthma, the determination of the allergenic causes must be made through histories recommended in this volume by means of scratch tests, environmental control, and especially with accurate, adequate trial diets, especially with our elimination diets.

Necessary to reiterate is the fact that skin tests are often negative to foods causing clinical allergy, especially dermatitis, and that they also may be negative to pollen and other inhalant allergens productive of eczema, as stated in Chapter 2. Positive tests to foods and inhalants, moreover, always need the confirmation of provocation tests to determine their actual role in etiology. Frequently this is difficult to be certain about, and their underlying importance must be gradually decided by results of desensitization or elimination. This may require weeks and at times months, which emphasizes the absolute necessity of co-operation, study, and therapy for months or even several years, depending on the degree of chronicity of the patient's eczema or other allergic manifestations.

FOOD ALLERGY IN ALLERGIC DERMATITIS

Food allergy may produce allergic eczema throughout life. In infancy it is the usual cause, decreasing in importance as years advance. As in asthma, urticaria, or migraine, allergic eczema resulting from food may be cyclic, probably because of desensitization after attacks. The lesions in infancy especially are likely to be exudative. Scaling, dry lesions with lichenification and induration are more frequent in adolescent and adult years. Infants having acute facial eczema are likely to develop dermatitis on the flexures and neck in the second and third years. It may form the basis of increasing sensitization to many inhalants and possibly contact substances. Andrews (1930), White (1935), Knowles (1935), Shelmire (1933), MacDonald (1932), and especially Urbach (1932) and many allergists and other physicians have confirmed the great importance of food allergy in the etiology of allergic eczema. Hopkins, Waters, and Kesten (1931) found our elimination diets of special value in their diagnosis and treatment. Causative foods were positive by skin testing in 43 percent and were determined only by trial diets in 53 percent. Eggs, milk, and wheat were the most common causes. Hopkins and Kesten (1935) affirmed this importance of food allergy and pointed out the origin of increasing numbers of sensitizations of various foods and particularly to pollen, animal emanation, and dust allergens as age increases. Their confirmation of the value and necessity of elimination trial diets in the diagnosis of food allergy coincides with our experience since 1926. They looked on the positive skin reaction only as confirmatory evidence favoring food sensitization. No case in their series was relieved with the elimination of a few foods to which skin reactions were obtained. Diet trial was always necessary. They found allergic eczema in adults at times a result solely of food allergy, though it was usually complicated or overshadowed by inhalant or drug sensitizations. In seventy-five patients the foods which caused eczema in order of frequency were eggs, wheat, milk, oranges, spinach, oats, cod, potatoes, and others less frequently. White (1935) described discrete erythematopapular lesions on the right hand from ingested chocolate and a recurrent eczematoid eruption on the palms of both hands in a nurse relieved by elimination of peas, beans, and peaches. Another man suffered for several years from an erythematofollicular eruption of the extremities with recent purpura due to peas and wheat. Of interest was the observation of Avit-Scott (1934). A dyshidrotic eruption occurred on the fingers and hands when orange juice was taken after the orange had been peeled. If it were only drunk, prickling of the fingers arose. Ingestion and contact were necessary for maximum lesions. Wise and Wolfe (1936) also observed two cases of dyshidrosiform eruption on the palms

and fingers, suggesting a trichophytid resulting from ingested orange juice.

Baer (1934) reported erythematous maculopapules on the neck, shoulders, arms, and forearms, with scaling in other places from a green dye in ingested gelatin. This was also associated with a cramping distress two or three hours after eating, at times associated with diarrhea, indicating an intestinal allergy. Dutton (1935) described chronic eczema from some allergen contained in drinking water such as algae or other organic matter. Distilled water rendered desired relief. I have a patient who develops severe facial dermatitis from chlorine and possibly organic allergens in drinking water and the same lesions when she inhales chlorine from Clorox® used for cleaning. One other patient develops extensive dermatitis of the face, neck, and arms when she passes through a room in which chlorine solutions or powders are being used. Anderson (1935) studied a patient whose dermatitis on the arms and hands arose only when grapes were rubbed into the skin and also ingested.

Pruritus without definite lesions may occur, especially in old age from those allergenic causes, particularly from foods, which produce marked erythema and eczema in the more delicate active skin of children and young adults. Wynn (1927) reported senile pruritus in old people from wheat allergy. We have relieved such patients with elimination diets excluding wheat, milk, or other causative foods. Urbach (1932) also discussed such pruritus from the viewpoint of tea, coffee, and alcohol intake. M.B. Cohen (1931) reported generalized pruritus resulting from potato and buckwheat ingestion to which skin reactions occurred. Actual lesions may only result from scratching, trauma, or medication. It is important to remember that pruritus in adults and especially in old people may also result from absorption from an obscure tumor, local infection, or may be due to hypothyroidism. Horder (1935) emphasized diabetes, uremia, jaundice, organic nervous disease, and gout as causes of pruritus. Mittleman (1933) reported pruritus since infancy in a woman thirty-six years of age relieved with elimination diets. A psychoneurosis and the habit of producing self-inflicted excoriations had arisen from this unrelieved allergic pruritus.

From our records we have assembled forty-eight cases of allergic dermatitis (eczema) in which food was the sole or major cause. The statistics on these cases which were successfully controlled by the use of elimination diets, modified by definite skin reactions which were obtained in a few cases, are presented in Table XXVIII.

TABLE XXVIII

STATISTICS ON PATIENTS WITH ECZEMA PRIMARILY RESULTING FROM FOOD ALLERGY

Number of Cases—48

	%
Male	42
Female	58
Average age in years	26
Bronchial allergy	18
Nasal allergy	12
Eczema	100
Urticaria	29
Angioneurotic edema	3
Allergic headache	10
Abdominal allergy	29
Family history of allergy	71
Food dislikes or disagreements	46
Positive Skin Reactions	
Food	44
Animal emanations	33
Dust	12
Pollen	19
Miscellaneous	2
Duration of Symptoms	8 yrs (1/3-61)

The patients were all adults with the exception of a few adolescents. Eczema in infants and young children which is so frequently a result of food sensitization alone

has not been included, as it was my aim to indicate its occurrence in adults and show the frequency of other allergic manifestations and of skin reactions to inhalant as well as to food allergens. With food elimination these patients were relieved of their dermatoses which had had an average duration of eight years, varying from one-third to sixty-one years.

As already discussed in this book, elimination diets can well be used in most cases in the study of food allergy in the etiology of allergic dermatitis. As a rule, no uncooked fruit other than lemon or grapefruit should be allowed in the first trial diet. Moreover, certain patients may have to use various supplemental elimination diets (see Chapt. 3) before etiological foods are found.

Case 79: Thus a girl sixteen years of age who for years had had scaling eczema on the forehead, temples, around the mouth, upper eyelids, neck, over the clavicles, and in the cubital areas did not clear until she was given a diet of chicken, tapioca, carrots, beets, asparagus, olive oil, sugar, and salt. Enough calories in these foods were taken to prevent weight loss. Our routine elimination diets had first been used with indifferent results.

Elimination diets should not be used without a careful thorough study of the technique, precautions, and possible pitfalls described in Chapter 3. With prolonged use nutritional damage, as stressed in that chapter, must be prevented. The characteristic cutaneous and other tissue changes resulting from deficient vitamin intake must be kept in mind.

The use of Urbach's propeptans to desensitize against foods causative of eczema has been disappointing in America. Likewise, Cormia (1933), Cornbleet, Kaplan (1934), and others have obtained no results with urinary proteose therapy.

Food allergy in our experience is more important than inhalant and blood-borne drug allergies in the causation of perennial atopic dermatitis. This has been supported by us for over thirty years and is evidenced in our statistics on 105 adults relieved of atopic dermatitis resulting from food and pollen allergy. It is especially emphasized by our excellent results in the control of atopic eczema in infants and children reported in Chapter 25. It is more important than contact allergy in the usual practice of medicine or clinical allergy except in patients exposed to recognized vegetable and chemical allergenic contactants in their living or working environments. Failure to adequately study inhalant and especially food allergies accounts, in our opinion and that of other allergists, for the unwarranted skepticism of many dermatologists about the importance of food and inhalant allergy in atopic dermatitis (eczema). This unfortunate skepticism and nihilism are evidenced in textbooks on dermatology and in articles on atopic dermatitis in the literature. Clarke, in 1948, deplored the tardiness of dermatologists in making use of allergic methods of studying and treating atopic dermatitis.

Our increasing recognition of food allergy in the last forty years has been due to a) our realization of negative skin reactions to causative foods, b) the fallibility of many positive skin reactions as indicators of clinical allergy, and especially c) use of our CFE diet for the study of possible food allergy as discussed in this chapter, in Chapter 3, and throughout this volume.

Food allergy requires study when eczema is perennial and especially when it is exaggerated in the fall to early spring, particularly in the winter, and decreases or is quite absent in the summer.

Thus food allergy is the usual cause of winter eczema, as shown in Figure 15. It is the usual cause of eczema in infants. Though it decreases or even disappears in

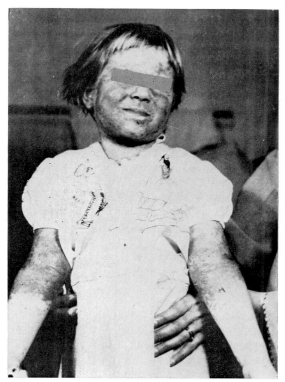

Figure 15. *Case 81:* Winter eczema resulting from milk, wheat, corn, and eggs, relieved with our CFE diet.

childhood, it often continues into adolescence or into adult life. Food allergy may also arise at any time during life, including old age. In infancy the face, neck, flexures, and (when severe) other areas are involved. At times the eczema is generalized, as discussed in our chapter on food allergy in children. Cradle cap and continued dermatitis with itching of the scalp during childhood and even in later years always require the study of possible food allergy. Erythema or dermatitis from contact of allergenic foods with the face and hands also must be recognized.

Thus we study possible food allergy in all cases of eczema or dermatitis except when it only occurs in the pollen seasons, affirming pollen allergy, or when obvious drug, chemical, or contact allergy is the evident cause. And even in these cases a mild or obscure food allergy may justify its study, especially if the treatment or control of the more apparent causes fails to reveal the causative allergies.

The distribution of eczema resulting from food allergy is also noted in this chapter.

INHALANT ALLERGIES

Next to food allergy, pollen allergy is of importance in the causation of allergic eczema. Pollen allergy especially needs emphasis when dermatitis occurs from early spring to late fall with marked or entire relief in the winter. If the eczema is caused by tree, grass, or fall pollens, its occurrence may be limited to or be exaggerated in those months when such pollens are in the air. In contrast to food allergy, definite, often marked skin reactions usually occur to the pollens.

Reactions occur to pollens in the air when eczema is present or to all pollens, though dermatitis may be due only to tree pollens or grass or fall pollens. In some patients reactions to other seasonal pollens indicate potential clinical allergy. Skin reactions to the causative pollens may be slight or even absent. The history of seasonal dermatitis therefore is of greater importance than skin testing in the diagnosis. Because of extreme allergy that often occurs to pollens responsible for allergic dermatitis, only scratch tests are done. Initial intradermal tests may produce a serious exacerbation of the eczema. Desensitization to pollens is advised later in this chapter.

DISTRIBUTION OF ECZEMA RESULTING FROM FOOD ALLERGY

In infancy eczema resulting from food allergy favors the face, scalp, neck, and flexures and is nearly always due to allergy to animal milk proteins, especially of the cow. Though allergy to mother's milk does occur, allergy may occur in an infant to the allergens of foods eaten by the mother which enter the milk, as discussed in Chapters 1 and 25.

When the skin is secondarily infected, especially with staphylococci, impetiginous eczema results. The scalp may be involved, causing "cradle cap." This eczema gradually may become generalized, resulting in erythematous, vesicular, oozing, crusting, and later scaling, thickened, and lichenified dermatitis. As foods other than milk are

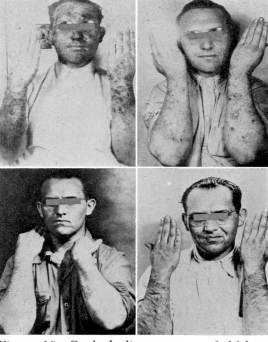

Figure 16. Gradual disappearance of lifelong allergic eczema in one year resulting from food allery alone because of strict adherence to our CFE diet. Photograph 2 in three months, 3 in six months (had worked for first time in life for 2 months), 4—complete control in one year. Note evident change in personality; similar strict cooperation for weeks or months is also required for tissue changes in the lungs from severe perennial bronchial asthma, chronic bronchitis, obstructive emphysema, or other chronic allergy resulting from food, as in chronic ulcerative colitis to disappear.

added to the diet, allergy to them must always be suspected. This eczema especially in the flexures, face, neck, and in other areas of the skin often continues into adolescence and adult life if allergenic foods continue in the diet.

Case 80: Such maximum atopic eczema resulting from food allergy is shown in the photographs in Figure 16. This eczema, present since infancy, had decreased in the summer for eight years but for fifteen years thereafter had been perennial, increased in degree, and prevented school attendance and employment. Depression and frustration resulted because of failure of treatment by several physicians and two dermatologists to control the eruption. With the study of food allergy with our CFE diet and no medication (cortisone and mycin antibiotics being unavailable in 1945), itching decreased in one month and dermatitis definitely decreased in three months, being practically absent in six months and entirely absent with the growth of normal hair on the arms in one year. These photographs show that the tissue changes resulting from longstanding allergy require weeks and at times several months to recede to a minimum without corticosteroids even though the causative foods are eliminated from the body in two to four weeks.

During the entire year our CFE diet was maintained with the addition of extra fruits, vegetables, fowl, and tea. No milk, eggs, chocolate, cereal grains, or coffee were added. The photographic evidence of the time required to relieve severe atopic eczema resulting from food allergy with only the elimination of foods would be difficult to duplicate today, since corticosteroids would be given by nearly all physicians even though the major role of food allergy may not be recognized.

As in bronchial asthma due to food allergy, this eczema often decreases or even disappears in the summer, being reactivated in the winter months. Parents or even adults report "winter eczema," which in our experience is usually a result of food allergy.

Case 81: Winter eczema is shown in Figure 15 in the photograph of a young girl whose mother stated that the eczema disappeared in the summer. With our CFE diet this eczema was absent in the winter but was reactivated by the addition of milk, wheat, corn, and eggs.

As a child grows older and enters adolescence, inhalant allergy especially to pollens as a sole cause and particularly associated with food allergy increases in frequency. The characteristics and control of pollen allergy are discussed later in this chapter.

In adult life food allergy produces perennial eczema often exaggerated in the winter half of the year in the face, neck, flexures and other areas of the skin as shown in Figure 16.

ECZEMA OF THE HANDS

The hands alone or in association with other areas of the skin are the site of eczema more frequently than any other localized area. Eczema of the hands occurs from food allergy in children and especially in adults, possibly because of greater irritation of the hands than of other skin areas. Young women after marriage often develop eczema of the hands from activation of potential eczema resulting from food allergy from washing dishes, clothes, and diapers and from irritation from cooking meals and doing housework. The first evidence of such hand eczema resulting from food allergy may be under the rings, with a gradual spread to all the fingers, the dorsa, and the palms of the hands. The irritation from the ring possibly because of accumulated soap under the ring activates potential eczema from ingested foods. The eczema then spreads to other areas of the fingers and hands, especially their dorsal surfaces, and continues as long as the causative foods are in the diet. The distribution of eczema resulting from food allergy in the fingers and hands and its occurrence in other areas of the skin in eight cases as reported by us in 1946 is shown in Table XXIX. Other statistics showing the age of onset, other involved skin areas, duration (average 7 years), personal and family history of allergy, fallibility of skin tests, the occurrence of associated pollen allergy (in 27%), the time required for benefit to be evident (in 2-9 weeks) from our CFE diet and the years of relief from adherence to the required diet (from 1-9 years) are included in this article.

NUMULAR ECZEMA

Numular eczema especially in the extremities and also on the torso, perennial in type, requires study of food allergy as exemplified in Figure 18. With such study an unknown etiology as stated by Helms and Berger in 1968 and in most textbooks may be modified or even reversed.

ECZEMA OF EARS AND EAR CANALS

This localized eczema resulting from food and/or pollen allergy with statistics on thirty cases in Chapter 13 is not discussed here.

Inhalant allergy especially to pollens was confirmed by Jillson and Piper in an article in 1955 in which twenty-two references were included.

HAND ECZEMA RESULTING FROM POLLEN ALLERGY AND CONTACT DERMATITIS

In an additional 102 cases of eczema of the hands, pollen allergy was the major factor in 22, as we reported in a separate

article on eczema of the hands resulting from pollen allergy in 1946.

In our practice only fifteen cases of contact allergy were identified—three to rubber in gloves, two to caine drugs in dentists, one to butesin picrate in ointment, one to a photo developer, one to toothpowder, one to ink, one to hand cream, and five from handling fruits and vegetables.

In addition, dermatitis of the hands was due to probable fungus infection in a limited number which was not well controlled because of unavailability of antifungicidal drugs such as Fulvicin® F in those years. Undetermined causes in other patients were probably due to contactants which we failed to recognize or the study of which was limited by poor cooperation by the patient. Contact allergy is seen more often by dermatologists than by us as allergists.

ECZEMA OF THE HANDS RESULTING FROM FOOD AND POLLEN ALLERGY

We confirmed eczema of the hands resulting from food allergy in fifty cases and resulting from pollen allergy in twenty cases in 1965 in the areas in Tables XXIX and XXX.

Failure of previous advice and treatment as shown in Table XXXI emphasizes the

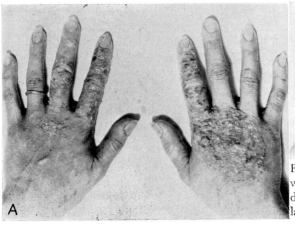

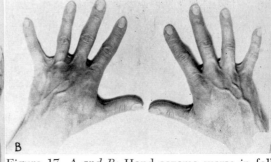

Figure 17. *A and B:* Hand eczema worse in fall, winter, and early spring, relieved with our CFE diet. This was to milk, cereal grains, and chocolate.

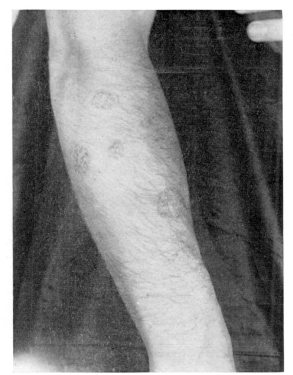

Figure 18. Numular eczema resulting from food allergy as determined by our CFE diet.

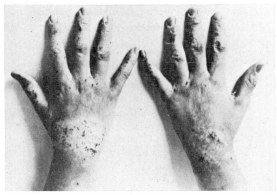

Figure 19. Hand eczema resulting from food allergy.

importance of eliminating allergenic foods and/or desensitization to causative pollens. The frequency of perennial nasal allergy, pollen hay fever, gastrointestinal symptoms, fatigue, and toxemia relieved by our antiallergic therapy is supported in this article.

TABLE XXIX

LOCATION OF ECZEMA OF HANDS

	Food Allergy 50 Cases		Pollen Allergy 20 Cases
Dorsa of hands	31		7
Dorsa of hands (alone)	5		0
Palms	15		9
Palms (alone)	0		6
Fingers (1-2)	4	often starting under rings	4
Fingers (3-5)	32		15
Hands and fingers only	12		8

Note: Other manifestations of atopic allergy occurred in Table XXX. Of interest was the greater frequency of perennial nasal, gastrointestinal indications of allergy in the food than in the pollen-sensitive patient.

TABLE XXX

PERSONAL HISTORY OF OTHER MANIFESTATIONS OF POSSIBLE CLINICAL ALLERGY

	Food Allergy 50 Cases		Pollen Allergy 20 Cases
Perennial nasal symptoms	9		1
Pollen hay fever	11		7
Bronchial asthma	16		2
Eczema (adult)	6	} 9	2
Eczema (infantile)	3		4
Headaches	9		3
GI symptoms	10		0
Fatigue and toxemia	8		0

Note: No clinical allergy (except eczema) in 30 of the 50 cases resulting from food and in 11 of the 20 cases resulting from pollen.

Case 82: A woman thirty-five years of age had had eczema on the back of the hands for thirteen years constantly increasing every month or so and worse in the fall and winter months. Vesiculation, itching, and crusting developed during an attack of four to five days—then dryness, cracking, scaling, and lichenification.

She had worked in fuse works for nineteen years handling black powder, asphalt, lead tubing, and cotton jute.

She had had sick headaches with nausea and vomiting since the early teens. She formerly had blurred vision and dazzling lights every two to four weeks. Between attacks she had gastric distress after eating, with some sour stomach. Then five years ago pain 1 to 1½ hours p.c. developed,

TABLE XXXI

DURATION OF RELIEF DETERMINED
BY FOLLOW-UP

	Food Allergy 50 Cases		Pollen Allergy 20 Cases	
½-1 year	8			
1-3 years	8		3	
3-5 years	9 ⎫	Good results in 34 cases	5 ⎫	Good results in 17 cases
5-10 years	15 ⎬	for 3 to over	8 ⎬	for 3 years to over
10 years (over)	10 ⎭	10 years	4 ⎭	10 years

Previous treatment:

By derma- tologists	27	8
By physicians	14	6
X-ray	14	7
Corticoids	15	4

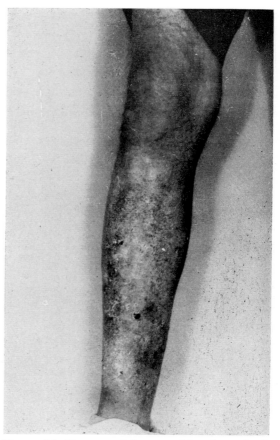

Figure 21. Eczema of legs resulting from foods determined with our CFE diet.

and dark blood was passed. A duodenal ulcer was found by x-ray. A milk diet was given with only partial relief.

Diet history revealed that she liked milk. Eggs caused burning one hour p.c. and nausea. Citrus fruits had soured her stomach for ten years.

Family history revealed that an uncle had asthma. A sister had sick headaches, and her mother had migraine.

Initial diet history: Milk, bananas, fresh apricots, and strawberries flared the eczema and caused migraine, sick headaches, and gastric distress. She recently had developed allergic gingivitis from fresh fruit.

Treatment and Results: Because of perennial hand eczema, recurrent sick headaches and indigestion, and the history of indigestion from citrus and other fresh fruits, our cereal-free elimination diet minus citrus and other fresh fruits was ordered in October of 1938. The headache and in-

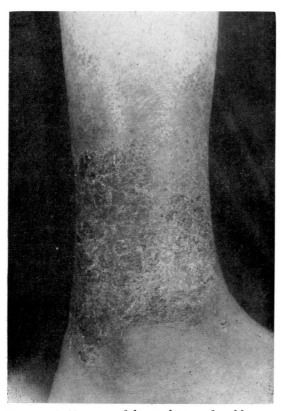

Figure 20. Eczema of lower legs and ankles resulting from food allergy.

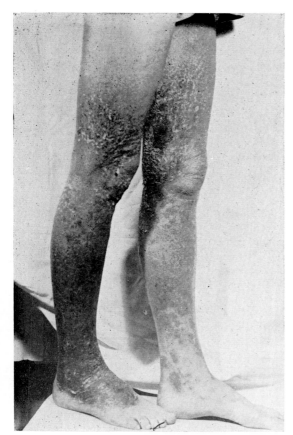

Figure 22. Eczema of the legs resulting from milk, cereal grains, and chocolate.

ECZEMA RESULTING FROM FOOD ALLERGY IN OLD AGE

Atopic dermatitis resulting from food allergy in old age is infrequently generalized and is limited to the face, neck, and flexures, as in children and adolescents. However, eczema on limited or extended areas of skin, especially on the torso and extremities, that persists or recurs perennially requires the study of possible food allergy. Such study is especially indicated if it is exaggerated in the winter and at times in late fall or early spring. Itching without definite dermatitis over limited or even the entire skin may occur from food allergy. Severe itching associated with varying degrees of dermatitis and usually excoriations on the legs and thighs is frequent in old age. Such dermatitis always requires study

digestion were absent for two months.

Though eczema of the hands decreased, moderate persistence was first attributed to working in an ammunition factory during the war. In February the eczema flared from bananas. Then with elimination of all fruit and spices, the eczema disappeared. In the thirty years since then eczema, headache, and indigestion have required the elimination of milk, veal, pork, and wheat to control headaches and eczema and entire elimination of all fruits, spices and flavors, tomatoes, and (of definite interest) peas.

Of importance is the control of these manifestations for twelve years before corticosteroids and in the twenty years since then, and this is one of the first cases which indicated the importance of our fruit-free and cereal-free elimination diet first published in the early forties.

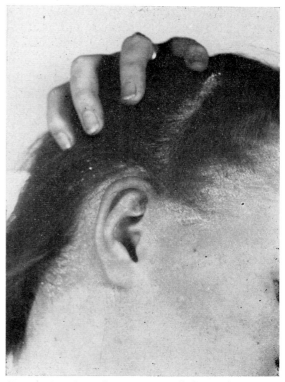

Figure 23. *Case 83:* Eczema of the scalp resulting from milk, eggs, and cereal grains.

of food allergy especially to wheat and cereal grains as well as to other foods. Relief develops in two to three weeks from such diet trial with strict adherence to the diet for one to two months, after which provocation tests with additional foods reveal the causative allergens when food allergy is the cause. Wynn, in 1927, reported senile pruritus and eczema especially from wheat and to other common allergenic foods. Such atopic eczema on the legs in an old man resulting from wheat and less so to other cereals is shown in Figure 22.

Diagnosis and treatment of eczema of other areas are discussed as follows: vulva and perineal tissues (Chapt. 21), in the ears (Chapt. 13), and in the eyelids (Chapt. 20).

ECZEMA OF SCALP

Eczema of the scalp after beginning with or preceded by cradle cap in infancy also continues through childhood and adolescence and may be exaggerated, reactivated, or occasionally develop for the first time in adult life. Though it may be confined to the scalp, other areas of the skin, especially the flexures, extremities, and upper back, may be involved.

When the eczema is perennial but exaggerated in the fall to late spring, especially in the winter, food allergy requires careful, adequate study with our CFE diet.

We have never encountered eczema limited to the scalp resulting from pollen allergy and thus improved or better in the winter. Eczema on the scalp from contact allergy to hatbands or fabrics is localized to contacted areas. Allergy to plastic sprays, dyes, medications, or "hair tonics" applied to the scalp including lotions and ointments containing mercury sulfonamides and other drugs or chemicals must be suspect and must be discontinued. In egg-sensitive patients, egg shampoos often cause dermatitis and edema associated with oozing and itching. It must be remembered that if a shampoo contains egg but less than 2 percent egg, federal regulations do not *allow* the mention of egg on the label.

Case 83: A woman fifty-two years of age had lifelong scaling, crusting, and thickening of the scalp, with constant itching. Former physicians had not inquired about seasonal occurrence. However, our questioning indicated exaggeration in the winter, which required consideration of food allergy (Chapt. 1). No other area of the skin was involved.

Favoring allergy to foods was the winter exaggeration and lifelong blocking of the nose with much postnasal mucoid discharge, frontal and sinal headaches, and former recurrent "head colds" without fever. Frequent depression, which often results in such food-sensitive patients, was present.

Diet history revealed no suspicion of food disagreements or dislikes. She gave one and two plus reactions to grass, fall, and tree pollens.

To study food allergy our FFCFE diet was ordered along with 12 mg of triamcinolone orally with its gradual elimination in two weeks.

In seven days there was "remarkable improvement." In four months she was entirely free of her scalp eczema. When pear and peach were added daily, moderate eczema recurred but was relieved in ten days with exclusion of fruits.

DIAGNOSIS AND TREATMENT OF FOOD ALLERGY

As already discussed, food allergy requires study as the sole cause, or associated with inhalant and drug allergies, of atopic eczema when it is perennial in occurrence and when it is recurrently exaggerated in the fall to early spring, especially in the winter. Its decrease or even its disappearance in the summer indicates food allergy. Though scratch testing with all ingested foods and important inhalants is routine in our practice, as advised in Chapter 2, allergenic foods causing the dermatitis infrequently are revealed thereby. The large reactions to foods producing immediate allergy especially in infancy and early childhood are important, although (as re-iterated in this volume) the clinical importance of all positive reactions has to be determined by provocation tests with the reacting foods in the symptom-free or definitely relieved patient. Thus the immediate use of our CFE diet rather than test-negative diets is nearly always advisable in office as well as in hospital patients for the study of possible food allergy. Directions for the ordering, preparation, modifications, and manipulation of the diet are detailed in Chapter 3. The accurate, strict, sufficient use of the gradually evolved diet must be emphasized.

Since it takes two or usually more weeks for previously eaten foods to leave the body and a longer period of time for the tissue changes especially from longstanding food allergy to disappear after the causative foods are excluded from the diet, initial relief from the itching, oozing, crusting, and thickening in the eczematous skin with medications is important. Corticosteroids available in the last twenty years give the greatest relief. In severe cases they can be given up to 30 to 50 mg daily by mouth, according to age. Parenteral decreasing doses of 12 to 40 mg of triamcinolone or Solu-Medrol can be administered three to even four times a day for two to three days until relief occurs. Then they can be continued by mouth up to 20 to 30 mg with rapid reduction or elimination in six to fifteen days according to the degree of resultant relief. Or if the eczema is moderate in degree, corticosteroids by mouth in initial doses of 10 to 40 mg of prednisone and lesser doses of the more active and often more effective corticosteroids suffice. If eczema is mild, relief of itching and gradual disappearance of the eruption may occur with the elimination of causative foods excluded from the elimination diet. Then rubbing into the skin of a cortico-steroid ointment such as Aristocort Cream or of Valisone® Cream, the latter being of marked efficiency in our practice, is advisable. Daily bathing with a mild soap and especially a lathering of the affected skin with pHisoHex® for six minutes if a secondary infection is present, complete removal of crusting and discharge by saline compresses, or prolonged saline baths along with antibiotics (especially Declomycin® or tetracycline by mouth) and the later rubbing in of an antibiotic ointment as of Achromycin is important. Corticosteroids parenterally and locally as advised above are also important.

KAPOSI'S ERUPTION RESULTING FROM VACCINIA VIRUS COMPLICAT-ING ALLERGIC DERMATITIS

Of great importance is the recognition of the varicelliform eruption of Kaposi resulting from vaccinia virus complicating atopic eczema, as emphasized by Fries *et al.* in 1948. Today the seriousness and former fatalities can be decreased or prevented by large doses of penicillin and of large and decreasing doses of corticosteroids as improvement occurs. The immediate control of probable food and/or inhalant allergy, the latter at first with strict environmental control is necessary.

Hence, vaccination for smallpox must not be done until all lesions of atopic eczema are absent.

The importance of controlling atopic dermatitis by determining and controlling the atopic causes, namely food, inhalant, and drug allergies, and recognizing and controlling contact allergy with or without atopic allergy rather than with the use of corticosteroid therapy alone must be emphasized. Dermatologists, allergists, and all other physicians must realize that control of atopic dermatitis, as we have reported for over thirty years, is the physicians' responsibility. Surrendering to the use of long-term corticosteroid therapy with its well-recognized resultant detrimental complications is contraindicated. The reader is referred to our discussion of corticosteroid therapy in Chapter 30.

If the eczema is severe, with oozing and crusting, warm salt or soda baths to remove serous discharge and crusting followed by lathering of the skin for five to seven minutes daily after the bath with pHisoHex to reduce secondary infection are indicated. Local compresses of solutions of 1:40 Burow's Solution two to three times a day on localized eczema are of help. Adrenalin 1:1000 0.4 to 0.4 cc according to age hypodermically every three hours for itching is justifiable.

When food allergy is the sole cause, the discomfort and lesions of the eczema decrease in three to seven days as allergenic foods leave the body with the use of our CFE diet and from antiallergic effect of the corticosteroids. The diet must be continued as advised in Chapter 3, and corticosteroids can be reduced to a minimum or eliminated in one to four weeks. As the patient and physician are assured that the diet has controlled the eczema for at least two months, other foods are gradually added, eliminating any which reactivates the eczema. It must always be remembered that foods tolerated in the summer may reactivate the eczema in the late fall and winter and requires the resumption of the initial CFE diet. The use of Urbach's propeptans to desensitize against foods causing eczema has been futile in our hands in the same way that urinary protein therapy advised in the 1930's was futile. In spite of this, propeptan therapy still is being heralded for relief of manifestations of food allergy, causing unwarranted expense and disappointment to the patient.

ANIMAL EMANATIONS AND MISCELLANEOUS INHALANTS

Allergic dermatitis resulting from animal emanations must be suspected if evidence is obtained from a careful environmental history and from positive scratch reactions to emanations of animals in the patient's environment. Such allergy of course requires study in patients who are around animals in homes, on farms, in recreation, in research laboratories, and in veterinary work. One patient had generalized dermatitis from the emanation of dogs. His allergy required the removal of all carpets in a recently purchased home in which dogs had been present. Another patient's dermatitis was due to emanations of a parakeet which had flown in the house for ten years. On the contrary, dermatitis attributed to emanations in a veterinarian had not been helped by desensitization to animal emanations but were entirely relieved when previously unrecognized food allergy was gradually controlled with our CFE diet.

Statistics on thirty cases of eczema resulting from inhalants and especially pollens, published in 1938, are to be found in Table XXXII.

Before synthetic fabrics largely replaced silk textiles, dermatitis, asthma, and at times other manifestations of clinical allergy resulted from the wearing and even the inhalation of its allergens. Larger scratch reactions usually occurred. Its disuse and at times desensitization beginning with extremely dilute silk antigens were important.

As in bronchial asthma, allergy to house dust plays a minor role in allergic dermatitis, and in our experience has never been a sole cause. When suspected, environmental control is important. When allergy to animal emanations is a definite factor, their presence as well as that of other environmental allergens and of possible unknown allergens must be considered. Strict environmental control is necessary. Possibly because of minimal dampness, moisture, and humidity in the western states, our experience evidences little or no allergy to spores of fungi as a sole cause of allergic dermatitis and even as a secondary factor.

POLLEN DERMATITIS

Pollen dermatitis usually starts on exposed skin areas during the pollen season. It decreases or disappears when causative pollens are out of the air and helped by ocean voyages or moving to high altitudes or districts where the specific pollens are absent. During succeeding years lesions increase in degree and extent, especially on exposed skin areas. At the height of the pollen season an involvement of the chest, abdomen, and back also may arise. Finally, all the skin may be involved, though the dermatitis is always worse on the face, neck, upper back, chest, and extremities. In chronic, very sensitive cases the entire skin may be the site of scaling, erythema, induration, thickening, and lichenification, which may be associated with exudation and with crusting in certain areas. Such pollinosis is not always associated with nasobronchial manifestations.

Diagnosis depends on history, especially activation in pollen seasons and scratch tests. Intradermal testing has activated the eczema in many patients and no longer is done.

Treatment with pollen allergens to which clinical sensitization exists is important. The preparation of antigens and choice of pollens have already been discussed in Chapters 4 and 12. When patients give slight or negative reactions and have symptoms throughout the summer and fall, treatment with antigens containing all important tree, grass, and fall pollens present in the air of the patient's environment must

be given. Pollens of cultivated flowers need definite consideration, especially if gardens are near the home or if the patient unavoidably contacts such flowers indoors. One patient had swelling and dermatitis of face and neck where pollen came through the open pattern of her dress from plum blossom pollens.

Pollen therapy needs to be specific. Good results denote proper antigens. If freedom from symptoms without therapy is desired, continuous administration of maximum tolerated doses at times for several years is necessary, for it is as necessary to gradually give as much pollen therapy to control dermatitis as is required for the satisfactory control of hay fever. In California there are many patients with severe localized and more generalized dermatitis resulting from inhalation of pollens. Treatment with pol-

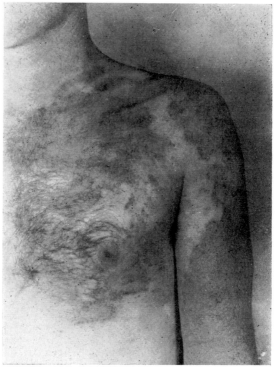

Figure 24. Allergic dermatitis resulting from multiple pollen allergy.

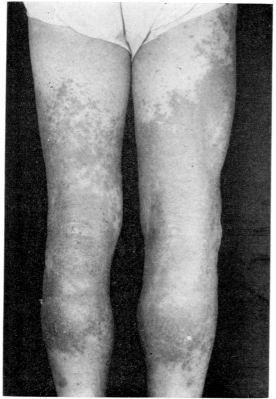

Figure 25. Allergic dermatitis resulting from multiple pollen allergy.

len antigens has been productive of many good results. Ramirez and Eller (1930) and Sulzberger reported good control of dermatitis on face, neck, and hands with injections of pollens to which skin reactions occurred. Contact dermatitis from pollen or leaf oils may arise as a primary or secondary problem as discussed on page 289.

STATISTICS INDICATING INHALANT ALLERGY IN ALLERGIC DERMATITIS

The statistics on thirty cases of allergic dermatitis in which inhalant allergy played a major role are reprinted from *Clinical Allergy,* published in 1937. Of great importance is the occurrence of good results with desensitization to pollens and environmental control up to 1937, twelve years before corticosteroids were available.

The ages varied from sixteen to sixty-two years, with an average of thirty-nine years. Several mild cases have been studied in young children and adolescents. Their data are not included in Table XXXII, since the problem usually becomes severe and chronic after puberty. The face, neck, arms, thighs, and legs are most frequently involved. Frequently the dermatosis originated on the neck, especially on the eyelids, and at times only involved the scalp, face, and neck in months or even in years. In many patients the entire skin and scalp were involved in varying degrees. The family history of allergy obtainable was not striking. That of other allergic manifestations in the patient was more definite, though nine patients apparently had no other clinical allergy. Though 30 percent of these patients reacted to foods, few gave many definite reactions, and in only a few

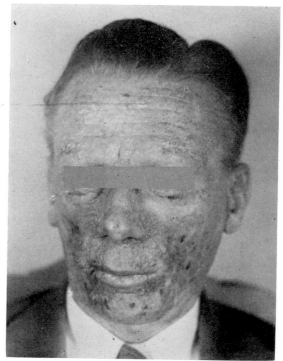

Figure 26. Seasonal facial eczema resulting from pollen allergy.

TABLE XXXII
STATISTICAL STUDY OF 30 CASES OF ALLERGIC DERMATITIS RESULTING FROM INHALANT ALLERGENS, ESPECIALLY POLLENS

Case No.	1	2	3	4	5	6	7	8	9	10	11	12	13	14	15	16	17	18	19	20	21	22	23	24	25	26	27	28	29	30	Total No.	%
Male	+		+		+	+	+	+	+		+		+	+		+	+			+				+			+				16	53
Female		+		+						+		+			+			+	+		+	+	+		+	+		+	+	+	14	47
Age	30	56	39	25	51	60	30	23	25	20	40	27	46	54	39	21	64	16	17	44	47	62	35	27	30	35	57	39	18	26	Av. age 39 yrs	
Duration of dermatitis	1	⅔	23	25	1	10	10	6	5	2	6	2	2	8	3	7	60	15	2	3	1	8	17	14	10	20	8	4	5	4	Av. dur. 11 yrs	
Exaggeration:																																
Spring	+		+	+	+				+				+	+	+	+	+			+		+	+	+	+	?		+		+		
Summer	+		+	+	+				+					+	+	+				+		+	+	+	+		+	+	+	+		
Fall	+								+					+	+				+	+	+	+	+	+	+	?	+	+		+		
Winter																																
Areas involved:																																
Scalp	+		+	+	+	+	+	+	+	+				+	+	+			+	+		+	+	+	+	+		+	+	+	18	60
Face	+	+	+	+	+	+	+	+	+	+	+	+	+	+	+	+	+	+	+	+	+	+	+	+	+	+	+	+	+	+	28	93
Neck	+	+	+	+	+	+	+	+	+	+	+	+	+	+	+	+	+	+	+	+	+	+	+	+	+	+	+	+	+	+	28	93
Hands	+	+	+	+	+	+	+	+	+		+		+	+	+	+	+	+	+	+				+	+	+	+	+	+		24	80
Arms	+	+	+	+	+		+	+	+					+	+	+			+					+	+	+		+	+		23	77
Back	+	+	+	+	+			+	+					+	+	+			+					+				+	+		13	43
Chest	+	+	+	+	+			+	+					+	+	+			+					+	+			+	+	+	15	50
Abdomen	+	+	+					+						+		+								+	+						8	27
Thighs	+	+	+	+	+	+		+	+	+	+	+	+	+	+	+	+	+	+	+	+	+	+	+	+	+	+	+	+	+	18	60
Legs	+	+	+	+	+	+			+					+	+	+	+	+	+	+	+	+	+	+	+	+	+	+	+	+	19	63
Family history:																																
Hay fever	+		+	+					+	+	+			+															+		6	20
Asthma			+	+	+		+		+																						8	27
Skin allergy	+		+		+		+	+								+	+	+						+	+	+					8	27
Gastrointestinal allergy											+																				1	3
Migraine						+																		+	+			+	+	+	4	13
Allergy in patient:																																
Hay fever	+		+	+			+		+	+		+	+			+	+	+	+	+			+					+	+	+	12	40
Asthma			+				+								+								+				+	+			9	30
Urticaria					+		+	+		+		+											+	+	+	+	+				9	30
Gastrointestinal allergy										+																					3	10
Migraine						+																									4	13
Skin reactions:																																
Foods (scratch)	1+	1+	1+						3+				1+	2+	2+	2+	1+	1+ 2+				2+			1+						9	30

TABLE XXXII (Cont'd)

Case No.	1	2	3	4	5	6	7	8	9	10	11	12	13	14	15	16	17	18	19	20	21	22	23	24	25	26	27	28	29	30	Total No.	%
Scratch and intradermal:																																
Pollens: Trees	4+						1+	1+	2+	2+		2+			4+	4+	2+	1+					1+	1+	1+			3+	1+		15	50
Grass	4+		1+	1+			2+	1+	2+	4+		3+	1+	1+	1+	2+	4+	4+			1+	1+	1+	1+	3+			3+	3+		21	70
Weeds	4+		1+	4+			2+	2+	3+	3+		1+	5+	3+	1+	5+	5+	3+			2+	2+		4+	5+			2+			19	63
Flowers	4+			2+			2+	1+	2+	2+		1+	2+		2+	4+	4+	2+						2+	3+	1+		1+	2+		16	53
Animal emanations	1+		1+	1+			1+	1+	1+	2+		1+			1+	3+	4+	1+	1+					2+	1+	1+		1+	2+		15	50
Silk				1+			3+										3+								5+			8+			4	13
Cottonseed			1+	1+			1+		2+				1+		1+	1+	3+								5+						7	23
Kapok				1+			1+	2+								4+	4+														5	17
Flaxseed				1+			1+		2+							3+	3+														4	13
Pyrethrum	1+						1+		1+	1+					3+	3+								1+							7	23
Glue								7+																							1	3
Orris				1+			1+	1+	1+	1+						1+	1+														7	23
House dust			1+	1+					1+						1+	2+	2+	1+						1+	1+		1+				9	30
Childhood eczema			+	+											+	+	+	+						+	+				+		7	23
Treatment:																																
Diet	+		+	+		+	+	+	+	+	+	+	+	+	+	+	+	+	+	+		+	+	+	+	+	+	+			11	37
Pollen		+	+	+	+	+	+	+	+	+	+	+	+	+	+	+	+	+	+	+	+	+	+	+	+	+	+	+	+	+	30	100
A.E.*			+	+		+	+	+									+							+	+	+		+	+		9	30
Miscellaneous			+			+	+	+								+								+	+	+			+		7	23
Dust				+			+	+															1								2	7
Environmental control		+	+	+	+	+	+	+	+	+					+	+	+	+							+			+	+		12	40
Duration of therapy	3	⅓	⅔	1½	1	½	⅔	1	3	3	1	2	3	1	4	2	2	1	1	1	1	3	1	2	1½	1½	½	3½	½	1		
Results:																																
Excellent	1		1	1	1		1	1	1	1				1	1		1			1	1	1									12	40
Good		1	1	1		1	1	1	1	1	1	1	1	1	1	1		1	1				1	1	1	1	1	1	1	1	13	43
Fair																							1			1					1	3
Failure																1	1	1	1	1	1										4	13
Coöperation:																																
Good	1	1	1	1			1	1	1	1	1	1	1	1	1	1	1	1		1	1	1	1	1	1	1	1	1	1	1	27	90
Fair																1	1														2	7
Poor																			1												1	3
Effect of therapy on skin reactions:																															av. 1.6 yrs.	
No reduction																			+				+								3	10
Moderate reduction	+		+			+	+			+					+	+	+					+		+	+	+					7	23
Marked reduction	+		+	+		+	+	+	+	+		+	+	+	+		+	+		+	+			+					+		11	37

Note: Patch tests with atriplex, artemesia, amaranth, acacia, and house dust oils were done on 18 patients. Positive results occurred in 5. In 3 cases excellent results arose from pollen desensitization. In 2 cases such therapy failed. No therapeutic oil was given.

* Animal emanations.

Published in Rowe, Albert H.: *Clinical Allergy.* Philadelphia, Lea and Febiger, 1938.

was food allergy found to be a definite factor, though its consideration always is necessary. Inhalant pollen therapy was of dominant influence in twenty-seven of the thirty cases. Glue, along with pollen and other inhalants, was of great importance in Case 8, and silk was a great factor in Cases 7, 26, and 29. Along with pollen allergy, camomile sensitization was especially important in Case 22 and a less definite factor in Case 20. A former article (1934) reported the frequency of positive patch scratch tests with camomile, though it seems of minor significance in the etiology of most cases of allergic dermatitis. In eight cases inhalant pollen allergy was of fundamental importance, even though skin tests were negative. In most cases etiologic pollen allergy was indicated by a history of seasonal exaggeration. In others, however, no seasonal variation existed, and pollen hyposensitization alone or with other specific therapy produced good or excellent results even in cases of dermatitis of years' duration. Of the eight patients with negative reactions, four received excellent and three good results from adequate pollen desensitization alone, except for additional animal emanation and miscellaneous desensitization in one case. Such patients who were benefited by pollen therapy did not necessarily show a history of exaggeration during the pollen seasons and often had a persistent or a recurrent perennial dermatitis. Dietary, hyposensitization therapy and environmental control were used as indications arose, but of all the measures prolonged adequate dosage of specific pollen allergens was adjudged most frequently important in obtaining the good and excellent results. Failure occurred in Case 18, who gave fair cooperation; in Case 19, whose cooperation was poor; and in Cases 21 and 23, who gave good cooperation but who probably had contact dermatitis arising from undiscovered contactants. The average length of therapy was 1.6 years. This did not indicate the ultimate amount of therapy each patient received. Even though well controlled, pollen therapy and in some patients hyposensitization to other inhalants and possibly to fungi or bacteria was considered a possibility.

Patch testing in nineteen patients was done with several local pollen or leaf oils; with flowers, leaves, pollens, cosmetics, dentifrices, foods, fabrics, and so on; and at times with routine groups advised by Sulzberger. Positive results occurred in five patients. In three of them hyposensitization with pollen extracts was successful without the use of specific oil desensitization. It may well be that some positive patch tests were nonspecific in nature.

On the basis of these results our optimistic attitude toward the control of dermatitis resulting from inhalant allergy developed in 1937 and has continued to be justified in the thirty years since then.

ADDITIONAL COMMENTS ON TREATMENT

The best results in allergic dermatitis have been in patients sensitive to pollens who have received prolonged desensitization with causative pollens over a period of more than one to two years, even up to twenty years.

Continued administration of large doses of the 1:50 or 1:100 dilution of pollen antigen every one to two weeks for several years, even for eight or more years, until evidence of dermatitis has been absent for two to five years is important. In the last twenty years the additional use of corticoids as advised in this chapter has been justifiable, providing specific desensitization to inhalants with or without strict control of existent food allergy is assured.

Some patients also gave positive skin

reactions to animal and miscellaneous inhalant allergens, environmental control and desensitization to which apparently contributed to the final result.

Case 84: One boy eight years of age had a generalized dermatitis always worse at night. Testing showed a slight reaction to kapok. Removal of his kapok mattress and desensitization with a kapok antigen cleared his eczema in about four months. His dermatitis originally was also dependent on a subordinate food sensitization not associated with skin reactions and controlled by our elimination diet.

Dermatitis resulting primarily from animal emanations, silk, and other miscellaneous sensitizations needs most careful environmental control if desensitization is to be successful. Many of these patients give large skin reactions and demand small doses of 1:5 million or even a more dilute antigen to prevent exaggeration of dermatitis at the start of therapy, with subsequent increase in doses into the 1:500 or if possible the 1:50 dilutions can be tolerated. Possible further sources of allergenic reactivity in the room even after most careful environmental control has been established must be considered. Certain patients are so sensitive to cottonseed or flaxseed that cotton or linen sheets cause difficulty. Ramirez and Eller (1930) recorded dermatitis on neck, chest, arms, legs, and abdomen of two years' duration because of rayon, to which a strong reaction was present.

The possibility of airborne allergens from silk, wool, or cotton clothing and from perfumes, cosmetics, hair lotions, or dyes used by friends, relatives, or nursery attendants of children must be thought of. Contact dermatitis of a severe or mild degree occasionally may exist along with allergic dermatitis. Thus local epidermal sensitization to special soaps, floor or furniture waxes or polishes, lacquers, varnishes, dentifrices, cosmetics, and any of the many substances discussed as causative of contact dermatitis in Chapter 30 must receive attention in obstinate problems. When dust and pollen filters supply air to rooms in which ideal environmental control is attempted, it is still possible that an allergenic or skin irritating substance might permeate through the filter into the patient's room. Urbach (1933) emphasized the frequency of animal emanations and other environmental allergens in the etiology of dermatitis and reported good results from remaining in allergen-free rooms in the home. Clues as to etiology were thereby obtained.

Wise and Sulzberger (1934) and Sulzberger and Goodman (1936) stated that hyposensitization in allergic dermatitis is not successful except in oil-sensitive individuals. Our experience, however, has justified an optimistic attitude toward the eventual control of marked cases of this type who may be sensitive to animal emanations, dust, many pollens, and even fungus allergens and often to foods providing a) unquestioning cooperation of the patient over a period of months or several years, if necessary, is obtained and b) gradual desensitization with antigens containing all specific allergens is given up to large tolerated doses and repeated until skin reactions are definitely reduced and relief occurs hopefully without corticoids. Environmental protection must be adequately executed, and causative food, drug and possibly fungoid or bacterial allergens controlled by measures discussed especially in Chapter 8.

When skin reactions are negative to inhalant allergens which are likely causes, desensitization with all such allergens and closely related ones over long periods of time, especially if improvement occurs, is as necessary as if positive tests had occurred.

Most of the unsatisfactory results in this

type of dermatosis, as in chronic bronchial asthma, are due to failure to recognize these requirements and to obtain cooperation of the patient over a period of years if necessary. Of great importance is the control of the problem by students of allergy who appreciate the difficulties, the persistency of allergenic effects, the resultant cellular and tissue changes, the necessity of an untiring attack on the dermatitis with therapeutic procedures already outlined, and the understanding cooperation of the patient. Reported failure from the use of the above measures indicates lack of use and persistence in the therapeutic procedures which have been outlined above and failure of strict adherence to an indicated elimination diet if necessary.

The foregoing discussion of the cases and statistics in Table XXXII are of special interest because of the reported results and could be used in all cases to hasten initial relief as advised in this chapter, concomitantly with the important study and control of the causative atopic and contact allergy. The importance of pollen and other inhalant allergy in cases similar to these in this series and the challenge of the control of specific allergies by environmental control and proper and continued desensitization to causative inhalants with the help of initial corticosteroids and their gradual reduction and elimination is today's challenge. That this is usually possible is stressed by the good results obtained in most of these patients fifteen to twenty years ago before corticosteroids were obtainable.

Allergic dermatitis resulting from pollen allergy may be erroneously diagnosed as "solar dermatitis" especially by dermatologists, as we have found in one case in particular.

STATISTICS ON 105 CASES OF ATOPIC DERMATITIS (ECZEMA) IN ADOLESCENTS AND ADULTS RELIEVED BY CONTROL OF FOOD AND/OR INHALANT ALLERGY, ESPECIALLY POLLEN

Statistics on 105 cases of atopic eczema in adolescents and adults resulting from allergy to foods and to a lesser degree to inhalants, especially to pollens, studied and relieved during the last fifteen years are summarized in Table XXXII. In contrast to the prevalence of boys in eczema in children, shown in Table XXXII, women dominated in this series of adults. Their ages when first seen averaged forty-eight years, varying from sixteen to seventy-nine years. The former duration of the eczema had been twelve years, varying from one to forty-three years. The exaggeration in the fall and winter in 38 percent as in the patient in Figure 20 emphasized food allergy in contrast to an increase in the eczema in the spring to late fall which emphasizes pollen allergy as discussed later in this chapter. The atopic dermatitis in the scalp, face, eyes, ears, neck, axillae, arms, cubital areas, forearms, hands, chest, abdomen, genitals and thighs, popliteal areas, legs, ankles and feet, and anus with generalization of eczema in 27 percent shows that all cutaneous areas are susceptible. Face, neck, arms, forearms, hands, popliteal areas, and legs were most frequently involved. Pruritus ani resulting from allergy is discussed in Chapter 5.

There was a personal history of asthma, perennial nasal allergy, hay fever, or headaches in only 3 to 4 percent, evidencing the skin as the major shock organ of allergy in these patients. Atopic allergy was indicated in 14 percent of the family histories. Relief depended on recognition and control of food allergy in 57 percent of the 105 patients and of pollen allergy in 55 percent.

TABLE XXXIII

STATISTICS ON 105 CASES OF ATOPIC
DERMATITIS (ECZEMA) IN ADOLESCENTS
AND ADULTS RELIEVED BY CONTROL OF
FOOD AND/OR INHALANT, ESPECIALLY
POLLEN ALLERGY

Total: 105 Cases

Age (years):	48 years average (16-79 range)
Sex: Male	41%
Female	59%
Duration:	12 years average (½ to 43 years)

	Number	%
Winter	19	18
Generalized	20	19
Scalp	9	9
Face	45	43
Eyes	21	20
Ears	12	10
Neck	47	43
Axilla	8	8
Cubital	23	22
Forearm	40	38
Arms	0	0
Hands	46	42
Chest	2	5
Back	16	16
Abdomen	6	6
Genitals (including pruritus ani)	4	4
Thighs	15	14
Popliteal	22	21
Legs	23	22
Ankles	11	10
Feet	14	13
Anus	10	9
Personal History		
Asthma	4	4
Hay fever	3	3
Headache	3	3
Migraine	0	0
Nasal allergy	15	14
Family History	15	14
Tests		
Food		
Animal emanations		
Pollen	33	31
Drugs		
Causes		
Foods	59	57
Pollens	56	55
Pollen oil contact	0	0
Vegetation contact	12	11
Foods alone	42	40
Pollen alone	36	34

Food allergy was the sole cause in 40 percent and pollen allergy the sole cause in 34 percent. Other inhalant allergens in the patient's environment were of minimal influence, though environmental control in the home to control such inhalant allergens was routine.

GRAIN AND OCCUPATIONAL INHALANT ALLERGENS IN ALLERGIC DERMATITIS

The inhalation of food, grain, and certain other occupational dusts apparently results in allergic dermatitis in certain patients. Large skin reactions to allergens of such substances may occur, and thorough and prolonged desensitization is warranted. In view of the marked localization of such dermatitis to the exposed skin areas, the possibility of contact dermatitis must always be considered. Patch tests, however, are frequently negative in the presence of positive skin reactions which favor the diagnosis of allergic dermatitis. As already stated, some of the allergen may reach the sensitized cell in upper layers of the cutis by way of hair follicles or sebaceous glands.

FUNGOID AND MICROBIC ALLERGENS IN ALLERGIC DERMATITIS

Dermatitis arising in sensitized cells of the cutis from allergens originating in distant foci of epidermophytosis or moniliasis or even from foci of bacterial infection is also an example of allergic dermatitis. Schwartz (1936) recently summarized evidence in the literature that fungus infection can spread through the vascular and lymphatic vessels to distant tissues of the body. Thus the allergen can also disseminate and give rise to the "id" reactions of allergy. Monilia especially even in the gastrointestinal tract may be responsible. Such allergens are more likely to produce lesions when other sensitizations, especially to drugs and particularly to arsenic, exist. In resistant dermatoses, therefore, it is necessary to consider all types of allergy in the etiology. The states of parallergy or metallergy may also enter the problem. The delayed tubercular type of skin reaction rather than the immediate wheal reaction usually occurs to antigens of such fungi or bacteria. Desensitization with trichophytin, oidiomycin and bacterial suspensions must be carefully executed, as Templeton (1934) pointed out, according to the method of pollen therapy. Kerr, Pascher, and Sulzberger (1934) confirmed their former opinion that desensitization with a combined oidiomycin-trichophytin solution was logical in persisting fungoid infections of the hands or feet, since both groups are omnipresent. Robinson and Grauer (1935) described the method of preparation of autogenous fungus extracts for the treatment of mycotic infections. A stock preparation was also used. That fungoid or bacterial infection, mild or severe in nature, may be superimposed on an allergic dermatitis from other causes is evident and was reported by White and Taub (1932), who listed a full bibliography on dermatitis resulting from fungi. Browning (1935) felt that epidermophytosis at times disappears when the allergic balance is reestablished by removal of ingestant allergens or control of other allergy. Pennington (1935) stressed the importance of desensitization with trichophytin or oidiomycin in chronic localized or disseminated eczema. In many patients the control of ingestant or inhalant allergies was also necessary for good results. Fungoid infections also may produce skin lesions which closely resemble allergic dermatitis. These possibilities complicate the problem but have to be recognized in a few individuals. Further discussion of the

fungoid allergy was given on page 89.

Andrews, Birkman, and Kelly (1934) have described a resistant pustular eruption on the palms and soles which was dependent on a focus of bacterial infection in distant tissue. MacDonald (1932) described a severe itching dermatitis apparently resulting from a chronic infected appendix. Mallory reported another instance of generalized dermatitis from a pyonephritic kidney. These and other reports emphasize the importance of foci of infection as causes of bacterial allergy in a few cases of allergic dermatitis. Dowling (1935), moreover, has reported dermatitis apparently from allergy to broken-down tissue products as formerly noted by Whitfield. Allergy to autogenous tissue products is further discussed on page 302.

PHYSICAL ALLERGY AS A CAUSE OF DERMATITIS

Dermatitis on the exposed areas of the skin may arise from hypersensitiveness to sunlight. This cause has been recognized for years. Bazin (1855) called its severe results hydroa vacciniforme and Hutchinson (1879) described a papulovesicular type, calling it summer prurigo. Light sensitization is so severe at times that the skin must be veiled when out of doors. Tolerance to light at times is increased by repeated exposures to small and increasing amounts. In addition, heat, wind, and marked changes in temperature may produce dermatitis in certain patients, suggesting that such agents activate an underlying potential allergy, as discussed on page 289. According to Bray, moreover, the literature indicated that roentgen rays or radium may produce allergic dermatoses and other manifestations of allergy. Cutaneous lesions from such allergy were recorded by Pardo-Castello (1936).

The possibility that the presence of

hematoporphyrin in the tissues is usually responsible for actinic sensitization is unlikely, as concluded by Templeton and Lunsford (1932) and others, in view of its absence in the majority of patients with this condition. Of interest is the fact that photosensitization may also arise after the use of barbituric drugs; certain photoactive chemicals such as Trypaflavine®, erythrosin, eosin, or acridine compounds.

Urticaria resulting from physical agents is discussed on page 302.

SECONDARY CAUSES OF ALLERGIC DERMATITIS

Stokes (1930, 1932, 1935) especially has considered allergy as only one of the several exciting causes of eczema. External irritants, local bacterial and parasitical infections, trauma, and nervous and mental disturbances were found to be of primary or secondary importance. The effect of organic, metabolic, or infectious disease must also be recognized. Scholtz (1933) discussed such alterations in reactivity of the skin from internal causes and not necessarily from allergy. Urbach (1932) commented on various dermatoses resulting from or associated with gout or disturbed uric acid metabolism. The states of parallergy and metallergy discussed on page 287 must be kept in mind. Stokes emphasized the nervous and mental components in the causation of eczema, urticaria, angioneurotic edema, and other cutaneous diseases through the production of neurovascular imbalance, disturbances in the sweat and sebaceous glands, and in pigmentation, hair growth, and even proper function of cutaneous nerves. The well-known effect of hysteria anxieties, depression, hallucinations, tension, and other psychotic states on the neurovascular equilibrium of the skin was stressed. Pusey thirty years ago stated

that emphasis on psychic rather than allergic causes of dermatitis was a backward step in dermatology. Of greater importance were the effects of hereditary predisposition, ichthyosis, seborrheic tendencies, primary or secondary pyogenic and mycotic infections, toxic states, and metabolic imbalance. Way (1932) has emphasized the effect of poor circulation in the legs arising from varicose veins and arteriosclerosis. That trauma, rubbing, scratching, and bacterial, fungoid, and yeast infections exaggerate skin lesions arising from allergy is obvious. White and Taub (1932) reported that such infections may predispose to the origin of food or other sensitization in the involved skin.

All of these factors undoubtedly operate in certain patients and probably explain some cases of apparent allergic dermatitis which fail to respond to prolonged therapy based on the conception of sensitization. Thus the possibilities of all these factors considered by Stokes, Becker, and other dermatologists must receive constant attention. However, the challenge of the discovery of unrecognized hidden allergic causes of the more successful desensitization and elimination of the recognized existent sources of allergy must constantly be faced. Too much emphasis on the psychic and neurotic state of the patient is unfortunate, especially for the patient. It too often justifies a static or hopeless attitude by the physician toward the patient's problem, which prevents the eventual control of his dermatitis. Mittelmann (1933) reported a case in point of pruritus since infancy in a woman thirty-six years of age. A family and personal history of allergy was present. Because of the constant itching and generalized dermatitis, she had produced excoriated lesions in the skin of the extremities and body and even the nose with needles, scissors, and finger nails for many years. A psychoneurosis had developed which failed to respond to prolonged psychotherapy because of the continued bodily discomfort. No skin reactions were obtained to any food, inhalant, or other allergens, but with the use of elimination diets, foods were found causative of the pruritus. After the relief of the pruritus, six months were required to gradually break the habit of self mutilation. Sulzberger has emphasized that neurovascular instability, scratching, and trauma intensity dermatitis but that nervousness is never the fundamental cause. He and Goodman (1936) found no definite evidence of an underlying psychoneurogenic etiology in fifty cases of atopic dermatitis. Rattner and Pusey (1932) reported another case of a man who developed a severe dermatitis soon after marriage. It was first ascribed to a neurosis associated with matrimony but was later found to be due to cosmetics and perfumes used by the wife. Pusey aptly stated that diligent search for specific causes of dermatitis will show that nervous and metabolic imbalances are rarely to blame. As the allergic status is eradicated through specific measures already discussed in this book, the secondary physical, irritant, and nervous factors have diminishing effects and finally may exert no more influence than on a normal skin.

CLIMATIC INFLUENCES ON ALLERGIC DERMATITIS

Improvement attributed to climatic changes is often due to escape from specific contact or inhalant sensitizations or possibly from ingestant allergens, the nature of which patient and physician are unaware. However, climatic disturbances undoubtedly affect dermatoses as they do other allergic manifestations, as discussed on pages 302 and 303. Light itself may act as an excitant on the sensitized skin. Kohn (1935) noted exaggeration of eczema in March and October in Berlin. Though atmospheric pressure varied little, its fall was associated with irritating winds carrying dust and pollen. Sudden declines of temperature in the autumn and rises in the spring produced cutaneous disturbances. Changes in relative humidity and the amount of light intensity and electrical potential also were considered. This indicates some possible influences of climate on dermatoses. As Wise and Sulzberger stated, however, there is no final conclusion or agreement possible from the various studies available.

DRUGS IN THE ETIOLOGY OF ALLERGIC DERMATITIS

The importance of allergy to drugs in the causation of allergic dermatitis requires constant realization, as evidenced by the enumeration of such possible dermatosis in the brochures of an increasing number of drugs of all types distributed by the many pharmaceutical manufacturers in the last thirty years. It also justifies the reprinting in the appendix of this volume a discussion of such dermatitis arising from drugs and medicaments used in the first third of this century, published in *Clinical Allergy* in 1937.

For the many dermatoses arising from most new drugs in varying degrees used by the profession in the last thirty years, reference to the brochures and information in books, especially the *Physicians' Desk Reference* must be read by the prescribing physician.

CONTACT DERMATITIS RESULTING FROM OILS AND RESINS OF POLLENS AND VEGETATIONS

Contact dermatitis resulting from oils and resins of the leaves of vegetations and of their pollens must be recognized when the eruption occurs during the spring or summer and especially in the early fall from ragweed and other fall vegetations. Patch tests with the oily extracts of vegetations which are known to cause such allergy in the patient's living area are indicated. Though some patients who give positive reactions also give large reactions to their respective or other pollens, reactions to the plant oils only may occur. The most common oils of vegetations causing such contact allergy are those of poison oak and poison ivy. Though the diagnosis of such allergy is usually made through history and not necessarily by patch tests, oils of the ambrosias (ragweed), artemesias (sage brush), Xanthium (cocklebur), chrysanthemums, other compositae, and less often those of other wild and cultivated vegetations and flowers which come in contact with the patient's skin must be suspected. Apparently on hot days the oils of vegetations evaporate into the air and may result in dermatitis without actual contact of the skin with the plants themselves. Relief from this contact dermatitis often results from the oral administration of the causative oils, starting with one to two drops of the 1:10,000 or even 1:100,000 dilution in a vegetable oil such as cottonseed or sesame, with a gradual increase in the dose up to ten drops daily and continued administration of stronger dilutions in similar drops up to the 1:1000 or even the 1:100 dilution as tolerated.

When patients react to the pollens as well as the oils of vegetation, hypodermic desensitization with the increasing doses of pollen antigen is also beneficial. Such hyposensitization is especially advisable, of course, if hay fever, asthma, or other manifestations of such pollen allergy are probable.

In the investigation of possible contact allergies, it must be remembered that allergy to ingested foods and less often to inhalants, as discussed above, and at times to medicaments taken by mouth or given parenterally may be responsible for the dermatitis rather than the suspected contactants. The recognition and control of such atopic allergy have revealed the causes and terminated disability and unemployment insurance in patients referred to us.

CONTACT ALLERGY

Atopic as well as contact allergy requires consideration in industrial dermatoses by dermatologists as well as by allergists.

The many causes of contact dermatitis as reported in our 1937 book and since then are in the Appendix.

CONTACT DERMATITIS RESULTING FROM CAUSES OTHER THAN OILS OF POLLENS AND VEGETATIONS

Since the lesions of contact dermatitis are similar to those of allergic eczema, the possibility of allergy to contactants always needs study. Cosmetics, dyes, toilet articles, drugs and medicaments, soaps, detergents, woods, varnishes, paints, polishes, waxes, and other chemicals used in the home; ingredients and chemicals in wearing apparel, bedding, and furnishings; and materials and chemicals encountered in any of the many industries, in agriculture, or in the patient's occupation and recreation may produce contact allergy. Many of these were discussed in *Clinical Allergy* in 1937 and have received extended consideration in many articles and several monographs and textbooks by various dermatologists. Methods of patch testing with a limited number of such possible allergens to determine specific causes or indications of possible contact allergy and of individual possible allergens contacted in the patient's home, recreational, and working environments, especially in many of to-day's industries, are advised in the literature.

A limited list of chemicals, dyes, and other contactants which need consideration in many patients, positive reactions to which indicate possible susceptibility to other contactants, has long been published by Sulzberger and other dermatologists.

FOOD ALLERGY IN OTHER DERMATOSES

For over forty years we have studied food allergy as a possible or associated cause in psoriasis. As we stated in our book in 1937, "marked relief of lesions characteristic of psoriasis has occurred in a few patients when other manifestations of food allergy were benefited by my elimination diets." Such benefit, however, has not been apparent in many other cases. That some psoriasis has an eczematous component resulting from allergy especially to foods, possibly to pollens or other inhalants, especially if large skin reactions to inhalants occur, is a possibility. And the marked relief from topical corticosteroids applied on covered areas of the skin and from large initial and gradually reduced doses of oral corticosteroids suggests an allergic cause. Thus the study of possible food allergy with our CFE diet along with our suggested administration of oral corticosteroids may be of benefit.

DERMATITIS HERPETIFORMIS

Sammis, in 1935, reported food and drug allergies as possible causes of dermatitis herpetiformis. Relief occurred with the elimination of specific foods determined with trial diets. Sulzberger also reported eosinophilia and indications of food allergy in some of these patients. The recent report of Fry *et al.* of marked relief in three patients from a gluten-free diet justifies

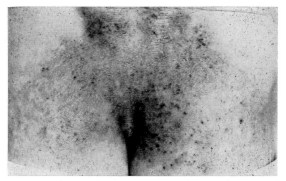

Figure 27. *Case 85:* Dermatitis herpetiformis relieved by our CFE diet and vaccine therapy.

continued study of the indicated role of food allergy. Benefit from a gluten-free diet plus sulfonamides was reported recently by Marks and Whittle in London.

During the last twenty years we have relieved a limited number of patients with definite dermatitis herpetiformis with the study and control of possible food allergy with our CFE diet along with concomitant desensitization to a vaccine containing hemolytic streptococci, staphylococci, and respiratory bacteria. In one patient 5 mg of prednisone a day was also required for relief. Previously, sulfapyridine had been given in most of these cases. One of our relieved patients received no benefit at all at a teaching hospital after conferences and studies by ten physicians, and prolonged oral sulfapyridine and other therapy were advised.

We opine at this time that bacterial allergy seems indicated by the apparent major benefit of this vaccine therapy continued at weekly intervals for two to five years in these cases. Along with the vaccine administration, there has been adherence to our CFE diet to which additional foods gradually have been added as determined by provocation tests. Marked or excellent relief, which has been so gratifying to these patients, justifies the consideration of such treatment by other physicians.

Case 85: A man forty-five years of age had had for two years a diffuse, punctate, itching, excoriated dermatitis over his legs, buttocks, lower back and moderately over the upper back and scapular and upper lateral areas.

No other clinical allergy had occurred.

Though he disliked milk, he had eaten ice cream and butter.

Drug allergy had been evident.

A dog was in the house for two months.

He smoked one package of cigarettes daily.

Physical examination was negative except for the above dermatitis. Blood, urine, Kline, and sedimentation rate tests were negative.

Scratch testing gave two plus reactions to spring and fall pollens, rabbit hair, and house dust.

Treatment and Results: Dermatitis herpetiformis was diagnosed. According to our experience, food and at times inhalant allergy need study.

Thus our cereal-free elimination diet was advised, and desensitization to a multiple antigen was ordered containing tree, spring, and fall pollens along with immunization to an antigen containing streptococci. This has continued for eight years with good relief. Aristocort 2 mg for one or two days has been necessary for increased symptoms because of slight breaks in the diet. Stopping tobacco had no apparent effect on improvement.

ACNE

In our books in 1931 and 1937, we reported food allergy as a possible cause of acne similar to acne resulting from allergy to the halogens and some other drugs, especially iodides.

Since then we have realized that the relief was due to the decrease of fats and oils from adherence to our elimination diets. Fat and oil reduction is effected by the entire elimination of milk and all of its products, the yolk of eggs, chocolate, nuts, pastries, and other fat-containing foods which are eaten in a general diet. The accumulation of fat from the blood in the sebaceous glands of the back, chest, face, and at times on the buttocks which occurs in susceptible adolescents and continues into adult years necessitates nearly complete elimination of fats and oils from the diet in order to obtain desired relief. With such a near fat-free diet suggested below, excellent control of even the most severe cases has resulted. Relief of the acne, of course, does not result in disappearance of the scars which have resulted from long-continued acne, especially of the pustular type.

Acne develops in adolescence when the appetite especially for fat-containing foods increases, when spending money is available to purchase such foods, and when milk and its products are often ingested in very large amounts. That not all adolescents do develop acne in spite of the ingestion of large amounts of fatty foods is indicative of a predisposition to acne which is often evidenced in the family history.

When secondary infection of the acneiform lesions occurs, gradually increasing doses of an autogenous vaccine, usually of staphylococci, is advised for several months. Cleansing of the affected skin by lathering with pHisoHex for five minutes two times a day and administration of tetracycline for five to seven days at indicated intervals are advisable. The strict maintenance of the fat-free diet is of paramount importance and is required not only for a few months until the acne is controlled but for a varying number of years thereafter in order to prevent recurrences from the ingestion of fats and oils even in minute amounts. The low-fat diet being advised in our practice is detailed below.

With this diet and our advised control of secondary infection, excellent results gradually evolve, as evidenced in Figure 28.

That drug and chemical allergies may produce acneiform lesions must also be remembered. Possible allergy to halogens in-

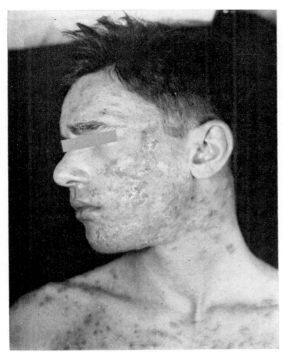
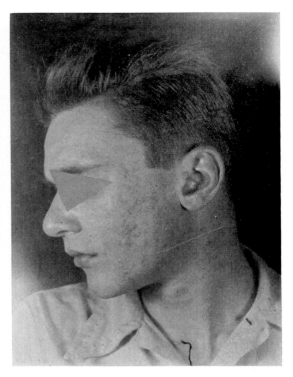

Figure 28. Relief of pustular acne from our fat-free diet and autogenous staphylococcic vaccine.

dicates the substitution of plain rather than iodized salt in food and cooking. It is important to avoid medications containing iodine or bromine, such as bromides and meprobamates, and to eliminate bromine in baking powder and food preservatives. Bromoseltzer and other bromine-containing medications sold over the counter have to be avoided. That many other medications including corticosteroids may be causative of an acneiform eruption must also be remembered.

DIRECTIONS FOR FAT-FREE AND OIL-FREE DIET

This diet excludes all oil, fat, shortening, mayonnaise, salad dressing which contains oil, drippings from the cooked meat (particularly bacon and ham), all milk, cream, butter, margarine, and yolks of eggs. This requires the elimination of all bakery products which either contain fat in the recipes

or fat in the crust or outer surfaces or which might contain grease or oil absorbed from the pans in which they are baked. The only allowed bakery products are listed below. Pie crust particularly must not be eaten. Nuts and avocado may not be used because of high fat content. All meat, fish, or food should be boiled or baked and should not be basted with oil or butter or margarine. Before eating, all fat should be cut away from such meat, fish, and fowl, and the fat in the meat itself should be entirely removed. Vitamin F is available from the small amount of fat which cannot be separated from the meat.

Ice cream and sherbet (which contains milk) and all other frozen preparations and puddings containing milk, cream, and the yolks of eggs are excluded. Bakery products which are allowed are Rye Krisp or special breads containing no fat or milk such as Hollywood Bread, Profile Bread or Sour French Bread.

Plenty of rice should be eaten without salt or sugar, or if desired, with plenty of sugar and salted to taste or possibly with fresh fruit or fruit juice. The rice can be used as a substitute for bread. White and sweet potatoes as desired can also be utilized.

Calories and adequate nourishment can be assured by eating plenty of the rice and white and sweet potatoes either boiled or baked (never fried), corn either canned or on the cob and of course without butter but with salt if desired, and corn meal or other corn products such as hominy and cane or beet sugar either for sweetening fruit drinks or eaten as cube sugar. All types of dry cereals served with sugar or fruit and its juices are allowed.

Since milk and the yolks of eggs are excluded, *adequate protein* must be obtained from meats, fish, and fowl cooked as noted above without oil or fat or from legumes such as dried peas, lima beans, or other types of beans cooked of course without bacon or any fat. For salads all type of fruits and vegetables with lemon or vinegar dressing without oil and with a moderate amount of various condiments and herbs are allowed. For dessert all types of fresh or cooked fruits may be used. Rice or tapioca pudding cooked with sugar and fruits or with the whites of eggs are permitted. A moderate amount of Angel Food cake, made of course without any milk products and only with the whites of eggs can be eaten. Candies made with cane sugar, beet sugar, or corn sugar and of course with no cream or milk or chocolate can be eaten. Chocolate in all forms is excluded.

Allowed beverages are tea, coffee (without cream) and all types of bottled, carbonated fruit drinks other than frequent Cola beverages. Homemade drinks of fruit juice with plenty of sugar or glucose made with ordinary iced tap water or iced carbonated water can be taken.

The object of this diet therefore is to eliminate all fats, oils, and all foods containing any traces thereof and also to eat enough of the allowed foods to maintain a satisfactory weight and nutrition. Synthetic multiple vitamins should be taken daily.

When definite relief of the malady for which this diet is prescribed develops, fat-free milk either in the liquid or dried preparations may be allowed through our advice.

SUMMARY

1. Atopic dermatitis (eczema) resulting from food, inhalant, and especially pollen, drug, and chemical allergies is discussed. Contact allergy from many allergenic agents including vegetations is reported.

2. Food allergy causes eczema in localized cutaneous areas usually exaggerated in the fall to late spring. At times it is associated with pollen and other inhalant allergies in its causation. The hands, face, scalp, upper and lower extremities, torso, and genitals are involved either alone or together in varying degrees. Pollen allergy may be the sole cause or associated with food allergy. Exaggeration in the spring to early fall emphasizes pollen allergy as a sole cause or associated with food allergy. Other inhalant allergies are indicated by history and skin tests.

3. Statistics on 105 cases of eczema in varying cutaneous areas resulting from foods and in 30 cases resulting from pollen allergy and less often to other inhalants are tabulated in Tables XXXII and XXXIII.

4. Evidence of bacterial and food allergy in dermatitis herpetiformis is presented along with a case report.

5. The importance of ingested fats as a cause of acne is evidenced by good results

from strict adherence to a fat-free diet. When pustular acne is present, immunization with stock or autogenous staphylococci vaccine is advised. Our fat-free diet is included in the Appendix of this volume.

6. The control of food allergy with adequate, strict use of our elimination diets and of inhalant allergy with indicated environmental control and necessary desensitization is advised. Adjunctive drug and corticosteroid therapy is important until causative allergies are controlled.

Chapter 15

Urticaria—Its Allergic Causes

Food allergy is the most frequent cause of urticaria in childhood and continues in nearly equal importance to drug and chemical allergies in adolescence and adult life, decreasing in old age. Allergy to medications increases in adolescence, and in adults it becomes of equal or even greater importance than food allergy. Though rare in children, pollen allergy produces hives in some children and increasingly in adults in many cutaneous areas during the pollen seasons. Since inhaled pollens cause urticaria, allergy to other inhalants must be kept in mind. Urticaria, moreover, does occur at times in the oral mucosa, has been observed in the esophagus, and is reported in the bronchi as a probability.

PATHOGENESIS AND CHARACTERIS- TICS OF URTICARIA

The lesions arise from allergy in the capillaries in the skin. The allergy causes vascular dilatation of the capillaries and resulting erythema which are associated with increased permeability of the capillaries and exudation of serum, giving rise to wheals. Associated with these hives, there may also be localized edemas because of increased permeability of the larger blood vessels in the lower layers in the skin, as discussed later in this chapter. Intense itching occurs, causing scratching and rubbing of the skin, which in turn result in additional hives. Vesicular hives suggesting chicken pox may occur, especially in children.

The hives usually decrease and disap-

pear in a few hours and recur often during the night usually in other areas. When severe, hives may recur for a few days, weeks, or even months until the causative allergens are eliminated. In some patients areas of erythema and localized edemas are associated with the urticaria. When urticaria is severe, small punctate or larger lesions coalesce into large edematous, erythematous, irregular areas varying from four to twelve or more inches in diameter. Hives may occur in the oral or pharyngeal mucosa or as stated above, in the airways because of the same localized vascular allergy which in our opinion is responsible for canker sores.

FOOD ALLERGY

The frequency of allergy to fruits, condiments, spices, eggs, fish, chocolate, milk, and to a lesser extent other foods makes food allergy the most frequent cause of urticaria. In childhood, allergy most often occurs from fruits after their ingestion on several occasions even in moderate amounts. In adult life hives often develop after the ingestion of large amounts of fruit, especially when uncooked. In adult life hives also may arise from fin and more often shellfish, nuts, chocolate, coffee, and to a lesser degree to other foods. Since urticaria can develop from most foods, failure of relief from the initial elimination of fruits or other suspected foods or if long-standing urticaria is present requires the study of food allergy with our FFCFE diet, which excludes the foods which cause

296

urticaria in varying degrees. If the diet does not reveal the causative allergenic foods, then the use of our minimal elimination diet as advised in our later discussion of the control of food allergy in this chapter is important. It must be remembered, moreover, that urticaria and cutaneous edemas which arise from ingested foods may also develop when their odors are inhaled. The inhaled air-borne osmyls of the foods, especially of fruit, fish, onion, garlic, and other odoriferous foods, are responsible. One man we observed had hives when he smelled vegetables of the cabbage group. Vallery-Radot (1930) reported them from the odor of crab.

MEDICAMENT ALLERGIES

The frequency of urticaria from many medicaments justifies their entire elimination in the initial study of causative allergies in chronic urticaria. As discussed below, this elimination must continue for two, three, or even more weeks until the hives disappear because of the slowness with which medicaments disappear from the body. The sole use of corticosteroids or epinephrine for the control of the symptoms of urticaria is justified because of the infrequency of allergy to these medications, as we discuss later in this chapter.

Penicillin causes more urticaria today than does other medication, superseding aspirin which was formerly the main drug to cause urticaria. Allergic reactions to penicillin develop after its previous injection or oral administration. In spite of common parenteral and oral administration to infants and young children, hives and especially severe and at times fatal anaphylaxis rarely occur in this age group. Such reactions always have to be anticipated in adults. Deaths within a few minutes after parenterally given penicillin have been reported. Though the newer penicillins are heralded as infrequent causes of allergy, reaction is always possible. Thus the use of antibiotics other than penicillin, except in infections in which it is particularly indicated, is routine in our practice. This avoidance is especially advisable in children. When it is used, an initial dose by mouth to ascertain possible allergy is advisable, though fatal anaphylaxis has been reported from small oral doses. Because of the persistence of the antibodies to penicillin in the body, chronic urticaria can continue for weeks or months. Traces of penicillin may remain for such periods.

When chronic urticaria is present in addition to the elimination of all medications and antibiotics, the entire exclusion of all milk, which often contains traces of penicillin, and of fruits and uncooked vegetables, which also may contain penicillin, is important. This elimination is accomplished with the use of our FFCFE diet as advised in our discussion of the control of food allergy. Because of the uncertain dependability of skin tests to reveal penicillin allergy and the contraindications for its use in urticaria, intradermal testing with penicillin is not advisable.

Aspirin allergy is a common cause of urticaria. Its entire elimination as such as in the dozens of medications containing aspirin which are advised for the relief of headaches, pain, fever, and body distress is mandatory. Possible allergy to other coal tar derivative drugs and chemicals used as preservatives or dyes in foods or in lotions or sprays applied to the skin or even inhaled requires consideration in hives of obscure origin. For example, one patient had hives from a chemical in one toothpaste and six years later from a chemical in a newly used deodorant.

Though the administration of animal immune serum because of diphtheria and tetanus is rarely necessary, varying degrees of serum sickness, anaphylactic shock, and occasional death, so common before immunization with toxoids of diphtheria and tetanus became routine, must be remembered. Testing for allergy to animal sera and knowledge about the manifestations of serum sickness and anaphylaxis must be kept in mind by all physicians. This knowledge is imperative because of the occasional necessity of administering immune animal sera when the physician cannot be assured that adequate immunization to diphtheria and tetanus is present and the possibilities of these diseases exist. Animal immune sera are also required in the treatment of botulism and snake poisoning. Though the diagnosis, manifestations, and treatment of serum allergy are summarized in many medical articles and the compendiums on allergy, we have found no English dissertation on this important subject of serum allergy including the diagnosis and the clinical manifestations, especially in the meninges, cerebral, ocular, spinal, radicular, and other neural tissues, comparable to that written by Ratner in 140 pages of his excellent book, *Allergy, Anaphylaxis and Immunotherapy*, published in 1943 by Williams and Wilkins.

In addition, urticaria may arise from hormones or organic extracts of pituitary, as from ACTH; extracts of ovary, thyroid, adrenal, liver, insulin, and trypsin; and extracts of pancreatic origin. Cutaneous allergy producing papules which result in necrotic lesions of the Arthus type occasionally arise to every injection of epinephrine, as we and others have reported.

As already stated, moreover, the possibility of urticaria and other cutaneous allergy from the oral or parenteral administration or injection into the body cavities of any medication requires discontinuance of all such medications until chronic urticaria is controlled. The discontinuance of toothpaste, mouthwashes, and nasal, sinal, rectal, and vaginal medications, even of vinegar douches, which have caused continued urticaria and other manifestations of allergy to fruits and condiments is important. Though all older and recently synthesized medications must be suspected, aspirin and other coal tar derivatives, quinine, and belladonna are to be remembered as of great importance.

POLLEN ALLERGY AS A CAUSE OF URTICARIA

Urticaria occurs from inhaled pollens, as Rackemann, White, Taub, and we had reported before 1938. Its occurrence to ragweed pollen also necessitates study of allergy to other fall pollens and also to tree, grass, and various cultivated flower pollens. Thus hives occurring during the pollen seasons, decreasing or absent in the winter, suggest allergy to the pollens in the air during the months when the hives occur. Though scratch tests to pollens usually are present and often are large, pollen allergy must be assumed, and specific desensitization is indicated when hives only occur or are exaggerated in the pollen seasons. Such desensitization is required even when skin tests to pollens are negative, as they are in 10 to 15 percent of pollen-sensitive patients. When skin tests to pollens are positive, if the hives occur only during the winter, pollen allergy as a cause of the hives can be excluded. Then food, drug, and other environmental allergens are the possible causes. Food and drug allergies along with pollen allergy may be responsible for perennial urticaria, which is exaggerated during the pollen seasons. Erythema at times may be associated with the urticaria, as in one patient who developed diffuse fiery erythema with initial urticaria during the grass season, causing edema and severe diffuse pain in both legs during the pollen seasons necessitating hospitalization and large doses of corticosteroids and prolonged immersion in warm water for resultant gradual relief. Desensitization to grass and tree pollens in her vicinity to which moderate scratch reactions occurred continued perennially for two years and prevented its recurrence during the three subsequent years. Then slight urticaria and erythema recurred and required resumption of desensitization for several months.

In our book in 1931 we reported urticaria on the neck, face, and hands during the summer and spring for three years in a man thirty-two years of age. Dermatologists had attributed it to solar radiation. Skin tests were positive to grass pollens, and pollen therapy for two years gave complete relief. Allergic dermatitis resulting from pollen allergy formerly attributed to solar radiation is also reported in Chapter 14.

Because pollen allergy is a cause of urticaria, allergy to other inhalants, including animal emanations; miscellaneous airborne allergens such as pyrethrum, cottonseed, flaxseed, castor bean; occupational and recreational and house dusts; perfumes; and chemicals in sprays and those inhaled in industries and other areas requires consideration as possible cause of urticaria. Though no evidence of urticaria from such causes has been recognized in our practice, its possibility must be remembered.

Definite evidence of allergy to airborne spores of fungi as a cause of urticaria has not occurred in our practice. Hives on the feet from *Tricophyton*, however, was reported by Sulzberger and Kerr in 1930 and from penicillin in a mattress by Ramirez and Eller in 1930. Remembering the frequency of hives from penicillin given by mouth and especially parenterally, hives from airborne spores of penicillin and other fungi need further consideration.

Urticaria and cutaneous edemas for many weeks exaggerated during the night were relieved when foam rubber in the bedroom which was being used to fill cushions and pillows was removed from the room. This patient also had nasobronchial allergy from petroleum fumes, especially from exhausts of automobiles which evidences his susceptibility to chemical allergy, many aspects and phases of which have been reported for many years by Randolph.

CONTACT ALLERGY AS A CAUSE OF URTICARIA

Contact allergy from animal emanations, furs, or animal hair (including goat's hair in mohair) and rabbit hair, silk, chemicals and dyes (especially formaldehyde in fabrics and other chemicals used in the finishing of cloth and fabrics) black and brown dyes, hair dyes, ingredients in perfumes, cosmetics (especially orris root which is incorporated in cosmetics less than in former years), and almond cream may produce contact urticaria. Of interest was the urticaria from almond cream in a patient who gave a four plus reaction to almond allergen as an illustration of the many possible causes. In this category is contact with pollens of grasses or flowers which produces multitudinous urticarial skin reactions in patients who give positive reactions to the pollens and who grow or are in contact with flowers in the garden. Since such allergy is usually easily recognized and avoided by the patient, it is not a common cause of chronic urticaria.

URTICARIA ARISING FROM ALLERGY TO PARASITES

Eyerman and Strauss, in 1929, and Rackemann, in 1931, incriminated malarial protein as a cause. Urticaria from hydatid cyst fluids, *Ascaris, Lumbricus, Strongy-*

loides, Oxyuris, hookworm, parasites, and especially from trichinosis have been described especially by Vallery-Radot (1930). Laboratory workers developed urticaria and other allergic manifestations from parasites during their study.

TABLE XXXIV

CHARACTERISTIC INFORMATION ABOUT URTICARIA IN 35 PATIENTS RELIEVED BY THE CONTROL OF ALLERGY TO FOODS, INHALANTS, ESPECIALLY TO POLLENS, AND MEDICAMENTS FOR 1 TO 20 YEARS (AVERAGE FOUR YEARS)

Ages	*Patients With Urticaria*
0-10 years	12%
10-20 years	16%
20-50 years	33%
50-75 years	39%
Male	51%
Female	49%
Duration of hives	in 22 cases (2-6 months) average 3 / in 13 cases (1-20 yrs) average 4
Generalized	18%
Former hives	5%
Associated swellings	34%
Eczema or dermatitis	6%
Nasal allergy	14%
Chronic bronchitis	6%
Asthma	2%
Headaches	17%
Nervousness and tension	15%
GI symptoms	10%
Years of cooperation	1-20 (average 4 yrs)
Suspected foods	34%
Skin tests:	
Foods	43% (1-2+)
Pollens	53% (1-6+)
Miscellaneous	5%
Causes:	
Foods alone	58%
Foods and pollens	16%
Pollens alone	14%
Drugs and medicaments	12%

DISCUSSION

Of interest is the moderate infrequency of urticaria in patients of an increased age, even in the group from fifty to seventy-five years. Males and females were equal in number. More patients (63%) had hives for two to six months, with an average of three months, than patients (37%) with hives from one to twenty years, with an average of four years. These long-continued hives had persisted in spite of efforts of many physicians to determine the causative allergens. Though moderate hives were diffusely generalized, marked exaggeration in 12 percent required treatment in the hospital.

Though urticaria was a major manifestation of allergy, localized swellings, especially in the eyes and face and less often in other cutaneous areas, occurred in 34 percent in comparison to the predominance of swellings over hives as indicated in Table XXXVII in Chapter 16 on angioneurotic edema.

The frequency of other past or present manifestations of clinical allergy was less frequent except for probable nasal allergy than in patients with some other manifestations of allergy as evidenced in statistics in other chapters of this volume.

Though food allergy was an assured cause in 74 percent, as determined by cooperating patients for one to twenty years for an average of four years, food allergy had been suspected by only 34 percent of the patients and never to all of the foods responsible for the clinical allergy. This emphasizes the important use of our elimination diets which exclude most foods, especially fruits, condiments, chocolate, spices, coffee, and other common allergenic foods we have found most often responsible for hives as advised in this chapter and in Chapter 3. Thus severe urticaria and localized swellings and gastrointestinal symptoms for twenty-four years occurred from even small amounts of celery, which allergy was not evidenced by scratch reaction, in one patient. Urticaria, moreover, occurred to ingested olives, which allergy was indicated by a five plus reaction to olive pollen but not by positive reactions to the allergen of the olive itself.

Though food allergy was incriminated as a major or minor cause of hives in 74 percent, positive reactions to foods occurred in only 34 percent. Many positive reactions, moreover, were present to nonallergenic foods. This evidences the fallibility of skin reactions to soluble food allergens as emphasized in Chapter 2 and throughout this volume.

Hives from medicaments (including aspirin), penicillin, iodides, quinine, and at times to other drugs is generally recognized by history and not by skin tests. Of definite interest was the severe generalized urticaria resulting from ACTH given intramuscularly first because of urticaria to fruit, the persisting urticaria being due to continued administration of ACTH every one to three days for two months.

Hives in one patient were due to allergy to protamine zinc insulin relieved by the administration of regular insulin. As stated in this chapter, allergy to crystalline zinc insulin also occurs. Hives in another patient resulted from crude liver extract given parenterally and continued for several weeks and not from other associated food allergies. This emphasizes clinical allergy to other tissue extracts, as noted on page 94.

Thus the importance of considering allergy to drugs and other medicaments as an important cause of urticaria and in other manifestations of clinical allergy must be remembered.

That allergy to drugs may be associated with food and inhalant allergy always needs consideration, as in one patient who for ten years developed hives from asparagus, artichokes, as well as to aspirin and iodides.

Inhaled chemicals, as from petroleum or paints, may cause urticaria. Chlorine and vegetations in drinking water also have been incriminated.

ALLERGY TO BITES OF INSECTS

Urticaria and other manifestations of allergy arise from sensitization to allergens injected into the skin through the bites of insects, fleas, mosquitoes, and probably lice, bedbugs, and scabies. Urticaria, cutaneous erythema, and other manifestations of allergy including anaphylaxis and sudden death from allergens of venom injected into the skin by bees, yellow jackets, and wasps are frequent. Desensitization to the allergens of insects and especially the venom of hymenoptera is usually successful and an important therapeutic measure. Though May and other lake flies cause asthma and nasal allergy through inhalation, especially of their pulverized bodies, urticaria is a rare or absent result.

HIVES FROM TRANSFUSIONS

Urticaria during or after transfusions is not infrequent. Brem *et al.* (1928) recognized allergic reactions, including hives, from food allergens in the blood and advised using fasting donors. Holder and Diefenboch (1932) used a donor who had urticaria from strawberries. For three months thereafter when the patient ate strawberries, hives occurred after which it did not occur because of the exhaustion of the passively transferred antibodies to strawberries by the transfusion. Today, fasting the donor to prevent allergy in the recipient from a transfusion is not as important as formerly, since administration of corticoids for a few days and if necessary, immediate adrenalin 1:1000 hypodermically will control the resultant allergy.

BACTERIAL ALLERGY

In 1937 we discussed bacterial allergy as an important possible cause of chronic urticaria. Since then we have found decreasing evidence of its occurrence, possibly because of the decrease in chronic infections since the advent of antibiotics, the better recognition and if necessary, surgical control of such infections, and the relative infrequency of infection in gums and around teeth. Moreover, our better control of food and pollen allergies and of the many drug and chemical allergies has in our opinion relieved much chronic urticaria in which bacterial allergy in former years would have been studied.

In spite of decreasing evidence of bacterial allergy, indications of it as a cause of chronic urticaria which we reported in 1937 are summarized. Danysz, and Barber previous to 1923 reported urticaria from infection in tonsils, gallbladder, and appendix. Cooke (1935) found hives resulting from infected sinuses. One of our patients apparently was relieved of hives by removal of a fecal fistula, another by removal of a chronically infected gallbladder, and another after tonsillectomy. Urticaria and severe angioneurotic edema associated with cutaneous and visceral manifestations of allergy also were relieved by removal of several infected teeth. Moreover, the administration of autogenous streptococci and colon bacilli in gradually increasing doses was associated with gradual relief of urticaria as reported by Emmett and Logan (1933) and Niles and Torrey (1934). Mateer (1935) reported relief in some urticaria from hypodermic administration of stock colon bacilli.

In addition, in 1937 we discussed the possible origin of urticaria from allergens in pathological tissues. Though allergy to bacteria and allergens in diseased tissues is a possible cause of urticaria, our adequate study and control of food, drug, chemical, and pollen allergies have greatly decreased the likelihood of this cause of chronic urticaria.

PHYSICAL ALLERGY

Duke, in 1924 and thereafter, reported urticaria and localized edemas from physical agents such as cold, heat, light, and injury. Such causes of urticaria has been reported especially to cold for many decades. In 1937 we commented on articles in the decade up to 1935.

Hypersensitivity to the electromagnetic radiation in the visible and ultraviolet spectral ranges is recognized as a common cause of eruptions in the skin. The mechanism is immunological in some cases of light urticaria and photocontact dermatitis. That other photosensitive eruptions are based on nonimmunological phototoxic reactions, as in porphyrin, phototoxic contact allergy, or drug reactions were also discussed by Baer and Harber in 1965. The rapid onset of light urticaria in one-half to three minutes after exposure to light causing a solid area of urticarial edema which is confined to the area exposed to light, its disappearance in one to four hours, and systemic reactions such as asthma or even collapse that may occur are reported by Baer and Harber. They also propose a classification of light urticaria according to wave lengths of light. They discuss the mechanism of photoallergic reactions to drugs such as certain sulfonamides and chlorothiazides and the nonimmunological phototoxic reactions in the skin from psoralen, various coal tar derivatives, and tetracyclines. The possible mechanism of rare localized heat urticaria also receives comment.

Cold urticaria has been studied by many investigators, as recently discussed by Rose in 1965. The familial and more frequently acquired form of edema of the skin and even of the lips and tongue from cold foods and the occurrence of an atopic predisposition in about one-third of the cases of cold urticaria are noted by Rose. Increased release of histamine in the plasma in five of ten subjects reported by Rose supports the role of histamine in cold urticaria as formerly reported by Thomas Lewis. In other cases other vasodilator substances such as acetylcholine and less frequently serotonin may be causative. Though cold urticaria can be passively transferred into a recipient's skin, the sensitizing factor is unknown.

That physical agents may be secondary activators of a basic causal allergy to foods, inhalants, drugs, or other allergenic causes needs definite consideration. This thesis is exemplified by the relief of urticaria arising from light after the control of milk allergy as reported by Hill in 1931. One of our patients was gradually relieved of dermographia by continued control of food allergy with our FFCFE diet.

Thus the possibility of atopic allergy being activated by heat, cold, light, or trauma must always be in mind. The study of possible food allergy especially with our FFCFE diet for at least six to eight weeks to determine possible decrease or disappearance of the former urticarial response to a physical agent is justifiable. Such atopic allergy may be the cause of a clinical allergy formerly attributed to a physical agent, as exemplified in the case of pollen dermatitis attributed to solar radiation by two dermatologists, as we reported on page 285.

DERMOGRAPHIA OR URTICARIA FACTITIA

Dermographia or urticaria factitia and recently termed *traumatic urticaria* is characterized by linear or irregular wheals of different sizes arising from varying degrees of pressure on the skin. Such wheals occur from stroking the skin, pressure under girdles, clothing, and belts. Moderate injury

of the skin will produce dermographia in susceptible patients. Erythema may also arise in varying degrees around the wheals in dermographia. Lehner and Rajka (1930) and Mendolsohn (1934) reported passive transfer of the whealing agent in the blood serum of patients with dermographia into skins of normal individuals. The whealing results from the rapid and normal release of histamine from the affected cells, as suggested by studies of Lewis *et al.* in 1924 and 1927. Wise and Wolf found that dermographia would not appear on stroked, heated skin but arose after applications of ice, indicating that heat dissipated the histamine released into the skin by pressure or stroking.

That this whealing reaction to pressure requires the study of longstanding uncontrolled atopic allergy as a possible cause has been emphasized in our practice for years. With the adequate and strict control of possible food allergy, especially with our FFCFE diet, the whealing response to pressure or on stroking the skin has gradually decreased and even disappeared in some cooperating patients. And when inhalant allergy is indicated, especially by history and at times by skin reactions, desensitization with multiple antigens with or without antigens containing environmental inhalants and airborne fungi has produced similar relief.

GENERALIZED PRURITUS

Itching of the skin with or without slight dermatitis or urticaria and in the absence of constitutional causes, especially new growths or hepatic, hematologic, or thyroid disease, requires the study of allergy to contactants, drugs, and especially to foods.

Pruritus, often with dry, indurated, discolored dermatitis especially of the legs in old age, as shown in Figure 22 with or without itching in other areas requires the study of food, as advised in Chapter 3. Allergy as a cause is indicated by the generalized itching, especially in guinea pigs during anaphylactic shock. Contact allergy to medications and inhalants also needs consideration. Itching and varying dermatitis from contact allergy and from its many causes as summarized in Chapter 14 requires consideration.

Dermographia occurring from pressure, rubbing, or scrubbing of the skin also requires adequate, sufficient study of atopic allergy, especially to foods, as advised in Chapter 3. Other clinical manifestations of such allergy may not be present. Attributing the cause to nervousness rather than allergy is easy for the doctor but unjustified from the patient's viewpoint. Inhalant allergy to pollens needs consideration if the dermographia occasionally is exaggerated or only occurs in the pollen seasons.

Pruritus resulting from nonreacting food allergens, especially to ingested corn, and not from allergy to skin reacting pollens occurred in the following history:

Case 86: A woman fifty-one years of age had had generalized pruritus, especially on the forearms, and diarrhea three to five times a day two to three days each week for eighteen years and nearly every day for two years. For three years scattered hives over her body had occurred. Advice from five physicians had failed. Eczema, especially in flexures, frequently had occurred from infancy to her twentieth year. Nervousness, irritability, and depression had been present. She "walked the floor at night." Her sister and father had asthma. Her diet history revealed no disagreements or dislikes for foods. Blood and urine analyses were normal. Scratch tests gave three plus reactions to grass, fall and tree pollens, and a one plus reaction to cedar, ash, birch and walnut pollens, and house dust. Reactions to foods were negative.

Because of perennial symptoms, food allergy was studied with our FFCFE diet. In two weeks itching, scattered hives, and diarrhea had disappeared. After continued relief for two more weeks, provocation feeding tests with all other foods gradually were made. When corn and later its starch and sugar were added, itching, hives and diarrhea occurred. Marshmallows covered with powdered sugar containing corn starch and containing corn glucose reproduced diarrhea. Similar symptoms have recurred after eating moderate amounts of water-packed pear, peach, and citrus fruits. Rice and oatmeal gave no symptoms. Adherence to her corn, fruit, flavor, and condiment-free diet has controlled pruritus and lessened hives and diarrhea for three years.

HISTORIES OF URTICARIA

Case 87: Urticaria resulting from food allergy.

A boy eleven years of age had had continued hives for many months with no previous history of cutaneous allergy. On four occasions he had had marked spells of urticaria lasting from two to three weeks. They especially annoyed him during school and at night. They occurred particularly on the arms, legs, and abdomen, varying in size from a pinhead to one-half inch in diameter, being irregular in shape and surrounded with an erythematous area. Mild nasal congestion exaggerated by inhalation of dust had occurred. There were no food disagreements. His appetite had always been normal. No digestive symptoms had ever been present since infancy, when colic occurred. His father had chronic indigestion and headaches. Milk caused definite gaseous unrest. With our FFCFE diet hives gradually disappeared within two weeks. Subsequently it was found that oranges and eggs produced hives. Leukopenic index studies showed a decrease in the white count of 500 after the ingestion of orange and of 450 after the ingestion of eggs. However, a fall of 400 after eating peaches and of 1400 after eating apricots occurred, and no urticaria arose from the ingestion of such foods.

Case 88: Urticaria, headaches, bronchial urticaria causing cough in patient with tuberculosis.

A man forty-six years of age had had generalized urticaria for five months. These lesions had been increasing in number and extent of distribution especially during the mid-day. For several weeks he had had undoubted urticarial lesions in the bronchial tract, causing marked coughing which had distressed him greatly because of active pulmonary tuberculosis. For two weeks a swelling had occurred on his lips, tongue, and in his larynx. His eyes had been increasingly puffy. For ten years he had had right-sided head-aches, recurring every two or three months and lasting for four or five days. There were no food dislikes or disagreements. His family history was negative for allergy. He had had pleurisy in 1919, and during the last year pulmonary tuber-culosis had developed. His scratch tests by the cutaneous method were positive to wheat, eggs, apricots, bananas, and plums. Slight reactions occurred to a few animal emanation allergens as well as to a few spring and fall pollens. During three years as a result of our elimination method of diet trial, milk alone was responsible.

Comment: This is especially interesting because of the forced feeding with milk during his treat-ment of tuberculosis in 1935 and the negative reactions to foods. It is possible that milk allergy either established itself or was intensified as a result of this overfeeding with milk. The foods which gave positive reactions have been eaten without any allergic manifestation.

This record also illustrates the production of a cough and bronchial irritation by urticarial lesions in the larynx and bronchi, which was a serious complication because of his active tuberculosis. His former migraine was another manifestation of his food sensitization.

Case 89: A boy ten years of age had had severe attacks of giant urticaria three to four times yearly for four years. They developed in one to two hours after the ingestion of any fruits, including vitamin C as such; fish, particularly when fried in peanut oil; and after insect bites from fleas, mosquitoes, and especially bees. The swellings gradually disappeared in three to ten days. Recent hospitalization was required for five days because of swelling in the throat which caused shortness of breath. Parenteral epinephrine, corticosteroids, and inhaled oxygen were required for relief.

There has been no seasonal variation. Neither has there been any other manifestation of allergy except for moderate headaches during the attacks of urticaria.

Drug history revealed urticaria twice from penicillin on two different occasions. There was no evident clinical allergy to pollens from trees and grasses in his area.

Family history revealed asthma in the mother.

Skin testing revealed two plus reactions to most grass, several fruit, and shade tree pollens. These reactions did not harmonize with his clini-cal allergy. Slight reactions occurred to eggs and milk. Reactions were negative to peanuts and fish. He gave a four plus reaction to bee venom.

His blood count was negative except for 7 per-cent eosinophilia.

Treatment and results: Because of his history of allergy to the citrus fruits, crab, fish, peanuts, and pork, they were eliminated entirely. In addition, the mother was instructed in the administration of 0.5 cc of adrenalin 1:1000 hypodermically if severe urticaria and particularly if swelling of the throat and larynx developed. She was in-structed to repeat the dose every twenty to thirty minutes until advice from us is obtained.

No urticaria occurred during the fall months. In late December generalized hives and swellings from "head to foot" with swelling of the left eye and lips were attributed by the mother to the odor of smoked ham. This attack justified his admittance to a hospital where our fruit-free and cereal-free elimination diet and adrenalin 1:1000, 0.5 cc hy-podermically as necessary, for relief of edema was given every three hours. In addition, Aristo-cort, 8 mg three times each day, was given for two days, eliminating it gradually in one week. Because of this severe attack of urticaria, allergy to fruit in jello and to ice cream was the suspected cause.

During the last year and a half, with the con-tinued elimination of all fruits, vitamin C, pork, peanuts, and milk, no urticaria has occurred ex-cept for severe hives in a few hours after eating two teaspoons of ice cream. In addition to the elimination of fruits, all spices, condiments and flavors have been omitted since then. No recur-rence of laryngeal edema and resultant difficult breathing has occurred since our initial study.

CONTROL OF URTICARIA

Because of the frequency of food and drug (including chemical) allergies as the cause of most urticaria, either acute, peren-nial or chronic, both of these causes require immediate study. When the urticaria is exaggerated in the pollen seasons, pollen may be the sole cause. Associated food or drug allergy also needs to be considered.

DRUG AND CHEMICAL ALLERGY

To study possible drug and chemical al-lergies, especially in adults, all drugs and chemicals must be entirely prevented from entering the body by mouth, inhalation, parenterally, or by injection into oral cavities. Patients must be told that it takes days, weeks, or even longer periods for drugs to leave the body entirely. The fact that allergy to injected penicillin, serum, or other injectants usually does not develop for seven to fourteen days, providing it has not been given by mouth or parenterally before, and the days and weeks that the urticaria continues after such injection emphasize the length of time drugs may remain in the body. Penicillin in foods, especially in milk as reported by Reisman and Arbesman in 1969 must be remembered.

To be sure that drugs and chemicals are eliminated, toothpastes, mouthwashes, body sprays, deodorants, medicated soaps, hair lotions and dyes, douches, birth control pills, contraceptives, and other medicaments including cathartics must be excluded. Only after the urticaria is absent for three to four weeks is it advisable to resume cautiously individual toilet articles and indicated medicaments, one daily for three to five days, eliminating any that reproduces urticaria.

If allergy to insulin is suspected, administration of an insulin of a different animal source or crystalline insulin as advised in current medical texts is indicated when diabetes is severe. That protamine in PZ insulin comes from the sperm of salmon must be remembered, as noted by Hughes and McAlester in 1945. If the elimination of Dilantin or other anticonvulsant drugs, digitalis, or other drugs is hazardous to the patient's health, the drug can be continued temporarily, hoping that the exclusion of all other medicaments and the control of food and indicated pollen allergy will relieve the hives. If allergy to pollens of castor beans occurs, clinical allergy to its oil given by mouth may occur, as reported by Blank in 1945. If suspicion of

these medicaments continues, other similar ones which have not been given previously may be substituted, hoping that allergy to them is not present.

FOOD ALLERGY

Food allergy, which is the most common cause of hives in young children, always requires adequate, strict, and persistent consideration by the physician in older children and adults. It must be studied in all patients with trial diet except when allergy to medications and chemicals or to pollens is the obvious cause.

Though it is generally agreed that positive skin tests to foods causing urticaria are very infrequent and that positive tests that may occur rarely indicate the foods which cause hives, scratch tests with foods ingested by the patient, especially in the days before the development of urticaria, are routine in our practice.

Because of the many false and nonspecific reactions which occur with the intradermal tests, only scratch testing is done. When a patient develops hives or other manifestations of allergy immediately after eating a food, definite positive scratch tests may occur which in part justifies routine testing. However, as in most chronic food allergy, foods causing hives for days or weeks or even months rarely give positive tests, making diet trial, especially with our FFCFE diet, of mandatory importance. And, as stressed throughout this book, especially in Chapter 3, the clinical importance of a definite scratch test must be proven by positive provocation ingestion tests with the reacting food done in the patient when he is free of urticaria for a much longer time than that of previous periods of relief.

If large scratch tests to one or more foods occur or if hives had occurred after the ingestion of foods such as eggs, shell or fin fish, or one of several fruits, the total elimination of that food for one to two weeks may relieve the urticaria without any antihistamine or corticosteroid therapy. Unfortunately such relief from the elimination of one or several such foods is infrequent, especially when persistent or chonic urticaria is the problem.

Therefore, our experience emphasizes that the role of possible food allergy in chronic urticaria is best studied with our FFCFE diet as advised in Chapter 3 except when individual foods are indicated as discussed above. This diet eliminates all fruits, condiments, spices, all shell and fin fish, all beverages, all milk, eggs, wheat, and cereal grains but allows a few cooked vegetables. Soy-potato bakery products are advised. If they are disliked or disagree, they must be omitted entirely or in part, as advised in Chapter 3. Since rice is not a common cause of hives as it is of bronchonasal allergy, allergic headaches, and eczema, rice or rice-potato bakery products may be substituted for soy products but only if soy or lima products are refused or disagree.

Since flavors and condiments are not allowed in this diet, flavored toothpastes, mouthwashes, denture fixers, and cleansers are not allowed. Teeth can be brushed with water alone or with a little baking soda or water and salt. Soda in water can be used as a mouthwash. Urticaria and other clinical allergy resulting from fruits have been activated by vaginal vinegar douches. Cigarettes are forbidden because of the allergens in tobacco and flavors or at times fruit juices mixed with the tobacco.

The frequency of allergy to fruits, flavors, and spices in causing hives does not mean that other foods known to produce other manifestations of allergy require little or no consideration. Emphasizing this were the diffuse coalescing welts on the calves and especially on the lips and face in four

hours after the ingestion of eggs in a woman forty years of age. Another woman forty-six years of age developed diffuse urticaria in four hours after ingestion of even small amounts of milk. No skin reactions had occurred in either case. Such food allergy to non-skin-reacting foods justifies the initial strict and expertise use of our FFCFE diet for the study of food allergy, since this diet not only eliminates fruits and condiments but also milk, wheat, other cereals, eggs, beverages, and other foods which most commonly cause clinical allergy.

As advised in the directions for our FFCFE diet, no trace of a food excluded from the diet is allowed. The patient is told that previously ingested foods remain in the body for one to two weeks or even a longer period of time and that a maximum degree of allergy must be assumed which would prevent relief or reproduce urticaria if traces of eliminated allergenic foods are taken even one to two times a week.

As emphasized in the directions for the preparation and maintenance of elimination diets in Chapter 3, advised weight and maintenance of nutrition are necessary.

If relief of urticaria continues for a period definitely longer than previous relief without the use of antihistamines or corticosteroids, individual foods can be added, one every three to five days, as advised in Chapter 3, eliminating any which reproduces urticaria or other associated allergy.

The good results we report in the control of urticaria usually of the chronic type have required the patient's strict, unswerving adherence to our recommendations for the study and control of drug and food allergies. It requires effort, determination, and self-control by the patient and continued direction and supervision by the concerned physician usually over a period of three or more months.

URTICARIA RESULTING FROM POLLEN

Though of lesser frequency than food and drug allergies, pollen allergy as already discussed is of definite and not infrequent importance. The history of urticaria starting in a pollen season, absent in the winter, with or without positive skin reactions to pollens or other manifestations of pollen allergy, requires the adequate and sufficient study and control of pollen allergy.

Desensitization to pollens is indicated according to our advice detailed in Chapter 14 for the control of allergic dermatitis resulting from pollen allergy and also in Chapter 4. Desensitization should be continued up to maximum tolerated doses of proper antigens until hives have been absent during two or more seasons.

As noted above, pollens may be the sole cause or associated with drug, chemical, or food allergy. Thus chronic urticaria resulting from food may continue through the year and may be definitely exaggerated during the tree, grass, or fall season or through all three seasons.

CONTROL OF URTICARIA RESULTING FROM INHALANTS OTHER THAN POLLEN

The reader is referred to our discussion of urticaria from other various inhalants. Such urticaria undoubtedly occasionally occurs. It must be suspected if scratch reactions occur to such inhalants. It is possible that we have not become aware of such allergy because of our usual advice to maintain modified dust control in the living and working environments and to sleep on Dacron or at times on foam pillows. If evidence definitely favors animal emanation or home, working, or recrea-

tional dust allergy, environmental control and desensitization with antigens containing the suspected inhalants which cannot be eliminated from the patient's environment may be advisable. But in our practice, hives from such inhalants, including airborne fungi, have not been definitely substantiated.

BACTERIAL ALLERGY

Though bacterial allergy in our practice seems an infrequent cause of urticaria, its possibility must be considered, especially if adequate study of food, drug, chemical, and pollen allergies has not revealed the allergic causes and given relief and if foci of infection are found in the patient. The study and control of possible bacteria allergy has already been discussed.

EMOTIONAL CAUSES

Psychic and emotional stress probably aggravates urticaria. There is no definite evidence, however, that they are primary causes. Their influences, when present, must be secondary in nature. As the causes of urticaria are recognized and controlled, associated nervous and psychological symptoms gradually subside. Because of possible allergy to drugs, sedatives, and tranquilizers, they are contraindicated. Adrenalin 1:1000 and corticosteroids, to which allergy very rarely occurs, given to control urticaria will relieve tension and nervousness.

INSURANCE AND LEGAL ASPECTS OF CHRONIC URTICARIA

Chronic urticaria which occurs in people who have private, union, government, or other types of insurance or are eligible for Medicare may present various challenges to the physician. Whether the urticaria develops after the injection of penicillin or after the oral or parenteral administration of other medications or from possible allergy to chemical or organic substances entering the body in some industrial, agricultural, or recreational occupation, the patient often insists that medical and at times hopsital charges and disability insurance, if available, be paid until the urticaria and other manifestations of allergy have been absent for weeks or even months.

Since such continued urticaria may not be due to the original or apparent cause and since the possibilities of drug, food, and inhalant or other possible allergies are difficult for many physicians to solve, chronic urticaria in these patients may continue for months or even years as the patient continues to go from one physician to another. This results in continued payment by insurance and welfare funds to cover medical bills and disability.

If the patient, however, is receiving disability insurance because of urticaria which he is controlling at times without the physician's knowledge with antihistamines or even corticosteroids, he intentionally may not cooperate in the strict and necessary dieting or the elimination of possible chemical causes, may even take foods or drugs or medications which are definitely responsible for his urticaria, or may expose himself to chemicals or other allergens in his working environment so that hives will continue and disability insurance will not stop. In doing so, his symptoms continue because of which he unjustifiably demands payments for medical services and disability.

On the other hand, if the patient sincerely wishes to control the cause, this can gradually be determined by the physician, who is experienced in the study of clinical allergy. Such determination of causes requires adequate study of the factors discussed in this chapter and unswerving cooperation of the patient during a two to even a six-month period.

TEMPORARY RELIEF OF URTICARIA BY MEDICATIONS

While the food, drug, chemical, pollen, or possible infectant allergies are being studied and until they are controlled as discussed and advised in this chapter, the distressing symptoms, especially the itching, burning, and swellings of the skin must be controlled by the following medications:

1. Epinephrine (adrenalin) 1:1000 hypodermically is the most important medication for the relief of marked or severe itching, erythema, cutaneous swelling and edema of urticaria, and (if present) of localized swellings of angioneurotic edema. The dose varies from 0.1 to 0.25 cc in children according to age and weight up to seventy-five pounds. For adolescents and adults the dose varies from 0.3 to 0.5 cc hypodermically. If moderate to definite relief does not occur in ten to fifteen minutes, another dose can be given. The relief should continue for one to several hours. Recurrence of urticaria and resultant distress justify repetition of the epinephrine hypodermically every one to twelve hours. The necessity of frequent doses in severe urticaria will decrease as antihistamines and especially the corticosteroids next advised counteract the allergic reaction.

Until causes of severe urticaria are recognized and controlled, patients or parents should be taught to give epinephrine 1:1000. This instruction is mandatory if the tissue swellings of urticaria and especially of angioneurotic edema may occur or have occurred around the mouth, in the pharynx, and especially in the larynx, which can cause suffocation and death as emphasized in our discussion of the control of localized swellings in this chapter. Three 1 cc vials of 1:1000 epinephrine and three disposable sterile 1 cc syringes with 25-

gauge hypodermic needles should always be carried by the patient.

2. Corticosteroids parenterally or orally cannot relieve the allergic reaction in a few minutes and cannot supplant epinephrine 1:1000 hypodermically for the rapid relief of severe urticaria or life-endangering swellings in the throat or larynx.

When hives or swellings are marked, however, 20 to 40 mg of triamcinolone or equivalent doses of other corticoids can be given intramuscularly after the immediate administration of epinephrine hypodermically. Prednisone, 5 mg two to six times a day or comparable doses of more concentrated corticosteroids such as triamcinolone can be continued by mouth, gradually reducing and eliminating them in three to ten days as the allergenic causes are controlled with relief of the cutaneous allergy. When allergies require study and attempted control for weeks or even two to three months, it is justifiable to continue 2 to 5 mg of a corticosteroid one to two times a day but only for one to three months until the allergic causes are determined and controlled.

SUMMARY OF THE DIAGNOSIS AND CONTROL OF URTICARIA

Food allergy, especially to fruits, condiments, flavors, nuts, and chocolate, is the usual cause of hives in young children. As age increases, medicaments and other foods and to a lesser degree pollen allergy always needs study and control. Infectant allergy must be in mind as a rare possible cause.

1. Food allergy is rarely indicated by dependable skin tests and must be controlled by total elimination of suspected foods. Foods responsible for chronic urticaria must be studied and controlled, especially with our FFCFE diet. Allergy to fruits, condiments and spices, and other

common allergenic foods excluded from our elimination diet must be studied as advised in Chapter 3.

2. When urticaria has developed after medicaments and chemicals have entered the body (orally or by injection, inhalation, or even cutaneous application), their entire elimination for one to four weeks often relieves the allergy. When allergy to several medicaments and chemicals is possible, total elimination of all of them, as advised in this chapter, is necessary. Our advised control of prolonged urticaria after parenteral penicillin, animal sera, or after some other parenteral medicament must be remembered.

3. Pollen allergy may be the sole cause of urticaria present from early March to late November. It may be associated with food or medicament allergy which causes urticaria in other seasons. Its recognition, especially by history, and its control by desensitization are discussed in this chapter.

4. Urticaria or other manifestations of atopic allergy attributed to cold, heat, or pressure allergy may be due to activation of unrecognized food, inhalant, or drug allergy as the cause rather than physical allergy, as in dermographia and dermatitis resulting from pollen, formerly attributed to solar dermatitis.

5. For the control of severe urticaria and especially of associated swellings, particularly in the larynx and throat, epinephrine 1:1000 hypodermically must be given and repeated to render relief as necessary. Corticosteroids produce delayed and continued relief, providing the allergenic causes gradually are being controlled. Antihistamines also may control mild hives and are justified for continued relief but only if the allergic causes are gradually being controlled.

6. Antihistamines parenterally will con-

trol moderate urticaria more rapidly than corticosteroids but less rapidly than epinephrine 1:1000 hypodermically, which, as emphasized above, must be used for rapid control of severe hives and especially for localized edema in larynx or throat. When given hypodermically, antihistamines, especially Benadryl, Chlor-Trimeton, or Polaramine®, produce relief more rapidly than parenteral corticosteroids. The use of Periactin® instead of antihistamines has been disappointing in our practice.

When such hives are due to foods such as fruits, nuts, or at times fish or chocolate, the discontinuance of the foods by mouth or by inhalation of their odors along with antihistamines for a few days may control the allergy without epinephrine hypodermically or corticosteroids. But severe hives from foods, drugs (including penicillin) and serum had marked pollen sensitivity infrequently will be adequately controlled with antihistamines alone.

Antihistamines in moderate doses are indicated for relief of mild or localized hives in oral doses recommended for each antihistamine. The relieving dose can be repeated according to printed directions of the manufacturers. Antihistamines cannot replace epinephrine for severe diffuse urticaria or swellings of the larynx or throat. The effect of antihistamines on other large swellings is uncertain.

SUMMARY

1. Urticaria or hives must be studied for possible food, drug, and chemical allergies and also inhalant allergy, especially to pollens if exaggeration occurs in the pollen seasons.

2. Allergy occurs in the superficial capillaries and lymphatics in the skin in contrast to allergy in the larger subcutaneous vasculature which causes angioneurotic edema or localized swellings.

3. Allergy to common allergenic foods, especially to fruits, condiments, spices, and flavors, is the most common cause.

4. Since skin tests to causative foods are too often absent or fallible, test-negative diets rarely give relief.

5. Usually our fruit-free and cereal-free elimination diet used in a strict, adequate manner as advised in this and in Chapter 3 is required for the study and control of food allergy.

6. Allergy to drugs and medicaments, especially to aspirin and penicillin, is common. Their total elimination for two to four weeks is advised in this chapter.

7. Inhalant allergy, especially to pollens, is indicated by history with or without positive skin tests.

8. Possible allergy to intestinal parasites, insect venoms, and rarely to bacteria must be remembered.

9. Physical allergy requires study of food and less often of drug allergy activated by cold and heat.

10. Dermographia requires study of chronic food or drug allergy activated by pressure on the skin.

11. Generalized pruritis without urticaria requires similar study of such allergies, as we advise in dermographia.

12. Histories of urticaria resulting from food and at times from pollen allergy are summarized. One case complicated by cough resulting from bronchial hives and one with laryngeal edema are included.

13. Control of drug, food, and inhalant allergy, especially to pollens, is advised.

14. Temporary relief from epinephrine, corticosteroids, and antihistamines until allergic causes are controlled is important.

Chapter 16

Acute Localized Edema (Angioneurotic Edema)

Acute localized edema, as we stated in 1931 and 1937, always requires the study of atopic allergy as the cause. Osler suggested "anaphylaxis" as the probable cause in 1914. Since then, increasing evidence in the literature has indicated that foods, medicaments, inhalant (especially pollen), and possibly bacterial allergies are responsible. We have especially emphasized the importance of food sensitizations in its etiology for many years. Vaughan and Hawke, Figley, Menagh, Dorst, and Hopphan added confirmation to the allergic hypothesis. These and other contributions are reviewed in our summary of the literature in Chapter 26.

Since allergy is a probable cause of angioneurotic edema described originally by Quincke, a better term for the manifestation might be *recurrent allergic localized edema*. The name *acute circumscribed edema* first used by Quincke in 1882, by Oppenheimer in 1898, and later by Cassier in 1901 when he reported 160 cases from the literature is a more acceptable term than angioneurotic edema. The implication that a neurosis is in part responsible for such edema arose from failure to explain it satisfactorily prior to the acquisition of our present knowledge of allergy. Some still hold that nervousness is the fundamental cause but have failed to study their patients in the exhaustive and thorough manner which we advise for investigation of allergic manifestations.

These localized edemas may occur in most tissues of the body. Most commonly they arise in the skin, especially on the face, hands, and feet. The eyes, lips, tongue, and nose are frequent sites. Edemas may arise in the esophagus and mediastinum (causing sensations called globus hystericus or substernal pressure), the stomach, intestines, and probably in other abdominal tissues, giving rise to acute digestive symptoms, abdominal pain, and even signs of intestinal obstruction.

In our discussion of chronic urticaria in Chapter 15, it was noted that acute localized edema frequently occurs with urticaria, at times with erythema, and often with other common allergic disturbances. In contrast to urticaria, these swellings themselves are infrequently associated with itching. It has been suggested that these localized edemas result from allergic reactions in the large cutaneous and subcutaneous arterioles and that urticaria is due to involvement of the superficial cutaneous capillaries. Dilatation and increased permeability of such blood vessels lead to subcutaneous or cutaneous edema. As in the symptoms of all types of allergy, the swelling may be brief or may persist for hours, days, or even a week or more. It may be of mild or severe degree and may be slow or rapid in onset. When a marked degree of sensitization is present, pressure on the cutaneous tissues of the hands, feet, or other cutaneous areas; the use of joints, such as those involved in eating; or the movement of other tissues will give rise to swellings. This also occurs in dermographia from stroking the skin. In such patients, moreover, heat, cold, emotion, or injury of tissues may activate the allergy and produce the edema. As in bronchial asthma and headaches, regular recurrent attacks with moderate or total interim relief indicate food allergy.

LITERATURE ON ANGIONEUROTIC EDEMA

Our review of the literature emphasizes the occurrence of acute localized edema in the larynx leading to death through suffocation, in the bronchi and lung parenchyma, in various parts of the urogenital tract (including the uterus and tubes), in the meninges of the brain and spinal cord, in the sheaths of the peripheral nerves, and possibly in the nervous tissues of the brain and cord leading to varying degrees and types of reactions in central and peripheral nervous systems including paresthesias, pareses, or paralyses. Nervousness, irritability, fear, and vasomotor and emotional instability may accompany attacks and suggest the occurrence of varying degrees of such edema in nervous tissue. Slight edemas occur in ocular tissues, as reported in Chapter 20. Symptoms of an epileptic equivalent at times resulting from allergy can be relieved occasionally almost miraculously by use of oral Dilantin. Such swellings, moreover, may occur in synovial membranes of joints and tendons, as we report in Chapter 23. Talley, in 1900, described angioneurotic edema of the salivary glands, four examples of which we have studied. Mild localized edemas resulting from or associated with varying degrees of allergic vasculitis may arise in the tissues of the heart, liver, spleen, kidney, and other organs. Some confirmation of such edema is found in the literature (especially German), as reviewed in Hansen's prestigious book on allergy as noted in Chapter 26. The association of acute localized edema with erythema, erythema exudativum or nodosum, and purpura, as reported by Osler, and the occurrence of hemoglobinuria, hematuria, and other idiopathic hemorrhages with attacks of such edemas, as noted by Joseph and Cassier, Packard, Holmes, Chittenden, and others, indicate that such symptoms may arise from allergy. The simulation of conditions usually demanding surgery, such as intestinal obstruction, perforated peptic ulcers (see Chapt. 5), appendicitis, renal or gallstone colic, hydronephrosis, and tabetic crises was stressed many years ago by Osler. Wiehl (1912) described severe abdominal pain and intestinal symptoms in five patients with angioneurotic edema. Bogart (1915) found edemas in the ileum and jejunum and blood-stained fluid in the peritoneal cavity in such patients with symptoms of intestinal obstruction. Vallery-Radot and Blamoutier (1931) recorded remarkable severe gastric pain, nausea, and vomiting every week for twenty-six years associated with laryngeal edemas, fatigue, and finally death. Food allergy was never studied as we advise. The reader is referred to Chapter 27 for further discussion of the surgical aspects of angioneurotic edema.

The predisposition to develop these localized swellings tends to run in families and is often associated with other allergic manifestations. A review of the evidence of such familial transmission was included in the article of Dunlap and Lemon (1929). Their record revealed a history of edema in twenty-four members of the family, six of whom had died suddenly, two from edema of the glottis, two from obscure causes, and one from severe intestinal colic.

For those physicians who are interested in the gradual evolution of knowledge about acute localized edema, we have summarized the literature during the last one hundred years in Chapter 26. This summary evidences the varied, bizarre, and often remarkable types of localized edemas, especially in the skin and also in other body tissues including the abdomen, brain, throat, larynx, abdominal organs, and even the peripheral nervous tissues.

LITERATURE SUGGESTING AN ALLERGIC CAUSE

In the last fifty years increasing evidence of an allergic etiology in acute localized edema has been reported. In 1916 Osler predicted that the cause of these edemas would be opened with "the key of anaphylaxis." Austrian (1919) presented evidence that such edema was allergic, reporting one case resulting from lobster and pork, others to different foods, and one apparently from bacterial allergy from infected teeth, evidence of which however was not very conclusive. Turrettini (1922) reported angioneurotic edema from allergy to cereals and eggs. Phillips (1922) described angioneurotic edema in a dog from pork and in another dog from fish. Edema in a man thirty-seven years of age also arose from pork. Kennedy (1926) reported giant swellings in a girl two years of age which were associated with severe pain in the head, recurring three or four times a day. Epileptic convulsions gradually developed. Skin tests to milk were positive, and its elimination relieved all symptoms. Evidence that allergy was responsible for other edemas in the tissues of the nervous system was presented. He described transient swellings of the optic nerve and retina, brain stem, and cord as possible results of allergy. One man had four attacks of hemiplegia with loss of vision, severe pain in the head, aphonia, difficulty in swallowing, and incontinence of urine and stool. He gave a history of asthma in childhood, and his mother had had urticaria from fish. In

1929 Kennedy again discussed the transient nervous symptoms often associated with angioneurotic edema.

Wason (1926) recorded severe abdominal pain and bloody vomiting. He attributed the edema to allergy and correctly stated that the magnitude of the part allergy plays in the production of such symptoms was as yet "only dimly recognized." Food allergy was not studied as advised in this volume. Crawford (1934) reported angioneurotic edema in a child eight months of age in the face, lips, and eyes from oranges, peas, and probably from wheat and egg.

POSSIBLE BACTERIAL ALLERGY

In addition to these cases of localized edemas from food allergy, we commented on several patients in 1938 in whom bacterial allergy from foci of infection seemed to be responsible. Barber, of Guy's Hospital, emphasized this possible cause. Two of his cases were relieved by extraction of infected teeth, another was cured after two operations on the maxillary and frontal sinuses, and another by tonsillectomy. Davis, as reported by Drysdale, felt that hidden sepsis was the most likely cause of chronic urticaria and angioneurotic edema, and Oberndorf reported such edema cured by removal of an infected appendix.

Additional evidence that bacterial allergy at times causes angioneurotic edema exists in the article by Dorst and Hopphan (1932). One male thirty-eight years of age was relieved of acute localized swellings of three years' duration by therapy with a vaccine of hemolytic staphylococci obtained from the ethmoids. A woman forty-five years of age with symptoms for six months was gradually benefited by desensitization with a vaccine of hemolytic coli. The skin reactions also gradually disappeared. A woman forty years of age with swellings for two years, was relieved after desensitization with *E coli cummunior* and later with *B mucosus capsulatus*. Small and gradually increasing doses of vaccine for prolonged periods were important.

In all of these cases attributed to bacterial allergy, the duration of follow-ups was not reported. Thus other types of allergy, especially to foods or medications, cannot be excluded.

Bacterial allergy may also explain such chronic edema reported by Stevens (1933) and New and Kirch (1933). Stevens recorded such chronic edema in the face after repeated attacks of erysipelas. Several patients had infected antra or ethmoids. Definite focal reaction arose with subcutaneous injection of filtrates from growths of autogenous staphylococci and streptococci. Gradual decrease in the edema with increasing doses of such filtrates led to desensitization in the affected tissues.

Allergy from parasites as discussed in relation to urticaria in Chapter 15 must also be remembered. Tenani (1912) reported angioneurotic edema because of malaria in a girl twenty-five years of age, though allergy to quinine or other drugs was not excluded.

HEREDITARY ANGIONEUROTIC EDEMA

Austen and Sheffer, in 1965, reported their study of the rare hereditary form of angioneurotic edema first recognized by Osler in 1888 with transmission as a mendelian dominant with irregular penetrance. The writers stated that of 530 reported cases in six families, in only two-thirds was there an adequate family history to place them in this rare category. It is characterized by recurrent, acute, localized, transient, nonpitting, nonitching, subepithelial edema of the skin or of the mucosa of the upper respiratory or gastrointestinal tracts

and the skin of face or extremities. Unusual edema in localized areas of the mucosa in the gastrointestinal and upper respiratory tracts causing vomiting and cramping and especially laryngeal edema resulting at times in fatal asphyxiation occurs. In 1965 Austen stated that according to the literature, death had varied from 6 to 54 percent in the different family kindreds.

Austen reported a deficiency in a normal serum inhibitor of activated first component of human complement C'1 esterase in the members of these families harboring this hereditary tendency. This information is important so that such individuals can be warned about possible mortality from laryngeal edema and being advised about prevention of serious or fatal results by the administration by medical personnel or by the patient himself of epinephrine hypodermically.

Since it is generally agreed and emphasized through our experience that the usual angioneurotic edema is due to atopic allergy, especially food allergy and at times drug allergy, its possible role in this rare hereditary type must be considered. Our review of fifty cases of the hereditary type in the literature indicates the following: since dietary history and skin reactions to foods causing allergy are often negative and the causative foods usually can be eaten between attacks with no symptoms, possible food allergy in these patients' hereditary angioneurotic edema should be adequately studied before its possibility is denied. There might be an inheritance not only of C'1 inhibitor deficiency but also of recurrently activated food allergy and the inherited tendency to localization of the allergic reaction.

Atopic allergy, especially to foods, activated possibly by injury or other cause should be studied accurately and adequately for over a period of six months as we advise. Moreover, all patients with this inherited type of angioneurotic edema as well as those with angioneurotic edema resulting from food or other allergy should be instructed in the self-administration of 1:1000 adrenalin 0.5 cc hypodermically, repeating the dose in five to ten minutes and every one-half to two hours thereafter until a physician is consulted. He can then advise further administration of adrenalin and indicated corticosteroid therapy and also perform a tracheotomy if necessary to prevent suffocation and death.

STUDIES OF ALLERGY IN ACUTE LOCALIZED EDEMAS

From our records, statistics have been compiled on thirty-eight cases of localized edemas we published in 1938 and on an additional twenty cases studied and treated in the last thirty years.

The frequency of acute localized edemas in adult life, especially from the age of twenty to fifty years, its predominance in females as in urticaria, and the occurrence of other manifestations of clinical allergy are shown in Table XXXVII. One or more such manifestations long with the acute edemas occurred in every case. Of interest was the fact that urticaria was of minor importance in 43 percent, as were acute edemas of minor occurrence in 34 percent of the cases of chronic urticaria as shown in Table XXXIV. Nasal allergy next to urticaria occurred in 30 percent (Table XXXVII), less than the occurrence of urticaria. The great frequency with which these edemas occur in the eyes, face, lips, and throat shown in Table XXXV, must be remembered. It is necessary to instruct patients in the self-administration of adrenalin 1:1000, 0.3 to 0.5 cc, to relieve laryngeal edema.

Food allergy was the incriminated cause

in eighteen (90%) of the twenty cases (Table XXXV). In comparison to urticaria in which pollen allergy was the sole cause in 5 percent (Table XXXIV), pollen as the sole cause was responsible in only one of the presently tabulated twenty cases and was associated with food allergy in only one case.

Specific foods causing these acute localized edemas as determined by provocation tests are listed in Table XXXVI. This list of foods does not rule out the less frequent possibility of acute ademas arising from other ingested foods.

Drug allergy, especially to aspirin and to penicillin, is a more frequent cause of acute edemas than has been evidenced in our practice. This is probably due to the recognition of such allergies by most physicians who do not refer such cases to us as allergists.

The average duration of the recurrent acute localized edemas before consulting us for the study of allergic causes was 1.8 years. In the last twenty years patients have consulted us sooner after onset of symptoms. This early allergic consultation is probably due to the increasing realization that the swellings require the study of allergy and possibly because of the increasing concern about the occurrence of edemas in the lips, throat, and their possible development in the larynx. Edema in the larynx necessitates adrenalin therapy as advised above.

DETERMINATION AND CONTROL OF THE CAUSES OF ACUTE LOCALIZED EDEMAS
Control of Possible Drug or Chemical Allergy

Though food allergy is the usual cause of acute localized edema, its less frequent origin from aspirin, penicillin, parenteral animal sera, and extracts as occurs in urti-

TABLE XXXV

STATISTICS ON 20 CASES OF ACUTE LOCALIZED EDEMA STUDIED IN THE LAST 40 YEARS

Male .... 9 ⎫
Female .... 11 ⎭ *Total:* 20 cases

Duration average .... 1.8 years (1/12 to 10 years except one recurring for 35 years)

Location of edemas:

Face .... 10 ⎫
Eyes .... 8 ⎬ 1 or both in 14 (70%)
Lips .... 14 ⎭

Tongue .... 5 ⎫
Throat .... 7 ⎭ 1 or both in 8 (40%)

Larynx 1
Ears 1
Abdomen 2
Arms 6
Hands 6
Axilla 1
Feet ⎫
Ankles ⎭ 6

Skin tests:
Slight reactions to foods 6
Pollens: large 3
          moderate 2

Causes:
Foods 18
Pollens alone 1
Pollens with foods 1
Aspirin° 1

°The reader is referred to our discussion of oral and parenteral allergy to drugs, sera, and other medicaments.

TABLE XXXVI

FOODS CAUSING LOCALIZED EDEMAS AS DETERMINED BY PROVOCATION FEEDING TESTS

(Listed Alphabetically)

Chocolate
Coffee
Condiments
Corn
Eggs
Fish
Flavors
Fruits
Milk
Pork
Rice
Shellfish
Wheat

Note: To a lesser extent other foods in additional tabulated cases were responsible.

Possible food allergy is best studied with our FFCFE diet rather than one eliminating the above foods, all of which are excluded from the FFCFE diet.

TABLE XXXVII

STATISTICS ON 60 CASES OF ACUTE LOCALIZED EDEMA SEEN IN THE LAST 40 YEARS

Male	32%
Female	68%
Average age	36 yrs (5-31 yrs)
Swellings	100%
Urticaria	43%
Nasal allergy	30%
Bronchial asthma	11%
Eczema	0
Headaches	14%
Abdominal distress (allergy?)	25%
Family history of allergy	37%
Food dislikes and disagreements	32%

caria must receive immediate consideration. If the edemas have originated immediately after the administration of such medications, indicating previous allergy, or in seven to twenty days after the administration of drugs by mouth or parenterally, such allergy especially needs study. In addition to the drugs noted above, various organ and tissue extracts as of pituitary or liver, quinine, and to a lesser degree many other drugs and medications can produce acute localized edemas. As we have advised in the control of urticaria, all medications should be discontinued while the causes of acute localized edemas are being investigated. The exception is epinephrine 1:1000

for the rapid control of severe edema and the diminishing doses of corticosteroids by mouth if the edemas are recurring or persisting every one to three days. If the edemas, however, are occurring every ten or more days with no associated or interim urticaria, then epinephrine hypodermically with no corticosteroids will usually control these intermittent edemas. If drug or chemical allergies are responsible, the entire elimination of all of them will gradually prevent additional subsequent edemas. It must be remembered, however, that drugs and chemicals remain in the body for one to three or four weeks or even a longer time. If the swellings continue in spite of the elimination of all medications, food, pollen, and rarely bacterial allergy must be studied as next advised.

Control of Possible Food Allergy

If the history indicates that one or several individual foods may be the causes of these acute edemas, their total elimination for one to three or four weeks may prevent further swellings. Allergy to foods, however, infrequently is proven by elimination except at times to walnuts, peanuts, fish, eggs, or specific fruits. Scratch tests, moreover, practically never reveal the causative foods. As in urticaria, therefore, diet trial with our FFCFE diet is indicated.

The reader is referred to our discussion of the control of food allergy in urticaria (Chapt. 15) for directions for the ordering, preparation, and the necessary time for strict maintenance and additions to the diet after relief of the cutaneous allergy is assured.

After the separate foods responsible for the edemas are found, it may be necessary to eliminate them entirely for months or even years before tolerance to them is established. Even after relief, reactivated food allergies may again cause hives, edema, or other manifestations of food allergy in three, five, fifteen, or more years.

To obtain such relief, strict adherence to the prescribed diets is absolutely necessary along with vigorous cooperation with the physician with no deviations from the diet, even to a slight degree. After relief is assured, it is the physician's responsibility to add gradually other individual foods, eliminating those that reproduce edemas (see Chapt. 3 and 30). However, if the interim between the swellings is two, four, or eight weeks in duration, complete relief must continue for at least twice the time of the interim period for one to be reasonably certain that the allergenic foods are being excluded from the diet. Good results depend in large part on the physician's directions and supervision based on his long, successful use of our elimination diets for the control of the many manifestations of food allergy.

Pollen Allergy as a Cause of Acute Localized Edemas

Pollen allergy as a cause is infrequent compared to its frequency in chronic urticaria, as indicated in Table XXXIV. Our statistics from twenty cases of acute localized edema revealed pollen as a sole cause in only one child of six years. In 1938 we also reported swellings during the spring to late fall as a result of pollen allergy. If the history indicates such allergy, desensitization as advised in its discussion in urticaria (Chapt. 15) is important. Skin tests to pollens may be absent, the diagnosis necessarily being made by history of the occurrence of swellings during the pollen seasons.

Bacterial Allergy

Though we have had no evidence in recent years of bacterial allergy, especially from a focus of infection, as a sole or even associated cause of these acute localized edemas, its consideration is justified, especially if strict, persistent, and adequate study of food, drug, chemical, and pollen allergies does not reveal the allergenic causes. This possible bacterial allergy has been discussed in Chapter 15.

Physical Allergies

Physical allergies, especially to cold, cause localized edemas as noted in our discussion of urticaria. Such allergy is evident in the history and avoidance of the cause gives relief.

TEMPORARY RELIEF OF ACUTE LOCALIZED EDEMAS

The paramount importance of epinephrine 1:1000 and the use of corticosteroids for delayed and more lasting relief if edemas are recurring every day or so are important as advised in our discussion on the control of urticaria.

As already stated, if the swellings are recurring every seven to ten or more days, relief from epinephrine alone is sufficient until drug, food, or inhalant allergy is studied and controlled. If the edemas recur every two to three days and especially if urticaria of secondary importance is present, corticosteroids in initial large and subsequent reduced dosage during a seven- to fourteen-day period are indicated. Long-term corticosteroid therapy without adequate study and control of the underlying causes of acute localized edemas, however, is rarely justified. Such control with corticosteroids has been unnecessary in our practice because of our persistent study of the causative allergies.

Antihistamines usually are of less temporary relief than in urticaria. The possibility of allergy to one or more of them and their questionable benefit militate against their frequent use.

SUMMARIES OF HISTORIES AND CAUSES OF ACUTE LOCALIZED EDEMAS

Case 90: A man twenty years of age had recurrent nonseasonal swellings of the eyes, mouth, tongue and throat with hoarseness and rhinorrhea every 2½ months for ten years. The maternal grandmother disliked eggs. The maternal grandfather vomited milk all of his life. There was no other history of allergy in the patient. Scratch testing gave large pollen reactions and no reactions to foods.

With the use of our FFCFE diet, milk, fruits, and spices were found responsible. There was no clinical allergy to pollens, though large reactions occurred.

Case 91: A boy ten years of age had recurrent swellings in the eyes, lips, face, arms, legs, and hands subsiding in a week, recurring nonseasonally during 1½ years. Along with these swellings there were nervousness, weakness, and headaches, indicating probable cerebral allergy. He has vomited milk in childhood and had been "raised on barley water." The mother also had vomited milk all of her life.

Adherence to our FFCFE diet revealed milk as the main cause, with coffee, chocolate, and Coca Cola® as minor causes.

Case 92: A woman eighty-one years of age had had attacks of edema in the face, lips, eyes, submaxillary glands, and tongue lasting for one to two days at intervals during a thirty-five year period. She had had relief for two to five years. The edemas had occurred every month or two for three years and several times a month for six months. There was no preceding itching. Antihistamines three times a day had decreased the severity but had not eliminated the edemas. Heartburn, always suggestive of possible food allergy especially to fruits, flavors, and condiments, had been present on and off for eight years. There was no history of familial allergies. Milk, fruits, flavors, and spices were found responsible. Former constipation was relieved with this diet. Recurrence of symptoms indicated food allergy.

This case shows that food allergy can develop in old age.

Case 93: A girl seventeen years of age had nonitching swelling of the eyes and lips for six months. The joints of the fingers and palms of the hands especially had been involved especially in school and when she had had her hands in water. Eczema had occurred for several years. Physical examination and laboratory tests were negative, and her scratch tests on two occasions with all important food allergens were negative.

By our eliminiation method, it was found that wheat was the sole cause of angioneurotic edema. She was given hypodermic desensitization to a wheat extract which was not beneficial.

GENERALIZED EDEMA

Edema involving the entire body or large areas of the body with or without urticaria resulting from allergy nearly always to foods is not infrequent. Such edema may not be evident and is never pitting in type. It is associated with sudden increases in weight from five to twenty pounds and is usually accompanied by marked nervous, psychic, and vasomotor disturbances and loss of strength such as those described from angioneurotic edema and from allergic toxemia (Chapt. 19).

Duke, in 1922, described such a case:

A woman, age thirty-five years, came into my office complaining of weakness, loss of energy, recent gain in weight (15 pounds), which symptoms apparently dated back six months or more. Upon examination were noticed mental apathy, pallid, waxy appearance of the skin, puffiness of the face suggesting myxedema and reduced blood pressure. We treated the patient for some months with little relief until she chanced to have an attack of bladder disorder with no evidence of infection in the urine or other adequate cause of these symptoms. A history of asthma in her father was then elicited, and she was immediately tested and found to be very sensitive to several vegetables, which she had been eating frequently. Her rapid recovery upon the discontinuance of these vegetables and with the use of a few doses of adrenalin was most interesting. Within a few days she gained her strength, energy, usual vivacity, and good color and rapidly lost her excessive weight.

Eyermann studied a patient whose weight increased seven pounds with the ingestion of one peanut. I have records of several patients whose weight varies according to the control of their ingestant or inhalant allergies. Diethelm (1905), Bernoulli (1910), and Schorer (1925) reported cases of generalized edema probably resulting from allergy. It is possible that the generalized edema only at menstruation recorded by Thomas (1933) with marked diuresis of 4500 cc with recovery may have been due to food allergy activated by menstruation (Chapt. 21). Other causes of water retention must also be considered.

Other causes of generalized edema as reported by Longcope (1934), such as inanition, protein starvation, chronic anemia, and hypothyroidism must be remembered.

Allergic edema may affect localized areas of the body and as such might better be termed chronic allergic edema, though the generalized edema is probably identical in etiology to the localized type. Such a case of extensive edema involving large and varying areas of the body we reported in 1928, as discussed in the previous section of this chapter. Other instances of localized edemas have been reported. It is possible that the generalized edema which Rose described and the cases of edema in the literature which he discussed may have been due to unrecognized allergy.

Case 94: Generalized edema of the entire body was associated with vomiting for nine years, sick headaches, dysentery from specific foods, an allergic cough for eight years, hives, canker sores, a white film on the gums, and a persisting soreness in the nostrils. This remarkable array of manifestations resulting from food allergy is worthy of attention as evidencing the fact that food allergy can affect nearly all the tissues of the body, as noted in Chapter 26. We have had an unequaled opportunity to observe this patient, and all of her symptoms, including the generalized edema, are controlled with proper "elimination diet." Generalized bloating of the body with sudden increases and reductions in weight because of food allergy has occurred in two other women who have been under our care.

Case 95: Generalized edema and swelling of the body associated with headaches, sore throat, and nasal congestion had been present in a woman thirty-eight years of age.

She had had vomiting one to two hours after nearly every meal for nine years since the birth of twins, at which time she overate greatly. For two years she had had sick headaches, lasting four or five days every one to two weeks. Tomatoes, berries, and to a lesser extent fruit made her mouth raw. Corn produced dysentery. Generalized swelling of the entire body especially of the hands, arms, feet, face, and abdomen had been present nearly constantly for eight years. Her nostrils had been sore and swollen especially at night up to three years previously, and she had coated lips for years. Frequent canker sores had also occurred. Hives were present nearly constantly in childhood. Itching and bleeding piles were frequent. Her bowels were usually loose and foamy. Other allergy was not present in the patient's history. The mother, whom we interviewed, had had practically the same symptoms most of her life. Physical examination was negative except for the diffuse firm swelling of the extremities and to a lesser extent the rest of the body. Laboratory tests, including stomach, stool, and food tests, were negative.

With the FFCFE diet relief gradually occurred in two months. After relief was maintained for one month, provocation feeding tests produced symptoms after the trials of wheat, eggs, milk, pork, cottonseed oil, figs, and bananas. The exclusion of these foods eradicated the nausea, cough, headaches, mucous colitis, and especially the generalized swelling of the body for 2½ years.

SUMMARY

1. Angioneurotic edema (localized swellings) is due to allergic reactions in large subcutaneous vascular channels compared with that in capillaries in urticaria.

2. As in urticaria, allergy to foods, inhalants (including tobacco), drugs (including animal sera), and bacteria are causative.

3. Review of the literature before the recognition of allergy as the cause in the early twenties and increasing reports indicating allergy, especially to foods, as the cause are summarized.

4. In contrast to other clinical allergy, evidence of occasional bacterial allergy is discussed.

5. Even though a deficiency of the inhibitor of serum complement C'1 esterase is reported in all patients suffering with rare hereditary angioneurotic edema, atopic allergy especially to foods might be a concomitant and activating factor. Its study as we advise therefore may be of benefit.

6. The areas of edema, the duration before our study and control, fallibility of scratch tests, and the importance of food compared with pollen allergy and the frequency of other clinical allergies are shown in the statistics in these twenty cooperating patients with angioneurotic edema resulting from atopic allergy.

7. Control of drug, food, infrequent pollen allergies, and possible bacterial and physical allergy is advised.

8. Records of informative cases resulting from food allergy are included in this chapter.

9. Generalized edema at times increased in the extremities or torso requires study of food and rarely of inhalant or drug allergy as advised in this chapter.

Chapter 17

Allergic Headache and Migraine

Migraine is a term derived from the Greek spavia, hemicrania. It is used by Germans (migrane), the French (migraine), and the English (megrim) to denote recurrent headaches of formerly unknown etiology.

Allergy to foods and at times to pollens according to our experience requires study as the cause of recurrent or persistent headaches and migraine. Though cyclic headaches, which are our challenge in this chapter, are rarely if ever due to the following causes, their absence must be assured. These include acute or chronic infections, especially in nasal sinuses; ocular, aural, menstrual, or ductless gland disease or dysfunction; hepatic, cardiovascular, or renal disease; intracranial tumors; disease or dysfunction of the nervous system; trauma; arthritis; or other toxic or nervous states. In the first edition of this book in 1931 we wrote "Food allergy has to receive serious consideration as the most common cause of migraine." Though allergic headaches usually occur with other manifestations of clinical allergy, occasionally they may be the sole manifestation of atopic allergy.

The necessity of an adequate history, physical examination, and all indicated laboratory and x-ray studies to recognize all possible causes of headache before or when allergy is being studied must be emphasized.

Allergic headaches occur in all parts of the head, often with radiation of chest pain into the neck, shoulders, arms, or upper chest and at times into the back. Allergy in the peripheral nerves may be present. They are frequently associated with nausea, vomiting, dizziness, and visual disturbances resulting from cerebral allergy or concomitant gastrointestinal allergy, as exemplified in our tabulation of symptoms in one hundred cases (Table XXXIX) in which our study indicated allergy as the probable cause. This relief justifies the accurate and sufficient study of allergy to foods and less often to pollens in all of these patients as advised in this chapter and in Chapter 4. In this group of patients with allergic headaches, approximately 20 percent had symptoms typical of migraine. One or more symptoms indicating probable migraine occurred in a similar number.

We wrote in 1937: It is important to realize that all degrees and variations of the severe classical migraine exist. For every severe case there are many mild ones which may or may not be associated with cranial, gastrointestinal, or toxic disturbances. Critchley and Ferguson (1933) stressed the occurrence of the bilious, ocular, menstrual, and cerebral types of symptoms of migraine and stated that one or more of the typical symptoms are frequently absent. Woltman (1925) in an excellent article also emphasized the mild and severe types of migraine, possibly evidencing itself only in a dull headache or transient scotoma, hemianopsia, and at times temporary mental depression, inertia or transient pareses, paresthesia, or aphesias. He felt that most so-called gastric or bilious headaches are migrainous in type.

Thus headaches alone or associated with nausea, vomiting, visual, or other neurological symptoms may be evidence of the migrainous predisposition and should be studied for possible allergy as the cause, especially if other recognized causes of headaches are not evident or even before such questionable possibilities are extensively investigated. This would save many ocular, nasal, and gastrointestinal examinations and even needless surgery. Other pathological causes of headache besides allergy are important to recognize. They should not be assumed as causes of migraine or allergic headaches until allergy has been studied in an adequate manner as we advise. Headaches in patients with seasonal or perennial hay fever or nasal allergy are not evidence of a migrainous prediposition.

PATHOGENESIS OF ALLERGIC HEADACHE AND MIGRAINE

The following tissue disturbances arising from allergic reactions may explain the symptoms characteristic of allergic migraine.

1. Localized edema of the meninges or possibly of the parenchyma of the brain itself may be responsible. Because of the sensitiveness of the dura as compared with the cortex, the pain of migraine is best explained by edema in the dural and meningeal membranes.

Quincke, in 1893, suggested angioneurotic edema of ependymal cells causing serous meningitis and resultant headache, atopic allergy being the best explanation of such edema. Of interest was Goltman's observation over a period of years of a patient with migraine who had been decompressed over the frontal area for relief. During his attacks edema and congestion of the pia and cortical tissue associated with vascular dilatation always occurred. This, however, was preceded by vasomotor spasm evidenced by blanching of the face, numbness,

and tingling of the body. Foster Kennedy (1933) favored meningeal edema, comparing it to urticaria on the skin. Such edema in one or more localized areas extending itself possibly into the crevices of the cerebrum and possibly involving the brain tissue can well explain the varying distribution of headache, the differing degrees of parasthesias, pareses, and cranial nerve disturbances which occur in this malady. Localized angioneurotic edema of the meninges has been observed during exploration of the brain because of severe pain suggestive of tumor. Quincke even described meningitis serosa resulting from such edema of the ependymal cells. Eyermann (1931) felt that edema was the best explanation of the headache, and Balyeat and Rinkel (1931) favored the possibility of urticarialike lesions. Such edema of the meninges and possibly of the tissues adjacent to the vascular walls through the brain itself may arise from allergic reactions in the walls of the blood vessels with changes in permeability, resulting in exudation of fluid into the surrounding tissues. Davidoff and Kopeloff (1934) have demonstrated local cerebral anaphylaxis in dogs whose cerebral tissues were sensitized to serum and egg white through craniotomy exposures. Subsequent intravenous injections yielded immediate motor disturbances.

2. Vascular spasm arising from smooth muscle contraction resulting from allergy in localized areas of various blood vessels could explain many symptoms of migraine. Such spasms moreover, might be accompanied by permeability changes and exudation of fluid, as noted above. Bassoe (1933) suggested that ophthalmic migraine may be due to spasm of the posterior cerebral artery, and Riley (1932) observed decrease in the size of retinal arteries during an attack. Kennedy (1933), on the other

hand, favored localized meningeal edema since he felt vascular spasm could not explain the bizarre and mixed symptoms of migraine.

Either or both of these lesions could explain the headache, the neuralgia, and the transient pareses, aphasia, visual, and other disturbances at times associated with migraine. The nausea and vomiting which accompany migraine may be of a central origin or may be due to a localized concomitant allergic reaction in the liver or the gastrointestinal tract. Cyclic recurrence of symptoms is characteristic of allergy.

Liver swelling accompanied by a mild icterus and evidences of hepatic dysfunction have been noted in cases of migraine by many writers, including Liveing, Brunton, McClure and Huntsinger, and others whom I have mentioned in my review of the literature on migraine. Such swelling could be due to a localized allergic reaction in the liver. In fact, it is quite likely that this organ is one of the shock organs in man, as it has been shown to be in certain animals, especially in the dog. The liver is the first organ that is influenced by the food proteins which pass through the intestinal mucosa, and it would be surprising if its tissue were not frequently subjected to allergic reactions. Alvarez (1934) suggested that nausea, vomiting, and dizziness in migraine may arise from cerebral irritation which produces a vagal stimulation and an upset of the intestinal gradient. The toxemia preceding or accompanying migraine which is reported throughout the literature is probably due in part to the impairment of the liver function as well as to a generalized allergic disturbance in other organs and tissues of the body. Whether such toxemia can cause headache without the assumption of a localized allergic reaction in the brain is difficult to say. This is possible, though it must be

remembered that migraine occurs at times without any other probable manifestations of allergy.

Migraine may be precipitated by psychic and emotional strain; fatigue; infections; gastrointestinal and other visceral disturbances; and by physical factors, including heat, cold, and even light, but it must be remembered they are of secondary importance. It is likely that symptoms may be prodromal manifestations of the oncoming allergic attack or may be secondary to the cellular disturbances present during the allergic reaction.

ROLE OF FOOD ALLERGY IN MIGRAINE

The following contributions have gradually placed the allergic etiology on a firm basis: Lesne and Richet Fils (1913) suggested migraine in youth might be due to milk or egg allergy. Rohrer (1915) according to Vaughan next suggested that migraine was of allergic origin. Pagniez, Vallery-Radot, and Nast (1919) suggested allergy as a possible cause of migraine and especially incriminated chocolate. Pagniez and Nast (1920) further discussed such etiology. Lubbers (1921) stated that the failure of migraine to develop with each ingestion of chocolate could be explained by the refractory state or desensitization which is generally recognized in allergy (Chapt. 1). He also recorded migraine from apricots.

Laing (1927) reviewed the possible causes of migraine, including anaphylaxis, and concluded it was due to a toxic neurosis. He commented on the relief obtained by a bowel movement or a cathartic. Nausea and vomiting were present in 120 of 146 cases, and constipation occurred in 131 cases. Females numbered 116 and males 29. A family history of migraine was present in 114 instances.

Hartsock (1927) minimized food allergy as a cause of migraine and laid emphasis on duodenal stasis and intestinal toxemia. His therapy excluded wheat, cereals, potatoes, eggs, and milk, as recommended by Brown. It is interesting that the diet eliminated foods commonly causative of clinical allergy. His recommendations of rest, sedatives, salines, mild mercurous chloride, and duodenal drainage have not been necessary to obtain relief from food allergy in our cases.

Rolleston (1927) in his interesting little book *Idiosyncrasies* stated that food allergy was a probable cause of certain cases of migraine.

In America Vaughan was first to report the control of migraine by the elimination of allergenic foods. He published two cases in 1922 and ten cases in 1927. Thereafter, he emphasized food allergy in migraine in several articles, especially in 1933, on results based on careful follow-up reports. Good results occurred in 50.8 percent, and sixty-two different foods were responsible in various degrees and combinations. In order of importance, wheat, milk, peanuts, chocolate, pork, peas, beans, onions, eggs, bananas, and so on were most frequently responsible. Patients at times were able to discover some causative foods which were ingested infrequently.

In 1935 he concluded that good results with the exclusion of allergenic foods should occur in 70 percent of all cases. Our contributions from 1927 to the present have already been summarized. Brown (1928) reported one case of a headache from food allergy. Balyeat (1928) cited one case and two other cases in 1929. In 1930 he published fifty-five cases of migraine resulting from food allergy. Balyeat and Rinkel (1931) studied 202 patients with migraine which started in the first decade in 27.7 percent and in the second decade in 30.6 percent. Cylic vomiting was felt to be allergic in origin and the forerunner of allergic migraine. In later publications Balyeat and Rinkel stated that allergic headaches may have all the symptoms of clinical migraines or may occur without cortical disturbances. Hunt (1933) studied patients with abdominal migraine and bilious attacks arising from food allergy. Eyermann (1931) reported good results in 69 percent of sixty-three patients with headaches. Slight or positive skin reactions determined the causative foods in contrast to our inability to demonstrate satisfactorily all etiological foods by such tests. Curschmann (1931) not only found migraine arising from food allergy but studied patients benefited in allergen-free rooms, indicating the probability of inhalant sensitizations. Vallery-Radot (1925) had reported migraine from perfumes of flowers, especially violets and roses. In addition to food allergy, Goltman (1932) found that the inhalation of "Fly-tox," of grass pollen, orris and feather allergens or cedar allergen from clothes in a cedar closet, and bacterial allergy were causative in other cases. Diets based on skin-reacting foods were ineffective. One of his patients had had a cranial decompression with no relief from migraine. Goltmann, in the discussion of Rinkel's article (1934), again stressed inhalant allergy in migraine. Berg (1928) also reported migraine, dizziness, nasobronchial allergy, or vomiting from apparent sensitization to inhaled tar fumes. Waldbott (1934) recorded severe migraine with ocular manifestations and numbness in the right arm with the accidental intravenous injection of a feather antigen. Waldbott also recorded an attack of migraine from an overdose of pollen, and we have observed a similar effect. De Gowin (1932) reviewed sixty cases of allergic migraine, of which 78 percent had received relief from test-negative diets. Of these only seven had ophthalmic symptoms. In discussion Phillips (1932) emphasized food allergy as a cause of migraine, the negative skin reactions to causative foods, and the value of "elimination diets" in diagnosis and control. Sison (1933) described ophthalmic migraine resulting from allergy and the occurrence of loss of vision, loss of sensation in the left arm and leg, and even loss of consciousness. A gradual return to normal in 1½ months occurred. Todd (1933) stressed food allergy in migraine and obtained good results in ten or twelve cases with elimination of specific foods. Andresen (1934) found that 58 percent of his cases with migraine were due to food sensitizations. Friedenwald and Morrison (1934) reported a typical migraine from milk and fish allergy. Westcott (1934) found allergic headache most frequently resulting from wheat, eggs, potatoes, oranges, tomatoes, veal, and peas. Forman (1933) ascribed to food allergy the cause of migraine and used elimination diets. In discussion, Steinberg stated that allergy should receive primary consideration in the study of all cases of migraine. Allan (1935) felt that food allergy at times released an underlying migrainous reaction. His lack of emphasis of diet trial and manipulation might explain his failure to find food allergy a frequent cause of migraine. Gerson (1932) encountered a case of migraine resulting in part from salt. Sheldon and Randolph (1935) benefited 60.8 percent of 127 cases of headache by eliminating allergenic foods. Sweetser (1934) reported relief in 62 percent of a similar series. Tuft (1935) confirmed the frequency of allergic migraine and the use of "elimination diets" modified by positive skin reactions. Contributions by Hamburger (1935) and Vallery-Radot and

Hamburger (1935) question the frequency of food allergy in the cause of migraine which was due (in our opinion) to their failure to use diet trial accurately over weeks and even months if necessary as discussed in Chapter 2. The persistency of allergic reactivity and probably of chronic tissue change, especially in nervous tissue with its marked susceptibility to slight cellular and metabolic disturbances, stresses the necessity of prolonged study and control, especially of food allergy. On the contrary, Vaughan, Balyeat, Rowe, and others have long contended that allergy is the most common cause of typical migraine and that allergic headaches without the cortical and gastrointestinal symptoms are due to the same type of reaction on the brain which causes the classical migraine.

Van Leeuwen (1925) stated that migraine and epilepsy might be due to allergy and that eggs and chocolate at times produced headache. He recalled the marked nervousness and irritability in anaphylactic guinea pigs, which suggested the plausability of allergy as a cause of cerebral reactions, as we emphasized in Chapter 18.

Tileston, in 1918, discussed "Migraine in Childhood" commenting on its association with epilepsy, its periodicity, its hereditary characteristics, and its motor or sensory symptoms. Its similarity to asthma and the lack of evidence that allergy causes migraine were noted. He doubted if migraine had ever been cured by correction of refractive errors, nasal troubles, or alterations in diet. A boy six years of age whose maternal grandmother and maternal aunt had had migraine, had had periodic headache and vomiting since the age of three years every one to three months. In winter migraine had recurred once a week. Definite allergy to eggs was determined, and elimination of eggs, meat, and fish gave definite relief. This case was probably due to food allergy.

Laroche, Richet, and Saint Girons (1919) opined that migraine might be due to food allergy. Curtis-Brown, in 1920 and again in 1925, stated that "protein poisoning" caused many conditions, including headache. Such symptoms were cyclic and occurred especially after cow's milk, meat, eggs, fruits, tomatoes, mushrooms, rhubarb, coffee, tea, and chocolate.

The foregoing articles on migraine and headache have been summarized for the following reasons: a) Those mentioned in the first paragraph indicate very markedly that food allergy is a definite cause of migraine; b) the other articles in a less definite manner point to such possible etiology or they suggest it even though the writers themselves were not cognizant of such a cause; and c) the relation between migraine, asthma, and epilepsy is stressed in certain articles and some suggestion of the varied manifestations. When headaches with or without other cerebral symptoms only occur or are exaggerated in the spring, summer, or fall, pollen allergy as later reported in this chapter requires adequate, accurate study.

Charted hemianopsia with migraine headache reported by Hansen is shown in Chapter 20.

PERSONAL STUDIES OF ALLERGY, ESPECIALLY TO FOODS, IN MIGRAINE AND HEADACHE IN FORTY YEARS

That food allergy necessitates paramount consideration as the most common cause of migraine has been evidenced by my confirmation of this with the use of our elimination diets reported in medical articles since 1928, in the first edition of this book in 1931, in *Clinical Allergy* in 1937, and in *Elimination Diets* in 1944. The following summary of these studies indicating the importance of food allergy summarizes our study up to 1938.

Food allergy necessitates paramount consideration as the most common cause of migraine. The possibility that inhalant and bacterial allergies are at times responsible is evident in the literature, as noted on page 353, and has had occasional confirmation in our work. In 1928 we first reported a series of thirty patients who had migraine as a major complaint and eighteen patients who had it as a minor symptom. All forty-eight patients obtained complete or nearly complete relief from their headaches with elimination diets. In 1931 86 cases of migraine which had been relieved by trial diets were reported, and in 1932 we presented statistics on 139 private patients with headaches. In them, good results were obtained with elimination diets in 73.1 percent, fair results in 6.9 percent, and failures in 20 percent. However, only fair or poor cooperation was given in 21 percent. Good cooperation was obtained in fourteen patients who failed to respond to diet manipulation, but these individuals had also failed to respond to former medical, surgical, and psychotherapeutic therapy. In this chapter another analysis of 247 consecutive private cases of headache will be found in Table XXXVIII. Of interest was the family history of headaches in nearly 50 percent of all patients and the frequency of nasal congestion, chronic indigestion, and constipation.

In this volume presently tabulated statistics on an additional one hundred cooperating cases of allergic headache and migraine are presented. Since good cooperation occurred in all patients, no fail-

TABLE XXXVIII

STATISTICS ON 247 PRIVATE PATIENTS WITH HEADACHE AS A MAJOR COMPLAINT

	No. of Cases
Ages:	
1 to 15 yrs	3
15 to 35 yrs	72
35 to 55 yrs	135
55 up	37
Males	66
Females	181
Duration of symptoms:	
½ to 1 yr	23
1 to 5 yrs	40
Over 5 yrs	184
Family History:	
Headaches	113
Asthma	50
Hay fever	39
Eczema	8
Urticaria	12
Chronic indigestion	42
Skin reactions:	
Foods	68
Inhalants	45
Miscellaneous	26
Personal history:	
Nasal congestion	80
Hay fever	35
Asthma	25
Chronic indigestion	98
Nausea	130
Vomiting	91
Abdominal pain	47
Constipation	142
Diarrhea	24
Eczema	40
Urticaria	68

	No. of Cases	%
Results:		
Failure	43	17.0
Fair	49	19.5
Good	155	63.5
Cooperation:		
None	6	
Poor	15	19
Fair	26	
Good	200	81

ures from too brief or poor cooperation are included.

These statistics show that these allergic headaches occurred more frequently in adults than in children and adolescents and slightly more often in women than men.

TABLE XXXIX

INFORMATION ABOUT 100 CASES OF ALLERGIC HEADACHE AND MIGRAINE RELIEVED BY CONTROL OF ALLERGY

	%
Male	45
Female	55
Age:	
5-18 yrs	19
18-35 yrs	39
35-60 yrs	49
Duration of HA:	
1-5 yrs	23
5-15 yrs	31-36
15-50 yrs	35
Over 50 yrs	6
Length of HA:	
½ day	16
1 day	30
2-4 days	42
4-10 days	12
Recurring HA:	
every day	16
2-5 days	18
1-2 weeks	28
2-4 weeks	18
1-3 months	20
Worse during menstruation	18
Family History:	
Headaches	48
Asthma	12
Nasal allergy	10
Eczema	8
GI symptoms	8
Personal History:	
½ headache	14
Nausea	37
Lights in vision	16
Vomiting	28
Distorted vision	18
Dizziness	19
Pain	
occular	41
frontal	65
temples	28
occiput	32
nuchal	28
Nasal allergy	26
Hives	3
Eczema	14
Indigestion	22
Constipation	18
Indicated Causes:	
Food allergy	87
Food and pollen allergy	7
Pollen allergy alone	6

When the patients consulted us, the headaches usually had been present for five to even fifty years. They had continued for one day or less frequently or for two to even ten days. Their recurrence from daily to a few days, weeks, or even months is shown in the statistics. Nightly headaches at intervals for two years and every night at 2 to 3 AM for two months relieved by 10 grains of aspirin occurred for the first time in a man fifty-five years of age as a result of milk which had produced diarrhea for forty years. Though avoided as such, total elimination of it and all of its products was necessary to stop his headaches. The frequency of nausea and vomiting and the location of pain in or in back of one or both eyes, in the frontal, occipital, temporal, nuchal, and other adjoining areas in our cases is shown as is the frequency of other manifestations of allergy. The occurrence of dizziness, of half or distorted vision, and of colored or white lights or scotomata indicates that migraine or its equivalent was present which was relieved by our recognition and control of allergy, especially to foods. The occurrence of drowsiness, irritability, depression, body aching, and especially fatigue which we have long reported in the syndrome *allergic toxemia and fatigue* (Chapt. 19) in a considerable number of these patients suffering with allergic headaches or definite migraine needs emphasis. That allergy especially to foods and less often to pollens (in 6%) is the cause instead of the frequently blamed tension or psychoneurosis must be stressed. In the family history headache is the major manifestation of possible allergy in these cases (48%), as is asthma in the family history of asthmatics.

Since food allergy often causes resultant manifestations with interim relief as discussed in Chapter 2, headaches resulting from such allergy may be activated by menstrual periods, justifying study of such allergy as we advise. If this fails, allergy

to hormones with gonadotropic hormones as advised by Phillips in 1943 may be justified.

Ophthalmic migraine even with hemianopsia is discussed on pages 399 to 401 of Chapter 20.

TYPICAL CASES OF ALLERGIC HEADACHE AND MIGRAINE

These histories exemplify the frequency, duration, and location of pain; occurrence of gastrointestinal, ocular, and toxic symptoms; and the indicated allergic causes.

Case 96: A woman fifty-nine years of age had sudden recurrent, pulsating right-sided sick headaches for two to three days for forty years, recurring every three to four months, four having been present in the last three months. The father, sister, brother, and paternal aunt had similar headaches. The patient's headaches were relieved with our CFE diet. A typical headache occurred twenty minutes after eating salmon. Another occurred twenty-eight hours after the inhalation of the odor of fish meal fertilizer on a neighbor's lawn. Boysenberries caused headaches in twenty-four hours. Later on the inclusion of eggs produced headaches. These headaches were absent for three years until the smell of fish fertilizer on a lawn next door produced an extremely severe attack. With the elimination of wheat, milk, chocolate, corn, egg, fish, coffee, and spices, no headaches have occurred in six years.

Case 97: A woman forty-eight years of age had had monthly headaches with her periods for twelve years. They were bilateral, starting in the frontal or occipital area, and always associated with nausea and vomiting, each lasting three to four days with a gradual decrease in symptoms in seven days. Photophobia was marked. Fatigue and abdominal distention continued between the headaches. Canker and cold sores had been relieved by the elimination of fruit. The patient had found "wheat was poison." With a wheat, milk, egg, and fruit-free diet, the headaches and canker sores were relieved.

Case 98: A man thirty-eight years of age had bilious attacks associated with violent nausea and right frontal headache every month or two most of his life. Since the age of twenty years they had decreased in frequency. For two years he had

had sudden attacks of floating bodies before the eyes followed by impaired vision, inability to read fine print, tingling in the hands and feet, weakness, and marked faintness, followed by severe nausea and frontal headache. Increasing drowsiness and finally a heavy sleep for three to four hours had followed. For one year he had found that the attacks developed fourteen to sixteen hours after eating even a minute amount of garlic or a moderate amount of onion. The last attack resulted from eating three olives dipped in oil flavored with garlic! He had disliked onions, garlic, turnips, and tomatoes for years. No other food allergy was present in his personal history, though mild allergic manifestations were present in his family history.

Physical examination, laboratory tests, and skin reactions to foods were negative except for a delayed reaction to garlic. No gastrointestinal attacks or visual or mental disturbances have occurred for two years since the entire exclusion of garlic.

Comment: This case is of special interest because of the violent allergic reactions resulting from a minute amount of food—the mere flavor of garlic. The history of visual and nervous disturbances and drowsiness associated with migraine is not infrequent. This patient had eaten raw onions as he would apples in childhood and probably became sensitized to onions and garlic at the same time.

STUDY AND CONTROL OF FOOD ALLERGY

Chronic, especially recurrently activated headaches that are not due to the causes listed in the first paragraphs of this chapter require study of possible atopic allergy as the cause. If the headaches and associated symptoms (Table XXXIX) are perennial and especially if increased in the winter, food allergy must be adequately studied as advised below.

If headaches occur in the spring, summer, and fall and are less active or absent in the winter, pollen allergy may be the sole cause or associated with food allergy. Though definite reactions to pollens usually occur, they may be absent even if pollen allergy is responsible. Moreover, positive skin reactions to pollens may occur which play no etiological role in the headaches.

This occurrence of pollen allergy as a cause of recurrent or chronic headaches requires study of a similar role of other inhalants, including animal emanations; house, feed, and other occupational dusts; and other miscellaneous inhalants as possible causes. Confirmation of such allergies has occurred infrequently in our practice.

Because of the fallibility of skin testing in indicating clinical food allergies, diet trial, especially with the adequate and accurate use of our cereal-free elimination diet, is indicated as advised in Chapter 3 and reiterated throughout this volume. If a decrease or relief of the headaches and associated symptoms fails in two to three weeks, our fruit-free and cereal-free elimination diet may be ordered, especially if definite or possible fruit allergy is indicated in the patient's history. And if such diet trial does not relieve the symptoms in two to three weeks, a minimal diet containing a few foods which infrequently cause allergy should be used before food allergy is eliminated as a cause. If relief is evident and maintained with the diet for twice as long as previous periods of relief, individual foods can be added, eliminating those which have been included in the previous one to two weeks.

Such diet trial must be accurately maintained and strictly supervised by the physician. The gradual recognition of single or several foods which have been responsible for the headaches and the associated symptoms amply justifies the time and effort necessary to utilize diet trial in an accurate and strict manner. Without such recognition of food allergy, these recurrent headaches with varying degrees of invalidism, toxic symptoms, and impaired efficiency in life's activities and responsibilities will continue for months or years.

STUDY AND CONTROL OF POLLEN ALLERGY

When pollen allergy is indicated by history with or without skin tests, an antigen containing the important pollens in the air during the months when the headaches are present must be administered, starting with a dilution of the antigen below the weakest that gives a positive scratch test with gradually increased doses through the stronger dilutions up to a dose in the 1:5000 to a 1:100 which is tolerated without producing a general reaction. This procedure gave excellent relief in the following case.

SEASONAL HEADACHES FOR FIVE YEARS AS A RESULT OF POLLEN ALLERGY

Case 99: A man forty-eight years of age had had severe pain in the left temple awakening him during the night "as though he had been hit," lasting two to three minutes radiating into the surrounding face and scalp usually associated with nausea and at times vomiting for four to five minutes. Pain has continued for one to two hours. Help from heat was questionable. Cafergot® had helped in one-half hour. At times a second one was required to relieve pain in two to four hours. Bright lights increased pain. Irritability followed relief.

Of great importance was the onset of the headaches in mid-March, continuing nearly daily through spring and summer until November with no pain in the winters for six years. Pain was increased when he operated his railroad locomotive in country areas, especially on windy days. There was no history of any other manifestation of allergy, especially of hay fever or asthma.

Diet history suggestive of food allergy was negative. Neither was there a family history of clinical allergy. Examination and advice from "twenty-five doctors" and treatment in a railroad hospital had failed. Skin testing revealed one and two plus reactions to several grass, fall, and tree pollens by the scratch method. There was no clinical evidence of allergy to *Hormodendron*, to which a five plus scratch reaction occurred.

X-rays of the sinuses and skull were negative. Routine laboratory work was negative.

Treatment and Results: Since allergy to the spring, summer, and fall pollens was indicated by history and skin reactions, desensitization to a multiple antigen containing such pollens in his living and working environments was started with a 1:500 million dilution which failed to react by a scratch test. The injections were given two times a week during the summer. Oral Aristocort 4 mg t.i.d. for four days was gradually eliminated in three weeks. In three months he was tolerating 0.3 cc of the 1:100 dilution. His headaches had been absent for two months in spite of operating his locomotive in the country where pain was severe before our treatment.

Since then, weekly injections of 0.7 cc of 1:100 of his antigen were given for two years and every two weeks for four years. No headaches have occurred for five years.

Comment: This seasonal history of cerebral allergy would have required desensitization to the pollens even if scratch tests had been absent.

This case emphasizes the important inquiry about seasonal occurrence which "25 previous physicians" had failed to do.

Though allergy to foods is the usual cause of allergic headaches, their daily absence in the winter excluded its probability.

Three of our patients relieved by pollen therapy reported previous excruciating headaches during the height of the pollen season which had prevented work and necessitated bed rest and much pain-relieving medication. Along with pollen desensitization, environmental control of airborne pollens with efficient air filtration and environmental control in the living and working environments is indicated. Such control will minimize inhalation of dusts which may contain pollens as well as other inhalant allergens to which actual or unsuspected allergy may be present.

As stated above, the possibility of headaches from animal emanations, fungi, and miscellaneous environmental and occupational inhalants is suggested by the headaches resulting from pollen allergy. Our failure to recognize such allergy does not rule out its possibility.

Seven additional case histories (53 to 59) of migraine with gastrointestinal symptoms, toxemia and vasomotor disturbances are summarized in the first edition of this book in 1931 and also in Cases 20, 21, 22, 23, 24, 25, 26, 31, 32, and 36 in *Clinical Allergy* in 1937.

HISTAMINE HEADACHES

Histaminic or Horton's headaches are unilateral, severe, and throbbing usually in the eye, forehead, or temple, lasting up to sixty minutes. Unilateral nasal and conjunctival congestion and lacrimation and flushing of face are frequent. They may occur daily for three to seven days, recurring in weeks or months, often awakening the patient at 3 to 4 AM. They are due to dilation of the extracranial arteries and develop after the hypodermic injection of histamine base.

Ergotamine drugs given parenterally or rectally may relieve the pain.

Desensitization to histamine often decreases or relieves the susceptibility to these headaches. Starting with the hypodermic injection of .05 cc of a solution of 0.25 mg histamine acid phosphate in 1 cc of sterile water (0.1 mg of histamine base), the dose is increased by 0.05 cc every twelve hours until flushing of the face or a mild headache occurs, the dose varying between 0.3 to 0.8 cc. The dose is then decreased to a slightly reactive dose which is repeated daily for two to four weeks, providing relief of the headache has occurred. Then the injection can be given every two to four days, especially if headaches tend to recur.

This histamine desensitization may relieve headaches, moreover, that have been partially benefited by control of food allergy as discussed in the last paragraphs of this chapter.

TREATMENT OF THE SYMPTOMS OF ALLERGIC HEADACHE AND MIGRAINE

Until the headaches and associated symptoms are relieved by the control of causative food and less often pollen allergies, the following medications are advised for the control of pain.

1. Aspirin 5 to 10 grains with or without phenacetin 2 to 3 grains every four to eight hours relieves some of the moderate pain. Allergy to aspirin causing severe bronchial asthma, urticaria, or gastrointestinal bleeding and other symptoms must be remembered. Toxic effects arise at times to continued phenacetin.

2. Codeine ¼ to ½ grains by mouth with or without aspirin every four to eight hours is often remedial.

3. Other drugs are advised for the relief of pain with or without codeine by various pharmaceutical companies, including Darvon® and Equagesic®. However, they infrequently relieve typical migraine.

Methyl sergide (Sansert®) 2 mg three times a day prevents migraine in some cases, but because of possible resultant retroperitoneal fibrosis, its continued use may be hazardous.

4. Ergotamine tartrate (Gynergen® or Cafergot) advised for the control of migraine headaches since 1932 apparently causes a dilatation of the cerebral arterioles resulting in a depression of sympathetic ennervation.

An initial subcutaneous injection of 0.25 mg may be effective. If relief fails, 0.5 mg every two to three hours may be given. An initial intravenous injection of 0.25 mg may be advisable. The effect, moreover, varies and at times decreases if given for weeks or months. This emphasizes the importance of determining and controlling the allergic causes.

It is also advised in doses of 1 to 2 mg by mouth followed by 1 mg doses every fifteen minutes for not more than 5 to 6 mg. Migral® containing ergotamine, caffeine, and an antiemetic cyclizine may be effective. Cafergot rectal suppositories containing 2 mg ergotamine may be beneficial.

Gangrene of the feet and even death in one patient have been reported from repeated use of ergotamine tartrate. This was caused by occlusion of small arteries and arterioles from constriction and thromboses. The drug should not be used in patients with vascular disease, including arteriosclerosis and especially in Buerger's disease. Because of its effect on the uterine muscle, it should not be used in pregnancy.

5. Since desensitization to histamine helps and relieves the throbbing headaches described by Horton, this therapy has been given to patients with headaches being studied for possible allergy which do not respond satisfactorily to various elimination diets. This subcutaneous injection of histamine has produced relief in some patients, indicating a probable histamine type of headache. In some patients the elimination of specific foods as well as histamine desensitization has given the desired relief.

SUMMARY

1. The importance of the study of atopic allergy, especially to foods, as the cause of migraine and recurrent headaches has been confirmed by us for forty years.

2. Allergic headache and migraine require strict, adequate, expertised study of food allergy as indicated especially by recurrent attacks which are marked indications of food allergy (Chapt. 1). Other manifestations of food allergy in the personal and family histories emphasize this challenge.

3. The pathogenesis of allergic migraine is discussed. Literature since 1919 indicating food allergy is summarized.

4. The frequency and duration of clinical allergy in the family history, the location of pain, the ocular symptoms, and the predominance of food allergy over pollen allergy in the etiology of one hundred relieved cases are tabulated.

5. Informative records of seven of our several hundred patients relieved by our study and control of food allergy in the last forty years are summarized.

6. The record of severe headaches for six years as a result of allergy unrelieved by advice from "twenty-five physicians" emphasizes the importance of a seasonal history, as in this case of headaches occurring only during the spring, summer, and fall months and absent in the winter.

7. Importance of control of indicated food and infrequent pollen allergy and of medications for preliminary relief, including histamine therapy when indicated, until relief of food allergy and (when indicated) inhalant allergy occurs are emphasized.

Chapter 18

Cerebral and Neural Allergy

In the last fifty years increasing reports have been published of symptoms and disabilities arising from allergic reactions in the brain, spinal cord, and cranial and peripheral nerves relieved by the elimination of foods and by the control of inhalant, especially pollen allergy and at times by the control of drug and chemical allergies. This relief has been attributed to the control of cerebral and neural allergy. Cerebral and neural allergy resulting from allergy to animal sera, sulfonamides, and also to penicillin, other drugs, and even to viruses is reported by Ratner in his excellent book in 1943. He reported aphasia, ataxia, and paralysis of cranial and peripheral nerves. Many manifestations of cerebral allergy discussed by Davison are summarized later in this chapter.

Physicians considering allergy as a cause of headache, vomiting, dizziness, Meniere's syndrome, convulsions, epilepsy, transient paralysis, and recurrent psychosis can benefit by reading Clarke's articles in 1944 and 1950.

In his excellent article on the historical development of allergy in the nervous system, Speer, in 1958, stated: "As the physician . . . recognizes that the allergic reaction knows no bounds of tissue or organ including the central nervous system, he will find himself in a position to bring relief to many sufferers from nervous conditions." He quotes Foster Kennedy's prediction in his discussion of CNS allergy in 1936: "The solution of many epilepsies, migraine, and other paroxysmal disorders including, I believe, many psychoses are behind the locked doors of which we pick at." As I emphasized in Chapter 2, paroxysmal recurrent manifestations always require study of food allergy as a very likely cause.

EXPERIMENTALLY PRODUCED ALLERGY IN THE CENTRAL NERVOUS SYSTEM

That the tissues of the central nervous system are susceptible to allergic reactions has long been evidenced in experimentally produced allergy in animals. Vascular allergy producing perivascular round cell infiltration, hemorrhages, and occasional thromboses with diffuse degeneration of nerve cells in the parenchyma of cerebral tissues occur in experimentally produced anaphylactic shock. When it is prolonged, areas of encephalomalacia occur. Davidoff and Kopeloff applied an antigen to the motor area of a dog's brain with no reaction. Intravenous injection of the antigen days later caused weakness in the muscles on the opposite side, followed by convulsions. Alexander and Campbell sensitized guinea pigs intraperitoneally. Later intracerebral injections caused localized hemorrhage, edema, leukocytic infiltration, and serum exudation. Jervis *et al.* found necroses in the center of the lesions of Arthus phenomena in such animals with varying destruction in myelin sheaths and lesser involvement in the axis cylinders and glia of nerve fibers in the periphery of the lesions. These were scattered through the brain, cerebellum, and medulla, containing glitter cells, few blood elements, and peculiar giant cells. The authors suggested that brain-specific antibodies were operative.

For an informative and further discussion of the pathological changes from experimental anaphylaxis in animals, the reader is referred to its discussion by Urbach and Gottlieb in 1946.

ALLERGIC TOXEMIA AND FATIGUE

Allergic toxemia and fatigue are next to headache the most frequent manifestations of cerebral and neural allergy. We first reported the symptoms of and named this syndrome in 1928 and in the first edition of this book in 1931. It now has received extended discussion in Chapter 19.

TRANSIENT CEREBRAL ALLERGY

Food allergy and less often pollen or other inhalant and occasionally bacterial allergies are recognized causes of cerebral reactions causing stupor, confusion, headache, unconsciousness or convulsions, transient paresis, paralyses or paresthesias, and cranial nerve involvements. Bizarre combinations occur, indicating scattered reactions of varying degrees and persistence. Multiple sclerosis may be simulated or possibly arise, as discussed later in this chapter. Persistent allergic reactions, moreover, might produce gliosis in nervous tissues, as suggested by Cooke in 1936. The frequency of transient cerebral and neural allergy from animal sera is also noted later in this chapter.

Davison, in 1949, in an excellent article on Cerebral Allergy especially to foods, reported paresthesias, twitchings, jerking, weakness and paralysis, faintness, vertigo, loss of consciousness (at times with convulsions), and headaches (especially from allergy to milk, chocolate, eggs, fish, shell-fish, onions, cabbage, nuts, apples, and less to other foods). He also confirmed many of the cerebral symptoms in the syndrome *Allergic Fatigue and Toxemia* first reported in 1931 and in subsequent books and articles, as summarized in Chapter 19 of this volume. In discussion of Davison's article Rinkel, Huber, and Thomas confirmed such cerebral allergy.

These transient dysfunctions in nervous tissues often (but not necessarily) occur when urticaria and especially localized edema in nervous and other tissues are present.

Quincke, Osler, and Oppenheim have reported transient hemiplegia and other disturbances in nerve function in patients with angioneurotic edema which, it is generally agreed, is due to vascular allergy especially to foods and less often to drugs, inhalants, physical agents, and possibly to bacteria. Bassoe reported recurrent aphasia and right hemianopsia with right-sided paresis in such a patient. Two exploratory craniotomies were performed. One revealed a soft hyperemic swelling of the brain. Kennedy especially reported cases of this type. One patient also had had deep, painful swellings of the muscles and skin for five years. Transient drowsiness, headache, impaired speech, decreased or absent vision or hearing, and even incontinence of feces and urine recurred with the swellings. Milk and veal allergy was suspected. Pardee and Winkelman recorded similar cases. Vaughan and Hawke reported meningismus with cephalic pain and various peripheral nerve disturbances and vasomotor instability in a patient with angioneurotic edema. Intermittent hydroarthrosis and bronchial symptoms also were present. Egg and tomato allergy were responsible. Staffiere, Dentiolila, and Levit (1952) reported right hemiparesis in a girl twenty-nine years of age who also had asthma, both relieved by the elimination of wheat. Kennedy reported a girl two years of age with giant urticaria and screaming three to four times a day with later convulsions and unconsciousness. With the elimination of milk there was no recurrence in twelve years.

The challenge of studying food allergy as we advise as a concomitant cause of fever and convulsions in febrile seizures when they recur is also noted in Chapter 24 on Allergic Fever and Chapter 25 on Allergy in Infants and Children.

PERSONAL CASES

Case 100: A man forty-six years of age had had swellings of his neck, face, tongue, pharynx, abdomen, and especially his feet occurring every one to four weeks for twenty-two years. For two years he had also had severe nuchal headaches, spreading to the occipital, temporal, and ocular areas; a staggering gait; inability to focus his eyes; mental stupor; pain in the abdomen and bladder; drowsiness; and a deep sleep for one to three days. Epinephrine hypodermically alleviated his headaches and drowsiness.

Sick headaches every two to four weeks had been experienced for ten years. Constipation for twenty years had occurred. Nervousness, dullness, and a "dumb, stupid feeling" had interfered with his teaching.

Skin reactions to all important foods and inhalant allergens were negative by the scratch tests.

With an elimination diet his severe headaches have disappeared. His stupor and staggering gait and other symptoms are absent, though twelve hours after eating celery drowsiness occurred for thirty-six hours, and a slight swelling in his right foot developed. His bowels are normal for the first time in twenty years. Provocation feeding tests revealed that wheat, corn, rye, milk, eggs, fish, celery, and all fruits and condiments caused his symptoms.

As stated above, allergic reactions may occur in the nervous tissues with no obvious history of hives or localized swellings, asthma, or other manifestations of clinical allergy. Foster Kennedy, in 1938, reported attacks of blindness in either eye and a normal plantar reflex and disturbances in

sensation of the thalmic type from probable pork allergy.

Mathieu reported great fatigue, dizziness, and coma for twelve hours with delirium, vomiting, flaccid paralysis of the right arm, and absent deep reflexes along with giant hives on the torso and extremities from allergy to pork. After the hives and swellings disappeared, normal sensations required one month to return!

Varying degrees of headache and dizziness from late February to early November because of tree, grass and fall pollens in our bay area for six years were controlled by desensitization to seasonal pollens.

ALLERGIC EPILEPSY

In the first edition of this book in 1931 and in *Clinical Allergy* in 1938, we stated that "allergy as a cause of certain cases of epilepsy is being recognized with increasing frequency." Such cases have been reported by Pagniez and Lieutand (1919). Ward (1922, 1927), Howell (1923), and Wallis, Nicol, and Craig (1923) studied many epileptics from the viewpoint of food allergy. Gracie (1924) studied two patients with epilepsy who had the purpura, urticaria, and abdominal symptoms of Henoch's syndrome. He stated that the convulsions were probably due to urticarial-like lesions in the meninges or cerebral cortex or to sudden temporary vascular spasms.

Epilepsy resulting from pollen allergy was first reported by us in 1927. We agree with Foster Kennedy, who wrote: "The evidence that many cases of epilepsy constitute a sensitization disease cannot be safely ignored." Allergic inflammation and spasm in the vascular tissues with edema, cellular infiltration, and changes in the adjacent tissues may occur in any part of the brain, the brain stem, or even in the cord. Thus the recurring alternations in consciousness with or without terminal convulsions and the varying degrees of paresthesia; visual and cranial nerve disturbances; fainting; or vasomotor, sudomotor, or cardiac symptoms may be explained. These tissue reactions from localized allergy could produce anoxemia, altered conductivity of the nerve fibers, and changed membrane permeability, recognized by Cobb as underlying causes of the fits. The reactions persist for different times and even may cause irreversible tissue changes.

Favoring allergy as one cause is the common familial association of epilepsy with migraine and sick headaches which are so often due to allergy, as noted in Chapter 17. The good results, moreover, reported from ketogenic and starvation diets suggest the possible exclusion of foods to which the patient was allergic.

Miller long maintained that allergy is a frequent cause of epilepsy and in 1924 wrote an excellent and important article on "Evidence that Idiopathic Epilepsy is a Sensitization Disease." Van Leeuwen (1925) stated that epilepsy and migraine were at times a result of allergy. Duke, in 1923 and in his book (1926), described a case of convulsions, coma, and transitory paralysis resulting from food allergy. In 1927 we reported two cases of epilepsy controlled by pollen therapy, summarized in our article on Allergy in *CNS Tissues* in 1944. Kennedy (1931) recorded an interesting instance of epilepsy and urticaria resulting from milk allergy. Balyeat (1928) reported two cases of epilepsy resulting from food allergy and in various publications since then has recorded other cases. Moore relieved one child of epilepsy of five years' duration by the exclusion of egg. Rowe and Richet (1930) recorded epilepsy in a woman thirty-seven years of age existent for seventeen years, occurring one to two times a week with interim mild spells for seven years. In addition, a nocturnal spasmodic cough was present. Wheat was the causative factor as determined by our "elimination diets." Weisenburg, Yaskin,

and Pleasants (1931) recorded epilepsy in a boy twelve years of age in whom an appendectomy and exploratory operation because of cecal stasis were performed who was not relieved until the mother eliminated milk from the diet. Levin (1931) found cheese as a cause of epilepsy in a child three years of age. One of our patients had recurrent attacks even at the table after eating pork. Wilson and Hadden (1931) reported Jacksonian epilepsy resulting from wheat. Forman (1934) relieved five cases with test-negative diets and one other case with "elimination diets." Perez-Moreno described an epilepticlike attack arising from food allergy. Guglielmini and Molinari (1935) reported epileptiform syndrome from ascaris allergy.

Of special interest was the report of Wilmer and Miller (1934) of epilepsy for nineteen years in a man thirty-four years of age. Sudden nausea, headache, dizziness, and mental confusion initiated his attacks. Gradual recovery occurred, though visual disturbances persisted. Later sleepiness, languor, and slight jaundice returned, and one week later a generalized convulsion in his sleep occurred. At college he had difficulty in thinking clearly. Seven months later a second convulsion arose. Drowsiness set in, and three months later he had a third convulsion during sleep. Nervousness, depression, reduced sexual power, headache, and recurrent seizures continued for three months. Psychoneurosis was diagnosed. Fatigue and headache persisted. In one year, because of another convulsion, an exploratory craniotomy with negative findings was done. For five years symptoms continued. He had paresthesias in the left hand. With severe pains, convulsions occurred. Finally allergy was considered. Test-negative diets were ineffective, but with Rowe's Elimination Diet No. 1, with milk, tomato, and cod-liver oil, his symptoms were controlled.

All of this emphasizes food allergy and the importance of diet trial in the study of idiopathic epilepsy and toxemia.

McQuarrie (1932, 1934), Peterman (1934), Talbot (1930), and other students of epilepsy have emphasized the necessity of considering the many possible causes of convulsions such as acute infections, cerebral birth injuries, meningitis, brain tumors and cysts, chronic encephalitis, congenital brain defects, hydrocephalus, tetany, brain injury, intracranial vascular lesions, lues, pertussis, malaria, and gastrointestinal disturbances. In the presence of Jacksonian epilepsy Fincher and Dowman (1931) have stressed the necessity of ruling out brain tumor, localized scars in the brain from trauma, thickened meninges with adhesions, cystic formations, organized subdural clots, cerebral atrophy with collections of fluid, birth trauma, cerebral atrophy, syphilis, arteriosclerosis, and other less frequent causes.

In 1938 Kennedy reported epilepsy in a boy thirteen years of age relieved by the elimination of milk and in a man by the elimination of milk and eggs. Davison (1949) reported convulsions arising from food allergy. Leney (1957) reported five cases of epilepsy resulting, in his opinion, from food allergy.

Dees and Lowenbach (1951) reported evidence in EEG tracings of epilepsy relieved by the control of allergy to foods. Occipital dysrhythmia occurred in fifteen of twenty-two allergic children with convulsive disorders without evidence of clinical allergy. Occipital dysrhythmia occurred in eleven, frontal dysrhythmia in four, and a spike wave pattern in two. The absence of other manifestations of allergy in the latter group indicates that the tissues in the brain may have been the only shock areas of allergy as are nasal tissues in some patients with hay fever and the lungs in some

patients with bronchial asthma. Therefore, EEG occipital dysrhythmia occurred in 73 percent of thirty-seven allergic children with convulsive disorders compared with the occurrence in only 45 percent of sixty-three allergic children with no convulsive disorders. Thus occipital dysrhythmia is not definitely diagnostic of epilepsy as is the low spike and wave arising from petit mal or the high voltage fast wave from grand mal.

The following case is illustrative of other cases reported by Dees and Lowenbach.

Case 101: A boy ten years of age had grand mal seizures for three years with moderate hay fever. EEG showed dysrhythmia and spikes in all six waves. With an elimination diet and desensitization to pollens, no seizures occurred for one year. Without the diet or pollen therapy, however, marked nervousness and inattention in his school occurred. With their resumption, convulsions, tensions, and inattention in school work disappeared.

Comment: The relief of epilepsy with practically normal EEG tracing evidences the importance of studying atopic allergy as an important cause by all physicians.

Summaries of three cases of convulsive seizures reported from an article on neurological allergy by M. B. Campbell in 1968 follow:

1. A nineteen-year-old woman had petit mal-like attacks with vertigo and epigastric distress since the age of seven years. The EEG showed dysrhythmia with bursts of activity indicting petit mal. Analeptic drugs failed to control symptoms. Confusion with dilated pupils for forty-five minutes biweekly were attributed to petit mal. Epigastric distress continued. Rhinorrhea for years indicated nasal allergy. With an elimination diet all symptoms gradually disappeared. Milk and chocolate proved responsible.

2. An eight-year-old girl had petit mal attacks with vertigo at times associated with a severe headache and episodes of macropsia and micropsia. Her EEG showed diffuse dysrhythmia with bursts of polymorphic nonspecific seizure activity. Medications caused a rash. Confusion and disorientation with frequent petit mal status developed which caused difficulty in eating meals. Elimina-

tion diets and provocation tests showed that tomatoes, oranges, peanuts, and chocolate caused rashes, irritability, confusion, and other cerebral symptoms. Skin tests showed marked reactions to pollens and dust. Desensitization to inhalants and elimination of allergenic foods gave marked relief from petit mal, vertigo, headaches, and other cerebral symptoms.

3. A man of twenty-four years of age had convulsive seizures from the age of twelve to sixteen years associated with left deviation of the head and upward deviation of the eyes associated with vertigo. The EEG showed a diffuse paroxysmal pattern with random bursts of polymorphic wave activity. An aunt had grand mal seizures. Brief amnesia and headache occurred with vertigo after which the patient found himself in unfamiliar areas. With an elimination diet marked improvement occurred. Wheat and tobacco smoke caused vertigo, confusion, and disorientation. Green beans especially caused severe agitation and depression for several hours. Fein and Kamin, in 1968, discussed convulsive disorders and epilepsy resulting from allergy to foods and especially to pollens, dusts, and fungi.

CASES OF EPILEPSY IN OUR PRACTICE RELIEVED BY CONTROL OF ATOPIC ALLERGY

Case 102: A boy sixteen years of age had had Jacksonian epileptic grand mal attacks every two to six weeks for six or seven years. Forewarning of tingling and twitching in the right fifth finger also occurred at times with no convulsive seizures. He had seasonal hay fever but no other allergic manifestations. His family history was negative for epilepsy, migraine, or other allergic manifestations. Skin testing showed several reactions to foods as shown by intradermal testing. With elimination diets his Jacksonian epilepsy disappeared and later only recurred when egg was eaten. Of interest was the fact that foods giving positive intradermal skin tests were tolerated without difficulty. Egg, which caused his epilepsy, gave no skin reactions. The young man graduated from college, played tennis strenuously, and is a teacher of music in school. Twenty years later ingested egg still caused convulsions.

Case 103: A girl eleven years of age had had petit mal attacks for about six years. She could never be alone and had them in school as well as home. Her mother had had hay fever. Skin tests

gave positive reactions to cat, horse, and rabbit hair proteins. Desensitization to horse hair and removal of her hair mattress has resulted in complete relief from her attacks for over two year.

DIAGNOSIS AND CONTROL OF ATOPIC ALLERGY IN EPILEPSY

As advised at the end of this chapter, the reader is referred to our Chapters 2 and 3 on the diagnosis and control of allergy to foods, inhalants, and other allergies. This advice, moreover, is summarized in Chapter 17 on Allergic Headache and Migraine and Chapter 19 on Allergic Fatigue and Toxemia.

When petit or grand mal or equivalents of epilepsy are present or possible, information from EEG studies and if indicated brain scans, x-ray studies (including possible spinal fluid examinations) to rule out other pathological causes is important.

Even when allergy is a sole or major cause, until its entire control is attained, anticonvulsive medications, especially Dilantin, Mebaral®, or others advised by neurologists, are indicated. Benefit may result from adjunctive and reducing doses of corticosteroids. As control of the atopic allergy increases, the above medications can be reduced and at times eliminated. Until they are stopped, toxic and allergic complications from the medication must be anticipated, and indicated laboratory tests must be performed.

MENTAL AND EMOTIONAL SYMPTOMS RESULTING FROM FOOD ALLERGY

Psychological and emotional deviations from normal frequently arise from cerebral allergy to foods and at times to inhalants, especially pollens. Allergic edema and vascular inflammation with associated and resultant changes in the tissues of the meninges and especially in the frontal lobes probably occur. In addition to the loginess, drowsiness, impaired ability to concentrate, confusion, depression, tenseness, and emotional instability in the syndrome, allergic fatigue and toxemia, which we first reported in 1928 and 1931 and which we have extensively discussed in Chapter 19, irritability, rebelliousness, continued crying, tantrums, and screaming may occur in children. Whether allergy in the cerebral or other body tissues is responsible for the marked fatigue, localized and generalized body aching, fever and occasionally night sweats, chilling, and goose flesh which occur in some patients afflicted with this syndrome cannot be definitely answered.

This syndrome has increasingly been confirmed by other allergists, especially by Randolph, Clarke, Davison, and Steer. Crook has stressed its frequency in the practice of pediatrics and has noted the dark circles under the eyes, the yellow complexion, the lack of interest in play and school, fatigue, as well as other symptoms which we originally reported in 1930 in the first edition of this book. He states that these symptoms resulting from allergy, especially to foods, are often incorrectly attributed to psychoneurosis, cerebral palsy, hypothyroidism, rheumatic fever, mental retardation, and even to trichinosis.

Control of many marked psychological and physical symptoms justifying the diagnosis of allergic toxemia and fatigue by the elimination of foods excluded from our CFE diet is reported in the following letters from the children's mothers.

Case 104: Mental and emotional symptoms in a boy eight years of age. "After being strictly on your CFE diet for four months, dramatic changes both physical and mental have occurred, some in a matter of days:

1. Constant nasal drip stopped and sores in mouth are gone.
2. Mouth breathing and snoring stopped.
3. Bad breath stopped.
4. Night sweating and occasional night fever stopped.
5. Extreme head sweating stopped (drenched pillow completely through).
6. Sleeps normally now (previously could not be aroused by light, noise, or shaking).
7. Requires only normal hours of sleep for age (always slept the clock around before).
8. Awakens bright-eyed and cheerful.
9. Before diet, eyes were very swollen on awakening, and swelling existed all day. Child was very irritable.
10. Teeth are straightening since sleeping with closed mouth (retainer used at night because of protruding front teeth).
11. Infantile speech because of tongue thrust caused by sore throat is rapidly improving.
12. Sense of smell is gradually improving. Was lost completely.
13. He is gaining weight.
14. Has lost fanatic craving for sweets.
15. Has slowed down to normal. Does not have the uncontrollable destructive energy that drove him into a frenzy and then left him unapproachable and exhausted.
16. He never cried before and could not be reached. He now sheds a tear and is eager for affection.
17. Car-sickness has abated. Since infancy he became nauseated only a few blocks away from home. Now he holds food down on long trips.
18. Does not have chills during the day. Insisted on wearing a jacket and hat during the warmest days.
19. Feet do not perspire. Had to change socks often, as feet would blister and peel. Dripped with perspiration at slightest activity (which was almost constant). Hair had to be washed daily as it had an odd sour odor.
20. Body itched all over (still does to some extent on back). Ears bled from infancy from scratching. Itch has subsided, and ears are free from scabs.
21. Is no longer vicious. Does not hate the boys with whom he competes. Seems more secure and less jealous. Concentrates much better. Always has been bright in school studies but failed socially. Is now being accepted by other children. Can play games without cheating and beating up the winner. Accepts responsibility. Has confidence in himself and can now play games and accept winning or losing gracefully.

"His teachers reported that the children were afraid of him, as he had such a desire to fight. He would injure his classmates. He was a spoil-sport and took joy in ruining one game after another. His excuse for fighting was that they were trying to push him around. They could not reach him. I was requested by the school to put him under psychiatric treatment.

"Within the last few months he has adjusted so well his teacher has nothing but praise, and his cry has changed from, 'I hate them, they are always pushing me around,' to a happy shout of 'They like me, Ma, I'm the leader.'"

The relief has continued during the last eight years.

Case 105: Mental and emotional symptoms in a boy six years of age.

"Up to age two our boy seemed normal and healthy. He had an excellent disposition and would sit and play for hours, singing to himself. At age two he became irritable, and we assumed he was entering the frustrating two-year-old period psychologists talk about. This condition continued until age 6½ when he went on your elimination diet.

"During the ages two to five he developed many persistent colds with no cough. Two pediatricians stated that his colds were caused by allergy, but no attempt was made to find a specific cause. He perspired freely at night.

"At age three he was in a nursery school. He did not get along with the children. Temper tantrums and fights were the norm. The director said that he did not feel well enough to fit into a group. He insisted on doing what he wanted to do. Spanking annoyed him but was ineffective. His attention was very brief. He often awoke complaining of headaches. He could not adjust to kindergarten. He threw tantrums. He was not popular with the other children. He seemed unable to change easily from one activity to another. Headaches became more frequent. He came home from kindergarten dragging. He was unhappy at home.

"His first-grade teacher reported that he was too nervous to learn. His voice would quaver and his hands would tremble when he tried to respond in class. She said his tantrums did not result from discipline but rather from nervous frustration. He would set his goals impossibly high, fail, and go into a screaming, kicking, destructive, irrational state. His coordination was so poor that learning to write was almost impossible. He woke up with headaches three times

a week. Bedwetting has continued all through life.

"The family doctor recommended tranquilizers, which helped considerably, but they were not the long-range solution. Psychiatric care was recommended, but we decided to test for allergy first.

"Your elimination diet was begun January 4, 1961. In two weeks' time headaches stopped. The tranquilizers were discontinued. In three to four weeks he was completely changed. There was a sparkle in his eyes that we had not seen in years. He had a calm outlook on life, not belligerent as before. He began to play with other boys, and they began to like him and include him in their play. He no longer wets the bed at night.

"Six weeks after the start of the diet we began to add other foods. Some gave immediate reactions, such as eggs (diarrhea), applesauce, pepper (added by mistake), and grapefruit (tantrums and bedwetting). Others seemed all right for a week, but then frustration began. The slow responders were oatmeal, corn, and rice. The symptoms we look for are headaches in the morning, irritability, a far-away look in his eyes, and a wet bed.

"It has now been almost eight months since our son started on the elimination diet which successfully relieved his symptoms. After three months of such relief, we tried to add other foods carefully one at a time every two to four weeks and later at six-week intervals. The only food we have successfully added to the basic diet over the entire year is banana.

"We want you to know that we appreciate what you have done. You have supplied with your elimination diet the means by which a very difficult situation has been controlled."

PERIPHERAL NERVE ALLERGY TO ANIMAL SERA

Nervous tissue allergy in man is especially evidenced by various cerebral, sensory, and motor disturbances arising from serum allergy, as extensively reviewed by Ratner in 1943. Headaches, neuralgia with associated urticaria and localized edema, nausea and vomiting so frequent in serum sickness, the less common evidences of meningitis and the rare aphasia, hemiplegia, loss of consciousness, and similar manifestations indicate cerebral or meningeal involvement. Paresis and paralysis are dramatic and not uncommon results of serum allergy in the peripheral nerves. Though the brachial plexus is most frequently affected, any of the peripheral or cranial nerves may be involved.

Evidence of allergic involvement of the tissues of the nervous system arises in serum allergy either from prophylactic or therapeutic serum therapy. Such nervous complications have been reported for years since the original report of Von Pirquet and Schick (1905). F. Kennedy (1929) reported one patient with fulminating cerebral symptoms during serum sickness, two patients with involvement of the brachial plexus and circumflex nerves suggestive of a poliomyelitis with a gradual disappearance of symptoms, two patients with sustained unilateral paralysis of the long thoracic nerves, and one with edema of the retina and meninges. One had generalized polyneuritis, moreover, after antityphoid vaccine. Kennedy (1936) also noted aphasia, right hemiplegia, hemianopia (with swollen nerve heads), fourteen lymphocytes in the spinal fluid, and recovery only after four weeks in a child four years of age from serum sickness. Many similar reports are in the literature, as noted by Kammerer (1934). Doyle (1933) found forty-seven reports in the literature of pareses and paralyses especially involving the brachial plexus from serum sickness. One case of urticarial edema of the brain and meninges, one of optic neuritis, and seven with involvement of the radial nerve and one of the long thoracic nerve were of interest. Sensory disturbances occurred in about one-third of the patients. Most articles were in the French literature. One of the best reviews of the literature on allergy of the central nervous system and especially the cranial and peripheral nerves was by Ratner in 1943. Of interest was the report of Sheldon (1933) that a papilledema associated with a scarlatiniform rash, pain, and effusion in joints and relieved by drainage of a peritoneal streptococcal abscess arose from streptococcal allergy arising during preceding tonsillitis.

Allergy directly or indirectly produces various types of nervous disturbances either by the production of allergic reactions in the tissues of the brain, spinal cord, and nerves themselves or possibly by the effects of allergic toxemia on the functions of the nerve structures of the body. That localized allergic edema may occur in the meninges of the brain or spinal cord, in the nerve sheaths, and probably in the vascular and perivascular tissues in the brain, cord, and nerve structure itself has already been pointed out in the discussions of angioneurotic edema and migraine. Moreover, experimental work with serum and with other allergens has demonstrated the origin of hyperergic arteritis and inflammation of the veins in the meninges and dura similar to the lesions of periarteritis nodosa and leading to microscopic necroses and cellular infiltration of surrounding tissues as reported by Ssolowjew and Ariel (1935). Such vascular changes in cerebral arteries could well explain disturbances in cerebral function occurring in clinical allergy. Vascular allergy, of course, need not be as extreme as that observed in such experiments and may only lead to increased permeability, endothelial congestion, and possibly slight cellular proliferation with surrounding tissue edema and infiltration as seen in urticarial lesions. Quincke years ago described meningitis serosa as an example of localized angioneurotic edema. Oharo (1933) discussed Quincke's edema in the brain productive of muscular contractions in the leg followed by dizziness and unconsciousness. Edema and paresthesia of the left hand occurred. He stated that repeated attacks might lead to tissue thickening as seen in cutaneous allergy and resultant chronic cerebral symptoms. Other cerebral symptoms from angioneurotic edema are noted on page 339. It is also probable that spasm of the smooth muscles in the blood vessels of the brain and cord may result from localized allergic reactions and be responsible for some of the nervous disturbances to be discussed, thus producing many obscure manifestations including meningismus with cephalic pain, peripheral nerve disturbances, Meniere's syndrome, amblyopia, nystagmus, and other symptoms.

The occurrence of transient aphasia, amblyopia, aphonia, paresis, and paresthesia in allergic individuals with migraine is presumptive evidence of localized allergic reactions in the brain itself. The profound nervous disturbances which characterize the syndrome we have described as allergic toxemia resulting from food allergy are evidences in part of a generalized reversible disturbance of the cerebral functions. It is probable that many vague nervous feelings, including heaviness in the head, confusion, irritability, or neuralgia may be due to food allergy as suggested in this chapter. The various nervous disturbances resulting from chronic food allergy will be discussed later. That inhalant, drug, and chemical allergies also need consideration must be remembered.

PERIPHERAL NERVE ALLERGY TO FOODS

That neuralgic pains are at times due to food allergy as we reported in 1931 has been confirmed by us and other allergists since then. Such pains relieved by the elimination of specific foods may occur in any part of the body, though our experience indicates that the head, neck, and shoulders are most afflicted. Neuralgia of allergic origin occurs most frequently in obviously allergic patients, that is, in those who have marked eczema, asthma, allergic migraine, or gastrointestinal allergy. The cause of the pain may be localized edema and resultant anemia of the nerves or near their nuclei. That angioneurotic edema might be the cause of trigeminal neuralgia in certain cases was suggested by Bassoe. Vaughan, in 1930, reported two cases of trigeminal neuralgia relieved by the elimination of specific foods.

Whether the important relief of herpes zoster from high doses of Prednisone advised by Elliott in 1964 is due to control of infection or of associated allergy is unanswered at present.

CASE REPORTS

Campbell reported a man forty-five years of age who had had back and leg aches after a fall. Many tests by several physicians were done, including myelography and discography. Laminectomy failed. Other physicians in several clinics failed to relieve causative deep pain in the right abdomen and leg, with weakness and paresthesias in the right leg, hyperflexia, and decreased vibratory sensation in his legs. Uric acid was 7.3 mg %. With Colbenemid and a meat-free diet, pain decreased and neurological examination was normal. Later ingestion of beef activated his symptoms which gradually disappeared with elimination of beef. With exclusion of beef, personality and health were normal. Relief depended on control of allergy to beef with elimination from his diet.

Case 106: A man twenty-nine years of age during the last three years had had pain in both hips and in the lumbar and sacroiliac regions. During the last three years his back had been painful and with any change in position, sharp, shooting pains in his hips had occurred. A roentgen ray of his back and hips had shown no abnormality. Medical treatment by specialists had failed. For seven months he had worn a supporting brace on his back with no relief. The pain had been so severe, especially in the early mornings, that sleep had infrequently been impossible.

During the last three months he had found that the daily use of enemas had ameliorated the pain! He had been suspicious that milk had increased his symptoms.

There was no personal or family history of allergy. His physical examination was negative, and his laboratory tests were negative.

Food allergy was studied with our CFE diet. In one day the pain disappeared, and he has been according to Campbell practically free ever since. Since then it was found that milk and eggs definitely produced the severe pain in the back and hips. After taking milk for two days, the pain in his back began in the early morning. He continued the milk for four more days, and pain became steadily worse. After discontinuing the milk, pain disappeared in one day. After being free from pain for three weeks, one egg was taken, and that night severe pain in the back and hips recurred. A few days later another egg was taken, and the same pain resulted. Wheat to which a positive scratch reaction occurred caused no pain. Relief continued with a milk-free and egg-free diet. This emphasizes the occurrence of negative skin reactions to allergenic foods (Chapt. 2).

Comment: The pain was definitely shown to be due to food allergy. There was little in the history to indicate its presence. The patient found that he can take all foods to which positive reactions occurred without any difficulty and that his pain was due to eggs and milk to which negative cutaneous reactions occurred. This case illustrates the occurrence of negative skin reactions to allergenic foods emphasized in this volume and especially in Chapters 2 and 3.

Randolph, in 1948 and 1950, reported food allergy as one cause of torticollis, or "wryneck," and especially of nuchal myalgia resulting in stiffness and deep soreness in the muscles of the neck, shoulders, and upper back muscles. Other symptoms of allergic toxemia occurred in varying combinations and degrees.

In 1951 Randolph again wrote an informative article on myalgia allergy, especially in the posterior cervical and trapezius muscles. Less often soreness, pain, and tautness occurred in pectoral, intercostal, abdominal, lumbar, ham string, and calf muscles because of allergy especially to foods. At times the generalized aching in muscles and joints, as reported in Chapter 23, occurred. Pulling, drawing, tightness, aching, and soreness, especially in the cervical muscles, had been designated as tension headaches—attributed to nerve tension and not to the causative allergies. Tender nodules were reported in the involved muscles in the neck and even in the calf or other skeletal muscles, with frequent muscular cramping. Randolph found house dust causative in some patients.

PERSONAL CASE

Case 107: A man thirty-five years of age had had very severe neuralgia in the right lumbar back whenever he took any Worcestershire sauce. He gave a history of having drunk a cup of such sauce in youth. He had had many other allergic manifestations, including eczema, over a period of thirty years, with marked headaches, fatigue, and indigestion. He gave large scratch reactions to wheat, eggs, milk, oats, corn, many fruits, vegetables, fish, and dusts.

Comment: This case illustrates the specific effect that some ingredient in the sauce had in causing severe pain in his back. The other reacting foods produced his migraine, fatigue, and indigestion and had no doubt caused his eczema.

TRIGEMINAL NEURALGIA

We have observed severe pain in the neck and jaw of two women who also had longstanding toxemia, nausea, vomiting, dizziness, mental confusion, and sluggishness of thought because of food allergy.

A severe case of trigeminal neuralgia relieved with an elimination diet is summarized below.

Case 108: A man thirty-nine years of age had had lifelong recurrent left-sided headaches and facial neuralgia every five to seven days, with nausea and vomiting especially severe for ten years. A gastroenterostomy had been done because of vomiting, with no help. For one year excruciating left-sided facial neuralgia and headaches had lasted three to fourteen days. All treatment, including six injections of alcohol into the fifth nerve, had failed. Scratch tests to foods were negative.

Food allergy was studied with our CFE diet plus rice and rye. In two months he reported no headaches or neuralgia. Appetite was "ravenous," and he was working hard. Wheat, milk, and eggs were added, with a recurrence of headache. With elimination of these foods, relief continued.

PERIPHERAL NERVE ALLERGY RESULTING FROM POLLENS

That pain and paresthesias in the extremities arise in the peripheral nerves at times from pollen allergy is illustrated in the following case.

Case 109: A woman twenty-five years of age in August developed edema of the hands with pain first in the right arm, extending into the forearm and the third and fourth fingers. In one week lesser pain began in the left forearm and hand. It increased until the rains in November. It was also relieved for two weeks in September when corticosteroids were taken by mouth. Pain was exaggerated from 2 to 3 AM. Aching also continued during the day.

Pain disappeared in December, January, and early February. Then it recurred and became very severe. Arteriograms and a myelogram were negative. Two weeks before we saw her, surgical exploration of blood vessels in the arms and neck had been scheduled.

Hay fever has occurred for four years from early spring to October, with some wheezing in September for four years.

Bronchial asthma from the age of three to seven years had been relieved with our CFE diet. Scratch reactions to pollens had been negative.

Diet history revealed vomiting and asthma from milk, wheat, and eggs in infancy, with abdominal cramping from eggs since that time.

Desensitization to the tree, grass, summer, and fall pollens in her area to most of which scratch reactions were positive in gradually increasing doses up to 0.6 cc of the 1:100 dilution repeated at weekly intervals for one year and every two weeks for two years has given excellent relief for five years. Oral corticosteroids given in the first two months have been discontinued since then.

VERTIGO AND DIZZINESS

Though vertigo and dizziness resulting from allergy as to foods usually result from edema in the inner ear, as discussed especially in Chapter 13, such symptoms can arise from allergy in other tissues of the equilibrium apparatus. Since sodium retention disturbing neurocirculation is an important possibility, a salt-free and later a salt-poor diet are important to consider this possibility. Moreover, calcium deficiency when milk is long excluded may be causative and requires calcium carbonate ½ teaspoonful daily as advised in Chapter 3.

Thus vertigo associated with petit mal attacks in Cases 1. and 2. in this chapter can be explained by allergy causing dysfunction in cerebral tissues or in the tissues of the equilibrium apparatus other than in the middle ear. The dizziness and vertigo in patients with symptoms resulting from gastrointestinal allergy or with allergic headaches or migraine especially when nausea and vomiting occur can be explained by allergy with resultant disturbed function in the equilibrium apparatus or other tissues rather than those in the middle ear. Before attacks of angioneurotic edema relieved by the elimination of wheat, milk, corn, and chocolate, one of our patients developed nervousness, dizziness, irritability, sleeplessness, fatigue, and "felt sore all over."

Study of dizziness of peripheral origin must be studied as advised by neurologists and discussed by Elia (1968) in *The Dizzy Patient* if symptoms persist.

MULTIPLE SCLEROSIS

Since allergy in the brain, spinal cord, and cranial and peripheral nerves to animal sera, foods, and at times inhalants causes symptoms which are similar to those occurring in multiple sclerosis (MS), the possibility that MS may be due to allergic reactivity in the tissues of the nervous system needs consideration. Experimental evidence and the pathology in the nervous tissues correlated with symptoms of MS favoring an allergic etiology with 110 references are in an informative article by Prigal (1956).

Food allergy, moreover, needs consideration, since transient pareses, paralyses, and paresthesias have been reported from such allergy as already noted in our discussion of allergic headache and migraine, convulsive seizures, and peripheral neural allergy. And since persistent allergic reactions in nervous tissue may cause irreversible changes or gliosis, as suggested by Cooke and others, consideration of allergy as the initial and continued cause of chronic MS is justified. A discussion of the possible role of allergy in MS in this volume in which food allergy receives major consideration can be considered, especially because of the opinion of Jonez that the study and control of possible food allergy with our elimination diets were of benefit in his treatment of MS. Moreover, if allergy is considered as a possible cause of any symptom, food allergy along with inhalant, drug, and possible bacterial allergies must be studied.

In 1944 Ferraro stated that allergic reactions in the tissues of the CNS was a probable cause of MS because of varying degrees of improvement from parenteral histamine therapy. Many other workers also reported such improvement.

Horten *et al.*, in 1944, gave daily intravenous injections of 2.75 mg of histamine diphosphate in 250 cc of isotonic solution of sodium chloride to 102 cases of MS. He reported varying improvement in 50 percent of the cases.

Jonez, in 1948, reported his study and treatment of MS during the preceding several years. Histamine subcutaneously and intravenously at first with prostigmine and later with d-tubocurarine with muscle re-education and management of possible food and inhalant allergies were used in 124 cases. The usual age of onset was between twenty and forty years. The average duration had been approximately ten years. Objective freedom of symptoms occurred in thirteen cases, there being marked improvement in twenty, definite improvement in thirty-eight, and slight improvement in thirty-three. There was no improvement in twenty. In some cases improvement was delayed three months. He advised continued intravenous histamine in all cases for one or more years.

His most important article on MS from the allergic viewpoint should be carefully studied by physicians who share or have the responsibility of treating this usually progressive disease. This report contains published evidence of cerebroneural allergy in the etiology of MS, his method of study and control of possible inhalant and especially of food allergy as we advise, the eradication of possible foci of infection, and especially the methods of histamine therapy according to Horton's method with injections of d-tubocurarine in oil and wax and the results of such therapy in sixty-two patients. References to fifty-one significant articles are printed.

Whereas no case was cured, Jonez reported objective improvement in the majority of his cases. This treatment was given in a sanitarium where patients were supervised and treated and cared for daily by Doctor Jonez and his staff.

Prigal, in 1951, reviewed the experimental evidence correlated with histories of demyelination of nerves and brain damage as the cause. Bacterial allergy and autotissue sensitivity were discussed. Atopic allergy to foods and inhalants were considered, but method of study or evidence favoring such allergy had not been reported. The recurrence of attacks is in part suggestive of food allergy. References of interest, 111 in number, are included in the article.

During the last ten years we have studied allergy as a possible cause of MS in several patients. In spite of strict adherence to the CFE diet and in some patients the later elimination of all fruits and spices and condiments and treatment of indicated pollen allergy, no definite benefit occurred.

Still impressed with the probability of allergy, possible bacterial allergy received our consideration. This had been emphasized to us since the excellent provocative article of E. C. Rosenow, in 1948, on "Bacteriological Studies of Multiple Sclerosis," in which he reported the isolation of a green-producing or alpha type of streptococcus from the nasopharynx, tonsils, and infected teeth in these patients and the production of symptoms of MS in animals after the intracerebral inoculation of pure cultures of these streptococci. The spotty distribution in the brain and cord of hemorrhage, edema, and demyelination and other vascular lesions from intracerebral injection of this vaccine in experimental animals is similar to those in patients with early MS. The importance of his studies justifies, we opine, reprinting his summary and comments in the Appendix (Chapt. 30) of this book.

Since autogenous and stock vaccines given to some of these patients had not been helpful, possible benefit from desensitizing miniscule doses of a similar streptococcic vaccine, which was reported of definite benefit when given by vein by Doctor Small in rheumatoid arthritis, along with the study of possible food allergy with our CFE diet have been continued.

The excellent results from such consideration of streptococcal and food allergy with or without histamine therapy, as advised by Horton, are reported in Cases 110 and 111 which justify its continuation in other patients with MS. Its use in severely incapacitated patients has not been encouraging, though we opine that its continuance for at least two years would be justifiable.

POSSIBLE ROLE OF ALLERGY TO STREPTOCOCCUS ANTIGEN IN THE CAUSATION OF MS

Kennedy, in 1938, reported symptoms indicating MS in a girl twenty years of age. She had had recurrent attacks of partial or total blindness in one or both eyes lasting one-half to four days because of retrobulbar neuritis. Abdominal reflexes were brisk and equal. Eczema had occurred in childhood. Asthma had also resulted from allergy to rabbit emanations. The diagnosis of MS had been accepted two years previously. Relief occurred after removal of tonsils from which *Streptococcus viridans* was cultured. Of marked importance was the evidence of the role of a green-producing or alpha type of streptococcus in producing neurological lesions in experimental animals similar to those in patients with MS reported by Rosenow of the Mayo Clinic. This finding indicated allergy to streptococcus as the possible cause of her MS, as discussed in Chapter 30.

With this in mind, our study and control of possible food allergy with our CFE diet were initiated, have been continued in the following case, and have been conducted in the last ten years with a remission of symptoms in a few months, continuing until the present time.

Case 110: A man twenty-eight years of age

developed numbness in the right thigh and lateral chest with burning in scattered skin areas in February, 1960, for three weeks. It recurred more severely for a week in June. In two months thereafter blurred vision and in two days loss of three-fourths of his central vision developed. These symptoms continued until we saw him six months later. Increasing burning and tightness in the right thigh and leg with weakness in both legs had continued. MS had been diagnosed by a neurologist and ophthalmologist.

Frontal and ocular headaches had also developed with his visual symptoms along with a "strained feeling in the eyes." Spinal puncture aggravated these complaints.

Nasal congestion and postnasal mucus had been present for many years. Eczema on his right hand and fingers had continued for two years up to three years before he was first seen. Diarrhea two to three times a day had occurred every one to two weeks for five years.

He gave no history of dislikes or disagreements for foods.

His family history revealed headaches and dizziness in the mother for five years.

The patient had had recurrent tonsillitis for six years.

Skin tests with important foods and inhalants were negative. X-ray of the lungs and sinuses were negative. Blood, urine, sedimentation rate, and Kline tests were negative.

Treatment: Because of a possible extreme allergy to streptococcus, as suggested by the relief of MS by Kennedy reported above, desensitization with a dilution of 10^{-17} intravenously was started on January 6, 1961. In one hour he developed a sudden chill, palpitations, and sweating, with fever lasting for eight hours. In one week his loss of vision had decreased. In ten days 0.2 cc of the vaccine 10^{-19} was given by vein. In twelve hours chilling occurred for one hour after walking in an upright position. Profuse sweating and palpitation occurred. The next day he was weak and had general malaise with temperatures of 100 to 101 F. In ten days 0.2 cc of sterile water was given by vein with no reaction. Steady clearing of vision occurred. Decadron, 4 mg twice a day, was given for one month to counteract possible neural allergy.

No injections were given for one month during which time vision improved and made reading possible. Paresthesias had decreased, but his legs

remained slightly weak. On March 14 0.2 of sterile water was given, with no reaction.

On March 18 0.15 cc of streptococcus vaccine 10^{-22} was given by vein and caused initial chills, weakness, and fever up to 102 F for three days. Thereafter, he had no evidence of MS except some "fatigue."

No injections were given for 2½ months when he returned to the office asking for injections of the vaccine because of a slight return of paresthesias in his right arm and leg. Because of the severe reaction to the 10^{-22} dilution, 0.15 cc of the 10^{-26} dilution was given by vein. At weekly intervals thereafter 0.15 cc of the 10^{-28} dilution was given. Slight malaise still occurred because of which 0.15 cc of the 10^{-30} dilution was given with no ascertainable disturbance. This dose was repeated at weekly intervals for one month. In two months because of recurrent infection in his tonsils, they were removed on September 9, 1961.

Since then intravenous injections of the streptococcus vaccine have been given as follows: 0.3 cc of the 10^{-30} dilution at two-week intervals during September and 0.2 cc of the 10^{-28} dilution every two weeks during October and November.

On December 5 he stated he had had slight paresthesias in his hands and feet at intervals for two to three weeks. Then at two-week to four-week intervals the intravenous vaccine was gradually increased from the 10^{-27} to the 10^{-23} during a five-month period. During 1962 and 1963 there was an entire absence of any indication of MS. During 1964 and 1965 injections were continued with the 10^{-22} dilution at monthly intervals. In 1966 and 1967 monthly injections of the 10^{-21} dilution were given.

The alert reader will have noticed that 10^{-30} is greater than Avogadro's number, which gives the number of molecules in a mole of substance. Because no attempt to change sterile syringes with each successive dilution was made, these dilutions expressed as exponents of 10 should be regarded as identifying numbers only.

There have been no neurological symptoms except slight numbness in the upper extremities and on the right lateral abdomen and lumbar area with loss of equilibrium for two to three weeks in November, 1966, relieved by the elimination of penicillin by another physician.

During these ten years he has adhered to our CFE diet except for the addition of all fruits and vegetables except for onions and garlic.

Comment: An extreme degree of allergy to the streptococcus best explains the severe reactions from its initial injections. The marked unanticipated improvement in the MS is also explained by gradual desensitization as tolerance for stronger doses developed.

Benefit from our elimination diet previously reported by Jonez is difficult to determine, though evidence of clinical allergy has occurred as additional common allergenic foods have been ingested.

Long-term spontaneous remissions with MS have been observed, but this remission for ten years correlated with desensitization treatments to streptococcus concurrent with elimination of all allergenic foods is nevertheless most significant.

CASE HISTORIES

Case 111: A woman fifty-seven years of age. When first seen in 1960 she had numbness, aching, and tingling in the left leg and incontinence of urine, complete at times, for seven to ten days during the last eight years. Hesitant speech, fatigue in talking (especially when frequent headaches were present), "great fatigue," and at times inability to sleep, blurring of vision, and walking "as if she were drunk" increasingly present during the preceding ten years led to a diagnosis of MS by a specialist. This diagnosis was confirmed in Tacoma in 1958, where she was placed on our CFE diet, given histamine intravenously, and desensitized with pollens.

When first seen she was eliminating a number of foods. She was using histamine by bronchoporosis. She was receiving an antigen every week. Though recurrent severe headaches for fourteen years had been benefited by the above therapy, a constant headache had continued for five years. Parennial nasal allergy with considerable postnasal mucoid discharge and nasal congestion for twenty-five years indicated food allergy as the cause.

When first seen, flashes of light were frequent, associated with blurring of vision. She felt fatigued and exhausted. Lifelong constipation persisted. As stated above, loss of control of urination and actual incontinence for hours or days still occurred.

Diet history revealed increased nasal mucus from milk and particularly from ice cream. Personal and family history indicating other clinical allergies was negative.

Our scratch tests revealed slight reactions to several grass pollens but no reactions to any other inhalant or food. Routine laboratory tests and x-rays of chest and sinuses were negative.

Treatment and Results: When first seen in 1960 she was placed on our FFCFE diet from which peas were excluded and tea and rice added. Desensitization with a multiple inhalant antigen in the 1:5 million dilution was given.

During 1962 and 1963 the diet was continued. She was still having headaches. Manifestations of MS had decreased, though in January, 1964, she complained of malaise, nausea, fatigue, and contractions in the legs and ankles. She had found that soy products produced headaches.

At that time intravenous injections of 10^{-17} hemolytic streptococcus vaccine were started, and in one month she was "less exhausted and felt better generally." At that time she was on a diet of rice, potato chips, corn chips, corn, ham, beef, chicken, turkey, vegetables other than legumes, bananas, cooked apples, coffee, sugar, salt, and a Unicap® tablet daily. Because of pus in the urine, Gantrisin® was given, 1 gm four times a day for five days and one four times a day for four days. Two weeks later she reported that trial ingestion of wheat, legumes, cereals, and strawberries had caused headaches. Raw apples produced bladder irritation, necessitating the wearing of a napkin because of slight incontinence.

The intravenous streptococci vaccine 10^{-17} was continued at weekly intervals through 1964, during which previously taken Equanil® 100 mg daily was continued. In October, 1964, she reported marked improvement, especially in the fatigue which had made her "lie down most of the time before." This improvement continued in spite of final fatal illness of her husband.

In January, 1965, she was still receiving streptococcic vaccine 10^{-17} intravenously and B_{12}. A marked improvement continued, making it possible for her to walk steadily and with increasing strength. Because of abdominal pains, fruits were entirely eliminated in the spring of 1965. In the fall improvement continued. She was still receiving 0.25 cc of the 10^{-17} streptococcic vaccine intravenously along with 300 µg of B_{12} every day and continued pollen desensitization with a #5 dilution every week along with 300 µg of B_{12} hypodermically every two weeks.

During 1966 this treatment continued. In the spring she developed a cold, requiring Declomycin. Her blood count and urinalysis were normal in the fall. X-rays of her lungs were negative. BEI was 3.8 μg%.

In 1965 she continued to be well controlled. Traces of fruit were found to cause involuntary urination which had been present for years. Her injections of pollen antigen, B_{12}, and 0.3 cc streptococcic vaccine 10^{-12} were continued during 1967 and 1968.

In the spring of 1969 she walked twenty blocks to the office with no difficulty. Rice was tolerated in her diet. White potato gave severe headache. Fruit caused bladder incontinence. Soy also continued to produce headaches. Her diet consisted of rice, beef, spinach, carrots, sugar, salt, tapioca, and Wesson oil. In October, 1968, chicken was eaten, and she had a generalized headache and slight nausea. Fish caused nausea.

In 1969 treatment has continued with 0.05 cc of respiratory vaccine given at weekly intervals along with 200 mg of B_{12}, 0.2 cc of #1 dilution of her pollen antigen, and 0.3 cc of the 10^{-16} streptococcic antigen. In June she reported that her MS was under good control.

Comment: Though marked evidence of allergy to the streptococcus similar to that in the above Case 110 did not arise, definite benefit from gradually increasing doses of the vaccine has developed with increased tolerance to the streptoccus and as control of clinical food allergies has occurred with our elimination diet.

The benefit from the treatment used in these cases justifies its utilization by other physicians, especially in patients with early or noninvaliding† MS.

PSYCHIC DISTURBANCES

We have observed certain patients with profound psychic disturbances because of food allergy. With such recognition of marked disturbances, it is evident that many milder symptoms probably occur. Pasteur Vallery-Radot (1931) reported establishment of depressed maniacal spells with urticaria and found that a depression of the white count occurred indicating sensitization. Mental confusion, inability to concentrate or think clearly, lack of ambition, irritability, spells of violent temper, nervousness, dazed states, fatigue, insomnia, and melancholia have already been

discussed in Chapter 19 on allergic toxemia resulting from food allergy. The increasing recognition of the allergic toxemia and fatigue syndrome, first reported by us in 1928 and 1931 and by other allergists since that time, has been noted. Hoobler felt that reactions in human beings and especially in children similar to the marked stimulation of the peripheral nerve endings which result in anaphylactic reactions in animals may account in part for the many nervous reactions from allergy. Duke, in his book on allergy as well as in a separate article (1927), described the psychic and nervous disturbances in allergic patients. In 1926, as reported by Rolleston, Craig, and Beaton, violent toxic psychoses in patients sensitive to mushrooms, shellfish, and pork were recognized.

Since 1931 and 1938 we have studied many patients with allergic toxemia, as reported in Chapter 19 associated with marked depression, confusion, and other nervous symptoms resulting from food allergy. The severity and persistency of such symptoms and the long period required to bring about improvement and at times to initiate such relief make one suspicious of the presence of severe and even irreversible allergic tissue changes associated with possible allergic arteritis as described by many students, especially by Rossle and by Kline and Young. As noted in Chapter 19, though food allergy is the most common cause of these psychological symptoms, inhalant allergy is also responsible. One patient had had uncontrollable crying, exhaustion, and nervousness all through the spring, summer, and fall months relieved by desensitization to pollens to which skin reactions did not occur. Another patient had had depression, nervousness and fatigue for several years after mid-July. Hyposensitization therapy with fall pollens and especially with cultivated flower pollens was necessary for effective relief. Another woman had marked mental depression whenever excessive amounts of house dust, animal emanations, or pollens were inhaled to which allergy existed. That pollen allergy can produce peripheral neuralgias, as in the arm, without cerebral allergy is reported in Case 109 in this chapter.

It is possible that many so-called psychoneurotic disturbances are fundamentally a result of cerebral allergy. Moreover, longstanding unrelieved nasobronchial, gastrointestinal, and especially cutaneous symptoms which are associated with pruritus are prone to make the patient introspective, nervous, irritable, and depressed. Years ago many patients with bronchial asthma were dubbed neurotics. Nervousness as a cause of eczema, dermatitis, and cutaneous edemas was evidenced in the term *neurodermatitis*. As stated in Chapter 14, we feel that the nervous symptoms are the result rather than the cause of such uncontrolled asthma and dermatoses. A confrere told us of a severe psychoneurosis of years' duration which arose from an allergy to cat hair. Because of such allergy, a marked phobia to cats developed in childhood. She feared other animals, began to mistrust herself, and became psychically incapacitated. Marked increased sensitivity in all the special senses developed. Recognition of the original cause made it possible for the psychiatrist to gradually unravel the pyramided causes of the nervous problem with benefit to the patient.

The question naturally arises whether some of the recurrent mental symptoms such as depression, melancholia, and personality changes may not be allergic in origin. Experienced, adequate study especially of food and inhalant allergies as major or complicating causes of psychoses, particularly when clinical allergy is evidenced in the history or physical examination and laboratory tests, is of great importance. Sulzberger has reported alcoholic psychosis which arose only when rye whiskey was taken. Rowe and Richet (1930) opined that many recurrent psychic disturbances should be studied from their allergic possibilities. The recurrent nature of such symptoms somewhat favors allergic causes. The cyclic characteristics of many of the well-recognized manifestations of food allergy, such as bronchial asthma, especially in infancy, and at times eczema and urticaria are important to keep in mind in this study of mental states of varying frequency and degree.

The confirmation of the psychological disturbances from allergy especially to foods which have been recognized for fifty years were included in our report of the syndrome *Allergic Toxemia and Fatigue* in 1928 and in the first edition of this book as by several allergists including Clarke and Speer.

Randolph especially has recognized and emphasized this syndrome and has extended his studies in other ecological influences in alcoholic and psychiatric patients.

Illustrative of mental disturbances arising from beet sugar in a food-sensitive patient from the ingestion of beet sugar is Randolph's report of marked resultant symptoms from cerebral allergy in his informative article "Clinical Ecology as It Affects the Psychiatric Patient" in 1966. This article and many others by Randolph and other allergists are in the list of references.

It must be pointed out that we realize neuroses in themselves are frequently the cause of many mental and gastrointestinal symptoms which may also be due to food allergy. We have increasingly realized through the last four decades, however, that certain allergic patients with chronic or severe food allergy may have many nervous symptoms resulting from localized allergic cerebral edema or vascular spasm. They also often become introspective, analytical, and neurasthenic because of their constant unrelieved distress as well as their self-analysis. Such minute analysis is usually carried out with the hope of finding some relief for their symptoms of allergic toxemia or other manifestations of food allergy such as those in the nervous, gastrointestinal, bronchial, bladder, and cutaneous tissues for which physicians have been unable to offer any relief.

RELATION OF ALLERGY TO CHARACTER PROBLEMS IN CHILDREN

Clarke's discussion, in 1950, of character and personality changes which we reported in the discussion of Allergic Fatigue and Toxemia in the first edition of this volume in 1931 not only in children but also in adults is of special importance, particularly to pediatricians, allergists, and psychiatrists. Because of this important information, we have reprinted Clarke's article with the necessary permission so that it can be available for reading by physicians who request it.

In his twenty-four case reports the study, recognition, and control of specific food and less often inhalant allergies have relieved the irritable, fussy, restless, unhappy, stubborn, unfriendly, uncooperative, antagonistic, at times angry, inattentive, tense, crying, recessive, somnolent, disliked, and at times enuretic children. These children have been fortunately and at times dramatically relieved of varying numbers of the above symptoms. Clarke's report of relief of attacks of excitement and a destructive desire in a boy about to be sent to a mental hospital by the elimination of wheat and oats to which allergy was demonstrated helped in part by desensitization

to inhalants, evidences the challenge of adequate study of atopic allergy especially to foods and when indicated to inhalants. In many patients even in mental hospitals, especially if a history of possible or definite clinical allergy is obtained, control of possible allergy constitutes one of the main challenges in the important endeavor to relieve chronic atopic allergy which occurs in practically all tissues of the body, thereby hoping to reduce economic loss of institutional care as well as loss to society of an individual.

Increasing evidence that cerebral allergy causes psychological symptoms similar to those included in the syndrome Allergic Fatigue and Toxemia that we first reported in 1928 and in the first edition of this book in 1931 arising from allergy, especially to foods and less often to inhalants, requires consideration of such allergy as a possible cause of psychological disturbances in children and adults. These symptoms, including psychoses, as reported by Randolph and increasingly by other allergists, have been summarized in Chapter 19, in this chapter, and in recent articles as one of Kittler and Baldwin, in 1970, on the role of allergy in causing minimal brain dysfunctions.

CONTROL OF CEREBRAL AND NEURAL ALLERGY

For the study and control of allergy as the cause of these symptoms, the reader is referred to our chapters on the elimination diets and on allergic headaches as well as on allergic toxemia. We must reemphasize that the discovery and successful control of food allergy demand a thorough knowledge of the principles of general as well as allergic diagnoses described in this volume and a willingness on the doctor's part to personally supervise the diet in more than a few cooperating patients in accordance with our elimination method for a period of several weeks and usually for months. Successful study requires time, patience, and meticulous supervision.

MIGRAINE, TRANSIENT BLINDNESS, NAUSEA, VOMITING

Case 112: A man thirty years of age had had sour stomach and belching for ten years associated with a great deal of intestinal gas which he had had all his life. He had had headaches recurring from two to four times a week and lasting from four to twelve hours, usually in the frontal region, since the age of ten years. With these headaches nausea and at times vomiting had occurred. Apples, tomatoes, oranges, bananas, butter, and bacon had produced indigestion. For twelve years spells of temporary blindness lasting from fifteen to thirty minutes, initiated by a whirling black spot in the center of vision, had recurred every few weeks, increasing in frequency to fortnightly intervals in the last two years. These blind spells were always followed by headaches and soreness in the side of his head lasting at times for two days. No other allergy was present in his personal and family history. A physical examination, laboratory test, and roentgen ray studies of his sella and of his gastrointestinal tract were normal. An "elimination diet," excluding milk, corn, strawberries, oranges, bananas, and pork, has eradicated the indigestion, headaches, and blind spells for one year, except when the diet has been broken.

MIGRAINE, VISUAL DISTURBANCES, PARESTHESIAS, DIZZINESS, DROWSINESS

Case 113: A man thirty-eight years of age had had bilious attacks associated with violent nausea and right frontal headaches every month or two most of his life. Since the age of twenty they had decreased in frequency. For two years he had had sudden attacks of floating bodies before the eyes followed by impaired vision, inability to read fine print, tingling in the hands and feet, weakness, marked faintness, followed by severe nausea and frontal headache. Increasing drowsiness and finally a heavy sleep for three or four hours had followed. For one year he had traced these attacks to garlic and had found that they came fourteen to sixteen hours after eating even a minute amount. The last attack resulted from

eating three olives dipped in oil flavored with garlic! He had disliked onions, garlic, turnips, and tomatoes for years. No other food allergy was present in his personal history, though mild allergic manifestations were present in his family history. Physical examination, laboratory tests, and skin reactions to foods were negative, except for a delayed reaction to garlic. No gastrointestinal attacks or visual and mental disturbances have occurred for two years since the exclusion of garlic.

Comment: This case is of special interest because of the violent allergic reactions resulting from a minute amount of food—the mere flavor of garlic. The delay in the appearance of the manifestations from fourteen to sixteen hours after the ingestion of the garlic suggested the presence of an area of increased permeability in the lower colon or a definite localization of sensitized membrane in that region. The history of visual and nervous disturbances and drowsiness associated with migraine is not infrequent. This patient had eaten raw onions as he would apples in childhood and probably became sensitized to them at that time.

NEURALGIA

Neuralgic pains are at times due to food allergy, and it may be that neuralgic pain resulting from bacterial infection may be due to bacterial allergy. Such pains resulting from food sensitization may occur in any part of the body, though our experience indicates that the head, neck, and shoulders are most often afflicted. Neuralgia of allergic origin occurs most frequently in obviously allergic patients, that is, in those who have marked eczema, asthma, allergic migraine, or gastrointestinal allergy. The cause of the pain may be localized edema or anemia of the nerves or their nuclei. That angioneurotic edema might be the cause of trigeminal neuralgia in certain cases was suggested by Bassoe. We have observed severe pain in the neck and jaw of two women who also had longstanding toxemia, nausea, vomiting, dizziness, mental confusion, and sluggishness of thought because of chronic food allergy.

We have recently relieved a severe case of trigeminal neuralgia with our elimination diets, a summary of which is given below. Brown suggested that neuralgia and possibly trifacial neuralgia was due to food allergy. Vaughan, in 1930, also reported two cases of trigeminal neuralgia relieved by the elimination of specific foods. The remarkable localization of pain in a patient with longstanding allergy, the pain being produced by a few drops of Worcestershire sauce, is recorded in Case 107.

Case 114: A man thirty-four years of age had had since his earliest memory recurrent migraine on the left side of his head at least once a week, nearly always associated with nausea and vomiting. For the last ten years his headaches had become very severe, and four years ago a gastroenterostomy was done because of nausea and vomiting. For a few months afterward on a restricted diet he was better, but since then his symptoms have been as bad as ever. During the last year his headaches have been excruciating, lasting from three days to two weeks. He had had all types of examinations and roentgen ray studies of his sinuses without any help. Six alcoholic injections in his trigeminal nerve had given no relief. His skin tests were negative to all types of food.

Treatment: On our elimination diet he has been practically free from his severe headaches, nausea and vomiting. In two months he reported that he was working hard and had had absolutely no headache for five weeks, which was the first time in ten months that he had gone over four days without a headache. He had a ravenous appetite and felt better than he ever had in his life. Since then milk, wheat, and eggs were gradually added. No symptoms occurred for one month, when a severe headache began. Since eliminating these foods again he has been entirely relieved for two months. The separate activity of these foods has not been determined.

Comment: This patient had such severe headaches and neuralgia in the left face that alcoholic injections were tried on six occasions but with no relief. The marked help obtained with the use of our elimination diet demonstrates food allergy as the cause of his longstanding symptoms.

SUMMARY

1. Evidence of clinical allergy from its activity in the cerebral and neural tissues has steadily increased, as predicted by Foster Kennedy in 1936.

2. The experimental evidence of such neural and cerebral allergy is summarized in this chapter.

3. Involvement of the CNS with allergic reactions from serum allergy has long been recognized.

4. Allergy to foods and to a lesser extent pollens best explains migraine and many otherwise idiopathic headaches as reported in Chapter 17.

5. Transient pareses, paralyses, paresthesias, and stupors resulting from allergy in the cranial and at times in peripheral nerves particularly to foods have been recorded as a result of edema and other tissue allergies.

6. Allergy as a cause of idiopathic epilepsy to foods reported since 1922, and to pollens, as we first reported in 1926, has been increasingly recognized by many physicians.

7. Evidence in encephalograms of relief of epilepsy from the control of food and pollen allergy has been reported by Dees and Lowenbach in 1951 as shown in Figure 31.

8. Mental and emotional symptoms in children and adults with other symptoms of allergic fatigue and toxemia resulting from food allergy are discussed in this chapter and are evidenced in two important case reports.

9. Allergy in the cranial and peripheral nerves arises from allergy to serum, foods, and to pollens.

10. A unique report of neural allergy to pollens in Case 109 is entitled to special emphasis.

11. Other case reports by Campbell of

instructive cases of neural allergy are included.

12. Food and other atopic allergies deserve study in trigeminal neuralgia, as illustrated in a case report.

13. Vertigo and dizziness require study of allergy, especially to foods, as advised in **Chapter 13.**

14. Allergy to foods and possibly to inhalants and drugs and to bacteria, especially streptococcus, is indicated in reports of two greatly benefitted patients with multiple sclerosis. Our reported benefit from the control of atopic allergy especially to foods and from desensitization to streptococci deserves further consideration.

Chapter 19

Allergic Fatigue and Toxemia Resulting From Food Allergy

Allergic fatigue and toxemia were first reported by us as a syndrome of symptoms in 1928 and 1930. This syndrome is characterized by fatigue, weakness, "not rested on arising," lack of energy and ambition, drowsiness, loginess, depression, inability to think and concentrate, and at times chilling and night sweats occurring in varying combinations, degrees, and frequency. Temper tantrums, irritability, and emotional instability may also be present. We reported this syndrome with case histories in the first edition of this book in 1931 and in three other books and several articles on food allergy since then.

In 1950 we published the following statistics on seventy patients, predominantly females, with histories of allergic fatigue and toxemia. Food allergy alone was incriminated in sixty-three (90%) patients, food and pollen in one, and pollen alone in four patients. Pollen allergy as a cause of toxemia in children was first reported by Kabin in 1927.

All of these patients were relieved of their various symptoms by the elimination of allergenic foods. All other possible causes were studied by us or by referring physicians. Psychiatric and psychosomatic study and treatment had been resorted to by eight patients.

Many additional patients with various other manifestations of food and inhalant allergy had mild or moderate fatigue and other symptoms of this toxemia. Moreover, many patients with severe sick headaches or migraine preceded or associated with fatigue and exhaustion were not included. Finally, the many patients with ulcerative colitis, fundamentally resulting in our opinion from food and at times to pollen allergy, in whom marked exhaustion, fatigue, and depression and other symptoms occurred, were omitted.

The onset was at any age from ten to seventy years, the condition having lasted one to forty years with an average duration of 9.4 years.

On skin testing there were a few reactions to foods. These reactions rarely revealed actual clinical allergy. Neither did they harmonize with the causative food allergies which were found responsible in 93 percent of the patients. It did reveal "slight" to "definite" pollen reactions in most of the pollen-sensitive patients.

These symptoms and associated fever up to 104 F both in children and adults were illustrated in a boy 2½ years old, whose parents reported "head colds," listlessness, sleepiness at times for three days, as well as general physical inactivity. Subnormal mentality had been diagnosed. Normal energy and alertness resulted from elimination of allergenic foods. Fever resulting from food allergy receives important discussion in Chapter 24 and especially in bronchial asthma resulting from food allergy in Chapters 8 and 25.

356

TABLE XL
ALLERGIC TOXEMIA AND FATIGUE
IN 70 PATIENTS

		%
Average age	42 (10-70 years)	
Male		28
Female		72
Duration of toxemia	9.4 years (1-40)	
Toxic symptoms:		
Fatigue		94
Not rested on arising		57
Lack of energy		66
Aching in joints		47
Aching in muscles		36
Aching in chest		10
Loginess, listlessness, drowsiness		37
Disability in concentration		27
Confusion		17
Depression		30
Irritability		20
Nervous tension		34
Emotional instability		6
Insomnia		11
Fever		10
Night sweats		3
Chilling and gooseflesh		3
Tachycardia		10
Manifestations of allergy other than toxemia:		
Gastrointestinal allergy		63
Headache (including nuchal pain)		50
Eczema		10
Hives and swellings		16
Hay fever		9
Nasal allergy		34
Bronchial asthma		6
Urogenital allergy		4
Epilepsy		3
Family history of allergy:		
Bronchial asthma		23
Nasal allergy		9
Hay fever		11
Eczema		7
Hives and swellings		7
Headaches		17
Gastrointestinal symptoms		19
Skin testing		
Positive reactions to:		
Pollens		20
Animal emanations		11
Dusts		10
Miscellaneous inhalants		11
Foods		21
Roentgen ray studies of gastrointestinal tract negative in		27
Roentgen ray studies of gallbladder negative in		23
Stomach analysis negative in		16
Achylia in		4
Positive dietary history		40
Causes:		
Food allergy		90
Food and pollen allergy		1
Pollen allergy alone		6

ILLUSTRATIVE CASES

Case 115: A girl seven years of age had "sinus attacks" with fever up to 105 F every four to eight weeks. She was listless, inefficient in school, refused to play, and disliked most foods. She stated: "I feel like a rag doll." Adherence to her elimination diet resulted in a normal, active, happy, hungry child.

Comment: Fatigue and weakness resulting from allergy may be most evident in the mornings, even after a long night's rest or sleep. Patients hate to get up or may find it difficult to awaken. Often this fatigue continues throughout the day. One patient said, "I'm so tired I wonder how I get through the day." Another stated, "I get tired and achy doing nothing." Some have to lie down most of the time. This fatigue may increase in the late afternoon and evening, causing sleep, drowsiness, and inability to concentrate mentally after dinner. When allergy is controlled, these symptoms disappear. One relieved patient stated that now she is anxious to work; formerly all mental and physical effort had been forced. She can accomplish much at home, even in the evening, which she "hadn't been able to do for twenty years."

Loginess, mental confusion, and drowsiness probably because of cerebral allergy often are associated with fatigue. This leads to inefficiency, impaired accomplishment, and lack of ambition. These symptoms, along with irritability, tenseness, depression, and at times emotional instability, produce changes in personality that may be recognized by the patient but over which he has no control.

When these allergic symptoms occur in children, their true cause usually is overlooked.

Dreams, nightmares, and restlessness during the night may occur. Insomnia, especially on retiring or after 1 to 4 AM may be present in infants and children and especially in adults. Character and personality changes are reported especially by Clarke in Chapter 18.

Aching and soreness in the joints, tendons, and muscles often result from allergic reactivity, especially to foods. At times these symptoms are confined to a few joints or to limited areas such as the low midback, the nuchal or shoulder areas, or extremities. Several encouraging results in rheumatoid arthritis as well as in chronic or recurrent tendosynovitis have justified our study of food allergy along with its other allergic and commonly considered causes.

At times fever, chilling, goose flesh, and sweating apparently occur in varying degrees from food allergy. Resultant vascular allergy probably accounts for the hypotension and tachycardia which often arise from food and other allergy. Fever resulting from food allergy receives important discussion in Chapter 24.

All these symptoms may vary in degree. As in other manifestations of food allergy, such as asthma or recurrent headaches, this toxemia may occur in cyclic attacks. Usually it is persistent and exaggerated at regular intervals, especially in women during their menstrual periods. Because of the beneficial effect of the summer and also inland, dry areas on food allergy long reported by the writer, allergic toxemia may decrease in these months and in such regions. Exaggeration of symptoms during the spring, summer, and fall occurs in toxemia resulting from pollen allergy. Other manifestations of allergy, especially cerebral, gastrointestinal, and nasal, occur in these patients, as shown in Table XL.

Since the publication of these statistics in 1950, we have recognized and controlled this syndrome with the elimination of allergenic foods and with control of less frequent pollen allergy in many other patients in the last nineteen years. In 1959 we published a second article confirming the occurrence of the various symptoms in this syndrome with summaries of varying symptoms in seven illustrative cases. Moreover, many additional patients suffering with al-lergic headache and migraine, gastrointestinal allergy, chronic ulcerative colitis and other manifestations of clinical allergy demonstrate varying symptoms of allergic toxemia and fatigue as reported in Chapters 5, 6, and 17 of this volume.

ADDITIONAL LITERATURE

Shannon, in 1922, reported nervousness, restlessness, irritability, and constant crying in children resulting from food allergy. Constant crying and restless movements of the body for five months in an infant was relieved by the elimination of milk and wheat. Such crying and restlessness had been continuous night and day in a four-teen-month-old child, necessitating constant holding and soothing until relief occurred with our CFE diet. Such crying and restlessness usually occurs from infantile colic because of cow's milk allergy (see Chapt. 25), and gastrointestinal symptoms may be absent. Varying degrees of the symptoms in this syndrome, moreover, associated even with paralysis, paresis, paresthesias, delirium, and even unconsciousness were attributed to allergy in important articles by Foster Kennedy from 1926 to 1936. This subject receives further comment in Chapter 25.

Allergic fatigue and toxemia in adults and children were confirmed by Alvarez (1935), Ruiz-Moreno (1940 and 1943), and Mariante (1948).

Randolph especially has elucidated these manifestations of food allergy. In 1945 he stressed their frequent occurrence, usually attributed erroneously to psychosomatic causes or neurasthenia. In 1948 and 1949 he reported food allergy as one cause of torticollis and especially of nuchal myalgia and acute torticollis resulting in stiffness and deep soreness in the neck, shoulders, and upper back muscles. Other symptoms of allergic toxemia, as reported by us in 1931 and 1959, occurred in varying combinations and degrees. In 1950 he reported fatigue, joint pains, irritability, headaches, and other symptoms in our syndrome *allergic fatigue and toxemia* from cottonseed oil giving no skin reactions. In 1951 Randolph again wrote an informative article on myalgia resulting from food allergy especially in the posterior cervical and trapezius muscles. Less often soreness, pain, and tautness occurred in pectoral, intercostal, abdominal, lumbar, ham string, and calf muscles because of such allergy. At times generalized aching in muscles and joints, we previously reported, occurred. Pulling, drawing, tightness, aching, and soreness especially in the cervical muscles have been designated as tension headaches, attributed to nerve tension and not to the causative allergies. Food allergy causing reactions in muscles and joints is discussed in Chapter 23. Tender nodules were reported in the involved muscles in the neck and even in the calf or other skeletal muscles with frequent muscular cramping. In Randolph's article of 1945 he confirmed the many physical and psychological symptoms in allergic fatigue and toxemia we reported in 1931 and 1948. Five illustrative case histories were summarized, making the article important for perusal by physicians challenged with patients affected with this syndrome.

Speer, in 1954 and in 1958, reported allergic tension and fatigue in many patients. He confirms this again in a book in 1970. The term *toxemia* still seems preferable to *tension*. The former was first used by Kahn in 1927 and by us since 1930 because of its connotation of depression, dopiness, confusion, and inability to think and concentrate which are so frequent in these sufferers. In 1952 Davison reported speech disturbances, aphasia, and stuttering in allergic children along with other symptoms of allergic toxemia. Cavanaugh and Berman recently reported allergy as a probable cause of difficulty in reading and writing associated with some motor incoordination and inability to do "sequential tasks" in 8 to 10 percent of school children. Impaired hearing was present in 55 percent of these children in whom nasal allergy and a family history of clinical allergy were present. Though actual food and inhalant allergy were not proved by relief of symptoms in the 180 children, they were interviewed and studied, and the challenge of probable allergic etiology exists.

CASE HISTORIES

Case 116: A man thirty-four years of age had constant fatigue for fifteen years. After fourteen hours of sleep, confusion, dopiness, irritability, daydreaming, difficulty in thinking and concentration, and a dull frontal headache continued. Generalized aching, especially in the back of the neck, shoulders, and hip joints persisted.

Postnasal mucus, nasal congestion, and burning and fullness in the epigastrium occurred most of the time.

Diet history incriminated only eggs as one cause of headaches. Family history revealed toxicity and indigestion for forty years in the mother.

Laboratory and x-ray studies, skin tests for allergy, and physical examination were negative except for a boggy nasal mucosa.

With our FFCFE diet plus rice there was improvement in six days. In one month improvement increased. Soy products had caused distention. In two months he was entirely comfortable. In five years his symptoms were absent with the continued elimination of milk, wheat, fruits, flavors, and condiments.

Case 117: A woman thirty-four years of age had increasing fatigue, weakness, confusion, indecision, apprehension, depression, impaired memory, and emotional instability for five years. Weakness finally necessitated aid in walking. Sleep was restless and disturbed by dreams, especially of falling.

Hives and swellings, especially of the face, lips, feet, and hands, had recurred for five years. Headaches with nausea and frequent soreness and vomiting had been recurring since adolescence. Pain and soreness in the lower abdomen, elbows, shoulders, and knees had been helped by the elimination of tomatoes and fruits. Milk and eggs had increased the localized swellings. Penicillin and sulfonamide drugs had caused edema and nausea.

Physical examination and laboratory tests, including skin tests with foods and inhalants, were negative.

Food allergy was studied with a minimal diet containing tapioca, white and sweet potato, chicken, turkey, salt, and water along with multiple synthetic vitamins and calcium carbonate, one-half teaspoonful in water daily.

For the last five years all symptoms have been controlled using the above diet with the addition of rice, oats, and lamb, one to two times a week; squab and duck also have been tolerated. Milk, eggs, beef, pork, all fruits, condiments, and spices reproduced symptoms.

Case 118: A woman twenty-five years of age had had aching, soreness, and edema in the arms spreading to the shoulders, neck, upper back, and lateral chest with mild and occasional aching soreness in the thighs for fifteen months. She had been unable to use and raise her arms. Symptoms had been perennial but were exaggerated in the spring, summer, and fall. For two months in the summer she also had soreness and pain in the right eye, especially with upward vision. She also had pain under the sternum with swallowing. With these symptoms she had felt weak, stupid, groggy, nervous, and dizzy. Prednisone, 10 mg daily, had ameliorated the symptoms. For many years she had had postnasal mucus with morning hacking and coughing. Her diet and environmental histories suggested no allergy. Morphine and codeine had caused vomiting and headaches.

Physical examination, comprehensive laboratory studies, and x-ray studies of the lungs and upper gastrointestinal tract were noncontributory.

On skin testing there were slight reactions to several grass, fall, and tree pollens and one plus reaction to cow's milk and goat's milk.

Because of exaggerated symptoms during the pollen seasons, desensitization with a multiple all-season antigen was started, initiated with a 1:5 million dilution. It was gradually increased through the winter up to the 1:50 dilution, which was well tolerated. In two months near or complete relief had developed. Increasing relief had continued during the last five months. A temporary recurrence arose when 0.4 cc of the 1:50 dilution was administered. This difficulty was relieved by temporary reduction to the 1:500 dilution. Since then 0.6 cc of the 1:50 dilution has been given and tolerated without symptoms.

Food allergy was studied with our FFCFE diet with no resultant incriminations of foods except for exaggeration of nasal allergy from milk and abdominal cramping from pineapple.

Comment: Fatigue is the most common symptom of this syndrome resulting from allergy, especially to foods. It often persists on awakening even after sleep or rest for ten to twelve hours, as evidenced in most of the above case reports. A lack of energy and especially of initiative and enthusiasm occurs. Such symptoms became so marked in Case 117 that walking required support. Moderate and severe fatigue occurs to a degree in many patients with other manifestations of allergy not only resulting from foods but also to pollens and drugs. Thus fatigue is not an uncommon symptom resulting from pollen in hay fever. Whether this is due to a generalized allergic reaction throughout the body or mainly in the skeletal muscles is unknown.

Mental symptoms including drowsiness; loginess; disability in concentration, thinking, and memory; confusion; depression and irritability; emotional instability; and nervous tension in varying combinations and degrees are best explained by cerebral allergy (Chapt. 18) resulting from possible edema or other results of vascular or other tissue reactivity. Along with irritability, disturbed sleep from annoying dreams may occur. A successful, active lumber mill operator complained of depression and "feeling blue" along with his generalized fatigue.

Nuchal soreness, stiffness, and pain are designated as headaches by many patients. This distress in the back of the neck may extend into the cervical and shoulder muscles and in the arms. It prevented raising of the arms in Case 118. Most patients have had neck traction, often in hospitals, with no help. We have observed this nuchal allergy in mild degrees in many other patients, usually associated with various manifestations of allergy. Torticollis and "wry neck" resulting from food allergy have been reported in a helpful article by Randolph summarized in Chapter 18.

Chilling with or without goose flesh may also occur in these patients.

Pain, soreness, and stiffness may occur in other skeletal muscles. In Case 118 the aching, soreness, and mild edema in the arms, spreading to the shoulders, neck, upper back, and thighs for fifteen months and even the pain in the right eye with upward vision were relieved by desensitization to the pollens present in her area without any consideration of food allergy.

Postnasal mucus caused a hacking and clearing of mucus from the pharynx and a soreness of the throat in Case 116. Frequent occurrence of nasal allergy with the cerebral symptoms indicates a regional area of allergic reactivity in these adjoining affected tissues. Asthma occurs less frequently than nasal allergy.

Hives had recurred all through life in Case 117. Foods, and in another case penicillin and sulfonamide drugs, were responsible.

Diet histories in the cases in this chapter gave little information indicating the responsible food allergies.

Drug allergy was present in Case 117. In Case 118 morphine and codeine caused vomiting and headaches. In not one of the cases did fatigue and allergic toxemia arise from drug allergy.

Case 119: Fever with fatigue and aching in joints and muscles in a girl ten years of age had kept her in bed for eighteen months because of possible rheumatic fever. Sulfadiazine had been given for two years with no benefit. With the CFE diet fatigue and fever have been absent three years. Wheat, corn, and milk have been the incriminated allergens.

Though a diet history reveals foods that are disliked or disagree in patients with various manifestations of food allergy, such a history often is of special diagnostic importance in allergic toxemia and fatigue. Patients frequently report that specific foods cause various symptoms of this syndrome. Milk, eggs, wheat, some or even most fruits, spices, condiments, chocolate, and at times sugar are suspected, but their exclusion usually has not been complete, or all suspected foods have not been eliminated. Too often, commonly eaten foods responsible for the symptoms have not been recognized. In an attempt to control symptoms with elimination of suspected foods, the diet may be very restricted with resultant loss of weight and impaired nutrition.

PATHOGENESIS AND PATHOLOGY

The pathogenesis of this syndrome is not known. Randolph has reported atypical mononuclear cells resembling those found in infectious mononucleosis in patients with allergic toxemia. Other evidence of systemic disturbance is lacking. Chronic allergy, especially to foods, does not produce recognized changes in the blood except leukopenia after ingestion of allergenic foods, reported especially by Vaughan. Eosinophilia is not usual. The sedimentation rate has been increased in some of these patients in the absence of any demonstrable cause other than chronic food allergy.

The symptomatology depends on the tissues affected by the allergic reactivity. Vascular allergy is known to produce vascular inflammation, increased permeability, and local edema. The possibility of collagen disturbances, the maximum evidence of which has been demonstrated by Rich and others in periarteritis nodosa, has to be considered in patients with severe, longstanding allergic toxemia.

Information from tissue biopsies in these

patients would be of great interest, but the good prognosis in cooperating patients allows no postmortem examinations.

DIAGNOSIS AND CONTROL

Before or while allergy is being studied as a cause of fatigue and these various toxic symptoms, new growths and infectant, metabolic, endocrine, cardiovascular, genitourinary, and other less common causes must be carefully studied and excluded. It is to be stressed, moreover, that allergy must be ruled out by adequate and experienced study and treatment before psychosomatic causes, which place the blame on the patient, are ever incriminated.

FOOD ALLERGY

To study possible food allergy, trial diet with our elimination diet has been utilized for forty years. The test-negative diet rarely yields any relief. Usually our CFE diet has been prescribed. Foods suspected of possible allergy or those giving large scratch reactions may also be excluded. If legumes or other foods disagree, they are eliminated. The time required to obtain relief and the method of manipulation of the diet to obtain the desired results have been detailed in Chapter 3.

Relief may be evident in four to fourteen days, increasing in the following weeks. Thus in Case 116, it was apparent in six days, being increasingly evident in the next three weeks and complete in 2½ months. In other cases, convincing benefit of the dietary therapy was not seen until after 2½ to 3 months.

POLLEN ALLERGY

Pollen allergy must be recognized by exaggeration of symptoms during the pollen seasons. Though scratch reactions usually are positive, they may be slight or absent, pollen allergy being indicated only by the history. Food and pollen allergy may be associated and must be recognized. Summaries of cases resulting from pollen allergy follow:

Aching, soreness, and limitation of motion in the neck, shoulders, and arms and fatigue in Case 118 became absent or only slightly recurrent in two months as a result of pollen therapy alone. This relief has continued with brief recurrence for two years. Pollen desensitization is being continued.

Case 120: Another woman twenty-five years of age developed increasing pain first in the arms extending into her forearms and especially into her third and fourth fingers. The pain had developed in August and had increased until the rains. Symptoms recurred in early spring. Large scratch reactions occurred to grass, tree, and fall pollens. Pain was entirely relieved initially with corticosteroids and gradually with pollen desensitization alone. Before commencement of our study, surgical exploration of her blood vessels of the arms had been scheduled.

The final elimination diets which have been necessary for the continued relief of allergic fatigue and toxemia symptoms vary. In Case 116 milk, wheat, fruit, flavors, and condiments have been excluded for five years. As in all cases multiple vitamins have been given.

In another case, milk, eggs, beef, pork, wheat, fruit, spices, and condiments have been necessary to eliminate to control symptoms for five years. Rotation of several vegetables and at times of beef and wheat has allowed their ingestion with minimum difficulty.

As noted above, the aching, pains, and fatigue in Case 118 have been controlled with desensitization to pollens.

SUMMARY

1. The common occurrence of fatigue and allergic toxemia in children and adults arising from food and less often from pollen allergy requires recognition by all physicians.

2. Fatigue occurs in mild to severe degrees. This fatigue and toxemia may be so marked that physical and mental in-

capacitation may prevent actual work and efficiency in occupation, business, or home.

3. Allergic toxemia usually accompanies the fatigue. Loginess; listlessness; drowsiness; aching and soreness in skeletal muscles and joints, especially in the cervical, shoulder, and arm regions and less so in other muscles; irritability; tension; depression; insomnia; difficulty in concentration and thinking; and fever resulting from food and less often to pollen allergy occur.

4. Gastrointestinal and nasal allergy and less often hives, eczema, and urogenital symptoms may be accompanying allergic manifestations.

5. Nuchal and other muscular allergies associated with fatigue and varying numbers and degrees of the above symptoms may be distressing and invaliding.

6. This fatigue and toxemia are evidenced in illustrative cases.

7. With the accurate use of our elimination diets, relief is evidenced in one to two weeks and may be complete in one to three months. Typical final diets necessary for freedom from symptoms are detailed. Pollen desensitization alone relieved the symptoms in Case 118.

8. Allergy, along with all other possible causes of fatigue and toxemia must be excluded as an etiological factor before a diagnosis of psychoneurosis is justified.

Ocular Allergy

Though atopic allergy to foods and to inhalants, especially to pollens, is the major challenge in this chapter, contact allergy and autoimmune allergy to antigens in the lens and iris, along with infectant allergy and infection, will be discussed. Drug allergy which is elicited in the patient's history must be constantly in mind. When suspected, all drugs must be eliminated, as will be discussed later.

The occurrence of antibodies to various allergens in all tissues of the body explains allergic reactions in the skin of the lids, conjunctiva, sclera, cornea, uveal tract including the choroid, retina, and optic nerve of the eye. These manifestations reported by many ophthalmologists in the literature, as discussed by Theodore and Schlossman in 1958 in their admirable book on ocular allergy with our comments about other reports of ocular allergy in the literature since 1958, will be summarized in this chapter. Though allergy often occurs in more than one of these ocular tissues, its manifestations reported in the literature and observed and controlled in our practice of allergy will be discussed in single or joint structures of the eye.

DERMATITIS OF THE EYELIDS

Allergic dermatitis of the lids from inhalants, especially pollens, and from foods is a major challenge to allergists and ophthalmologists. Though it may only be on the upper lid, the lower lid is usually involved. The dermatitis often extends onto the cheeks, forehead, ears, neck, and at times it develops on other areas of the body as shown in Table XLI and in Chapter 14 on allergic dermatitis.

Next to contact and drug allergies discussed below, pollens and less often other inhalant and food allergies have caused lid dermatitis most frequently in our practice.

POLLEN ALLERGY

Pollen allergy is indicated by the onset of the dermatitis during the pollen seasons in the spring, summer, or fall, recurring or activated in these seasons each year with a disappearance or definite reduction in the winter. Statistics on fifteen such cases in our practice are in Table XLI.

The diagnosis and treatment of pollen allergy are summarized at the end of this chapter and discussed more fully in Chapters 2 and 4.

CASE HISTORIES

Case 121: One woman fifty-eight years of age developed an erythematous, itching dermatitis on the upper lids spreading on the cheeks and around the neck relieved by our CFE diet. The CFE diet incriminated allergenic foods which have had to be eliminated for its control during the last fourteen years.

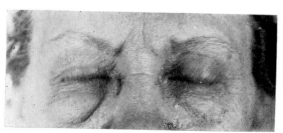

Figure 29.

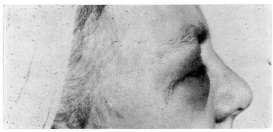

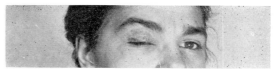

Figure 32.

Figure 30. Eyelid dermatitis resulting from pollen allergy and relieved by desensitization to causative pollens.

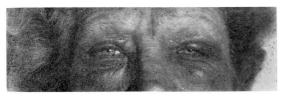

Figure 31.

Case 122: A boy sixteen years of age developed eczema on the left upper lid in December, spreading onto the ears, hairline, and cubital areas in a two-month period. Relief occurred and has continued with the use of our CFE diet.

Case 123: A man of fifty-seven years of age developed a dry dermatitis first on the right upper eyelid, extending around the mouth over the face and on both eyelids during a month's period. His dermatitis also was relieved with the above diet.

Case 124: Such origin on the upper lid appeared in a woman twenty-six years of age with the extension of dermatitis over the face within one month. With provocation feeding tests after relief was assured with our CFE diet, wheat, milk, and chocolate were found responsible.

DERMATITIS OF THE LIDS RESULTING FROM MEDICATIONS

The frequency of dermatitis resulting from drugs and chemicals in ointments, lotions, and eye medications is discussed and emphasized in many articles and books on ocular allergy. Usually there is concomitant, even severe allergic conjunctivitis resulting in dermatoconjunctivitis. Most drugs used by ophthalmologists can produce in varying degrees such allergic inflammation arising from a hapten reaction in which a chemical in the drug unites with the tissue protein to which combination antibodies in the lids develop. These in turn react with the chemical or drug if its application continues. In former years belladonna, atropin, quinine, chloral, cocaine, and other analgesics, mercurials, and the wool fat in lanolin were usual offenders. Since then sulfonamides, synthetic local anesthetics, and antibiotics, especially Neo-

TABLE XLI

BLEPHARITIS

Dermatitis of the Eyelids Because of Pollen

Number of Patients	15
Females	80%
Family History:	
Hay fever	20%
Asthma	33%
Years of Dermatitis (⅓ to 7 years) ..... av.	2½ yrs
Patient's Symptoms:	
Itching	100%
Erythema	90%
Edema	80%
Oozing	30%
Crusting	36%
Burning	30%
Other Areas of Dermatitis:	
Face	42%
Neck	36%
Ears	8%
Torso	14%
Genitalia	0.6%
Extremities	20%
Other Allergies in Patient:	
Nasal	36%
Asthma	0.6%
GI symptoms	13%
Skin Tests (positive) to Pollens	80%
Skin Tests (negative; diagnosis by history)	20%
Associated Food Allergy	20%
Pollen Therapy	100%
Relief obtained with the	
1:100 dilution	60%
1:500 dilution	20%
1:50,000 dilution	20%
Duration of treatment (½ to 3 years) av.	1.9 yrs

mycin, have become important causes. The reader is referred to the many listings of drugs and medications which can cause dermatoconjunctivitis recorded in the literature in separate articles and in various texts on ophthalmology. Ointments containing mercury and its derivatives are suspect. It is discussed in *Ocular Allergy* by Theodore and Schlossman.

The physician's challenge in relieving patients with such allergic dermatitis is to stop all medications being applied to the lids or instilled into the eye. Compresses of warm sterile water or weak boric acid solution, the instillation of a 1:2000 epinephrine solution, and when the dermatitis is severe, corticosteroid therapy is used as advised in this chapter. That medications require hours or even days to relieve the involved tissues must be remembered.

Since blood-borne medications given by mouth or parenterally cause allergic dermatitis which might intensify or rarely initiate the dermatoconjunctivitis, their discontinuance is justified until the dermatitis is controlled. Important medications which are necessary to control other disease as in the heart or in diabetes may be continued. After the ocular dermatitis is relieved for one to two months, other medications can be given by mouth, eliminating any which reproduces the dermatitis. Possible allergy to medications absorbed from the body orifices such as toothpaste, mouthwashes, nasal drops or spray, medications for headaches or indigestion, birth control pills, vaginal douches or enemas, and other medications must be known to the physician. Soaps, detergents, insecticides, and fertilizers used in gardening must be in mind. Contact allergy to oils and resins encountered in gardening, particularly if they are transmitted to the eyelids by the hands, may cause this dermatitis. Naphthalene in mothballs or pyrethrum in insecticides may be offenders.

CONTACT ALLERGY TO COSMETICS, DYES, AND PLASTICS ON EYELIDS

Allergy to various ingredients in cosmetics including perfumes, hair, eyebrow and eyelash dyes, orris root, and synthetic chemicals contained in such preparations must be suspected, as emphasized by Seinny in 1951. Nail polish and dye rubbed on the lids by fingers may also cause dermatitis. The many inflammations and dermatitis arising from contact allergy to drugs in ointments or solutions applied to the lid from cosmetics, especially those containing orris root; perfumes from dyes, especially paraphenyldiamine; mascara particularly in eyebrow pencils; and from plastics in spectacles including secondary infection and the results of collagen disease must be remembered, as reported and discussed in Theodore and Schlossman's excellent book on *Ocular Allergy*, which contains a list of over 140 ingredients in cosmetics, creams, hair preparations, lipsticks, nail polish, antiseptics, and miscellaneous substances.

One woman of sixty-five years of age had had moderate palpebral dermatitis for one year greatly exaggerated with involvement of her entire scalp after the use of a new plastic hair spray for about one week. With its discontinuance and with the use of corticoids by mouth, marked improvement occurred which was not complete until the plastic frames of her eyeglasses also were eliminated. Contact allergy to brown hair dye also occurred.

BLEPHARITIS AND GRANULATED LIDS AND STYES RESULTING FROM FOOD ALLERGY

Allergy in the edges of the lids with resultant granulation and inflammation with lacrimation and at times recurrent styes requires the study of possible food allergy especially if these manifestations are perennial and particularly if exaggerated in the winter (Chapt. 1). This may occur with little or no associated dermatitis of the lids or conjunctivitis which is usually present when pollen allergy is the cause. Associated eczema in the scalp, ears, face, and nostrils may occur especially because of allergy to milk in infants and young children.

CASE RECORDS

Case 125: A woman forty-one years of age had granulated lids with moderate conjunctival congestion and perennial nasal allergy which indicated study of food allergy. After relief arising from strict adherence to our CFE diet, provocation tests showed that wheat allergy was the sole cause.

Case 126: A woman thirty-eight years of age had marginal blepharitis with recurrent styes for ten years. Desensitization to pollens for nine years had given no relief. Skin tests to foods and inhalants were negative. Relief occurred with our CFE diet. Because of the improvement of food allergy during the summer, most foods were added, with resultant exaggeration of the symptoms in late September and October. During the fall and winter adherence to the CFE diet gave continued relief. Provocation tests in the winter to determine specific foods responsible for her allergy were refused.

Case 127: A woman thirty-nine years of age had had granulated eyelids with lacrimation and mucoid ocular discharge perennially for five years. The absence of itching and its perennial persistence suggested food allergy. Relief occurred with our CFE diet within three weeks' time. Provocation tests than showed that eggs, milk, wheat, and chocolate were responsible.

Case 128: A woman thirty-five years of age had marginal blepharitis and granulated lids and styes most of the time for five years. Treatment by several ophthalmologists with eye drops, ointments, scraping of the edges of the lids, and the administration of stock, and autogenous vaccines had failed.

She knew that milk, wheat, and tomatoes increased the eruption.

A diet eliminating corn, coffee, fish, olives, and peaches to which skin reactions had been obtained by an allergist had failed.

Relief occurred with our FFCFE diet. Then in two months with provocation feeding tests, cereals, milk, chocolate, coffee, and uncooked fruit proved responsible. Achromycin ointment was used locally to control secondary infection. No autogenous or stock vaccines were given.

Bothman reported blepharitis and chronic conjunctivitis and recurring chalazion of all lids usually because of ingested wheat. He also stated that blepharitis in infants and young children is often associated with eczema of scalp, ears, and cheeks resulting from milk allergy. He comments on Berneaud's report in 1932 of blepharoconjunctivitis and eczema of the lids resulting from primrose, oak sawdust, and even feathers and house dust.

EDEMA OF THE EYELIDS RESULTING FROM FOOD ALLERGY

Case 129: A woman thirty-seven years of age had had edema of the eyelids and congestion in the conjunctiva with a sandy feeling in the eyes for four years. Though perennial in occurrence, it was worse with periods, which suggests food allergy as noted in Chapter 21. For five months eczema had also been present on the right malar area. Frequent headaches had occurred.

With our CFE diet, as advised later in this chapter and also Chapter 3, relief from all these symptoms resulted. Provocation tests gradually showed that milk and eggs were the cause. Headaches, for example, occurred in twelve hours after the ingestion of milk.

Case 130: A woman fifty-nine years of age had edema of the eyelids with redness, burning, and a sandy feeling in the eyeballs with a clear mucoid discharge; a feeling of pressure in the eyes; and blurred vision for six years. These symptoms occurred for one to two weeks every month or so, especially in late December, January, and February, suggesting food allergy. The patient dated the onset of her symptoms after the administration of hormones, but there was no relief after their discontinuance. Since then moderate doses of estrogens had been taken, with no reaction. Fatigue associated with aching and weakness in her lower legs occurred with the ocular symptoms. Pain and soreness of the throat and in the left side of her neck extending down to the clavicle were present. For six months nausea had occurred before and after meals. Bowels were normal.

A diet history revealed ingestion of bakery products and fruits, causing a burning, itching, and sandy feeling in the eyes; an aversion for milk; and a dislike for cheese. Fish also was avoided. She stated that she "could not stand fruits." Family history revealed asthma in an uncle. Her physical examination and routine laboratory tests were all negative. X-rays of her sinuses showed slight cloudiness compatible with allergy in the mucosa. Skin testing revealed one to two plus reactions to grass, fall, and tree pollens and a six plus reaction to oak to which no clinical allergy existed.

Food allergy was definitely suggested by the recurrence of her symptoms every month, lasting for one to two weeks, with exaggeration during the winter months (see Chapt. 1). This history is comparable to the history of recurrent bronchial asthma because of food allergy summarized in Chapter 8.

To study food allergy, our FFCFE diet was ordered. Fruits were eliminated because of her history of aversion to fruits which frequently produce allergic fatigue (see Chapt. 19). All ocular symptoms, pain and soreness of the throat and neck, and marked fatigue disappeared within three weeks and remained absent for two months. Then with provocation tests, allergy to fruit was confirmed. Her ocular symptoms also were reactivated when wheat, rice, corn, oats, eggs, milk, and coffee were added to the diet. Her skin reactions to pollens were of no clinical significance, especially since symptoms were not exaggerated during pollen seasons!

In addition to blepharitis, this patient had allergy to the conjunctiva and possible allergic uveitis, accounting for the pressure in the eye and blurred vision. The pain in the left neck may have been due to neuritis resulting from food allergy as discussed in Chapter 18. Her relief from fatigue indicated that allergic fatigue and probable slight toxemia were present, as discussed in Chapter 19.

In addition to the above case of edema of the lids resulting from food allergy, we have controlled moderate or marked edemas of the lids in other patients suffering with marked urticaria, as in one young girl seventeen years of age who had had these symptoms for many months relieved with our FFCFE diet. After relief was assured, provocation tests showed that milk, eggs, and uncooked fruits were responsible. In addition, there are many patients who have localized swellings or angioneurotic edema of the eyelids extending onto the face, especially the lips, tongue, and at times the throat and larynx with or without localized or generalized urticaria resulting from food allergy or occurring in the pollen seasons because of pollen allergy. Drug allergy also always has to be considered. Such edema is discussed in Chapter 16.

Finally, other causes of edema of the lids must be remembered, including hypothyroidism, nephrosis, or cardiorenal disease.

Case 131: One patient, whose photograph is in Figure 33, had persistent edema of the right eyelid for five months. Previous investigations by several physicians had failed to explain the edema. Our study of possible localized edema resulting from foods or drug allergy was ineffectual. Finally, lupus erythematosis was suspected, and the administration of medications gave entire relief.

Bothman comments on palpebral edema resulting from allergy to ingested fish, as reported by Berneaud in 1932; lid edema with lacrimation and pruritus resulting from apricots reported by Strebel in 1936; and similar edema of the lids, face, and right arm and hand after the splashing of cat's blood in the above skin areas. Allergy to emanations of many animals was evidenced by positive skin reactions. Another case of edema of the eyelids, lips, and tongue because of allergy to ingested shrimp and lobster was reported by Bothman in 1941.

CONJUNCTIVAL ALLERGY TO FOODS

Atopic allergy to foods in comparison to pollens and less often to other inhalants has not been sufficiently recognized because of failure to realize its possibilities, arising from the failure of relief from diets

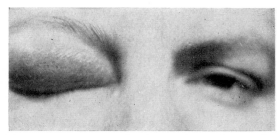

Figure 33. Edema of the eyelid relieved by drug therapy for lupus erythematosis.

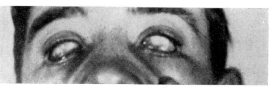

Figure 34.

based on positive skin tests and the failure to use diet trial, especially our elimination diets, without which our recognition of food allergy usually would have failed. The only cases reported by other investigators seem to be the following.

Conlon, in 1919, reported edema and hyperemia in the conjunctiva from tomatoes and strawberries. He also reported a man fifty-six years of age who had had congested conjunctivae with dilatation of the numerous capillaries in the conjunctivae, lacrimation, a feeling of sand in the eyes, and inability to use the eyes for five years. All of these symptoms were entirely relieved by the elimination of eggs, to which a positive skin reaction occurred. In 1938 Vail informed us of chronic conjunctivitis from cereal grains and from chocolate, occurring within one hour after their ingestion. Conjunctivitis occurred in another patient from a particle of lobster in the eye and in another patient from a particle of fin fish in the eye, as reported by Lundberg in 1937. Fish also caused gastrointestinal symptoms in the last patient. Thomas and Warren, in 1940, concluded that food allergy was responsible for conjunctivitis in five patients. In one patient eggs caused conjunctivitis and also paroxysmal nocturia.

PERSONAL CASES

In 1937 we reported conjunctival hemorrhages, hazy vision, and pain in the eye associated with allergic toxemia relieved by the final elimination of meat, cereals, citrus fruits, beans, and cranberry. Since then in the last twenty years the following cases of conjunctivitis have been relieved in our patients with our elimination diets.

Case 132: A woman twenty-nine years of age had had recurrent attacks of itching, redness, and smarting with enlarged blood vessels in the conjunctiva, indicating associated episcleritis, worse for one week at monthly intervals with moderate interim discomfort. There was generalized itching over the body, aching of the knees, and associated fatigue and exhaustion. Relief occurred with our CFE diet and continued for four months with the cooperation of the patient. Further contact with the patient was lost.

Case 133: A man thirty-four years of age had had redness in the conjunctiva and throbbing in one or both eyes continuing for four to six weeks every two to four months, occurring during the fall, winter, and spring with a decrease in the summer. Skin reactions to foods were negative. Relief occurred with our CFE diet. Because of large reactions to grass pollens, desensitization to them was given for four months with questionable benefit.

Food allergy was studied with the CFE diet because of the frequency with which food allergy produces recurrent attacks perennially, as of asthma, with interim relief (Chapt. 2). Recurrent attacks failed to occur for eight months as the diet was maintained. For ten years since

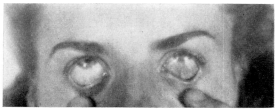

Figure 35. Conjunctivitis relieved with our CFE diet, wheat and milk being the major causes.

then the patient reports continued absence of symptoms with the entire elimination of milk, corn, and to a lesser extent eggs.

Case 134: A woman fifty-six years of age had burning, moderate lacrimation with blurred vision, soreness, and a sandy feeling in the eyes exaggerated during meals, reading, and driving. Discomfort lasted for fifteen to twenty minutes with moderate subsequent distress for one or two hours. At first this recurred every three to four weeks, but for six months it had recurred every one to four days. For twenty years headaches and vomiting had occurred once a month, the history of which always suggests possible food allergy (see Chapt. 17). The ocular symptoms and headaches were relieved with strict adherence to our CFE diet for six weeks, after which provocation tests showed that wheat, milk, corn, and coffee were offending foods.

CONJUNCTIVITIS BECAUSE OF POLLEN ALLERGY

Conjunctivitis because of pollen allergy occurs in the spring, summer, and fall, depending on the patient's sensitizations to tree, grass, or fall pollens. Its decrease or absence in the winter when pollens are not in the air is important evidence of allergy to pollens. Itching, at times intense, with redness and lacrimation usually but not necessarily is present. A case record with typical ocular symptoms in June and July in England was reported by Bostock in 1819 without his recognition of pollen allergy as the cause.

Though skin reactions to pollens causing this conjunctivitis varying from one to four plus by the scratch tests are usually present, they may be absent. Then the diagnosis of pollen allergy depends on the history of seasonal occurrence, the causative pollens being those in the air in the patient's environment when the conjunctivitis occurs. Surveys of all areas of the United States are published in textbooks, such as in ours entitled *Bronchial Asthma—Its Diagnosis and Treatment*, 1963.

It must be remembered that the con-

junctivae as well as the nasal, bronchial, cutaneous, or other tissues which become allergic to pollens may become sensitized to the pollens of cultivated flowers. Allergy to the pollens of fruit trees and even of insect pollinated shrubs in the immediate environment of the patient may be present. This indicates scratch tests with such pollens if suggested by history or if symptoms are not controlled with desensitization to wind-borne pollens.

It must be realized that conjunctivitis resulting from pollen allergy may occur in the absence of nasal manifestations of pollen allergy (hay fever). The conjunctiva with or without keratitis or other manifestations of ocular allergy may be the main or even the only shock organ of such allergy. Thus other manifestations of pollen or other causes of allergy may be present or absent.

Woods, in 1937, reported pollen as the cause in seven of eight cases. Lemoine, in 1929, also reported seven cases because of pollen allergy. Thomas and Warren, in 1940, reported conjunctivitis resulting from spring and fall pollens.

Bothman reported seven cases of allergic conjunctivitis, two due to feathers and pollens, one to molds, and three to pollens. He reported that beefy red conjunctivae with stringy secretion and thickened red lid margins had been present in two cases resulting from spring pollens.

Case 135: A woman thirty-five years of age had frequent marked redness, burning, and itching of the conjunctivae with photophobia during May and June for five years from February to November for seven successive years. Scratch tests to tree, grass, and fall pollens and to airborne fungi were negative. The seasonal history, however, indicated pollen allergy.

During the first five years allergy only to grass pollens was the indicated cause. In the last seven years symptoms from February to late November indicated an extension of her sensitization to the early grass pollens, especially *Poa Annua*, to the tree pollens present in the air during February, March, and early April and also continued sensitization to the fall pollens until the November rains. As stated above, scratch reactions to all of these pollens were negative.

Desensitization to antigens, one containing the pollens of the trees and early grasses and the second containing pollens of the late spring and summer grasses and fall pollens, relieved her conjunctivitis in two months. Continued perennial desensitization was advised (Chapt. 12) to maintain this control of her conjunctivitis during the next two years. Subsequent relief lasted for five years without desensitization.

Case 136: Another patient forty-three years of age had had red, congested conjunctivae with itching and mucoid discharge from March to November for eight years. Skin reactions to pollens also were negative. She had no nasal symptoms resulting from pollen allergy! Her conjunctivitis was relieved with pollen therapy similar to that given to the preceding patient. Excellent results and relief continued for five years while we were in communication with her.

CONJUNCTIVITIS RESULTING FROM POLLEN ALLERGY WITH POSITIVE SCRATCH REACTIONS

Other cases of conjunctivitis resulting from pollen allergy with positive skin reactions to pollens in the air during the months when the symptoms occur but with no evidence of nasal allergy because of skin-reacting pollens in the air when symptoms are absent are not infrequent. Relief in these patients requires desensitization only to the pollens which are in the air when the conjunctivitis occurs.

ALLERGIC CONJUNCTIVITIS ASSOCIATED WITH HAY FEVER RESULTING FROM POLLEN ALLERGY

Finally, allergic conjunctivitis associated with marked itching and lacrimation in patients with definite hay fever resulting from pollen allergy are most frequently encountered. Both ocular and nasal symptoms are distressing. In many patients aching of the eyes often occurs.

Scratch reactions to pollens are usually present and often are large. Positive scratch reactions may occur to practically all tree, grass, summer, and fall pollens, though clinical allergy may occur only in the spring or fall. In these patients reactions to pollens in the seasons when the ocular and nasal symptoms are absent indicate potential allergy to such pollens which may cause future symptoms.

In patients with severe ocular allergy, edema of the conjunctiva may be such that it protrudes even through the eyelids, causing a cupping of the cornea and iris in the base of the cup.

Case 137: I (Albert Rowe, Sr.) developed a beefy red itching conjunctivitis after scraping pollens from glass shelves on which blooming bunches of grasses and weeds were present. This allergy developed after I had harvested pollens during a six-year period before 1924 when pollens were not available for sale. This initial allergy to fall pollens spread to nearly all tree, grass, fall, and cultivated flower pollens, resulting in conjunctival congestion and burning except on rainy days here in California. Desensitization with a multiple pollen antigen has decreased the degree of allergy. This therapy has been required every one to three weeks during the last thirty-five years to prevent moderate activation of the conjunctivitis. Lasting desensitization has not been achieved.

CONJUNCTIVITIS RESULTING FROM INHALANTS OTHER THAN POLLENS

The occurrence of allergies to animal emanations, miscellaneous inhalants, fungi, and house and occupational dusts in the causation of nasal and bronchial allergy necessitates their consideration as a cause of conjunctivitis. This is especially necessary when conjunctivitis is not relieved with the accurate study and control of food and pollen allergy as advised in this chapter and in Chapters 8, 12, and 13. Allergy to these other inhalants may or may not be indicated by skin tests. The history of exaggeration of the conjunctivitis when these various inhalants are in the air of the patient's environment is important evidence of such inhalant allergy. Allergy to tobacco smoke is noted and discussed in Chapter 8.

Bothman notes reports by La Grange, in 1935, of conjunctivitis from house dust, cat emanations, and wool and oak dust; by Taub, in 1930, from silk allergy as a cause; by Balyeat and Bowen, in 1935, of orris root in hair oil and camphor balls causing conjunctivitis; and of Thomas and Warren, in 1940, of conjunctivitis from molds, pollens, or chemicals associated with other manifestations of allergy.

In our study of conjunctivitis, exaggerated particularly in the winter, these inhalants other than pollens have not been definitely demonstrated causes. This does not rule out this possibility, and we continue to keep such possible inhalant allergy in mind when relief from the control of food and pollen allergy is not satisfactory. Perennial conjunctivitis from allergy to the inhaled spores of fungi has been reported by Rinkel, Feinberg, Figley, Summers, and others in former years. Unless we obtain evidence in the patient's history of exaggeration of conjunctivitis occurring in damp or other areas where the spores of fungi are abundant, desensitization to suspected fungi, even to those giving positive scratch reactions, is not routine. We observe that desensitization to antigens containing spores of fungi by other physicians has usually been indicated by skin reactions rather than by evidence that clinical allergy actually exists to such fungi as discussed in Chapter 4.

CONJUNCTIVITIS BECAUSE OF CAUSES OTHER THAN FOOD, INHALANT, AND DRUG ALLERGIES

If the cause of chronic conjunctivitis is uncertain and is not relieved by the study of food, inhalant, and drug allergies, the opinion and treatment of an ophthalmologist are mandatory. Possible bacterial or viral infections may be the sole or associated cause. Recognition of herpetic conjunctivitis which may produce necroses and in the treatment of which corticosteroids are contraindicated is important. Conjunctivitis occurring in Reiter's and Bechet's syndrome makes its recognition by the ophthalmologists important. A probable allergic cause is indicated by marked relief from corticosteroids. As we review medical contributions on these syndromes, previous insufficient study of possible inhalant and especially of food allergy, particularly with our elimination diets, is evident. And recognition of the rare oculomucocutaneous syndromes of erythema multiforme and Stevens-Johnson Disease described by Theodore and Schlossman and many others is most important. Our advised study of possible atopic allergy in these diseases may be justified.

VERNAL CONJUNCTIVITIS

Vernal conjunctivitis is characterized by interstitial conjunctival inflammation of each eye exaggerated or occurring in the spring, summer, and fall and decreasing in the winter. Thus it has been called spring or summer conjunctivitis. Though this seasonal occurrence indicates possible pollen allergy, negative skin reactions and poor results from former pollen therapy usually have failed to support this cause. Theodore and Schlossman favored physical allergy to heat as a probable explanation. In the last decade pollen allergy is being supported by other students and by excellent results from pollen therapy. It usually occurs in boys from ages six to twenty years who usually have a personal or familiar history of allergy.

In our opinion allergy to pollens is the most logical cause of vernal conjunctivitis.

Its occurrence during one or all of the pollen seasons supports this likelihood. Absent scratch reactions to pollens as noted in Chapter 2 and in this chapter do not exclude pollen allergy. Favoring atopic allergy in these patients is the usual occurrence of a family and personal history of allergy with positive skin reactions to pollens, occurrence of eosinophiles in the conjunctival secretions, the relief from epinephrine instilled onto the conjunctiva, and the benefit derived from topical, oral, and parenteral corticosteroid therapy.

According to Bothman, in 1941, Pusey, in 1911, had first suggested pollen as a cause of vernal conjunctivitis or "catarrh." Lemoine reported six cases reacting to pollens or pollens and foods. Lehrfeld recorded reactions to pollens and reactions to pollens and foods in 46 of 102 cases. Bowen obtained pollen reactions in forty-six of one hundred cases. Martin, in 1943 reported four cases of severe vernal conjunctivitis treated with repeated large doses of 1:50 dilution of a spring, grass, tree, and fall pollen antigen, with excellent results. Weinstein, in 1931, reported thirty cases of vernal conjunctivitis, eight of which he attributed to pollen allergy. In some cases powderlike epithelial lesions occur in the cornea, and corneal dystrophias are rare complications. Allansmith and Frick, in 1963, reported clinical evidence and serum antibodies to grass pollens favoring pollen allergy as the cause, reaffirmed by Allansmith in 1969.

In 1969 she reported relief from corticosteroids and 80 percent relief from desensitization to multiple pollen antigens. If pollen therapy had been given up to maximum doses for two or three years, greater or complete relief would have occurred. This also would prevent complications, including possible glaucoma, cataracts, or corneal ulcer, from continued corticosteroid therapy.

Thus desensitization with a maximum tolerated dose should be repeated during a two-year or longer period of time. As relief increases from such pollen therapy, the corticosteroids should be reduced and gradually eliminated. The study and control of pollen allergy receives further discussion at the end of this chapter.

CASE REPORT

Case 138: A boy ten years of age had had burning and itching of the eyes for two years especially on bright days and less in the dark. This had increased and finally became continuous during the daylight for six to eight months. There had been definite improvement in the winter with reactivation when pollen returned to the air in the spring. In the day the discharge was watery and with very little mucus. However, the lids were stuck together on awakening, and the burning and discomfort were increased until the mucus was soaked away. Of importance was the fact that his symptoms had increased when he played in the grass or during windy days. In the daylight he kept his lids lowered to protect his eyes against light, walking with his eyes downward to decrease his ocular distress. This had interfered greatly with his ability to read and study. It had caused moodiness and unhappiness, especially because his playmates "made fun of me." The conjunctivae of the upper lids were red and papular. An ophthalmologist in a medical school had diagnosed vernal catarrah and advised no treatment, predicting that it would probably disappear in five years.

His family and personal history of other possible manifestations of allergy was negative. There was no history suggesting allergy to foods, drugs, or environmental allergies. Scratch tests revealed one plus reactions to grass, fall, and tree pollens. He also gave two plus reactions to corn, wheat, eggs, milk, string beans, and to *Alternaria.* Usual routine laboratory tests were negative. His nasal secretion contained 19 percent eosinophiles. His ocular mucus revealed no eosinophiles.

Treatment: Desensitization to a multiple pollen antigen containing all of the important tree, grass, fall, and summer pollens present in his area along with Prednisone 5 mg t.i.d. gave definite relief in two weeks. Flowers were not in the home. The strength of the antigen was gradually increased up to 0.60 cc of the 1:100 dilution, and it was repeated weekly for 1½ years and every two weeks for 2 years.

During the first four months our CFE diet was maintained. Other foods were gradually added with no reactivation of his vernal catarrh. During the last year a general diet has been eaten. Evidences of vernal catarrh are now absent, there being no plaques or cobblestone lesions in his conjunctival membranes.

ALLERGY OF THE CORNEA (KERATITIS, CORNEAL ULCERS)

Most keratitis, except that arising from trauma, infection, and dystrophic abnormalities, is due to allergy, in the opinion of most ophthalmologists, as stated by Theodore and Schlossman in their book in 1958. Contact or atopic allergy to drugs applied or instilled onto the eye causes mild to severe keratitis. Drugs and cosmetics which are common causes have been noted in our discussion of allergic conjunctivitis and possible allergic glaucoma. Keratoconjunctivitis because of allergy to the plastic in contact lenses must be remembered. In the seven million or more wearers of these lenses, such allergy fortunately is rare. Possible allergy to plastic ocular prostheses must also be in mind.

That keratoconjunctivitis with resultant scarring of the cornea and conjunctiva with a reduced vision to 20/100 may occur along with severe exfoliative dermatitis, especially on the face, from a drug given orally or parenterally is evidenced by its occurrence from a sulfonamide, as reported by Havener in 1959. Former dermatitis from this drug contraindicated its further use.

That no redness occurs in keratitis is due to the absence of blood vessels in the cornea. Its nutrition occurs through lymph spaces in and between the epithelial layers. Cloudiness of the corneal grafts also has

been attributed to allergy to the foreign tissue corneal protein. Delayed healing of wounds after corneal surgery or injury may arise from an autogenous tissue allergy or from an uncontrolled allergy to inhalants, even to drugs and especially to foods. Delayed healing of wounds from injury or surgery from food allergy was reported by us in Chapter 26, to which the reader is referred.

That the cornea is susceptible to allergy was indicated in animal experiments, as summarized by Theodore and Schlossman. This justified the study of corneal allergy in man, the manifestations of which will be our present challenge in this chapter.

Experimental evidence of keratitis in animals was first reported by Loeffler in 1881, later by Wessely in 1911, and by Von Szily and Schoenberg in 1914. This led to the study and recognition of the role of syphilis and tuberculosis in allergic keratitis, the frequency of which has been minimized so greatly by the remarkable benefit of drug therapy.

ATOPIC CORNEAL ALLERGY, ESPECIALLY TO FOODS

Though atopic allergy to foods and inhalants in the cornea in man has been reported in the literature for four decades, its recognition and control by ophthalmologists and allergists are too infrequent. Lemoine, in 1929, reported dendriticlike corneal ulcers from chocolate. Parlato, in 1935, also recorded such ulcers from orris root. Episcleritis from food allergy was recorded by Balyeat and Rinkel in 1932. Ruedemann, in 1934, controlled keratitis with the elimination of milk. He also attributed phlyctenular ulcers to foods and pollens in five cases. In 1938 we commented on the report by Moore of corneal ulcers for ten years resisting all therapy until fish and beef were eliminated from the diet. One of our patients had redness of the sclera and severe ocular pain every two to three months from allergy to eggs and milk for eight years. Another patient had phlyctenular keratitis from ingested tomato. Hansen, in 1950, noted three cases of superficial keratitis from allergy to eggs in one case, to chocolate in another, and to nuts in a third.

Bothman, in 1941, reported two cases of phlyctenular keratitis in children—one only from pollen allergy, one from pollens and foods—and two in adults—one from food allergy and one from food, pollen, and other inhaled allergens. In one case fish was a marked offender. The reader is referred to detailed histories in Bothman's article. In these patients there was recurrent palpebral conjunctivitis usually with folliculosis, ciliary infection with photophobia, and lacrimation. Minute or moderate phlyctenules were present in parts of the cornea or limbus.

The report of interstitial keratitis in six cases caused by food allergy by Dean, Dean, and McCutcheon in 1940 deserves special comment. The allergy first caused slight irritation and redness of the cornea with moderate discomfort and lacrimation varying in degree for several weeks. Increased haziness in vision occurred. When the allergic involvement increased, the central cornea was so involved that shadows only were seen by the patient. Pain usually was unbearable. One patient requested enucleation of the eye. At first, faint irregular gray or yellowish interstitial opacities and small vacuoles appeared in the cornea. Loops of scleral vessels developed, and conjunctival loops extended into the superficial corneal stroma. Opacities increased in the entire cornea. Scar tissue developed in the stromal layers, producing increased opacities and (at times) ulceration. Other ocular complications usually were absent.

When food allergy was suspected, its study and control resulted in a decrease of ciliary injection and pain in two to three days, and opacities decreased. But in severe corneal involvement scar tissue remained. Reingestion of allergenic foods reproduced mild symptoms in twenty-four hours. With such evidence of food allergy the strict elimination diet was maintained, and the severe keratitis did not recur.

Hogan, in 1953, in an excellent article on Atopic Keratoconjunctivitis reported five cases in patients who had had atopic dermatitis on face, neck, flexures, and extremities since childhood. There was redness and thickening of the bulbar and palpebral cornea. Vascularization of the corneal stroma occurred after recurrent exaggerations. In severe attacks the entire cornea was scarred and vascularized. Phlyctenulosis of the conjunctiva and cornea was often associated with this type of inflammation. These lesions were satisfactorily relieved with topical and oral corticosteroids.

If the allergenic causes of the ocular allergy in these cases had been studied for possible pollen and especially food allergy as advised in this chapter, the possible role of such allergies either individually or concomitantly probably would have been determined.

The determination and treatment of these allergies, moreover, gradually should diminish the allergic reaction so that long-term corticosteroid therapy even with intermittent use would be unnecessary.

KERATITIS FROM POLLEN ALLERGY

Woods, in 1924, relieved interstitial keratitis from corn pollen by desensitization therapy. Mauksch, in 1937, reported keratitis from pollen allergy. Bothman, in 1941, recorded keratoconjunctivitis from pollen allergy.

Bothman, in 1941, reported a man forty years of age with recurrent redness, lacrimation, and blurred vision in the spring and fall for three years. One or both eyes were affected. During attacks there was ciliary injection with edema and cloudiness of the cornea with a few punctate opacities and interlacing lines clearing in three to five weeks. In five years fine brown precipitates were on the posterior cornea, which cleared in two weeks. Desensitization to molds for one year gave relief. In two cases exacerbations seemed to occur after ingestion of listed foods.

Bothman also reported several cases of corneal edema usually in patients with urticaria, angioneurotic edema, or migraine, in all of which allergy to foods or drugs and less often to inhalants always needs study.

Anneberg, in 1938, reported keratitis from *Amaranthus* pollen (pigweed). Erythema, itching, and pain with moderate contraction of the iris was followed in two to three days by gray areas of infiltration in the border of the cornea, ½ to 1 mm in diameter. A diffuse haziness and stippling of the entire cornea occurred in three to five days in two cases, clearing in seven to ten days with no visual impairment. No corticoid therapy or desensitization was given. In one case peripheral infiltration led to ulceration complicated with secondary infection which healed after the infection around a tooth was controlled.

O'Brien and Allen, in 1943, reported recurrent corneal ulcers with subepithelial infiltrate and necrosis associated with mild iritis and palpebral and bulbar conjunctivitis in a boy of twenty years. This recurred on three occasions after orange juice was squirted into the eye, eating marmalade, and a third time ingesting orange. Along with this case there was a report of corneal ulcers from the instillation of Bu-

tyn® Sulfate and lanolin onto the conjunctivae.

PERSONAL CASES OF CORNEAL ULCERS FROM FOOD ALLERGY

Case 139: A man sixty-one years of age had had recurrent corneal ulcers every three to four months for eight years. A sandy feeling in the eyes with burning and lacrimation exaggerated before the ulcers developed and to a moderate degree between the ulcerations had occurred. Because of the recurrent ulcerations and the perennial symptoms, food allergy was indicated even though skin reactions to foods were negative (Chapt. 2). With adherence to our CFE diet the ulcers and other ocular symptoms remained absent.

Case 140: A woman thirty-eight years of age was seen in our allergy clinic at the University of California Medical School in 1942 because of keratoconjunctivitis and recurrent corneal ulcers in the left eye every two to three months for two years. Constant inflammatory keratitis gradually developed. In the last year conjunctival and corneal inflammation had increased in frequency, being constant for several months. Scarring of the cornea with loss of vision had developed. Extreme photophobia had necessitated being in a dark room for two months. No ray of light was tolerated, necessitating being guided into the clinic with eyes covered with a towel. Recurrent sick headaches had occurred for ten years before her keratitis developed which history along with a moderate dislike for milk indicated possible food allergy. Negative skin reactions to food and in-

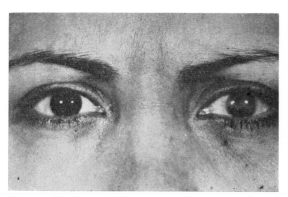

Figure 36. *Case 141:* Scarring keratitis reduced by elimination of allergenic foods determined with the CFE diet (Rowe).

halant allergens did not rule out allergy, especially to foods. Mucoid secretion from the conjunctiva showed a moderate number of eosinophiles. Study and treatment by ophthalmologists had given no relief. Corticosteroids were not available in 1947.

Because of the perennial inflammation, the recurrence of the ulcers, the history of recurrent sick headaches (see Chapt. 17), and the diet history, food allergy was studied with our CFE diet. No medications were given with the exception of a 1:2000 adrenalin, which was dropped into the eyes.

In one week inflammation and photophobia were reduced with strict adherence to the diet. Corneal ulcers and conjunctival inflammation and episcleritis had nearly disappeared in one month. This relief continued, but the scarring of the cornea persisted. Provocation feeding tests gradually revealed milk, wheat, corn, chocolate, and coffee as the causative allergens. There was no recurrence of the keratoconjunctivitis or corneal ulcers in the following year after which contact with the patient was lost. The persisting scarring of the cornea is shown in Figure 36.

No cases of keratitis or corneal ulcer have been studied by us in which inhalant allergy seemed to be the sole cause. This does not rule out such an etiology, since the number of patients referred with possible ocular allergy is limited.

Case 141: A woman thirty-three years of age first developed episcleritis and corneal ulcers thirteen years previously, continuing for five years. Relief then occurred in a dry area. Perennial episcleritis developed again five years before, along with recurrent styes. Then various foods were eliminated, with much relief for a period of two years. Episcleritis and recurrent corneal ulcers had continued since the spring four years before.

Severe frontal headaches recurring every two to seven days for fifteen years suggested possible food allergy. Diet history of possible food allergy and scratch tests with foods and inhalants were negative.

Treatment and results: Because of the perennial episcleritis and corneal ulcers, food allergy was studied with our CFE diet minus citrus fruits. In addition, desensitization with an antigen containing tree, grass, and fall pollens present in her local environment was given, starting with a 1:500 million dilution with a gradual increase every three to seven days up to a maximum

tolerated dose in the 1:50 dilution. Such pollen therapy is discussed at the end of this chapter and was indicated because of the exaggeration of her symptoms in the spring months in spite of negative reactions to pollens.

In one month there was definite improvement in the ocular allergy. Headaches of years' duration were relieved.

Since then provocation feeding tests with additional foods to those in the prescribed diet reproduced ocular symptoms and headaches when wheat, pork, fish, coconut, chocolate, and especially milk were added.

Pollen therapy was increased up to 0.60 cc of the 1:100 dilution of the pollen antigen. This was repeated at weekly intervals for two years.

Relief for five years thereafter with no pollen therapy indicated continued desensitization to the pollens.

For the last ten years ocular symptoms have been controlled with the entire elimination of milk and its products and pork. Traces of milk reproduce redness in the sclera and slight corneal distress but no ulcers. Milk also reproduces headaches.

SJOGREN'S SYNDROME—
FOOD ALLERGY AS A POSSIBLE
CAUSE

This syndrome of arthritis, keratoconjunctivitis, and dry mouth (usually in women over forty though its origin at present is not known) should be studied as we advise for atopic allergy particularly to foods because of its chronic perennial character. This is justified especially because of the role of food allergy reported by foregoing ophthalmologists and allergists, including ourselves. Such study, if done, would require the strict, sufficient use of diet trial as we advise and conjunctive and decreasing use of corticosteroids as recommended in this volume. Favorable results, as we have achieved in the detached retina as in Case 148 and in cases of conjunctivitis, corneal ulcer, and other ocular manifestations of atopic allergy, would justify additional adequate study of food allergy and of possible inhalant and drug allergy if indicated in the history indicative of this syndrome.

ALLERGIC SCLERITIS

Allergy best explains most inflammation of the sclera, as stated by Theodore and Schlossman and other ophthalmologists. It is important for other physicians to remember that the sclera is the outer fibrous layer of the eye, 1 mm thick, continuous with the cornea, and posteriorly with the dura of the optic nerve. Scleritis from tuberculosis, syphilis, and leprosy fortunately have decreased from modern drug therapy. A probable allergic mechanism as in collagen diseases is an assumed cause of scleritis occurring in rheumatoid arthritis and periarteritis nodosa.

ATOPIC ALLERGY IN SCLERITIS

Allergy to foods and inhalants needs emphasis especially in episcleritis. Its recognition and control are our challenge in this chapter. It may be diffuse and edematous in character or there may be tender, round, or oval purplish nodules in the superficial sclera over which there is free movement of the conjunctiva. Scar tissues replace the nodules, and the lesions tend to recur in the same area (episcleritis periodica fugax as named by Fuchs, according to Bothman in 1895). They may be associated with migraine or ciliary spasms causing transient myopia. As early as 1921 Sinsky, Levin, and Sachs opined that ingested foods were probable causes. Shoemaker, in 1924, decided that bread and cake were causative. Balyeat and Rinkel, in 1932, reported episcleritis in a patient allergic to foods, feathers, and pollens. Eating of suspected foods caused pain, lacrimation, and deep scleral injection for seven to fourteen days.

Superficial edematous involvement of the sclera is called episcleritis. Less frequent inflammation of all layers of the sclera causes scleritis. Varying degrees of vascular engorgement remaining after the relief of erythema and congestion in the conjunctiva from vasoconstrictors especially indicates scleritis. Localized purplish-red areas of edema occur, or a flat bulbar tender area of inflammation or firm nodules may develop in the sclera from allergic scleritis. Uveitis and secondary glaucoma may be associated with severe scleritis.

According to Theodore and Schlossman, scleral inflammation occurs especially in women. Pain and photophobia occur in severe cases. Recurrence of these symptoms may be present with the periods, each attack lasting two to eight weeks. As food allergy tends to recur in attacks often with menstrual periods in bronchial asthma, scleritis also tends to recur or be exaggerated with periods. These histories are always suggestive of allergy to foods (Chapt. 1).

Scleritis from atopic allergy, according to Theodore and Schlossman, arises from foods more often than from inhalants. The authors, however, only cite one case of scleritis in which allergy to foods (sea foods) was evident.

Moreover, they cite no reports in the literature of scleritis from food allergy.

In contrast, scleritis usually with involvement of the cornea, conjunctiva, and probably of the uveal tract has been controlled by the elimination of specific foods in several of our patients. Such food allergy has in some cases been suggested by a history of dislikes or disagreements for foods indicating the study of possible food allergy with our elimination diets as advised later in this chapter. The rarity of dependable, or any, positive scratch tests to allergenic foods requires diet trial especially with such diets. It is our opinion that ophthalmologists as well as allergists and other physicians will reveal and control food allergy as a quite frequent cause of allergic inflammation in the sclera as well as in other tissues of the eye with the strict, accurate use of the elimination diets as we advise.

Episcleritis with possible involvement of the upper layer of the sclera probably occurred in several of our seven patients with marked conjunctival allergy relieved with the use of our elimination diets already reported in this chapter. Varying degrees of scleritis were also associated with keratitis, especially with ulceration relieved with the elimination of specific foods. Episcleritis, keratitis and recurrent corneal ulcers present for thirteen years in Case 141 was relieved with the initial use of our CFE diet, with continued relief for ten years with the elimination of all products of milk and pork.

Case 142: A woman thirty-eight years of age had had attacks of sudden redness of the sclera with ocular pain, usually unilateral, every one to two months for five years. Pain lasted one day and redness for five to seven days. Interim inflammation and symptoms were absent. She had had perennial nasal allergy in childhood. Diet history revealed a long dislike for milk, some of which she forced herself to drink. She had been a finicky eater in childhood, which often is due to food allergy. Skin tests with foods and inhalants were negative. Family history was negative for allergy. Her recurrent perennial attacks and her diet history suggesting food allergy indicated its study with our CFE diet. After assured relief for three months, provocation tests showed that milk, wheat, corn, and pork were the sole causes.

In 1937 we reported ocular pain with episcleritis and gastrointestinal symptoms in a woman forty-nine years of age because of food allergy, especially to milk.

Case 143: A man forty years of age had attacks of episcleritis with edema in the lid and corneal ulcers associated with severe ocular pain in the right eye in the summer, lasting two to three weeks. This recurred two years later in August. Episcleritis and corneal ulcers recurred three times in the fall. It recurred again in July three years later when he was referred to us because of

his physician's opinion of a possible allergic cause. With recent attacks paralysis of the right medial rectus muscle occurred. The corneas showed bilateral nasal limbal craters. The fundae and fields were normal. Scratch tests gave one plus reactions to grass and summer pollens. This along with the summer recurrence of the scleritis and keratitis indicated pollen desensitization. Parenteral ACTH therapy two times a week for two weeks gradually relieved the inflammation.

In the last eight years pollen therapy has continued every one to two weeks. In the first three years two attacks recurred, relieved by ACTH. In the last four years attacks were absent except for slight recurrence only each spring relieved with one injection of ACTH.

ALLERGIC UVEITIS

Coles expressed the general opinion of ophthalmologists that allergy is operative in most endogenous, nongranulomatous uveitis. Because of major and usual initial susceptibility of vascular tissues to atopic allergy, the uveal tract, being the vascular layer of the eye, is especially susceptible to such allergy. Practically all nongranular endogenous allergic uveitis occurs in the anterior segment of the uveal tract. According to Coles, even in granulomatous uveitis arising from viable organisms of tuberculosis, syphilis, brucellosis, and leprosy; from filtrable virus; from protozoan infections, especially toxoplasmosis; from fungus infection causing actinomycosis; from blastomycosis; and from histoplasmosis resulting from nematodes and agents of unknown origin especially sarcoid, an allergic reaction to the causative organisms may aid the granulomatous response in preventing the invasion of the disease into normal surrounding tissues. The frequency of uveitis from these causes as found in 566 cases by ophthalmologists was noted by Van Metre. In contrast to our opinion and some evidence that atopic allergy to foods and inhalants requires study and control when present, he found no definite evidence of atopic allergy in causing uveitis. Van Metre discusses the allergic aspects of these causes of uveitis and their occurrence in 50 percent of cases of sarcoidosis.

Because of the importance of determining the type of uveitis and extent and degree of the involvement of the iris, ciliary body, and choroid and associated involvement of other ocular tissues, the study of allergy by the allergists should always be with the counsel and cooperation of an ophthalmologist with special interest and experience in disease of the uveal tract.

Our challenge in this chapter is endogenous uveitis from atopic allergy involving the iris, ciliary body, and choroid, each in varying degrees.

Though it is generally opined that such allergy explains practically all endogenous uveitis, the type of such allergy often has been obscure. It is our opinion that reports of allergy to inhalants, especially to pollens and even to animal emanations, dusts and other airborne allergens, will be increased when ophthalmologists consider its possibility and utilize adequate study, indicated environmental control, and desensitization therapy.

Study of possible atopic allergy is justified as a cause of uveitis in which bacterial allergy from demonstrated or possible foci of infection is not the confirmed cause. The benefit of fever therapy with intravenous injections of small doses of typhoid bacteria is explained by resultant increase in the circulating steroids as well as by capillary dilatation and increased cellular and antibody transudation into the uveal tissues which probably result from the fever from such therapy.

Study of atopic allergy to foods and inhalants is also justified as a cause of uveitis when tuberculin allergy resulting from allergens from a possible quiescent distant focus of tuberculosis has not been con-

firmed or assured. Against tuberculin allergy as a cause of uveitis is the report by Fritz, Thygeson, and Durham of no uveitis in two thousand Alaskan children with active TB. It is important to remember that a three plus reaction does not definitely indicate active TB as a cause of uveitis.

FOOD ALLERGY IN UVEITIS

Since food allergy has been recognized in our practice as a cause of allergic conjunctivitis, keratitis, corneal ulcer, scleritis, and also of dermatitis of the eyelids and blepharitis as well as in certain involvements of the retina and optic nerve and since it is the cause of many ocular symptoms in allergic headache and cerebral allergy, as we have reported in this chapter and in Chapters 17 and 18, inflammation in the uveal tract from food allergy is a definite probability. In our practice, however, we have had little opportunity to study food allergy in uveitis probably because of the failure of ophthalmologists to consider its possibility and to study it necessarily with trial diets. Coles comments on the scarcity of reports of uveitis from food allergy. He does cite iridocyclitis relieved by the elimination of egg and chicken in two patients by Parry in 1939, by the removal of egg from the diet by Potvin and Bossu in 1954, and also by Leopold and Leopold in 1955. Bothman, in 1941, stated that he had seen patients with attacks of serous iritis associated with pain, ciliary congestion, and fine keratitis, precipitates and cells in the anterior chamber preceded by a "head cold" with no fever. His suggestion that the "cold" was due to allergy is supported by our opinion that such nasal symptoms preceding manifestations as of recurrent bronchial asthma are usually due to recurrently activated food allergy. In addition, he summarized three cases with recurrent iritis attributed by him to allergy to molds or house dust. Favoring possible food allergy was the recurrence of attacks of uveitis which, as in recurrent bronchial asthma, headaches, and other manifestations of allergy, suggests possible food sensitization as a cause.

CASE REPORTS

Case 144: Allergic uveitis from food allergy can explain the dilated pupil causing marked blurring of vision associated with a "pressure behind the ears" in a boy nine years of age. This visual disturbance had caused absence from school during January and up to mid-February for two years. An ophthalmologist noted no change in the retina or optic discs and no congestion in the conjunctiva or sclera. There was marked irritability and nervous tension in the patient.

The occurrence of the dilated pupil and symptoms during the winter with entire relief after mid-March suggested food allergy, the activation of which during the fall and winter we have long reported, as noted in Chapter 1 and in other cases of ocular allergy and of various manifestations of food allergy throughout this volume. Also suggesting food allergy was the perennial nasal congestion and postnasal mucus which had been intensified in the winter. His mother, moreover, had recurrent headaches and chronic nasal allergy which are often due to food allergy. As noted in Chapter 2, absence of skin reactions to foods did not rule out food sensitization.

He was first seen in late February when slight dilatation and blurred vision were still present. Food allergy was studied immediately with our strict CFE diet with resultant relief in two weeks.

Then in mid-March other additional vegetables and fruits were first added to the diet, and in thirty-six hours after the ingestion of orange, moderate dilatation of the pupil and blurred vision arose. This disappeared about eight days after the exclusion of orange.

During the late spring, summer, and fall a general diet reproduced no ocular difficulty. Dilatation of pupils and blurred vision, however, returned in early December of 1967. The elimination diet was resumed, with relief in one week. There was no recurrence during February or March. A general diet was resumed in April and continued through the summer and fall.

Allergy to other foods, especially to milk, wheat, cereal grains, eggs, chocolate, and others eliminated from our CFE diet, could not be determined by using provocation tests (see Chapt. 3) after assured relief from the diet had continued for about a month in January of 1968.

Case 145: A man thirty-one years of age had recurrent attacks of iritis with pain, tearing of the eyes, and conjunctival congestion every one to two months for five years. With the attacks he had been depressed and fatigued. Because of the perennial, recurrent attacks, food allergy was assumed and studied with our CFE diet. Resultant relief continued for three months. Then other fruits and vegetables were added during a two-month period, with no resultant symptoms. At that time milk was added, with a recurrence of the iritis. The elimination of milk once again controlled the iritis. In a month one-half of a glass of mlk reproduced a red sclera in the right eye with moderate ocular pain which disappeared five days after milk again was excluded from the diet.

It is our opinion that if endogenous uveitis which has not been relieved by previous study and attempted treatment of infection or bacterial allergy by ophthalmologists were studied for possible food allergy, as advised in this chapter, evidence of the occurrence and probable frequency of food allergy would accumulate.

INHALANT ALLERGY IN UVEITIS

More evidence of uveitis from inhalant than to food allergy has been published, as noted by Coles in *Ocular Allergy* by Theodore and Schlossman. Coles commented on recurrent iritis attributed to inhalant allergy. Walker, in 1947, reported recurrent iritis for twenty years apparently from cat and other animal emanation inhalants. Desensitization to cat dander prevented recurrences of iritis. Kimura, Hogan, and Thygeson, in 1954, reported iritis relieved with the removal of a cat from the house. Leopold and Leopold, in 1955, reported uveitis from chicken feather emanations. Uveitis relieved by desensitization to house dust, feathers, and orris root along with a wheat-free diet was reported by Callaghan in 1955. Orris root was the reported cause of anterior uveitis by Good in 1955.

ANGIONEUROTIC EDEMA OF THE UVEA

As stated in Chapter 16, drug, other medicaments, food, and less often inhalant allergies and possible infectant allergy must be considered as a cause of infrequent angioneurotic edema of the eye, including the uveal tract.

1. Possible drug allergy can usually be suspected in a detailed history of present and recently taken drugs and various medications. To consider such allergy, all drugs given by mouth, into the body cavities, rubbed into the skin, or even by parenteral injection should be discontinued for one or two months.

2. Angioneurotic edema from allergy to a food may arise in minutes or in one to several hours after its ingestion. Positive scratch reactions to the proteins of causative foods are infrequent. After a decrease or a disappearance of the localized swelling in the ensuing one to five days, it may recur every one to two months thereafter, arising from the same food or foods eaten every day.

3. Inhalant allergy as a cause of angioneurotic edema is less frequent than drug and food allergies. When it is suggested by history with or without positive skin tests, it must be studied and controlled as advised at the end of this chapter and in Chapter 2.

4. Infectant allergy is rarely responsible for localized angioneurotic or localized edemas, though it must be considered if food and inhalant allergies are not demonstrated causes and if obvious foci of infection in teeth, tonsils, and other tissues as noted in Chapter 8 and throughout this volume are present.

Remembering the allergenic causes of angioneurotic edema, we opine that the above causes must be adequately studied when angioneurotic edema of the eyes, especially with probable involvement of the uvea, occurs.

With such study the causative allergies might have been determined in the following cases cited by Coles in 1958.

CASE REPORTS OF PAROXYSMAL INTRAOCULAR EDEMA WITH INVOLVEMENT OF THE UVEA BY COLES

Angioneurotic edema of the right eye, as reported by Weekers and Barrac in 1937, led to its enucleation. Iridocyclitis with increased tension in the left eye indicated iridectomy during a second attack one year later. Thereafter, recurrent angioneurotic edema in the left eye caused ciliary injection, corneal edema, hemorrhage in the iris, cloudy media, and moderate increased tension. These recurrent attacks especially favor food allergy as a possible cause.

Study, especially of food allergy, would have been important in another patient with recurrent uveitis associated with ocular edema and localized swellings in other tissues especially in the lips and face as reported by Hambresin in 1954, cited by Coles. Corneal edema, iridocyclitis, and increased intraocular tension occurred. Relief from antihistamines indicated allergy.

A case of recurrent unilateral edema of the lids with severe anterior uveitis and moderate intraocular tension reported by Coles could have been studied for possible food allergy because of the frequency with which food allergy produces its recurrent manifestations. The statement by Coles that "no allergen has been demonstrated" is not justified according to our experience until possible atopic allergy to foods has been studied with trial diet, especially with our strictly prepared and supervised CFE diet. In contrast to the statement by Coles that the causes of hives and localized edemas are rarely determined, the allergic causes of such edemas and urticaria can nearly always be demonstrated with our study and control of food, inhalant, and at times drug allergy as we advise at the end of this chapter and in Chapter 15.

LENS PROTEIN ALLERGY

Uhlenhuth (1903) first discovered that experimentally produced sensitization to lens protein is organ and not species specific—that is, the sensitized animal reacts to the protein of the lens of any animal. He and Hendel (1910) moreover sensitized an animal by incision of the lens of one eye, later killing the animal with injection of the lens protein of the remaining eye. This result was repeated by Von Szily and Arisawa (1913). Verhoeff and Lemoine (1922) first suggested that endophthalmitis anaphylactica may arise from sensitization to lens protein remaining after cataract operation or arising after second cataract operations. They reported positive skin reactions and beneficial desensitization with lens protein extracts. Lemoine and Macdonald (1924) found that such intraocular inflammation arose when any lens substance was left in the eye after cataract operations in 50 percent of all patients who showed positive skin reactions preoperatively to lens proteins. Courtney (1933) found that about one-sixth of all patients developed such positive skin reactivity after cataract removal. Burky and Woods (1931) agreed that reactions from absorption of lens substance were allergic and nontoxic in origin. Desensitization with lens extract prepared by their method (1931) was recommended preoperatively when positive skin reactions are present. The use of such extracts by oral or hypodermic administration without surgery were of no benefit to cataracts in their opinion. Burky (1934) by combining lens substance with staphylococcic toxin was able to sensitize rabbits to lens protein and concluded that concomitant action of bacterial toxin or infection probably explains intraocular inflammation or sympathetic ophthalmia after surgery. Burky (1934), moreover, obtained endophthalmitis from needling the lens of a rabbit previously sensitized to lens protein. This would indicate possible danger from needling of a lens after a previous cataract operation, especially if the skin reaction to lens substance is present. Lamb (1935), in experiments, found the corneal corpuscles transforming into macrophages. Courtney (1933) recommended lens protein skin testing especially before second cataract operations. Desensitization with lens extracts was advised in the presence of positive reactions. With such allergy intraocular tension was often increased. Burky and Woods (1931) again advised skin testing and such desensitization before surgery. Goodman (1935) stated that such lens allergy is rare but when present that desensitization should be continued until skin reactions are negative. An initial dose of 0.1 cc of a 2 percent extract of lens protein was suggested, with an increase every four to five days until 4 to 5 cc was given. Such dosage should vary, however, with each patient's sensitization and should proceed as with pollen desensitization therapy as discussed on pages 604 to 605. Of interest also was the report of Hobart (1933) of sensitization to vitreous protein. He recommended tests with it before second cataract operations and preliminary desensitization if tests are positive.

UVEAL PIGMENT ALLERGY

Elschnig (1910, 1911) first studied sensitization to uveal pigment and resultant sympathetic ophthalmia therefrom. Positive skin tests to such pigment were demonstrated. Woods (1933) reported positive skin reactions to uveal pigment especially after penetrating wounds of the eye. He found twelve cases of endophthalmitis associated with allergy to uveal pigment. Sympathetic ophthalmia, however, did not develop. He also used pigment extracts hypodermically with benefit in the therapy of twenty-one cases of sympathetic ophthalmia. Friedenwald (1934) also concluded that such pigment sensitization often explains sympathetic ophthalmia arising from ocular injury or cataract operation. Zerfoss (1935) stated that Gill confirmed such origin of sympathetic ophthalmia and suggested moreover that some recurrent iritis and uveitis might arise from pigment allergy.

Recently Woods (1936) has summarized the historical, clinical, and experimental aspects of allergy in relation to sympathetic ophthalmia. He demonstrated the organ-specific properties of uveal pigment, the antigenic action of uveal pigment in homologous animals, the experimental production of uveitis through the medium of uveal pigment antigenically, the occurrence of skin reactions to uveal pigment in patients who had absorbed uveal pigment after eye injuries, the presence of allergy to pigment in some patients after uveitis arising from injury or operation, and the occurrence of pigment allergy in all cases of sympathetic ophthalmia. The good results with pigment therapy in desensitization in cases of such ophthalmia and the identical histological findings in pigment allergy and sympathetic ophthalmia point very definitely to the role of allergy in this condition. However, Woods stated that pigment allergy may occur without sympathetic ophthalmia. Hence it is necessary to assume that such allergy is the predisposing cause necessary for the development of the dis-

ease. What other factors are required was difficult to determine. Friedenwald suggested that the proliferation of melanophores in the Dalen-Fuchs nodules is important in the development of the ophthalmia, the abnormal pigment being susceptible to autolysis from antibody-pigment union as compared with the pigment in normal cells. Woods suggested, moreover, nonspecific stimuli, toxic or bacterial in type, as active in setting off the ophthalmia when pigment allergy is present. Berens, in discussion, agreed with the findings and studies of Woods and felt that a bacterial toxin may be the exciting factor arising especially from the nasal sinuses. With this Burky* agreed and stated that the allergic hypothesis rather than an infectious one best explains sympathetic ophthalmia.

FOCAL INFECTION AND OCULAR ALLERGY

The discussion by Woods (1933) of bacterial allergy in relation to the eye is worthy of study. He cited the work of Swift and Derick (1928, 1930) and other experimental studies which demonstrated that bacterial infection of special types produces allergy in the ocular tissues. Animals sensitized to nonhemolytic streptococci developed interstitial keratitis when the bacterial cultures were instilled into the conjunctival sacs after scarification of the cornea. Woods pointed out the frequency of negative cultures from inflamed tissues in cases of iritis and uveitis and the frequent failure of improvement after removal of definite foci. These facts and experimental evidence indicated to Woods that bacterial allergy from distant foci rather than bacterial metastases into the ocular tissues accounts for many ocular lesions. The removal of foci in such cases must be followed by desensitization in addition to

---

*Personal communication.

an increased immunity. He outlined the indications for the use of nonspecific protein such as milk or intravenous typhoid bacilli injections. Other experimental studies of Brown, Julianelle, *et al.* and Scholtz emphasize bacterial ocular allergy. Woods stated that bacterial ocular allergy especially needs future study for the benefit of patients.

After a careful review of the literature on the relation of paranasal sinus disease to retrobulbar neuritis, Hansel (1936) concluded that many infections including syphilis, tuberculosis, acute infectious diseases, and infections of the paranasal sinuses may be responsible. Oliver and Crowe (1927) also listed toxic causes from kidney disease, burns, continued quinine, salicylate, arsenic and other drug therapy, methyl alcohol, tobacco, and multiple sclerosis. They studied ten cases of retrobulbar neuritis in which polypi and polypoid mucosa and cellular infiltration with eosinophiles suggested allergy. Beck (1923) also found edema of the ethmoids and infiltration with plasma cells and eosinophiles in cases of retrobulbar neuritis. Hansel studied six cases in which such neuritis was probably allergic. Polypi, edema of sinuses, and no evidence of infection were present. Thus Hansel concluded among the other causes noted above that infection or allergy alone or combined should be kept in mind. Vascular contraction may also occur and may be benefitted by intranasal operative procedures even in the absence of infection or by local heat to cervical sympathetics, displacement therapy in the posterior sinuses with warm saline solution, or even with fever therapy with typhoid vaccine.

ALLERGY IN SYPHILIS AND TUBERCULOSIS OF THE EYE

Woods (1933) has admirably reviewed the experimental and clinical studies on the effect of syphilis in the eye. After initial infections a general tissue immunity arises in which the eye tissues do not participate. Inoculation of the eye with spirochetes, moreover, does not produce immunity to reinoculation as occurs in other body tissues. Allergic reactions in the eye from syphilis are not frequent. However, it may produce interstitial keratitis, and iritis may arise in relapsed syphilis in insufficiently treated patients.

Woods (1933) also thoroughly reviewed the relation of immunity and allergy to tuberculosis of the eye. Intraocular tuberculosis must arise through lymph or blood channels or from extension from infections in nearby tissues. He reviewed studies on phlyctenular keratoconjunctivitis, tuberculosis of the cornea and sclera, and tuberculosis of the uveal tract and of retinal vessels. He favored tubercular allergy as the cause of phlyctenules on the cornea and conjunctiva. They may arise from small, early tubercular foci in the eye or from tubercular allergens from other foci in the body. Other antigens might also produce them. Woods concluded that there was no conclusive evidence of allergy as a cause of tubercular interstitial keratitis. He suggested that certain recurrent retinal hemorrhages might be due to allergy possibly to tubercular proteins. Urbach (1934) also discussed tuberculin allergy in relation to the eye in several articles.

Woods described his successful method of slow and careful desensitization with Davy's Bouillon filtrate in ocular allergy to tuberculin. His monograph should be consulted for details of therapy. He agreed with Rich and McCordock that desensitization rather than true focal reaction and resulting fibrosis best explains good results from such tuberculin treatment. Woods also considered trachoma from the viewpoint of allergy.

OTHER EXPERIMENTAL STUDIES IN OCULAR ALLERGY

Sattler (1909) first produced local ocular anaphylaxis with injections of serum into the eyes of sensitized animals. Wessely (1911) stated that interstitial keratitis was often allergic in origin. Among the recent experimental studies of many investigators, only a few will be mentioned. Seegal and Seegal (1930) was able to sensitize the eye by egg protein injections into the anterior chamber so that injection of egg intravenously two weeks later resulted in profuse lacrimation and hyperemia for twenty-four hours. Desensitization of the ocular tissues gradually arose with daily intravenous injections of the specific proteins but was only complete with large doses. Of interest in relation to the production of ocular allergy by food was the reaction which arose in the rabbit's eye after the ingestion of the specific food. Wessely (1933) produced allergic reactions with intracorneal injections of horse serum in rabbits and concluded that parenchymatous keratitis probably has an allergic etiology. Seegal *et al.* (1933) demonstrated remarkable general tissue sensitization with protein injections into the anterior chamber of the experimental animal's eye. Chambers (1933) confirmed Seegal's findings.

Reihm (1934) discussed the mechanism of allergic reactions in the eye in the light of the clinical inhalant, ingestant, and bacterial allergies already mentioned. Brown (1932) injected rabbits intraocularly with bacterial suspensions, egg whites, foreign erythrocytes, and other antigenic substances. Ten days later intravenous injections were given. In a few hours circumcorneal congestion, contraction of the pupil, vitreous opacities, and engorgement of the ciliary bodies and especially of the uveal tract arose. He concluded that uveitis often may be allergic. Brown and Dummer (1932) also sensitized the eye with injections of bacteria. Subsequent iridocyclitis arose with the intravenous injection of the same bacteria but also when egg albumen were used. After four or five instillations cloudiness of the cornea and then vascularization occurred. The corneal cell proliferation or a primary destruction of the cornea propria arose. Capillaries entered the cornea from adjoining conjunctival vessels and ran between the lamellae of the cornea propria from the periphery inward. The reaction extended even to the anterior chamber or iris. Opacity was even greater than the vascularization resulting from proliferation of the corneal cells and infiltration with large mononuclear cells, small lymphocytes, and plasma cells. Lagrange and Deethill (1933) emphasized the bacterial causes of ocular allergy. Scholtz (1932) reported a case of severe conjunctivitis, purpura, bronchitis, rhinitis, and oral membrane inflammation from allergy to a hemolytic streptococcus. Julianelle and Morris (1932) sensitized the corneae of rabbits with injections or by scarification and instillation of the antigen —either bacteria or egg white. After three or five weekly injections, vascularization of the cornea with a resulting pannus formation arose extending inward from the periphery. This gradually disappeared when instillations stopped, indicating again the possible effects of allergy.

UVEITIS RESULTING FROM SERUM ALLERGY

That serum allergy affects the uveal tissues is evidenced by iridocyclitis which may occur in generalized serum sickness. Theodore and Lewson, in 1939, as cited by Coles, were first to report bilateral iritis from such allergy. A fibrinous exudate "like cotton" occurred in the anterior chamber with minimal inflammation with recovery in a week. Sedan and Guillot, in 1955, reported bilateral iridocyclitis from allergy after injections of animal serum. Its original onset in this case in 1946 occurred in three days. The second attack in 1952 developed in ten hours and in a shorter time after the last injection. Increasing degree of allergy after successive injections of serum was indicated. Hoover, in 1956, reported unilateral uveitis in nine days after the injection of horse serum. Its later recurrence after the intradermal injection of a minute amount of such serum indicated the high degree of allergy present at the second injection. Bilateral anterior uevitis with cottonlike exudate, as in the case of Theodore and Lewson, also occurred in the anterior chamber of the eye in a patient in one month after the development of serum sickness.

Sedan and Guillot, in 1955, also reported severe uveitis in four days after implanting fresh placenta in a patient's abdomen. Injections of placental extract given one year previously for treatment of cataracts was blamed for this allergy.

POSSIBLE ROLE OF ALLERGY IN GLAUCOMA

Since allergy occurs in the uveal tract, the lens, and in other ocular tissues, allergic inflammation in the ciliary body and in its meshwork, elastic fibers, and interstices of the trabeculum and in Schlemm's canal as well as in its collecting canals and aqueous veins as a possible important factor in increasing or decreasing the volume of the aqueous fluid leading thereby to increased ocular pressure justifies consideration as one cause of glaucoma. Such consideration, moreover, is justified not only in open angle glaucoma occurring in 90 percent of primary glaucoma but also in acute narrow angle glaucoma and especially in secondary glaucoma.

Theodore and Schlossman, in 1958, noted glaucoma secondary to conjunctivitis and episcleritis from severe irritations and at times from allergy to drugs including atropine, pilocarpine, physostigmine salicylate, neostigmine, and similar drugs. Secondary glaucoma may also occur in angioneurotic edema of the eye which usually also occurs in cutaneous tissues, especially in the head, oral cavity, and neck with its varying occurrence in the respiratory, gastrointestinal, urogenital, and even in the cerebral tissues, as already noted in our discussion of angioneurotic edema in the eye. The study and control of food and less often of pollen allergy as the usual causes of such edemas are required as advised in Chapter 16.

Secondary glaucoma also results at times from allergic dermatitis and associated allergy in other ocular tissues from eyelash and eyebrow dyes and even from dyes for the hair on the scalp especially from paraphenylene diamine and similar coal tar dyes. Possible secondary glaucoma, moreover, may arise from severe dermatitis, conjunctivitis, episcleritis, keratitis, and uveitis from allergy to mascara, eye shadow, eyebrow pencils, creams, hair lacquers, shampoos, tonics, permanent wave preparations, nail polishes and other cosmetic aids as listed by Theodore and Schlossman and also by Schwartz and others. Such dermatitis may also arise from fabrics, dry cleaning chemicals, leather, rubber goods, furs, and jewelry, especially that containing nickel. Dermatitis from contact allergy from spectacles or from the nickel in the white gold spectacle frames or from plastics in such frames causing eyelid dermatitis and conjunctival, scleral, or corneal allergy in which chronic and severe uveitis and secondary glaucoma may occur is a rare possiiblity.

Contact dermatitis to the resins of vegetation including poison oak, Japanese lacquer, cashew nuts, primulas, geraniums, chrysanthemums, tulips, gladiolas, ragweed and cocklebur, and others are rare causes. The other causes of contact dermatitis such as varnish, shellac, pigments in paints, cleaning fluids, detergents, plastics and other household products have never been reported as causes of secondary glaucoma.

ATOPIC ALLERGY IN GLAUCOMA

Atopic allergy as a possible cause of glaucoma has received limited consideration by allergists or ophthalmologists. As already noted in our discussion of angioneurotic edema causing uveitis and resultant glaucoma, the study of atopic allergy to foods and less often to inhalants is very important. The statement of Theodore and Schlossman that "conjunctival, corneal, and especially uveal involvement with secondary glaucoma are sometimes of great magnitude" in the ocular manifestations of angioneurotic edema stresses the study of such atopic allergy in its etiology, as we have emphasized in Chapter 16. That such edema occurring in the eye may also occur in the spinal cord and meninges as well as in the cutaneous, respiratory, gastrointestinal, urogenital, and joint tissues has been noted in the previous and subsequent chapters.

ROLE OF ATOPIC OR DRUG ALLERGIES IN GLAUCOMA

The following reports in the literature indicate atopic allergy in the causation of glaucoma.

Transitory myopia may be associated with increased ocular tension, as reported by Schachne, according to Theodore and Schlossman, in a woman thirty-nine years of age. Sudden loss of vision developed in four days with five diopters of myopia. Anterior chambers were shallow, and ocular tension was 30 mm. Miotics reduced it to 14 mm and with PPZ vision returned to 20/20 with ocular tension of 16 mm. Angioneurotic edema from fish had occurred one year before after the ingestion of fish. Quinidine, however, was the present suspected cause.

Barkan, in 1919, reported recurrent localized edemas for seven years associated with congestive glaucoma. Tension rose over 40 mm Hg one-half hour after onset of edema of lips, tongue, and cheeks. Miotics controlled the pressure. Lack of cooperation would have prevented study of possible food allergy as we advise. Theodore and Schlossman opined narrow angle glaucoma developed during the localized edema. Posner and Schlossman, according to Bothman, opined that edema of the ciliary body caused closure of the narrow chamber angle by relaxing the zonule by shortening the ring of attachment.

Kraupa, in 1935, recorded unilateral intermittent glaucoma in four men. Large precipitates were on the posterior surfaces of the cornea. Previous therapy had failed. Finally, discontinuance of tobacco with the use of miotics controlled the pain.

Weekers, according to Bothman, reported two cases of anaphylaxis and migraine with edema of the globe of the eye in one and of the cornea and posterior synechiae in the other. Keratins in the vitreous and fibrin in the aqueous, he opined, may cause glaucoma. Along with migraine, gastrointestinal symptoms justify study of food allergy, especially with our CFE diet.

Weekers and Barac, in 1937, also reported probable Quincke's edema of the uveal tract causing weekly attacks of pain leading to enucleation of the right eye. Thereafter, similar attacks occurred in the left eye with ciliary congestion and keratitic precipitate.

Wiseman and Moore, in 1954, published an important article reporting recurrent attacks of redness, tearing, and pain in the left eye preceded for three hours with distention in a man sixty-seven years of age for six years, increasing to weekly intervals for one month. History and diet manipulation with feeding tests indicated orange as the chief offender, peaches and peas causing distention and to a lesser degree ocular symptoms. Ocular tension increased during attacks to 35 to 54 mm Hg. They refer to glaucoma resulting from food allergy in three cases reported by Behrens in 1947. Six other references are of interest.

This important challenge of atopic allergy in chronic simple glaucoma with six summaries of relieved cases and many references to pertinent articles in the literature was discussed by Raymond in 1961.

The estimate that blindness in over twelve thousand people in this country results from glaucoma justifies continued study of the degree to which atopic allergy is or may be the cause. As Raymond stated, the continued reduction of vision and visual fields occurring at times after initial relief from surgery indicates that the basic cause persists. This also justifies study of possible atopic allergy, especially to foods, as we advise.

Altered permeability of small blood vessels and congestion in the uveal tissue, vasospasm with microthrombus, and edema retarding outflow of the aqueous are explained by allergy in the tissues. The benefit of epinephrine in glaucoma and the effect of edema in the neural tissues from possible localized allergy are discussed. His emphasis of this role of atopic allergy is based on the benefit from his study and control of allergy, especially "with desensi-

tization" in 113 cases of chronic simple glaucoma.

His report justifies study and control of probable or definite atopic allergy as we advise.

When inhalant allergy is indicated in the environmental history to allergens in the home or area of occupation in winter and to pollens and other airborne allergens in the spring, summer, and fall, desensitization with indicated antigens is required, but also adequate, strict study of food allergy as we advise is indicated especially if symptoms persist or increase in the fall, winter, and early spring when such allergy is activated.

References to contributions of many students of the role of allergy in glaucoma are in this article by Raymond.

GLAUCOMATOCYCLITIC CRISES

This syndrome, described by Posner and Schlossman in 1948, is characterized by "recurrent acute noncongestive glaucoma usually with slight cyclitis in one eye." The pupil enlarges and the tension increases with slight visible ocular inflammation during a two-week period. Between the attacks tension and vision are normal.

Definite decrease in the length and degree of symptoms with corticosteroid therapy favors allergy as the cause as does the usual familial and personal history of clinical allergy. The cyclic recurrence throughout the year also favors food allergy as the cause, as discussed in Chapter 2. The ophthalmologist must make the diagnosis and must counsel with the allergist if study of possible allergy is indicated.

SPECIFIC THERAPY IN UVEITIS

As Coles states, the control of nongranulomatous uveitis by removal of foci of infection, which may cause possible bacterial allergy, increasingly has been disappointing. As we already opined, unrecognized food or less often inhalant allergy may be responsible for the inflammation and resultant symptoms in such cases. That marked cures, however, at times result from the elimination of such infection is important to remember. The use of stock or autogenous vaccine especially of different strains of streptococci, however, infrequently is of help.

When tubercular infection is present or probable in the uveal tissues, ioniazide, para-aminosalicylic acid and dihydrostreptomycin are indicated, as advised by Coles and by other students of such treatment. If allergy to tuberculin rather than actual infection is quite certain, steroid therapy with antitubercular drugs may be justifiable. Desensitization to tuberculin as previously stated is of questionable value. At times it activates the infection in other areas than the eye.

CORTICOSTEROID THERAPY IN UVEITIS

The beneficial and often dramatic results of corticosteroid therapy by instillation onto the conjunctivae and in severe cases by oral administration and parenteral injection has supplanted former foreign protein therapy already noted in this chapter. These corticosteroids have relieved and controlled the severe inflammation of single or recurrent attacks of nongranulomatous uveitis. Such relief enables the ophthalmologist and/or allergist to study the probable allergic causes. This relief, as emphasized by Coles and other ophthalmologists, does not eliminate the underlying allergic cause. Study and control of probable allergies, as discussed in this chapter, are required.

When granulomatous uveitis resulting from invasion of viable bacteria, viruses, or protozoa into the uveal tract, including the choroid, is present, corticosteroids are contraindicated because of resultant decrease in the normal resistance against infection. Coles states, however, that when the macular area is involved and resultant serious decrease in vision is threatened, corticosteroids are indicated until antibacterial drugs decrease the active infection.

Corticosteroids, at times in large amounts for months or even years, are indicated to control the severe inflammation of sympathetic ophthalmia. With its continued suppression Coles states that the disease "may burn itself out." He also states that corticosteroids should not be given in the first two weeks after a perforating eye injury. Unsatisfactory healing may be masked which might later require prophylactic enucleation of the eye.

Endophthalmitis phacoanaphylactica requires immediate local and parenteral corticoids. Lens removal should be by the intracapsular procedure with minimal injury to the lens and no release of lens allergens into the anterior chamber to prevent this complication.

ALLERGIC CATARACTS

Atopic cataracts occurring in patients with chronic allergic dermatitis are due to entrance into the lens through its permeable capsule of serum antibodies which have been responsible for the chronic atopic dermatitis. The union of these antibodies with blood-borne antigens to foods, inhalants, or possibly to foods or drugs which cause the dermatitis results in an allergic reaction in the lens which at times evolves into mature cataracts. Since the lens and the skin are ectodermal in origin, the allergy responsible for the atopic dermatitis can cause allergy in the lens resulting in cataracts. It is possible that control of atopic dermatitis especially on the face and eyelids and to a lesser extent on other parts of the body with indicated treatment of food and/or inhalant and at times drug allergy, as advised at the end of this chapter, may prevent initial lenticular opacities from increasing into mature cataracts or might cause a regression of the initial changes in the lens which (when uncontrolled) evolve into mature cataracts.

Opacities in the lens which eventuate into cataracts are preceded by atopic dermatitis especially on the face, eyelids, and neck with or without eczema in other cutaneous areas present for ten to thirty previous years. As Theodore and Schlossman state, the cataracts may also occur in months or even years after the dermatitis has disappeared. In rare cases these antibodies to the allergen may remain at times for years in the lens before a union with the allergenic antigen produces changes which increase and terminate in mature cataracts.

Cataracts in association with atopic dermatitis nearly always develop in the third decade. Cowan and Klauder report an average onset of 23.3 years, the youngest being 18 years, the oldest being 36 years. Cordes and Cordero-Moreno studied four cases, one being forty-nine years of age. Sack reported that eight out of thirty cases were unilateral. Allergic cataracts usually mature in one to two years. Cowan and Klauder and also Brunsting reported occurrence of cataracts in 8 to 10 percent of patients with definite uncontrolled allergic dermatitis. They found lenticular opacities in 28 percent of one hundred normal patients and in 26 percent of patients with atopic dermatitis. Cataracts, however, only involved in 8 to 10 percent of those patients with atopic dermatitis. This emphasizes the control of atopic eczema, especially on the face and upper extremities, as advised in Chapter 14.

The two types of allergic cataracts are

a) the classical cataract of atopic dermatitis described by Vogt and reported by Beetham in eight of eighteen cases and b) the complicated cataract. Differentiation must be made by the ophthalmologist and is not discussed by us as allergists.

In the classical type, irregular, white, or gray opacities develop in the anterior or posterior cortex followed by opacities of the whole lens. In contrast, in the complicated type opacity begins in the posterior pole of the lens spreading peripherally through the whole posterior subcapsular area. In both types the entire cortex becomes cloudy, forming a mature cataract. As stated above, final maturity occurs in one to two years.

The history of patients with atopic cataracts usually reveals a familial and personal history of various manifestations of allergy, which are noted in Chapter 1.

PERSONAL CASES OF ATOPIC CATARACTS

Atopic cataracts have occurred in two of our many patients with severe, disseminated lifelong atopic dermatitis studied and controlled in our practice during the last thirty years.

Case 146: A young man seventeen years of age had had atopic dermatitis especially on the face, eyelids, scalp, neck, flexures, and to a lesser extent over the rest of his body since infancy, as shown in Figure 37 (p. 392). Bronchial asthma had been present since the age of three months. Scratch testing gave three to five plus reactions to all tree, grass, fall, and most cultivated flower pollens. The exaggeration of his eczema in the winter, moreover, favored allergy to foods to which no scratch reactions occurred. Asthma and eczema were present in his family history.

When first seen, he had bilateral cataracts which only allowed perception of light. Ophthalmologists had refused to remove the cataracts because of the marked degree of his atopic eczema, especially on his eyelids, face, and scalp, and the assumed secondary infection in his skin. Our treatment of his dermatitis was initiated with the study and control of food allergy even in the absence of positive skin reactions to foods with our CFE diet (Chapt. 2). Control of pollen allergy was initiated with an injection of 1:500 million dilution of an antigen containing tree, grass, and fall pollens in the air of the patient's living area and to most of which positive reactions had been obtained. With the strict maintenance of the diet and the gradual increase in the doses of his pollen antigen, the dermatitis was controlled in four months. Then one cataract and in three months the other cataract were removed, with complete restitution of his vision. Glasses were required only for reading.

In the next five years while he was in communication with us, his dermatitis was controlled with the elimination of wheat, milk, eggs, chocolate, corn, and rye. Desensitization to pollens was continued for three years. The dermatitis did not recur, and good vision continued.

The speed of relief of his dermatitis would have been increased today with the proper use of corticosteroids which were not available when he was studied in 1947. Today, after initial and gradual reduction of corticosteroids, the control of food and pollen allergies, however, would still be mandatory. With little or no long-term corticosteroids to control the atopic dermatitis, such relief not only allows the ophthalmologist to operate with minimal or no complications and possible secondary infection but also prevents development of other manifestations of ocular allergy in the future.

Case 147: A woman twenty-seven years of age had gradually developed a mature cataract in the left eye in the previous year and had increasingly impaired vision from a maturing cataract in the right eye for eight months.

Atopic dermatitis present since the age of ten months had persisted perennially since then, generalized throughout the skin, being especially severe on the face, eyelids, neck, and flexures. There had been moderate control with oral corticosteroids taken continually for five years.

Bronchial asthma had been present perennially since the age of three years. Recurrent attacks

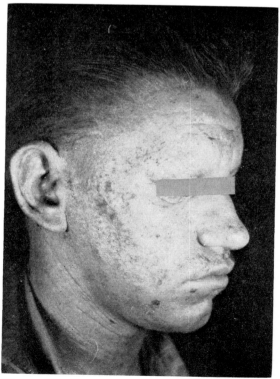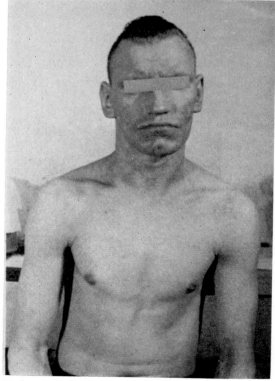

Figure 37. *Case 146: Left:* Allergic dermatitis from food associated with inhalant energy. *Right:* Relief of atopic dermatitis.

with moderate interim relief especially when corticoids were being taken had occurred.

Scratch tests revealed large reactions to grass and lesser reactions to fall and tree pollens. One to three plus reactions were obtained to eggs, milk, pork, and fish. Her initial blood count revealed 17,500 WBC and 22 percent eosinophiles. Physical examination showed a dry, scaling, excoriated dermatitis on the eyelids, face, neck, and flexures and a generalized dryness and scaling in the rest of her skin. Moderate diffuse wheezing was heard in the lungs. The lens of the left eye was opaque as was the right lens.

Treatment: Because of the diffuse eczema and asthma, she was hospitalized for thirteen days. Food allergy was studied with our CFE diet minus tomato and beef, to which she opined she was allergic. Corticosteroids which had been advised by mouth for five years were given parenterally in larger doses for three days. They were continued by mouth in reducing doses from 12 to 6 mg of Aristocort daily in twelve days. Desensitization to an antigen containing the important grass, tree, and fall pollens in amounts according to their frequency as determined by our survey of her area was initiated with a 1:5 billion dilution. As the strength was increased, exaggeration of the dermatitis occurred from this antigen, requiring a return to the 1:5 billion dilution. As the diet was continued, allergy to fruits and spices became apparent.

The excellent control of the eczema as well as the asthma for six months justified the surgical removal of the cataract in the left eye. In three months the cataract in the right eye also was removed. Healing was rapid, and excellent vision has continued during 2½ years. Contact lenses are worn during the day, glasses being used for reading.

Our FFCFE diet (see Chapt. 3) has been maintained to which cooked vegetables, excluded from the original diet, have been added. Rice, oats, corn, milk, and eggs have reactivated the dermatitis and continued to be excluded. The pollen antigen in the 1:5 million dilution is now tolerated without activation of the eczema. Multiple vitamins and calcium carbonate ½ teaspoonful daily are being administered.

Comment

That control of food, inhalant, and possibly drug allergies responsible for the marked longstanding atopic dermatitis in these cases may prevent the progression of incipient cataracts which are indicated by lenticular opacities revealed by the ophthalmologist's examination may be possible. Since we have not had the opportunity to study and treat such patients, the possibility of preventing the development and the maturing of atopic cataracts with our antiallergic therapy cannot be confirmed. Its possibility is a definite challenge. Once a mature atopic cataract has developed, however, antiallergic treatment cannot be expected to decrease the changes and to restore even fair vision.

Relief of atopic dermatitis especially on the lids and face with the control of food, inhalant, and (at times) drug allergies usually with decreasing corticosteroid therapy lessens the hesitation of the ophthalmologist to surgically remove atopic cataracts and minimizes possible subsequent allergic inflammation or occasional secondary infection in the uveal tissues. With the control of allergic inflammation, it is possible that there will be a definite and important reduction of the complications which are reported after cataract surgery, including retinal detachment, iridocyclitis, glaucoma, retinal edema, and hemorrhage, which Theodore and Schlossman state are more common after removal of atopic cataracts than of senile cataracts.

RETINAL AND OPTIC NERVE ALLERGY

That allergy can produce marked manifestations in the retina is evidenced especially by the retinitis, papillitis, and neuroretinitis which may occur from serum sickness arising during generalized allergic reactivity to animal sera. Mason, in 1922, reported edema, blurring of the disc margins, and small retinal hemorrhages along with fever and urticaria occurring nine days after antipneumonic horse serum had been given. Mild optic neuritis developed in four other patients during serum sickness. Brown, in 1925, reported serum sickness in seventy-five patients in nine of whom blurred vision, dilated pupils, and engorged arteries and veins in the conjunctiva and sclera occurred. Papilledema in varying degrees was noted when urticaria was most marked. Bedell, in 1935, published important photographs of the retina in a patient who had urticaria from serum sickness in which edematous white swellings obscured the nerve head. Enlarged veins and several hemorrhages also occurred in the retina. The retina returned to normal in seven weeks except for enlarged veins with yellowish deposits on the side of the disc and small remnants of edema in the vitreous in front of the macula. Kennedy, in 1936, reported hemianopsia, papilledema and edema of the retina along with aphasia and right hemiplegia during serum sickness in a boy of four years. This case was previously summarized in Chapter 18. Bothman, in 1940, reported preretinal edema, moderate papilledema, and hemorrhage in the macular area. This occurred twenty-four hours after the injection of horse serum, gradually decreasing in two months.

FOOD, INHALANT, AND DRUG ALLERGY IN THE RETINA AND OPTIC NERVE

Retinal and optic nerve allergy to foods, pollens, and drugs has been reported. Plummer, in 1937, reported blurred vision with congestion and haziness in the left macular area. Peanuts were judged to be responsible. A second attack occurred after their reingestion. Criep, in 1941, reported transient amblyopia and a blurred disc whenever the patient ate fish. Chocolate caused blurred vision and "spots" be-

fore the eyes associated with nausea, vomiting, and headache, as reported by Bothman in 1941. Blurring of the margins of the right disc and temporal hemianopsia occurred. The disc appeared normal in three weeks after the stopping of chocolate. Similar findings were reported by Ruedemann in 1930 after eating chocolate and nuts. Gallerani, in 1932, as noted by Theodore and Schlossman, reported transitory amblyopia, scintillating scotoma, and temporal amblyopia with blurring of the margin of the discs during attacks of migraine which occurred after ingestion of milk. Hayden and Cushman, in 1941, recorded impaired vision during attacks of recurrent bilateral optic neuritis resulting from marked allergy to milk and eggs. Optic atrophy resulted in one eye and less damage with a return to normal vision occurred in the other eye.

Ruedemann, in 1930, reported neuroretinitis during the pollen seasons and papillitis from primrose pollen. Though similar cases are not in the literature, the occurrence of allergic inflammation from pollen allergy in other tissues of the eye as reported in this chapter justifies the consideration of such pollen reactivity during pollen seasons in the retina and optic nerve. Possible allergy to animal emanations, miscellaneous inhalants including spores of fungi, house and other environmental airborne dusts, and other airborne allergens also must be considered. We opine that allergy to such inhalants, however, is not a common occurrence.

DRUG ALLERGY

That allergy to drugs as well as to the already discussed animal sera must be considered is emphasized by Bedell's report of impaired unilateral disturbed vision for eleven days in a woman fifty years of age from procaine allergy. Vision was 20/50.

Edema of the entire retina with many superficial striates and deep hemorrhages with an irregular dark oval macula surrounded by deep and petechial hemorrhages are shown in his published photographs of the retina. After gradual subsidence of the inflammation the same lesions and symptoms recurred after procaine local anesthesia given for the extraction of a tooth. Blood eosinophiles were 15 percent.

FOOD, INHALANT, AND DRUG ALLERGIES

These allergies must be studied as a cause of allergic edema in the retina and optic nerve. Bettman, in 1945, reported sudden edema of the macula with reduced vision to 20/200. Hay fever, nasal allergy, bronchial asthma, and keratoconjunctivitis had been present for a number of years. Epinephrine hypodermically improved vision to 20/50. Possible atopic allergy could have been studied as a cause, as we advise in this chapter and in Chapter 2.

Blurred vision occurred in a man reported by Kennedy, as already noted in Chapter 18 in this volume. Attacks lasted for a few days to one or two months. Discs were blurred as if "puffs of smoke" passed over the retina. Study of possible atopic allergy would have been justified.

Brickner reported two attacks of blindness associated with edema of the disc in another patient. Handwerck, in 1907, had observed two diopters of edema in the right disc in a woman seventy-five years of age concomitant with generalized urticaria and angioneurotic edema. Ullmann, in 1899, reported papillitis in a man when swellings of the hands, pharynx, and larynx and focal epilepsy from angioneurotic edema occurred. Bassoe, in 1926, reported increased intracranial pressure, headaches, vomiting, and choked discs because of which cranial decompression was done. The results and findings in this case were reported in Chapter 18 on epilepsy. Bassoe suggested that the previous choked disc could have been a primary evidence of allergy or the result of allergic edema in the meninges or brain resulting in increased intracranial pressure. Papillitis in a girl with localized swellings in the right face and on the following day similar symptoms in the left face was reported by Albracht. The retinal blood vessels and intracranial pressure were normal. In this case and in those summarized above, as in all patients with angioneurotic edema and in others with or without urticaria (see Chapt. 16), food, inhalant, and (at times) drug allergy need study as advised later in this chapter.

RETROBULBAR NEURITIS

As Theodore and Schlossman state, many cases of retrobulbar neuritis not resulting from involvement of the optic nerve by multiple sclerosis require consideration of infection in sinuses, encephalomyelitis, arteriosclerosis, vitamin deficiency, and allergy as possible causes. Allergic aspects of multiple sclerosis are discussed in Chapter 18 of this volume.

Because papillitis at times arises from allergy, retrobulbar neuritis because of allergic edema or inflammation needs consideration.

Kennedy reported several such cases suggestive of an allergic cause. Retrobulbar neuritis occurring with an acute cerebellar seizure and with a history of temporary right hemiplegia was attributed to probable pork allergy. Another patient with swellings in the skin developed a dull headache, ocular tenderness, and foggy vision followed by temporary blindness. A similar attack one year later lasted for two weeks. Study of possible atopic allergy would have been justified.

Frantz, in 1938, reported retrobulbar neuritis during one of four attacks of numbness and disturbed coordination in the extremities after eating chocolate and eggs. Allen and Seidelman, in 1949, reported retrobulbar neuritis in a woman sixty-three years of age which caused fogginess of vision and pain in the eyes during severe attacks of urticaria from strawberries. In one attack left scotoma for red developed. Avoidance of suspected food and inhalant allergens along with pyribenzamine by mouth prevented further attacks.

Wilder also reported attacks of urticaria, marked itching, and blindness during exposure to cold. In such cases it is justified to consider the possibility that cold activates allergy to foods and possibly to inhalants.

MICROBIALLERGIC REACTIONS IN THE RETINA

Though our major challenge of food, inhalant, and less frequent drug allergies is not operative in the following cases, the probable role of bacterial allergy justifies the inclusion of this information in this chapter. Theodore and Schlossman record the report of Weizenblatt in 1949 of bilateral neural retinitis and cyclitis with decreased vision because of allergy which developed five days after the intradermal injection of old tuberculin in a girl eighteen years of age. Edema and hemorrhages in the retina, including the macula, and in sheaths of the large vessels occurred. These symptoms indicating allergy recurred after a second injection of tuberculin.

Muncaster and Allen reported bilateral iridocyclitis and retinal periarteritis two weeks after a second tuberculin test with 0.005 mg of purified tuberculin. Kennedy, as noted in Chapter 18, reported unilateral blindness for four days possibly because of allergy to streptococcal antigen. The blind-

ness disappeared after removal of tonsils infected with streptococcus viridans.

PERIARTERITIS NODOSA IN THE RETINA AND CHOROID

Though the cause of this severe generalized vascular disease is not known, its probable allergic etiology justifies comment about the hypersensitive albuminuric retinopathy, the hemorrhagic neuroretinitis, and retinitic patches resulting mainly from the disease in the kidneys and cardiovascular tissues, as discussed by Theodore and Schlossman. Periarteritis occurring in the choroid and retina are comparatively uncommon.

Retinal detachment has occurred in this vascular disease possibly from periarteritis in the choroidal vessels and resultant exudation under the retina. The reader is referred to the discussion of the pathogenesis in periarteritis by Theodore and Schlossman and other ophthalmologists.

CENTRAL ANGIOSPASTIC SEROUS RETINOPATHY

As summarized by Theodore and Schlossman, there are evidences of allergy in the causation of this condition. Wolkowicz noted the similarity of its lesions to urticaria. Its sudden onset, its usual unilateral occurrence, the absence of retinal abnormalities except for minimal red-free light hemorrhages, and usual macular edema are reported.

The recurrent attacks in about 50 percent of the cases, as in other manifestations of food allergy, certainly suggests such allergy as a cause. Though recovery after an attack is usually complete, visual damage with changes in the pigment of the choroid at times may be lasting. Benefit from corticosteroids favors an allergic etiology.

Largely because of the suggestion of an urticarial-like lesion and especially because of the recurrence of the attacks, we opine that food allergy should be considered and studied with our elimination diets as advised at the end of this chapter and in Chapter 3.

When corticosteroids relieve any symptoms and the pathology in affected tissues, allergy (including that to inhalants and especially foods) is a justified possibility.

RETINAL DETACHMENT

Theodore and Schlossman doubt the possible role of allergy in the pathogenesis of typical retinal detachments with disinsertions and retinal breaks. That localized exudations from allergic inflammation or edema under the retina or that sneezing or coughing from hay fever or bronchial asthma might result in detachment is possible. Retinal detachments after surgical removal of atopic cataracts and when periarteritis nodosa or lupus erythematosus is present do occur, as noted in this chapter.

Prewitt, in 1937, reported bilateral detachment in a very allergic patient. Corrugation of the fundus developed after intracapsular removal of the lens. Allergic edema recurred three months afterward, with retinal detachment several months later, caused according to Prewitt by nodular swellings under the retina of probable allergic origin. The cause of the probable allergy was not determined, though food and animal emanatoid allergy were possible.

Balyeat, in 1937, reported bilateral detachment of the retina in a man twenty-one years of age who had had hay fever, asthma, and eczema activated by inhalation of silk allergens. He opined that the ectodermal origin of the retina made it susceptible to the causes of allergic dermatitis.

Appelbaum reported retinal detachments from possible allergy to pork insulin. Allergy to catgut used in eye surgery must be realized, as discussed by Aptstal in 1951 and by others as listed in the bibliography.

DETACHED RETINA PRECEDED BY EDEMA OF THE RIGHT EYELID AND OCULOMOTOR PARALYSIS

Case 148: A woman forty years of age in January, 1962, developed edema of the right eyelid with a moderate bulging of the eyes and double vision. (There was loss of vision except for light and shadow in the right eye.) "The right turned inward toward the tip of the nose." There were congested and enlarged blood vessels in the conjunctiva and sclera. There was a serous discharge from the conjunctiva causing a sticking together of the lids on awakening. Relief occurred in one week. Similar symptoms recurred four times with nearly complete interim relief for one to two weeks. She was then referred to an ophthalmologist, who found no abnormalities in the eye except the edema of the lids, congested and enlarged blood vessels in the sclera and conjunctiva, and an inward deviation of the right eye. Since there was no cause other than possible allergies, ACTH was given by vein for two days, followed by oral decreasing prednisone for three weeks with gradual relief. Edema and muscle paralysis recurred two more times in the spring and summer, relieved by oral prednisone given for one to two weeks.

During the fourth attack a detachment in the inner upper area of the right retina was found. Since there was no history of an injury, corticoids were given again, with relief of the edema with gradual reattachment of the retina in three to four weeks. After corticoids had been discontinued for one to two months, moderate retinal detachment recurred in the same area, causing blurring of vision. Edema of the eyelid and paralysis of the sixth nerve were absent. With corticoids, relief was reestablished. Detachment with similar relief occurred in three months. For two to three days during and after retinal detachments severe headaches in the temporal and occipital areas had occurred. "Dark circles" had been present under the eyes for four years.

The patient consulted us in May of 1967 for study of the possible allergic cause of the recurrent detachments. In addition to the ocular symptoms, nasal allergy with postnasal mucus had been present for two years. She had had migraine headaches and vomiting every two months, with photophobia, nervous tension, and fever up to 105 F for five to eight days from six to twenty years, the cause of which had not been determined.

Family history revealed her son was formerly allergic to eggs, cats, and dogs.

She had smoked one pack of cigarettes daily for twenty-one years.

Scratch tests gave one and two plus reactions to grass and fall pollens and two plus to egg. X-ray of the sinuses revealed slight cloudiness in the antra. Chest x-ray and blood and urine analyses were negative.

Because of the recurrent attacks of edema, oculomotor nerve paralysis, and (finally) detachment of the retina, study of possible food allergy was initiated with our CFE diet. Without cortisone but with strict adherence to this diet, relief of moderate blurring of vision indicated reattachment of the retina in two weeks.

Possible food allergy as a cause of the initial attacks of edema of the right eyelid, bulging and redness of the eye, paralysis of the right sixth nerve, and (finally) detachment of the right retina was studied with the CFE diet. Food allergy was indicated by the former history of perennial nasal allergy with postnasal mucus for two years and by the migraine headaches with vomiting possibly because of allergy every two months from six to twenty years of age. Her hay fever and the reactions to pollens, moreover, indicated her allergic status.

During the year and a half since then, no serious retinal detachment occurred. With the strict diet from June through the summer and fall, no edema of the lids, congestion of the conjunctiva, inward deviation of the eye, and fuzzy vision which had occurred with previous detachments developed. Finally, in November small amounts of wheat, milk, and eggs were included in the diet, with resultant engorgement of the blood vessels in the conjunctiva and sclera, fuzzy vision, and moderate pain in the eye, indicating mild recurrence of her detachment. With the return to the strict diet, particularly with the elimination of all traces of wheat and especially of milk and its products, evidence of detachment disappeared. During the winter and spring slight amounts of milk and cheese, corn, pork lard, and wheat at intervals of two to six weeks produced dilated blood vessels in the conjunctiva and sclera in six hours, with blurring of vision in the upper right visual field in twelve hours. When eaten in more than slight amounts, contrary to our orders, diarrhea, abdominal pain, and distention developed in the night, continuing in the following day. During June and July of 1968 slight to moderate amounts of these foods were eaten every one to two weeks, with no or less resultant symptoms until early October. Similar relief from edema and paralysis of the sixth nerve had occurred each summer since 1962. As emphasized in Chapter 1, this summer relief favors food allergy. No corticoids had been taken since our elimination diet was started in June of 1967.

In early October of 1968 she ate two ounces of ice cream. On the following morning there was marked redness in the inner side of the conjunctiva and sclera of the right eye associated with a moderate increase in mucoid secretion without edema of the eye lids or inward deviation of the eye. We advised the elimination of all traces of wheat. Eight milligrams of Aristocort were ordered three times a day for three days followed by 4 mg four times a day, reducing it and eliminating it in seven to twelve days. Because of the mild evidences of detachment and congestion of the conjunctiva which occurred during the previous spring and winter months when wheat and milk were added to the diet, she was convinced that these two foods had been responsible for her ocular symptoms.

MACULAR DEGENERATION

Bothman, in 1941, opined that allergy may be the cause of "the central disciform degeneration of the macula" which occurs in young adults. It starts in small retinal hemorrhages which after absorption leave a greenish-black or slate-colored area usually beneath the superior macular vessels. Recurring hemorrhages form retinal cysts, which may not disturb vision. Large, gray, irregular cysts, however, may involve the entire macula, which may evolve into yellow crystalline lesions.

Attacks from spring to late fall along with skin reactions to pollens justify desensitization to pollens. Similar lesions in one woman thirty-seven years of age, involving the macula, were benefitted by

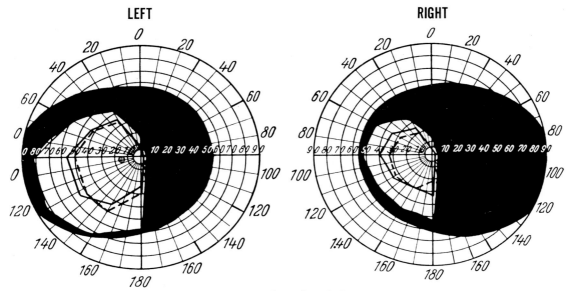

Figure 38. *Case 149:* Hemianopsia with right-sided trigeminal neuralgia and right facial hyperesthesia because of egg allergy (Hansen).

elimination of specific foods and desensitization to pollens and molds which prevented recurrences.

OPHTHALMIC MIGRAINE

In this chapter on ocular allergy the visual symptoms preceding the onset of migraine usually continuing during the headache and decreasing as the attack subsides require discussion. Though they do not arise in the ocular tissues, these symptoms are best explained by dilatation or spasm, with resulting edema in the blood vessels of the pia and cerebral cortex in localized areas of the occipital lobes from which nerves originate which pass forward, crossing in the optic chiasma and terminating in the retina. Since it is generally agreed that allergy to foods and at times to inhalants and probably to other allergens requires study in migraine, as discussed in Chapter 17, it is probable that allergic reactivity especially to foods in the occipital lobes of the brain is responsible for these visual disturbances which usually oc-

cur before and often during the actual migrainous attack. When such symptoms are present, the headaches and visual symptoms may be bilateral rather than unilateral.

The frequency of disturbances in vision has been reported by various students. In one hundred of our patients with allergic headaches or migraine, as shown in Table XXXIX in Chapter 17, visual disturbances occurred in 18 percent.

An early and important report of visual disturbances in migraine was published by Liveing in his classical treatise "On Megrim, Sick Headaches and Some Allied Disorders," published in London in 1873. In his sixty-seven cases of migraine forty-one had visual affections in contrast to disturbances in touch and "general sensibility" in twenty-two, vertigo usually moderate in ten, nausea in thirty-nine, and vomiting in fifty-three. These visual disturbances in individual patients were described by Liveing as follows: "Central obliteration at times centrifugal with sparkling and dazzling lights, dimness and dazzling and colored lights in the whole visual field, unilateral nebulous vision, general obscuration of vision, inability to read certain words or letters in words, blank whiteness, horizontal hemioptic obliteration followed by chromatic zig-zags, showers of sparks, transient loss of sight, intolerance to light and noise, hemioptic obscuration, central lateral obscuration and dazzling, partial loss of sight (½ hour before headache), visual field all alive, (and) unilateral dimness with zig-zag trembling spectrum." As reported by Liveing and others, half vision is absent in many patients with migraine.

Though the symptoms of migraine are explained by involvement of the sensory nervous tissues, occasional pareses or paralyses of ocular nerves relieved when the symptoms of ophthalmic migraine are controlled by antiallergic therapy suggests the possibility that such allergy was a primary or secondary cause of the involvement of the ocular tract.

Because of the frequency with which allergy especially to foods and at times to inhalants has been the demonstrated cause of ophthalmic migraine, such possible allergy always deserves careful and adequate study. As reported in Chapter 17, moreover, recurrent headaches with or without nausea and vomiting when ocular symptoms occur present the same challenge. In some patients frequent longstanding allergic headaches with or without other manifestations of clinical allergy may be present along with less frequent attacks of typical ophthalmic migraine, both of which may be due to the same allergies, especially to foods.

Pain in one or both eyes which initiate frontal or temporal headaches or is referred anteriorly into the eye after starting in the occipital or nuchal areas and are not associated with visual disturbances of typi-

cal migraine are best explained by referred pain resulting from vascular and possibly neural allergy in the pia or dura of the brain.

EXTRAOCULAR MUSCLES

Transient diplopia may occur with attacks of migraine. Duane, in 1923, reported paresis of the right abducins nerve before such attacks, disappearing in a week. A man fifty-eight years of age had partial or incomplete oculomotor paralysis without migraine involving the right superior and left inferior recti muscles. There was vertical diplopia on and off for several years. Lemoine, in 1925, recorded attacks of scintillating scotoma, vertigo, and diplopia relieved with omission of cheese in the diet. Criep reported vertical diplopia after eating eggs. Bothman, in 1941, observed a man fifty-two years of age who had had attacks of migraine all of his life and had paresis of the left inferior oblique nerve with a recent headache lasting for three days. The indicated cause of the former and present headaches was chocolate.

Since food allergy especially needs study in such headaches, as emphasized in Chapter 17, these pareses of the extraocular muscles also require consideration of such allergy.

Paralysis of ocular muscles temporarily in association with detached retina both relieved by control of food allergy is evidenced in Case 148.

RIGHT HEMIANOPSIA WITH RIGHT-SIDED TRIGEMINAL NEURALGIA AND HYPERESTHESIA RESULTING FROM FOOD ALLERGY

Hansen, in his prestigious book on allergy, reported the following case:

Case 149: A woman thirty years of age had had attacks of right-sided trigeminal neuralgia associated with right-sided hemianopsia hyperesthesia in the right face, and at times numbness in the right half of the body. The syndrome had developed during a period of one to twenty-four hours and had gradually terminated in three to eight days, the scotoma being last to disappear. Ringing in the ears with some right-sided deafness and disturbances in taste had occurred. Four major attacks and several moderate ones had recurred during the past year.

In addition, she had had recurrent corneal ulcers, which are best explained by recurrently activated food allergy as already noted in this chapter.

Her family history revealed asthma in the paternal grandfather, urticaria in the mother, and eczema in the sister. Diet history revealed a dislike for chocolate.

After intradermal skin tests with eggs and milk, a temperature of 37.9 C developed in the evening continuing at 38 C the next day (read Chapt. 24). In the first evening she felt sick and developed trigeminal neuralgia especially in its third branch, herpetiform eruptions in the right cornea increasing after the first hour following the test, a right-sided hemianopsia, and hyperesthesia for touch over the right side of the body even in the side of her tongue, resulting in disurbance in taste.

On the next day moderate ptosis of the right eyelid was attributed to slight edema or to lowering of the lid to protect the ulcerated cornea.

In five days the sensory disturbances and hemianopsia had disappeared, and the keratitis was healing.

In the following fifteen years as milk and especially eggs continued to be eliminated, the above symptoms did not recur except for slight symptoms three times when small amounts of egg had been ingested.

Doctor Hansen concluded that the right-sided hemianopsia, trigeminal neuralgia, right hemi-hyperesthesia, moderate involvement of the right acoustic nerve (cochlear), and impairment of taste were due to an allergic reaction, especially to eggs. He opined that a reversible reaction in the posterior inner capsule in an area supplied by the anterior choroid artery caused by vasospasm or edema was responsible.

This case was the only documented one of hemianopsia with trigeminal neuralgia, hyperesthesia, and with some cochlear involvement because of food allergy recorded by a dependable allergist in the literature.

TUNNEL VISION BECAUSE OF FOOD ALLERGY

Tunnel vision as diagnosed by ophthalmologists in one identical twin, both of whom had been relieved of recurrent serous otitis by adherence to an elimination diet for nine years, as reported in Case 65 in Chapter 13, occurred in September after wheat had been given for two months during the summer. To rule out an intracranial lesion, spinal fluid examinations and encephalograms were done in a university hospital.

When informed about the tunnel vision, we advised strict elimination of wheat and adherence to the CFE diet which had completely controlled the serous otitis media for nine years.

This tunnel vision had occurred in December two years before, being controlled by the elimination of wheat which he had eaten.

Decreasing doses of triamcinolone were given for five days, with its discontinuance in one week. In two weeks vision was normal, remaining so with no return of tunnel vision for three years since then, depending on strict adherence to the diet.

His tolerance for wheat in June, July, and August is similar to the former relief of serous otitis media in the summer because of inactivation of food allergy in many patients during the summer, as emphasized in Chapter 2.

Copies of his visual fields are in Figure 39. Since discontinuing wheat, the fields have been normal for three years.

Comment: Food allergy as a cause of tunnel vision on two occasions has not been reported previously.

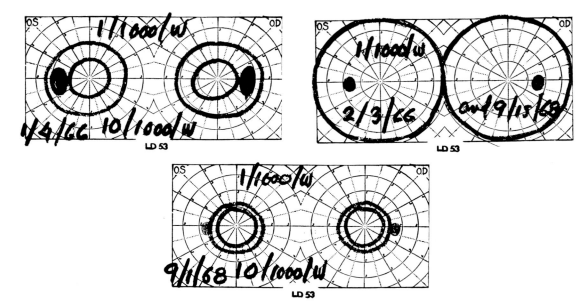

Figure 39. *Case 65:* Tunnel vision resulting from wheat in an adolescent with recurrent serous otitis media because of food allergy (Chapt. 12).

DIAGNOSIS AND CONTROL OF OCULAR ALLERGY TO DRUGS

A careful recorded history of all drugs and medicaments taken by the patient or medicaments used locally on the eyelids, conjunctiva, or cornea or absorbed from its application on any other skin area may be important from the point of view of allergy to drugs. Possible ocular allergy resulting from injections given parenterally or into body cavities, including the nasal sinuses, vagina, and rectum, may cause allergic inflammation in the ocular tissues if they are sensitized to such medications. Medications purchased by the patient or used by him or in home cabinets may be offenders. Possible allergy to medications being taken by mouth or parenterally or even in the previous one to four weeks may be important to consider as possible allergenic causes. Clinical and other medications given parenterally or less often by mouth must be listed. Until the type of

allergy responsible for the ocular allergy is determined, all drugs and medications should be entirely eliminated for two to four weeks. After relief is assured, medications necessary for the control of chronic disease other than allergy can be resumed, one by one, eliminating any which reestablishes manifestations of ocular allergy. Along with the elimination of medicaments, flavored toothpastes, fixatives for dentures, mouthwashes, and of course laxatives and birth control pills should be omitted until the underlying cause of allergic manifestations is determined. Possible allergy to vitamins, colored dyes, or other chemicals including chlorine in food or drinking water may be responsible.

Since it takes several days up to two to four weeks for medications to leave the body, total elimination must continue until a decision in regard to such possible allergy is made. Desensitization to drugs by mouth or parenterally is not possible.

DIAGNOSIS OF OCULAR ALLERGY FROM FOODS

Food allergy is easily and gradually controlled by any ophthalmologist or allergist or other physician, as we have summarized and discussed more fully in Chapter 3. Indications for such study of food allergy follow:

1. Perennial symptoms and possible allergic inflammation in any ocular tissue justify the study of possible food allergy, even though its following characteristics may be absent.

2. Recurrent activation of symptoms and inflammation for one to several days every two to eight weeks requires study of food allergy. Interim relief is explained by the union of specific antibodies to the causative food allergens in the tissues during the attack as discussed in Chapter 1. After gradual reaccumulation of antibodies to the causative food, the relief stops, and another attack occurs.

3. Ocular inflammation and symptoms often decrease or disappear in the summer, being exaggerated in the fall to late spring especially in the winter, as we have reported especially in asthma for forty years. Its probable explanation is in Chapter 1. Absence of this seasonal variation, however, does not rule out perennially active food allergy.

4. A diet history may reveal dislikes or disagreements to foods. Allergy thereto can only be determined by provocation feeding tests with such foods. This must be done, however, when the inflammation and symptoms from allergy have been controlled by the total elimination of suspected foods for twice as long as the previous relief (see discussion of provocation feeding tests in Chapt. 3).

The interpretation of diet histories and the failure of most diet diaries to aid in determining allergenic foods are discussed in Chapter 2.

5. Absent skin tests and the fallibility of slight, moderate, or even large reactions to allergenic foods greatly decrease or eliminate the value of skin testing in determining clinical food allergy. This lack of diagnostic value does not pertain to the large scratch reactions to foods causing definite allergic symptoms in minutes up to one to two hours. The possible occurrence of such positive reactions justifies routine scratch tests with foods, providing they are done by technicians supervised by the allergist or informed physician. Unless a history of immediate symptoms within one or two hours of the ingestion of large reacting foods is obtained, however, clinical allergy to such foods and also to foods giving slight or moderate reactions can only be determined by provocation feeding tests with those foods. Such tests necessarily have to be done in the symptom-free patient. The reader is referred to our discussion of the absent and fallible positive skin reactions in Chapter 2. Test-negative diets rarely reveal clinical food allergy. Thus failure of relief of symptoms with such diets does not rule out clinical food allergy.

CONTROL OF OCULAR ALLERGY TO FOODS WITH ELIMINATION DIETS

When one or more of the above characteristics of clinical food allergy indicate such possible allergy, its study and control are necessary as follows and as amplified in Chapter 3.

1. Strict elimination of foods giving large scratch reactions especially if they cause definite clinical allergy in any tissue of the body and the elimination of foods to which definite dislikes and idiosyncrasies exist relieve symptoms in a few patients. If dependable skin testing is not available, as in most office of ophthalmologists, or if

skin testing must be done in laboratories not supervised by the physician himself, a diet excluding foods which are disliked or which disagree with the patient may be tried. Rarely, however, does any relief occur.

2. Because of the usual failure of test-negative diets and of diets excluding foods suspected in the diet history, diet trial with the initial elimination of the most allergenic foods is necessary in practically all patients when food allergy is suspected.

For such diet trial our elimination diets as advised throughout this volume have been used with increasing success in revealing and controlling ocular allergy from food allergy. Their use has revealed the important and possible role of such allergy, as it has the equal or greater role of food than inhalant allergy in the many manifestations of clinical allergy occurring in most tissues of the body reported in this book.

Our CFE diet is most important for the initial study of possible food allergy. The allowed foods, detailed menus, and recipes for soy-potato bakery products, its ordering in a hospital, and its instruction and use by the patient after hospital discharge or in office patients at home are detailed in Chapter 3. The time required for its initial use, its manipulation after relief has been obtained by the physician, and the necessary maintenance of weight and nutrition are also discussed and advised.

Though food allergy is often the sole cause of ocular allergy, concomitant allergy to inhalants, drugs, and contact allergens even in the absence of food allergy must be remembered.

The importance of these studies of allergy, as evidenced in our reports, in most tissues of the eye and especially in the uveal tract is so great that the possibility of allergy should be studied by all ophthalmologists, we opine, as advised in this chapter and volume.

Our CFE diet with the use of our inexpensive elimination diet booklet can be explained and supervised by the ophthalmologist or by any physician. Nurses or secretaries can be easily trained for such instruction if they are supervised at all times by the physician. The physician and members of his office staff who may also explain the diets to patients should read our discussion of the diet in Chapter 3. Patients must understand that only those foods listed in the diet can be taken and that bakery products must be made by an honest baker supervised by the physician or at home. Such accurate and strict use of the diet and subsequent supervision by the physician, as advised in Chapter 3, become an easy routine after our discussion of the use and preparation of the diet are read and carefully followed and used in more than a few patients for at least two or more months. The discussion of this diet in our book *Bronchial Asthma—Its Diagnosis and Treatment* (1963) is of important help.

This recognition and control of food allergy is of such importance to ophthalmologists as well as to all physicians who are challenged with the study and control of the many other manifestations of food allergy that the study of these diets and their use should continue until it becomes an easy routine for the physician and his associates.

FRUIT-FREE, CEREAL-FREE ELIMINATION DIETS

As discussed in Chapter 3, some patients know that a few or even many fruits, spices, condiments, and at times vitamin C cause allergic symptoms. Fruit sensitivity especially occurs in urticaria, angioneurotic edema, gastrointestinal allergy, allergic toxemia, and bladder and joint allergies. At times patients may suspect that specific fruits cause or increase possible ocular allergy. Whereas we have not found that allergy to fruits is a common cause of ocular allergy, its possibility must be considered with the use of our FFCFE diet as advised in Chapter 3 if the history indicates possible fruit, condiment, or spice allergy and at times allergy to vitamin C as such. Unsuspected fruit allergy may be revealed with strict use of this diet if probable or definite food allergy is not controlled with the CFE diet containing fruit.

SOYBEAN OR LIMA BEAN ALLERGY

Though the CFE diet includes soy- or lima-potato bakery products, they must be eliminated if allergy to soybeans or lima beans is evidenced by history or by symptoms from ingestion of their products. If such products are not readily available, moreover, they may be omitted as they were by Kaplan in Johannesburg, who with the other foods in our CFE diet has confirmed the importance of this elimination diet for the relief of chronic asthma as reported by him in *Food Allergy—The Missing Link in Chronic Bronchial Asthma* in 1967 and in more recent publications. The CFE diet minus soy products is also advised in other countries where soy flour and potato starch are not available as they are in the United States (see Chapt. 3). Some patients tolerate lima beans and not soybeans because of which lima-potato bakery products are advised, recipes for which are in Chapter 3.

MINIMAL ELIMINATION DIETS

The possibility moreover that a broad-based type of food allergy to a great many foods, as discussed in Chapter 3, may be responsible for occasional cases of ocular allergy must be mentioned. Though we have no definite cases of ocular allergy which support the frequent occurrence of such multiple food allergies, their possibility must be kept in mind.

DIAGNOSIS AND CONTROL OF OCULAR ALLERGY FROM INHALANTS

Inhalant allergy, especially to pollen, has been demonstrated in our practice more frequently than food allergy. However, when food allergy has been studied as we advise in more cases of keratitis, recurrent corneal ulcers, scleritis, uveitis, and neuroretinitis, we opine that it will prove to be as frequent a cause as pollen allergy of perennial and at times recurrently activated allergic inflammation and resultant ocular symptoms.

Pollen allergy is indicated by ocular inflammation and resultant symptoms in one or all pollen seasons. Pollen as a cause of ocular allergy also frequently produces the following concomitant manifestations of pollen allergy: nasal, bronchial, aural, and at times gastrointestinal allergy and occasionally seasonal headaches, neuritis, arthritis, genitourinary, as well as eczema in other cutaneous areas than the eyelids. Adequate, proper desensitization to pollen as advised below is mandatory in vernal catarrh to obtain good and continued relief.

Skin testing, especially with the scratch method, gives positive reactions to allergenic pollens in approximately 85 percent of cases. That positive reactions often occur to pollens not productive of clinical allergy and that scratch reactions to pollens which cause ocular inflammation and symptoms are negative in about 15 percent of the cases must be remembered. Thus the diagnosis of pollen allergy depends on a seasonal history of ocular symptoms.

DESENSITIZATION TO POLLENS

Desensitization to pollens requires antigens containing the important pollens in the patient's environment, their amounts depending on their abundance in the air, and the patient's possible skin reactions thereto when the symptoms from pollen allergy are present. Desensitization to pollens of trees in the patient's environment, especially to the pollens of fruit and nut trees around the home and to pollens of cultivated flowers which are in the immediate environment, may be important, as discussed in Chapter 2 and especially in our book *Bronchial Asthma—Its Diagnosis and Treatment*, published in 1963. The results of pollen desensitization are evidenced in case reports throughout this chapter. More information about desensitization to pollen is in Chapters 8 and 12.

The importance of desensitization, as we have reported, is especially stressed in vernal conjunctivitis. For treatment of vernal conjunctivitis, antigens containing all important pollens in the patient's environment at times in two or even three separate combinations with a gradual increase up to large tolerated doses of the 1:100 or the 1:50 dilutions are given. These maximum doses are then repeated every one to two weeks perennially for two years, after which booster doses are then given for several more years. The benefit of such therapy has been emphasized in our discussion of vernal conjunctivitis in this chapter.

Inhalant allergy to animal emanations; house, occupational, and environmental dusts; miscellaneous inhalants; and airborne fungi may be indicated in a well-recorded environmental history. If skin testing first with scratch tests and later if indicated with intradermal tests give positive reactions, the clinical significance of such possible allergy to these allergens must be determined by relief resulting from environmental control or even by a limited course of desensitization with antigens containing such allergens. The clinical importance of such positive reactions in ocular or other tissue allergy must be confirmed by provocation tests through inhalation of the inhalants by the symptom-free patient.

Environmental control of the patient's living, working, and (if possible) his recreational environments where the above allergens are in the air or inhaled even in small but allergy-producing amounts often eliminates the allergenic inhalants so that the reactions in the ocular or other tissues and resultant symptoms are controlled. Animal emanations or other allergens or dusts on the clothes of members of the family or friends may produce symptoms in the patient allergic to them. Changing such outdoor clothes to clean house clothes before coming into the house of the patient may be necessary to prevent the development of allergic symptoms.

If, however, environmental control is ineffectual and the allergens of animal emanations, various dusts, allergens in tobacco smoke in room air, and other airborne allergens continue to be inhaled, causing ocular or other tissue allergy, then long-term desensitization to such allergens is indicated, as advised in Chapter 4.

While desensitization is proceeding, corticosteroids are justified to give temporary relief. Such corticosteroids, however, must be reduced in one to three weeks and discontinued after environmental control with or without specific desensitization therapy relieves allergic symptoms. Restraint in the use of corticosteroids and their gradual discontinuance in two to six weeks are important because of possible complications from their long-continued use, as emphasized in Chapter 30.

Desensitization to inhalants demonstrated as causes of ocular or other allergy is advised in greater detail in Chapters 8 and 12.

RELIEF OF SYMPTOMS FROM ALLERGIC INFLAMMATION BEFORE RECOGNITION AND CONTROL OF CAUSATIVE FOOD, INHALANT, DRUG, AND CHEMICAL ALLERGIES

Relief of allergic inflammation, itching, and dermatitis of the eyelids may require the following:

1. Warm or cold water or saline compresses.

2. Hydrocortisone, Aristocort, or especially Valisone Ointment.

3. If secondary infection is present or probable, Achromycin or other mycin ointments may be applied between applications of the corticosteroid ointment. Oral antibiotics may be advisable.

Relief of itching, burning, and inflammation arising from allergic conjunctivitis with or without keratitis may require the following:

1. Washing eyes with warm water to give temporary relief.

2. Epinephrine or adrenalin 1:1500 dropped onto the conjunctiva every hour if necessary.

3. Corticosteroid suspension as prepared by pharmaceutical companies and used as directed until control of allergenic causes gives relief.

4. Oral corticosteroids for limited periods.

5. These recommendations about relief of ocular allergy assume that bacterial and viral infection is being controlled or has been ruled out by the ophthalmologist or allergist.

Relief of pain, at times pressure, and of impairment of vision from uveitis, retinitis, optic nervitis and at times detachment of retina until control of causative food, inhalant, drug, or chemical allergies relieves the distress and other symptoms may require the following:

1. Corticosteroids by mouth or by intramuscular injection are indicated beginning with large doses as advised by pharmaceutical companies with their usual reduction and discontinuance in one to two weeks when the control of food, inhalant, or chemical allergies begins to relieve the allergy. ACTH is contraindicated because of frequent allergy to its pituitary protein.

The diagnosis and supervision of such treatment of ocular manifestations of possible allergy must be the responsibility of the ophthalmologist. Study of allergy by him or (if he so advises) in cooperation with an allergist is important. This study is especially necessary if allergy is studied as a possible cause of glaucoma in which the control of ocular pressure by mydriatics by the ophthalmologist is mandatory until hoped for possible relief from control of allergy occurs.

SUMMARY

1. Though pollen and to a lesser extent other inhalant, drug, and contact allergies are recognized causes of conjunctivitis, the allergic reactions to inhalants and especially to foods in all ocular tissues have not received sufficient recognition.

2. Information about blepharitis (lid dermatitis) from pollen in twenty cases is analyzed in Table XLI.

3. When symptoms are perennial and not due to contact allergy, food allergy requires special study and control as we advise especially if edema, granulated lids, and at times styes occur, as in six reported cases resulting from food allergy.

4. Conjunctivitis from food rather than inhalants persisting in the winter is reported in four cases, causing redness, itch-

ing, burning, and a granular sensation and mucoid discharge.

5. That pollen allergy at times with no skin reactions or associated hay fever needs recognition and control with desensitization to causative pollens is reported.

6. Vernal catarrh, exaggerated as it is during the pollen seasons, necessitates adequate, prolonged desensitization to pollens, as advised in this chapter and in Chapters 8 and 12. Dean *et al.* reported good results from such therapy, confirming our experience together with that of Kerbitch, as reported in this chapter.

7. The role of allergy to other inhalants and also foods is indicated in the literature and is illustrated in our controlled cases.

8. Allergy as an important cause of uveitis is emphasized by Coles and other ophthalmologists.

9. The recognition of other inflammation from chronic infection, fungi, sarcoid, and parasites as causes of uveitis must be remembered.

10. Benefit from corticosteroids in uveitis also favors probable allergy. Study and control of inhalant and food allergy will increase the recognition of such allergy, especially to foods.

11. Ophthalmia from autoimmunity to iris pigment and to lens allergens is emphasized in the literature and receives special comment in this chapter.

12. That atopic, drug, and contact allergies may cause glaucoma is indicated in the literature and by limited results in our practice.

13. Cataracts developing in patients with chronic allergic dermatitis are explained by the causes of such eczema, namely food in perennial cases and pollen when the eczema is exaggerated in the pollen seasons. Adequate control of such allergies in the future may reduce early evidences of cataracts, as it does concomitant eczema.

14. The role of food, inhalant, and drug allergies, as reported in the literature, in the retina and optic nerve is summarized.

15. Retinal detachment from vasculitis and resultant exudations between the retina and choroid from allergy, as suggested in the literature, is supported by good results in one cooperating patient whose frequent previous detachments have been terminated by our control of food and to a lesser extent pollen allergy.

16. Food allergy in ophthalmic migraine receives special comment as reported in Chapter 17.

17. Pareses of ocular muscles relieved by control of food allergy is discussed.

18. Our advised study and control of food and pollen allergy are summarized and receive extended discussion in Chapters 3 and 12. Relief of symptoms with medications until food, inhalant, and drug allergies are controlled is advised.

Chapter 21

Urogenital Allergy—Bladder Allergy

Duke, in 1922, reported bladder symptoms as a frequent result of food allergy, especially in patients who exhibited little or no pathology in the urinary tract. Frequent and painful urination, bladder tenesmus, incomplete emptying, varying degrees of pain, and soreness over the bladder and polypi from chronic allergic edema were emphasized by Duke as arising from food sensitization:

> The condition may vary in severity from slight discomfort to pain and tenesmus, which confines the patient to bed for months. Bladder allergy of long standing may be complicated by infection, in which case the symptoms of cystitis obscure the diagnosis. In one case it was complicated by polypi which surrounded the internal urethral meatus. This was thought to be the result of chronic edema (allergic) of the mucous membrane. In patients having chronic bladder allergy, frequently no pathology can be found by internists, urologists, neurologists, roentgenologists, or pathologists, except hypersensitiveness to foods. Frequently the case may be misdiagnosed as cystitis, trigonitis from unrecognized infection or irritation, urethral caruncle, misplaced uterus, or pelvic inflammatory disease. Treatment of such conditions often gives partial relief, but as a rule the bladder symptoms continue as severely as before.

He stated that bladder allergy was at times associated with pelvic as well as bladder pathology, and was frequently accompanied by generalized symptoms, including other allergic manifestations and toxemia. That bladder allergy can exist was substantiated by production of contractions in smooth muscle of the bladder as well as the uterus in sensitized rabbits by Manwaring and Marino in 1927.

During the last forty-seven years allergists and urologists have drawn attention to this manifestation in books and articles on urogenital allergy. Duke, in his book on allergy in 1925, reaffirmed such bladder allergy and reported five informative cases in women from the age of twenty-two to fifty-two years. Vaughan and Hawke (1931) described bladder irritability, Dietl's crisis, and urethral obstruction from allergic edema in the bladder with many nervous, cutaneous, and other disturbances from food allergy. Dutton mentioned a patient whose left ureter had been dilated at intervals for five years because of ureteral colic from food allergy. Some evidence points to interstitial cystitis arising from food, drug, or at times inhalant allergy. Search for eosinophiles in the urine should be routine in all patients suspected of such allergy as reported by Salen, Kutzne, Thomas and Wicksten, and others. Their absence does not rule out allergy. Along with urological allergy, burning, edema, pruritus, and resulting excoriations and possibly eczematouslike lesions of the vulva and vagina may occur, which will be discussed in this chapter.

Salen (1932) reported urticaria of the bladder, increased urinary frequency, and a sense of pressure in the bladder arising from food allergy. The urine in one case contained eosinophiles exclusively. Feinberg (1934) stated that bladder allergy to foods and drugs was not infrequent and reported one case with urinary frequency for thirty years because of wheat allergy. Westphal noted bladder and ureteral spasms with eosinophiles in the urine in a patient with allergic cystitis. In 1944 Thomas and Wicksten added evidence of urological allergy, including frequent urination and nycturia from eggs, cereal, and carrots and tenesmus from chocolate and grapefruit. Of special interest was the hematuria and allergic purpura in a boy sixteen years of age occurring four days after inhaling smoke from heated tar, allergy to which may have occurred from his chewing it in childhood. Nausea, vomiting, melena, edema of the face and feet, and joint pains also occurred. We opine that more evidences of food allergy causing Hunner's ulcers also may occur with its study as we advise.

Eisenstaedt (1954) reported dysuria with abundant eosinophiles in the urine from Brazil nuts, quoting Salen. In 1954 he reported hematuria from milk allergy in a worker in a creamery. Milk in any form was responsible. Hematuria from glomerulonephritis in patients with Henoch-Schonlein purpura was reported by Alexander and Eyerman, Brown, Alexander and Lazarus, and Hampton, attributed by the writers to food allergy as noted in Chapter 22. Kittredge also reported hematuria from milk in 1949. The possibility that food allergy may be one cause of urological symptoms in Reiter's Syndrome should be studied, especially with our fruit-free elimination diets.

Unger, Kubich, and Unger, in 1949, noted the failure of most physicians, including many urologists, to study urological allergy, especially "in all obscure cases of cystitis."

Case 150: A man forty-nine years of age had had urinary burning, dysuria, and urgency through a ten-year period, lasting two to three hours every week and associated with a rash on his face and hands. Cystoscopy revealed hyperemia of the bladder mucosa. Elimination of legumes and nuts controlled the urinary symptoms and dermatitis.

Increasing realization of urological allergy has occurred in the last twenty years, as reviewed by Powell in 1961. He emphasized a history of various clinical manifestations of allergy as favoring possible urological allergy, especially if the symptoms are not controlled by usual urological therapy. Indicating bladder allergy are cystoscopic findings of pale, edematous mucosa in the urethra or bladder with areas of hyperemia and oozing of blood with a reduced capacity and irritability of the bladder. Red blood cells, a few pus cells, and especially eosinophiles are usually found in the urine. With diet trial, allergy to foods was found, especially to fruits, condiments, chocolate, and nuts along with allergy to other foods.

Of special interest was Powell's report of interstitial cystitis illustrated by its occurrence in one patient for eight years relieved by the control of food and inhalant allergy. Thomas and Wicksten also reported interstitial cystitis relieved in six weeks with the elimination of allergenic foods along with desensitization to pollens.

ALLERGY TO IODIDES

The comments of Powell about allergic reactions from intravenous organic iodine dyes used for excretory urograms are important in this discussion of urological allergy. Fortunately these reactions are not numerous, and fatal reactions are very rare, having been reported in only 31 out of 3.8 million intravenous injections, according to Pendegrass (1955). Probable allergic and shock reactions not reported in the literature are more frequent. To forewarn about such possible allergy, saturated solution of iodine, ten drops in water, is given in our patients two times on the day before the urogram. If nasal congestion, headache, and especially swelling of the submaxillary glands occur in twelve hours, indicating iodine allergy, the urogram may be contra-indicated.

PERSONAL CASES OF BLADDER ALLERGY

Cases of clinical allergy in which bladder allergy was a major problem follow:

Case 151: Constant burning of the bladder and abdominal distress for thirteen years. A woman fifty-four years of age had had a burning, stinging discomfort in the bladder nearly constantly for thirteen years following a panhysterectomy. Marked frequency of urination had been present. She found by accident that a diet of meat and cooked vegetables, except for carrots, cabbage, and cauliflower, gave complete relief. Much medical and bladder therapy had not relieved her. Pain and tenderness over the bladder region for four years and severe constipation for thirty years had been present. Mucous colitis had been recurrent for a long time. Practically all fruits, wheat, milk, tea, chocolate, and melons had caused sour stomach and abdominal distress. The family history was negative for allergy. Sour stomach and abdominal disturbances have been entirely controlled on a diet consisting of lamb, white fish, chicken, asparagus, artichokes, squash, spinach, baked potatoes, and olive oil. Milk, fruits, nuts, melon, and tomatoes especially produced her symptoms. On her present diet she has also maintained her weight and strength.

Comment: The association of bladder and abdominal allergy is of special interest. As in Duke's patients with bladder symptoms, allergy to fruits was very definite. It is possible that her dysmenorrhea was due to an allergic reaction in the uterine tissues, which is described on page 419.

Case 152: A woman thirty-eight years of age had had unrelieved "bladder catarrh" for thirteen years. Marked burning in the bladder, pain over the lower abdomen, tenesmus, and frequent urination had been present. She felt that foods were responsible, but physicians had not considered such a possibility. She had had urticaria continuously in childhood. Recurrent sick headaches had occurred. Eggs had always nauseated her. Dry beans, almonds, and apricots were known to cause epigastric burning. A maternal aunt had asthma. Her physical, laboratory, and urological examinations were negative. Skin reactions to various allergens were negative.

During the past two years the patient has been relieved of her bladder symptoms on an "elimination diet," which was gradually evolved by our diet trial. Then provocation feeding tests showed that wheat, citrus fruits, cabbage, cauliflower, almonds, beans, apricots, and apples caused bladder distress. On one occasion a half of a wheat cracker was taken. Frequent urination, spasms, and burning in the bladder occurred in eight hours. Pain all over the lower abdomen, and in the groins, vagina, and rectum was severe, and the vulval tissues were sore and associated with a burning feeling for several days afterwards.

Case 153: A woman fifty-eight years of age had had "cystitus" for two years unrelieved by urological therapy. Nausea and shivering with painful urination occurred several times a week. There was no personal history of allergy. Allergy to all fruits was responsible.

Case 154: A woman fifty years of age had pressure in the bladder and moderate hematuria in the last two springs. Hay fever had been present in the spring for thirty years. With our FFCFE diet relief occurred in three days. It was not due to pollen therapy, which in two months had relieved her hay fever. Fruits caused bladder symptoms in a half hour as did vitamin C in four days as reported in Chapter 29.

Pressure in the bladder and its impaired emptying require study of bladder allergy previously reported by Salen in 1932, as noted above.

Brief reports of other cases of bladder allergy in our practice follow:

Case 155: A woman forty-nine years of age had urgency and burning with urination for three to four days every one to two weeks. Cystoscopies, bladder irrigations, and antibiotics had failed. "Life was not worth living." With our FFCFE diet relief occurred.

Case 156: A woman fifty years of age had tenesmus and hematuria for two years unrelieved by urological study and therapy. Sick headaches every two months indicated possible food allergy. Elimination of wheat, fruits, alcohol, and spices gave relief. Pineapple in two hours caused burning, aching, and throbbing in the bladder, decreasing in six days.

Case 157: A woman fifty-eight years of age had burning, pain, and pressure in the bladder with vaginitis and dermatitis of vulva and groins for two years. Cystoscopy showed urethrotrigonitis. Eczema on the fingers in a sister was relieved by our CFE diet. Previous urological therapy had failed. She gave two to three plus scratch reactions to pollens. The FFCFE diet and pollen desensitization were required for relief.

Case 158: A woman fifty-five years of age, had burning, painful, urgent urination for twenty years. Irrigations, cauterizations with silver nitrate, and urethral dilatations every three to eight weeks had failed. Vulval and vaginal itching had been present for eight years. All symptoms continued to be relieved with a fruit-free, spice-free, and egg-free diet.

Case 159: A woman sixty-six years of age had had burning and pain in the bladder and frequent urination for thirty years. Urological therapy and elimination of condiments had failed. Relief occurred with our FFCFE diet. Fruits, spices, coffee, eggs, uncooked vegetables, and vitamin C by mouth and parenterally reproduced symptoms. Vitamin C allergy is discussed in Chapter 29.

Of particular interest are the history and cystoscopic findings in the following patients:

Case 160: A woman sixty years of age had developed pressure and aching in the lower mid-abdomen and hematuria with burning and urgency of urination six years ago. Oral canker sores for three years and vomiting of blood from a small duodenal ulcer and diffuse gastritis shown by x-ray twenty years ago had been controlled by our FFCFE diet, with the later demonstration of milk as the main cause.

With this fruit and milk-free diet winter bronchitis and gastrointestinal hemorrhage had been absent for twenty years except eight years ago, when dark, bloody stools occurred for three days after fruit had been eaten for one week (Chapt. 1).

Before this hematuria and urinary distress occurred six years ago, fruit had been eaten on and off for ten days. With resumption of the fruit-free diet, no hematuria has recurred since then.

Cystoscopy when hematuria was present showed thirty to forty 1 to 2 cm erythematous areas in which dilated and bleeding capillaries were present visualized by cystoscopy and seen by us. Distention of the bladder with fluid caused increased bleeding. There was no evidence of infection in the bladder or urine.

Such cystoscopic findings have also been reported by Kindall and Nichols (1949). The onset of bladder allergy after difficult childbirths, pelvic surgery, or injury to the lower abdomen suggests that potential allergy, as to foods, may be activated in the urological tissues by such localized tissue stress.

Case 161: Bladder retention, attacks of hematuria, urethral soreness.

For six years since her second childbirth, a woman forty years of age stated that her bladder had not emptied completely. Attacks of soreness in the urethra with blood and at times clots had been passed for two to three days, one to three times a year. Soreness in the urethra for two to three days also had occurred every one to two months. Though infection in the bladder had been questionable, antibiotics and dilation of the urethra had been routine with brief benefit. Incomplete emptying of the bladder had persisted. Recent cystoscopy revealed engorgement of the bladder mucosa, and cauterization was advised. Six urologists had not given satisfactory relief.

Marked nervousness and emotional instability from these symptoms had occurred.

Possible food allergy was indicated by perennial nasal allergy, postnasal mucus, and a geographic tongue.

Diet history revealed postnasal mucus from milk. Inflammation of the tongue occurred from walnuts.

Penicillin produced urticaria. Other medicines given to relieve bladder symptoms were tolerated.

She was a nonsmoker.

Family history revealed asthma from food allergy in the father and nasal allergy in the mother.

Scratch tests were positive to grass, fruit, and tree pollens. She gave a five plus reaction to walnut. Physical examination, blood count, and urinalysis were negative.

Treatment: Food allergy was studied with our FFCFE diet. Aristocort in reducing doses was given orally, eliminating it in seven days. In one week emptying of the bladder was improved. In one month emptying of the bladder had been complete for one week. In two months relief continued. For the first time in six years desensitization to reacting pollens was not necessary to obtain the former, slight, brief relief of bladder distress. No dilatators or medications had been taken.

Case 162: A woman forty-eight years of age developed burning in the bladder and urethra and frequent urination twenty-eight years ago. Symptoms increased in degree and frequency, necessitating urination every hour night and day, making her a "nervous wreck." Since advice from over ten physicians, including four urologists, had been ineffectual, other physicians were not consulted until we studied and relieved her bronchial asthma. Several cystoscopies, pyelograms, dilatations of urethra, and antibiotics, including a vaginal hysterectomy and repair of a cystocele, had yielded no relief. One physician denied the possibility of bladder allergy. These symptoms made her an "emotional cripple" because of constant distress and inability to find the cause.

Bronchial asthma for two years at first in attacks every two weeks, becoming incapacitating and constant in December and January and less severe but constant in the preceding two months had occurred. Recurrent attacks, especially in winter, indicated food allergy (Chapt. 1).

Diet history revealed that she disliked and avoided milk. However, she took it in butter, cream, and other foods.

Drug history revealed that morphine caused nausea. Bronchodilators were of little help.

Environmental history did not indicate allergic causes.

Family history revealed that two brothers and two sons have nasal allergies.

Laboratory tests including pulmonary function tests were negative. Scratch tests gave large reactions to grass and lesser reactions to summer and fall pollens and a few questionable reactions to foods.

X-rays of the lungs were negative, except for slightly flattened diaphragms.

Treatment and results: With the FFCFE diet bladder symptoms and asthma gradually were controlled. Relief of bladder symptoms has required elimination of all fruits, spices, and condiments, including the odors of fruits.

Asthma also was controlled with the diet and desensitization to an antigen, containing tree, grass, and fall pollens in her Nevada area.

NEPHROTIC SYNDROME

The nephrotic syndrome is reported in Chapter 25 resulting from pollen and probably food allergy.

RENAL AND URETERAL ALLERGY

Experimentally produced allergic reactions in kidneys in guinea pigs and frogs by Letterer and others and especially by Masugi are reviewed by Urbach and Gottlieb, indicating probable allergic susceptibility of the kidney in man.

The following case of "renal colic" caused by foods and reported by Duke in 1922 is of marked interest:

A woman, age thirty-four, had had severe attacks of pain in her left flank for nine years, lasting one-half to one hour or more, and having recurred recently every two days. Many surgeons and specialists all over the United States, including six of the best known surgeons and urologists, had been consulted. Her pain started gradually in the left flank, increasing to a marked severity, radiating into the left costovertebral angle and down the inner side of the left thigh and even to the heel. Frequent painful urination, bladder tenesmus, and attacks of extensive purpura occurred with pain and urticaria frequently following the attacks. She was markedly sensitive to quinine. Painful menstruation was present. Her grandfather and nephew had asthma, and a sister was allergic to quinine. Her examination was negative, except for slight tenderness in the left flank and dermographia. Intracutaneous tests showed questionable reactions to a few food allergens. Her attacks were immediately relieved by Adrenalin.

Because of her unsatisfactory skin reactions, food trial was instituted, and beef, ham, bacon, oysters, tea, coffee, chocolate, cocoa, peas, and beans were found to cause attacks within 2½ hours after ingestion. With the exclusion of such foods her attacks which had required morphine for relief were controlled, and her menstruation became regular and free from pain. She gained ten pounds.

Hansen in his excellent chapter on Urological Allergy in his prestigious book *Allergie* (1956), reported severe recurrent kidney colic in a woman thirty years of age for 3½ years. Migraine and tachycardia were present. The daughter had eczema and hives. Allergy to milk and wheat was responsible. He also reported hematuria from milk confirmed by provocation tests.

Vaughan and Hawke reported "renal colic" and urinary retention attributed to obstruction from edema of the urethra because of egg and tomato. Kern also reported renal pain with hematuria associated with symptoms indicative of Henoch's purpura from onion. Alexander and Eyerman found glomerulonephritis associated with Henoch's purpura attributed to food allergy.

Ureteral-like pain relieved by the elimination of meat, fruit, and beer was reported by Litzner and also by Gutman, as noted by Urbach and Gottlieb in their book on clinical allergy. Relief of such pain by epinephrine subcutaneously favored allergy as the cause.

PERSONAL CASES

We have studied several patients with abdominal pain suggestive of renal colic apparently from food allergy. The allergic reaction may produce edema in the mucosa of the kidney pelvis or ureter, spasm in smooth muscles of the ureter, or allergic reactions around the arterioles in the kidney substance.

Case 163: A man fifty years of age had pain in the mid-abdomen and upper abdomen radiating into the left lumbar region, recurring over a period of five years when he ate chicken and also guinea hen. Other foods produced a rash and gastric symptoms.

Case 164: A man fifty-seven years of age had typical renal colic associated with longstanding sour stomach, belching, and constipation. All laboratory tests and skin tests were negative. Milk proved the cause of all symptoms (allergy in the kidney is discussed on page 508).

Case 165: A man fifty years of age developed pain in his left upper abdomen and mid-abdomen

five years ago. It suggested renal colic. The pain radiated downward and into the left lumbar region. Examinations were negative. He knew that bananas had always disagreed and that strawberries gave a rash. Chicken had produced abdominal pain three times within the year. He has since found that avocado and shellfish gave him gastric symptoms. During the last five years his left abdominal pain has recurred with breaks in his prescribed diet, though a moderate tolerance to additional foods has developed which allows him more freedom in his diet. He has found that guinea hen is as bad as chicken.

Of special interest was the pain in the lower, mid, and left abdomen characteristic of renal colic with inflammation of the bladder from allergy to quinidine given for six weeks to control paroxysmal tachycardia in a woman forty-two years of age. This allergy had developed while the quinidine was discontinued for one month because of the absence of palpitation. When it recurred and the quinidine was given again, the pain in the mid abdomen and left abdomen developed. It was relieved when quinidine was discontinued.

Comment: Development of allergy when the drug is not given may justify the continuance of a small dose of a drug which is important for the relief of chronic symptoms every one to three days in order to prevent establishment of an allergy to a medication which may be required by the patient for months or even years.

BLADDER, ALLERGY, CANKER SORES, EPIGASTRIC DISTRESS, DISTENTION, AND BACKACHE

Case 166: A woman thirty-two years of age had had indigestion, consisting of gas, distention, and a heavy, full feeling in the epigastrium for three years. Associated with this there had been an aching and a deep soreness in the lower abdomen and back, together with general fatigue. Marked burning of the bladder and frequent urination of three years' duration had been unrelieved by bladder irrigations. The slightest bit of cantaloupe gave severe bladder distress. Beans, onions, melon, cauliflower, and cabbage produced nausea. Tomatoes increased her bladder symptoms, and chocolate caused a recurrent large canker sore on the lower lip, with marked swelling of the face. No other allergy was present in her personal or family history. Physical examination, laboratory tests, and food tests were negative, except for delayed reactions to wheat. An "elimination diet," excluding wheat, lettuce, tomato, cabbage, melon, beans, chocolate, and coffee, has controlled the indigestion as well as the severe bladder burning and lower abdominal soreness for a period of two years. The following letter from the patient is illuminating:

"Your history of my case will, I believe, show that wheat, coffee, and lettuce brought on cystitis and that chocolate was responsible for sores on the lip. I later found that cabbage and cauliflower also caused cystitis. During the past year, at least, I have eaten all the chocolate I desired and have abstained absolutely from eating any wheat, lettuce, coffee, and so forth, with the result that I have felt no ill effects whatever. I have assumed that the 'chocolate idiosyncrasy' was overcome. Last week I attended a wedding breakfast, and because I felt conspicuous in refusing everything and also because I thought I might have outgrown my trouble, I drank a cup of coffee and ate an average size piece of cake. This was about 11 A.M. The following morning the inside of my mouth was sore all around the gums, and I had a large sore on my lip. By 8 P.M. I had the beginning of such a bad case of bladder inflammation that I was awake nearly all that night. I am not yet over the attack, although it is receding. I was surprised greatly at the vehemence of the attack, although I have learned that even a very small trace of wheat will bring a trace of cystitis."

POLLEN ALLERGY

Physicians and urologists must also remember that pollen allergy can cause urological symptoms during the pollen seasons, as illustrated in our case. It is well known that bladder spasm, urgency, and even involuntary urination occur from too large doses of pollen or other inhalant allergens when anaphylactic reactions occur.

ALLERGIC VULVITIS AND VAGINITIS

Allergy often causes marked dermatitis in the vulva, perineum, or around the anus with varying edema, erythema, papulovesicular lesions, and (when severe) oozing, crusting, and secondary infection.

Vaginitis may also occur. Though pruritus ani only may be present, it is often associated with vulval allergy. Dermatitis also may occur on the adjacent inner thighs and inguinal areas or may be associated with dermatitis on other parts of the body, especially on the flexures and extremities.

Whereas food allergy may be entirely responsible, especially if the dermatitis only occurs or is definitely exaggerated in the fall, winter, and spring months, pollen and less often other inhalant allergies may be the sole cause, occurring or being exaggerated in the pollen seasons or in special environments, decreasing in the winter when pollen is not present in the air.

That allergy to medicaments given by mouth, parenterally, or locally may be primary causes or may be associated with food or inhalant allergy in the etiology must also be remembered.

Conjugal allergy and contact allergy from fabrics, medications applied to the genitals (intravaginally or intrarectally), and synthetic or natural rubber condoms must be remembered.

Study of atopic allergy as the cause of pruritus vulvae and ani is justified with control of the following:

1. Bacterial and fungus infection, especially *Candida*, Trichomonas, pediculosis, menopausal senile vaginitis, and associated pathology including prolapsed hemorrhoids, fissures, fistulae, and other recognized causes.

2. Contact allergy to silk, rubber, rayon dyes and finishes in fabrics, toilet articles including powder, perfume, and contraceptives used by the wife or husband, and drugs in douches and enemas. Allergy to cain ointment to relieve itching before the initial cause is eliminated should be considered.

3. If the many possible causes noted above and other less common causes re-

ported by dermatologists are not responsible, then a) Localized atopic allergy to foods must be studied, especially if its other possible manifestations as reported in this volume are present with or without a history of dislikes or disagreements for foods or positive scratch reactions. This study and control of food allergy is advised in Chapters 2 and 3 and also in Chapter 14 on allergic dermatitis from food allergy. b) Inhalant allergy to pollens as indicated by exaggeration of the dermatitis in the pollen seasons with or without scratch tests to pollens. If the dermatitis continues in the winter, environmental allergens as discussed in Chapters 1 and 14 as well as food allergy alone or jointly is the challenge. The control of such inhalant allergy is advised in Chapter 4. The recognition and control of secondary bacterial or mycotic infection as well as of the atopic dermatitis is important. In addition, local therapy advised in Chapter 14 including compresses with iced water saline solution, 1:40 Burrow's solution, and 1:3000 epinephrine in an absorbable ointment and especially a corticosteroid ointment are advised. Epinephrine .3 to .5 cc hypodermically in adults every two to six hours relieves itching. Control of a secondary bacterial, fungus, or parasitical infection is important as advised.

Case 167: A woman fifty-six years of age had had perineal itching, inflammation, and edema of the vulva and vagina and pruritus ani during the night for three years. Recently dermatitis had spread six inches down the inner thighs. For three years diarrhea had occurred.

She suspected coffee and peaches as exaggerants of the pruritus. Skin tests were negative.

With our FFCFE diet for three weeks it was practically gone, and diarrhea was absent. Since then elimination of fruit, milk, spices, and especially pepper has controlled the pruritus and the diarrhea.

Case 168: A girl seven years of age had had attacks of marked soreness, irritation, and excoriation of the vulva especially around the urethra, lasting about two weeks and recurring every four to eight weeks for two years. These attacks had always been associated with fever of 102 to 103 F during the first three days, with marked nausea and vomiting. Attacks were preceded by a marked nasal congestion and postnasal discharge. Between the attacks irritation of the vulva had constantly been present.

During the first ten months she had always had head colds and nasal congestion suggesting food allergy. Indigestion and constipation occurred in childhood. All laboratory, x-ray, and skin tests were negative.

Recently headaches had occurred during her attacks and severe hives all over the body. Eczema had been absent.

Her physical examination and laboratory tests were negative, except for marked redness and excoriation of her entire vulva. Scratch tests with all types of allergens were entirely negative.

With our CFE diet the vulval irritation and eczema were controlled, wheat and milk proving responsible.

Case 169: A child seven years of age had burning and excoriation of the vulva and the adjacent skin of the legs which came in contact with any urine and of the skin of the lower eyelids and cheeks which contacted tears. Acidity had been the only explanation offered by physicians. Skin reactions were present to kidney beans, spinach, squash, strawberries, and wheat. Wheat and kidney beans proved the only causes.

Case 170: A woman fifty-six years of age had had pruritus ani for twenty-five years with questionable benefit from two hemorrhoidectomies. For one year a vesicular, erythematous, edematous, papulovesicular oozing and crusting dermatitis had involved the vulva, perineum, and inner thighs, with a moderate itching dermatitis around the anus. For six months she had also had edema of the upper lip, mouth, and eyelids and hoarseness on two occasions. Relief occurred with our CFE diet. Milk, which she had always disliked, proved a major offender. Wheat and to a lesser extent eggs were of minor importance.

Case 171: A woman thirty-seven years of age had erythematous, edematous, crusting, itching eruption on the vulva on and off for fourteen years, exaggerated in the fall months when dermatitis also developed on her arms, axilla, feet, and legs. Hay fever had been present for ten years when living in the country. She gave marked reactions to grasses and lesser reactions to tree and fall pollens. Desensitization with a multiple antigen containing fall, grass, and tree pollens gradually gave excellent relief. The treatment was continued at weekly intervals for one year, and the dermatitis and vulvitis have been absent for four years.

Case 172: A woman fifty-three years of age had had an erythematous, edematous, nonoozing eruption on the vulva and perineum with moderate itching around the anus for six months. On five previous occasions she also had had hives and localized edema on her face, lips, and eyelids. She had found that celery and related parsley caused marked vaginal itching. The vulvitis and pruritus ani were controlled with our FFCFE diet. Fruits, celery, milk, and wheat also proved to be responsible.

Case 173: A woman fifty-seven years of age had itching and resultant excoriations in the axilla for twenty-five years. Relief during two successive summers suggested food allergy. It recurred on the outer vulva and inner thighs ten years later. Recurrent exaggerations in the axilla, inguinal, and vulval areas for three years again suggested food allergy. Then elimination of common allergenic foods was of help. Itching recurred with a regular diet, moderate relief occurring from application of 95 percent alcohol. It had continued for four years in spite of many local and oral medications. There was no history of other clinical allergy.

Diet history revealed suspicion of itching from chocolate and spices and slight relief from partial elimination of wheat, milk, and eggs, as advised by another allergist.

There was no knowledge of allergy to drugs or contactants. Familial allergy was not present.

Laboratory tests and physical examination were negative except for excoriated skin in the axillae, vulva, and inner thighs. Scratch tests were one to two plus to a few grass, fall, and tree pollens and negative to foods.

Treatment and results: Food allergy was indicated by perennial itching for twelve years, relief in the summer for the first two years, and also by moderate relief from former partial elimination of wheat, milk, eggs, and coffee.

Our FFCFE diet was ordered to study such allergy along with triamcinolone 8 mg t.i.d. for four days with a reduction to 4 mg daily in one week and to 2 mg a day for four days.

In two weeks itching and excoriations of skin were absent, though some itching and moderate dermatitis remained in the groins. A secondary fungus infection in the skin of the vulva indicated by relief of such itching by Tinactin® ointment locally for one week.

Addition of cooked fruit, wheat, corn, and chocolate reproduced itching.

In the last eight years continued elimination of milk, wheat, corn, chocolate, and uncooked fruits and vegetables has been necessary to prevent reactivated pruritus, confirming food allergy as the underlying cause with fungus infection as a former complicating factor. Estrogens by mouth are also taken five days a week.

GENITAL DERMATITIS FROM POLLEN ALLERGY

The following cases in our practice were due to pollen allergy. Mitchell, Sivon, and Mitchell also reported severe pruritus with no eruption in eight girls two to twelve years of age because of pollen allergy and relieved by desensitization. Bernard (1964) reported seasonal vulvovaginitis from pollen in sixteen of three hundred girls treated for hay fever because of ragweed.

Case 174: A man fifty-seven years of age had had an erythematous, itching oozing eruption on the scrotum extending ten inches down the adjacent thighs for four months. Pruritus ani had been present for one previous year. Scratch reactions were positive to grass and fall pollens. Desensitization starting with a 1:5 billion dilution with a gradual increase into the 1:5 million dilution over a period of six months, along with prednisone 5 mg one to three times a day gave relief. Continued relief was reported three years later without corticosteroids.

Case 175: A man twenty-six years of age had a marked itching dermatitis on the scrotum, penis, and inguinal areas. There also was an erythematous dermatitis of his face, eyes, neck, wrist, and feet. Though reactions to pollens were not present, its onset during the late spring and summer months justified desensitization to a pollen antigen containing grass and fall pollens. The dose was gradually increased into the 1:50 dilution over a period of several months when relief occurred. Continued desensitization with a 1:50 dilution for another year maintained the relief, which he now reports has continued during the last sixteen years.

Case 176: A woman fifty-three years of age seen in 1947 had dermatitis on the vulva, perineum, and around the anus, the inner thighs, groins, face, and moderately on the scalp for nine months. For fifteen years it had been on the eyelids in the spring, summer, and fall. Scratch tests were one and two plus to various grass, fall, and cultivated flower pollens. Desensitization starting with a 1:5 billion dilution with a gradual increase to 0.5 cc of the 1:100 dilution of an antigen containing all important pollens in her environment controlled the dermatitis in five months. With treatment for 1½ years, relief of dermatitis was still present in three years. No corticoids were ever given.

Case 177: A woman twenty-three years of age had erythema, edema, and crusting and itching of vulva, spreading to the mons veneris, down the inner thighs, and around the anus and buttocks for one year. Scaling and crusting were in the scalp and ear canals. Skin tests were negative. Because it was perennial, food allergy was studied with our CFE diet. Relief occurred during the winter while the diet was continued. Recurrence of severe dermatitis in the spring indicated pollen therapy. With continued pollen therapy and adherence to the diet, the dermatitis continued to be controlled.

Case 178: A woman forty-five years of age had had vulval erythematous, edematous, crusting dermatitis extending into the perineal and perianal areas for eight months. With our FFCFE diet and oral Aristocort limited to two weeks, the dermatitis disappeared in two months. As foods were added, eggs, spices, and all fruits reactivated the vulval and perianal eczema. Chocolate and nuts caused oral canker sores.

URETHRAL AND PROSTATIC ALLERGIC REACTIONS

It is probable that idiopathic urethritis at times is due to allergy. This may be comparable to the vulval irritation described above. The secretions might be studied for eosinophiles, and our elimination diets with the initial exclusion of fruits from the CFE diet might be used for diagnostic study.

CONTACT ALLERGY

The possibility of allergy from medications, contraceptives, condoms, or contact substances must be considered. Rattner (1935) reported nonspecific urethritis with dermatitis of the penis from a pure rubber condom.

POLLEN ALLERGY

Exaggeration in the pollen seasons would require consideration of pollen allergy. Davis (1934) reported prostatic and vesicular pain in one patient during hay fever attacks and in another patient only from home-brewed beer. Mickey and Montgomery reported six cases of eosinophilic granulomatous prostatitis. Food allergy might be causative.

The occurrence of allergic reactions in the parotids noted on page 502 suggests the probability of allergy in other glands including the prostate.

ORTHOSTATIC ALBUMINURIA FROM FOOD ALLERGY

Confirming Dees and Simmons' report of food allergy causing orthostatic albuminuria in 1951, Matsumara *et al.* reported milk, eggs, and soybean allergy in twelve of sixteen cases in 1966. In fourteen cases duodenal or gastric ulcers, migraine, abdominal epilepsy, hives, and pollakisuria along with dizziness, fatigue, and weakness in varying degrees were relieved with the elimination of allergenic foods.

NEPHROTIC SYNDROME

Pollen allergy and the necessity of studying food allergy in the etiology of this syndrome is noted in Chapter 25.

ENURESIS

The possibility that enuresis may be allergic in origin has been suggested by several allergists. In an article published with Richet (1930), we reported the following observation of Moore of Oregon. A child five years of age had enuresis and eczema. When eggs, to which reactions were obtained, were excluded from the diet, both complaints disappeared. Bray (1931) reported enuresis in five percent of eight hundred allergic children. In a boy five years of age wheat was to blame. An eleven-year-old boy gave large reactions to feathers and rabbit hair, the removal of which relieved longstanding enuresis for over one year after feathers, oatmeal, rice, and potatoes were eliminated.

Thus Bray counseled attention to ingestant and inhalant allergens in enuresis which do not respond to ordinary methods of control as advised in Chapter 25.

J. W. Gerrard favored us with a letter reporting a decrease in bladder spasm and enuresis in "probably a quarter of the (afflicted) children" with elimination of milk, eggs, citrus fruits, tomatoes, chocolate, and flavored colored drinks. If our FFCFE diet as advised in this chapter were used, more evidence of food allergy would occur. Improvement in the reduced bladder capacity in his patients from strict use of the diet would be important to record.

PERSONAL CASES

Case 179: A seven-year-old boy had had enuresis all of his life, uncontrolled by medical advice.

Canker sores had continued three to four times a week for one year.

Moderate nasal congestion and postnasal mucus had continued for four years.

He hated eggs and had avoided milk for two years. He had had a poor appetite for several years.

Family history revealed nasal and gastrointestinal allergy and edema in the mother.

Skin testing gave one plus reactions to two grasses, four fall, and three tree pollens and none to foods.

Physical examination was negative. Blood count and urinalysis were negative.

Treatment and Results: With our FFCFE diet

his canker sores, enuresis, and headaches disappeared in one month and remained absent for three months. Milk in the winter caused bronchitis. Fruit caused canker sores and enuresis.

In five days the mother reported that all symptoms were relieved on the original diet plus rice and any vegetable, except onion. Traces of fruit and wheat cause enuresis. Milk and eggs are still eliminated.

UTERINE ALLERGY

Uterine symptoms from food allergy need definite consideration. The abundance of smooth muscle and of mucous membrane in the tubes, uterus, and vagina emphasizes the probability that allergic reactions may occur in this tract. Food allergens after their entrance into the blood should be able to produce edema of mucous membrane and smooth muscle spasm in the female genital tissues as they do in the bronchial tract, where they result in bronchial asthma, or in the nervous system, where they produce migraine or neuralgia. Moreover, in experimental allergy, uterine strips have long been utilized for the graphic demonstration of specific sensitization in the guinea pig. Gynecological lesions of all types must be carefully ruled out in patients suspected of allergy. However, it should be remembered that allergic reactions may accompany other types of pathology. Important to remember is the fact that allergy to drugs occurs in obstetrical and gynecological practice. Simon and Ryder (1936) studied hypersensitivity to pituitary extracts which is present in a few individuals and found it occurred to an organ-specific substance common to the pituitary glands of animals and man.

LITERATURE

Duke, in 1923, first reported painful and frequent menstruation relieved by avoiding foods to which allergy existed. In 1928 we confirmed his opinion that food allergy could produce disturbed menstrual function, and early in 1931 we stated that we were "more convinced of the rather frequent occurrence of uterine discomfort and dysfunction due to food allergy." In the same publication we stressed the probability that certain menstrual symptoms in patients with migraine, urticaria, bronchial asthma, bladder allergy, hay fever, or gastrointestinal allergy might be due to food sensitizations. The fact that leukorrhea could result from food allergy in the same way that the mucous discharge in certain cases of perennial hay fever is due to such allergy was recorded. Since then Smith (1931) reported twelve patients with essential dysmenorrhea, leukorrhea, and irregular periods who were relieved by the elimination of specific foods. Dutta (1935) recorded three cases of dysmenorrhea from allergy, eosinophiles being found in the vaginal secretion in one case.

Uterine spasms and abnormal bleeding resulting from constitutional reactions from pollen therapy in two patients were first reported by Cooke (1922). Similar menstrual disturbances were later mentioned by Kahn (1928) and Robinson (1929). Thommen (1931) recorded laborlike pains followed by menstruation after a general pollen reaction. Cooke, in his original report of such disturbances, warned against the danger of abortion from constitutional reactions in pregnancy. These reactions are similar to the gastrointestinal symptoms from pollen therapy reported by Duke, Eyermann, Rackemann, and Cohen. We have also observed similar uterine and gastrointestinal symptoms from a constitutional pollen reaction in one patient. Robinson (1929) also reported laborlike abdominal pain with vertigo and weakness from an overdose of orris root extract.

Our studies continue to support food allergy as a cause of menstrual distur-

bances. Such allergy is most likely to occur in patients who have one or more other allergic disturbances, such as asthma, hay fever, migraine, headaches, neuralgia, cutaneous allergy, or gastrointestinal allergy. Most patients moreover, give a positive family history of allergy. However, as with other types of allergy, localization of sensitization in the genital tract may occur without a personal or family history of any other allergy. This necessitates its consideration in the differential diagnosis of all symptoms which are not obviously due to some other cause.

1. Menstrual allergy may produce painful, excessive, scanty, or irregular periods. Vaughan (1933) described severe dysmenorrhea and indigestion from wheat and a few other foods. A summary of a previously reported case follows:

A girl eighteen years of age had had extreme pain during the first four hours of her periods for several years. Her bowels had been constipated all her life, and for the last three years she had had attacks of pain in the lower right quadrant lasting three or four days, especially before her periods. As a baby she could not tolerate milk, and since then she had never cared for it, though in recent years she had tried to drink it to increase her weight. Her father had severe constipation and hay fever, and his father had had asthma. Her mother and the patient's sisters could never tolerate milk.

Her physical examination was negative except for an undernourished state and moderate tenderness over the lower right quadrant. No rigidity was found. Roentgen ray studies of her entire gastrointestinal tract were negative except for retarded motility in her ascending colon and moderate lack of mobility in her cecum. Skin tests were negative. With the use of our elimination diets her periods have been normal, her constipation has been relieved, and no further pain in the lower right quadrant has recurred in the last two years except when milk and wheat have been taken. Definite relief of a lifelong anorexia has resulted.

2. Painful periods accompanied by severe nausea or vomiting which may lead

to acidosis may occur from food allergy. One girl was relieved of painful, excessive periods, longstanding constipation, and severe abdominal and bearing down rectal pains before and during bowel movements. This patient, moreover, was extremely irritable and had recurrent epileptic attacks which were controlled by proper "elimination diets." Such patients may have cyclic vomiting during their childhood and during their teens and are subject to migraine after that time.

3. Prolonged abnormal menstruation may be due to food allergy, thus a woman twenty-eight years of age found that uterine bleeding occurred whenever she ate crab, to which there was no skin reaction. Bleeding from the intestinal tract and allergic purpura because of food allergy are discussed on page 426. The following case record illustrates this type of allergic bleeding.

Case 180: A woman thirty years of age had had constant vaginal bleeding between her periods since puberty. One year ago she had several actual hemorrhages. Curettement five years ago gave no help, and in spite of much medical study and therapy, no relief had ever occurred. Marked leukorrhea but no dysmenorrhea was present. Since her earliest memory she had had severe, sick headaches, usually two to three times a week.

Annoying mental confusion and slowness of thought were frequently present. For two years she had suffered with recurrent urticaria. She had had hay fever in the spring. Moderate bloating, distention, and canker sores had occurred. Her mother, her maternal aunt, and her grandmother, as well as her sister, had had migraine. She was not aware of any food idiosyncrasies. She had been married three years and had not been pregnant. Skin reactions were obtained to goose feathers and to a few spring and fall pollens.

With our CFE diet her vaginal bleeding, leukorrhea, urticaria, migraine, constipation, nasal congestion, and her allergic toxemia have been practically absent over a period of six months. Recently she ate a hard boiled egg and two sandwiches, which resulted in a severe headache within two hours and vaginal bleeding, which was not associated with a period, on the following morning, lasting two days. Milk, wheat, eggs, and chocolate have been found to reproduce her symptoms.

LEUKORRHEA FROM FOOD ALLERGY

4. Finally, leukorrhea may at times be due to food allergy, as reported in our former book on food allergy. Smith (1931) published several other instances of leukorrhea from food sensitization. We now have records of twelve women in whom leukorrhea was relieved by food elimination. Allergic reactions in the uterine tissues resulting in mucous discharge can be assumed as readily as can similar reactions in the nasal, bronchial, or gastrointestinal membrane. Other allergic disturbances, especially mucous colitis, constipation, and headaches, are frequently present in patients with leukorrhea from food allergy. One patient had had leukorrhea, swelling of her face and of other parts of her body, together with a general toxemia for many years because of milk. All of these symptoms returned in a few days with the addition of a few drops of diluted milk to her diet. Thomas and Wicksten (1944) reported eosinophiles in vaginal secretion and allergic rhinitis relieved by elimination of eggs and wheat and by pollen allergy. Another case of leukorrhea was controlled by pollen therapy.

Leukorrhea in childhood has been relieved by the elimination of allergy-producing foods in two patients, indicating that such a cause should be kept in mind when this symptom is present in children.

OTHER TYPES OF GENITAL ALLERGY

We have previously reported the occurrence of angioneurotic edema in Fallopian tubes as observed by Briggs in 1908. This led to an exploratory operation because of the severity of the pain. Such swellings were also reported by Lyon in 1928 in the labia as well as other regions of the body in a breast-fed infant six weeks old because of corn and beans in the mother's diet.

Vaughan and Fowlkes (1935) reported several cases of cohabitation allergy. Irritation in the vagina from rubber allergy or various drugs or powders is not very uncommon, as noted above.

INFLUENCE OF MENSTRUATION ON ALLERGIC REACTIONS

It is well known that some bronchial asthma, migraine, and other allergic reactions similar to eczema are precipitated or intensified by the menstrual period. Increased metabolism may be the cause of such exaggeration of symptoms. However, the fact that the elimination of the causative foods prevents the recurrence of the allergic reactions even during the periods shows that ovarian activity or menstruation are not the cause of the symptoms. Thus the termination of periods by means of surgery or radiation therapy is distinctly illogical for the relief of any condition which might be due to allergy and should not be done until thorough study of the patient with "elimination diets" of various types has been tried. In 1938 we reported two patients whose periods had been terminated unnecessarily and futilely in an attempt to stop migraine. Tuft (1935) reported two similar cases. In another patient hysterectomy because of a few fibroids was done with the hope that it would eradicate an urticaria. No allergic investigation whatsoever had been made in this woman. Hives in our patient continued during her period even from a trace of ingested fruit.

Finally, certain marked vasomotor disturbances associated with various allergic reactions are often attributed to ovarian dysfunction. Patients suffering with food allergy may have marked erythema of the face and neck.

Case 181: A woman sixty years of age had had swelling of various parts of her body, especially of the tongue, face, and hands for two years. Along with these swellings she had marked flushings of the face and neck which had been ascribed by several physicians to a prolonged menopause. All of her symptoms were relieved with the elimination of wheat and milk from her diet. Thus so-called "hot flushes" and other vasomotor disorders at times may be the indirect result of allergy.

Careful study of the patient with physical and laboratory examinations must be made so that all existing pathology is discovered. The determination of the role of food allergy in the etiology of the symptoms of patients suspected of food allergy has been described in our previous publications and in Chapter 2 of this book.

TOXEMIAS OF PREGNANCY

The possibility that pregnancy toxicoses may be due to maternal allergy to the products of fetal metabolism or glandular hormones has received consideration for several years, as by Seitz (1935), Jegerow (1934), and others. Jegerow particularly has pointed out the possibility of the allergic origin of early and late toxic states in pregnancy arising from sensitization to normal protein substances from the fetus, its membranes, and the placenta which are foreign to the mother. The early nausea and vomiting of pregnancy may even have an allergic origin. Moreover, the rapid rise and disappearance of edema and of changes in skin elasticity suggest allergy. The demonstration of vascular allergy by Rossle, Klinge, Gerlach, and others also suggested to Jegerow that the changes in arteries and veins and the tendency to thrombophlebitis may arise from such an underlying allergy developing during pregnancy. The fact that varicose enlargements are not always explainable by pelvic pressure alone may be due in part to such vascular allergy. The fact that nervous and mesenchymal tissues are always involved in allergy explained in his mind the various characteristics of these early and especially the late convulsive "allergoses of pregnancy." The increasing and at times fulminating character and the sudden termination with delivery of those disturbances favored this possibility. Moro and Keller, as noted by Kline and Young (1935), suggested that the hemorrhagic necrosis in the eclamptic liver may arise from the effect of the excessive pituitarylike hormone on the liver sensitized to another foreign protein. Thus it would be an example of parallergy or possibly of a Schwartzmanlike reaction. Knepper (1934) reproduced convulsions in rabbits by the injection of serum and pituitary substances simultaneously and concluded that the hepatic and renal changes in eclampsia were due to allergy. Kammerer (1934), discussing this subject, pointed out that placental proteins are foreign to the body and might lead to allergy particularly because of the digestive action that pregnant serum has on such placental proteins. He agreed that eclampsia resembles other allergic manifestations in definite respects, especially epilepsy and severe migraine which are being found due to allergy in varying numbers of cases (Chapter 18). It will be important to confirm the report that toxemias of pregnancy are more frequent near the ocean as are certain manifestations of allergy, as noted on page 168. Campbell (1937) reported one toxemia in every 250 pregnancies in private practice around San Francisco Bay as compared with one in every six hundred

deliveries in other regions. Could this be due to a local climatic influence increasing allergic susceptibility to products of fetal metabolism or bacterial, ingestant, or other allergens? Could the lessened toxemias in Germany during the World War be explained by the reduced intake of allergenic foods during that period? Continued study of the allergic possibilities of toxemias of pregnancy obviously is most necessary and will probably lead to lessening of their incidence and severity.

TREATMENT—STUDY AND CONTROL OF ALLERGY TO FOODS, INHALANTS, AND DRUGS

Since allergy to foods, inhalants, and drugs may cause reactions and resultant symptoms in any part of the urogenital tissues, it is necessary to remember its possibility especially if the cause is not evident and symptoms have not responded to other usual therapy. If the cause is not recognized, moreover, it may account for failure of desired relief after surgery or other urogenital procedures, as discussed in Chapter 27.

Allergy must be suspected if the patient gives a personal or family history of any manifestations of clinical allergy. Food allergy is indicated by recurrence or exaggeration of symptoms during the fall, winter, and spring with a decrease in the summer or a history of definite dislikes or disagreements to foods. Pollen allergy requires study of symptoms occurring or exaggerated in the pollen seasons. Scratch reactions to pollens usually but not necessarily are positive. Exaggeration of symptoms from the inhalation of environmental airborne substances in the living and working environment of the patient suggests other less frequent inhalant allergy. Finally, a history of present or past drug allergy necessitates consideration of drug allergy as a possible cause. If questioning of the patient gives any such information, a carefully recorded history of present and recent medications according to our recommendations in Chapter 2 is required.

If inhalant allergy is indicated, scratch tests with important pollens, animal emanations, fungi, dusts, and other inhalants suggested by the history are advisable, as recommended in Chapter 2. The patient's susceptibility to reacting inhalants as emphasized in Chapter 2 must be determined by undoubted clinical allergy thereto or by provocation inhalant tests necessarily done when the patient is symptom-free. That skin tests are negative in 10 to 15 percent of patients sensitive to inhalant allergens and that patients are not necessarily allergic to all reacting inhalants must be remembered.

Scratch tests with allergenic foods usually are negative, especially when cumulative allergy occurs (see Chapt. 2). Food allergy which produces immediate symptoms in minutes or one or two hours after ingestion of the foods is usually indicated by large scratch reactions. The clinical significance of these large reactions, however, unless confirmed by undoubted history of allergy to the specific foods, also must be determined by positive provocation tests with the ingestion of the reacting food and only when the patient is necessarily symptom-free without corticosteroid therapy. All of this is discussed in extenso in Chapter 2.

Control of Food Allergy

If food allergy requires study as a cause of possible urogenital allergy, our FFCFE diet is preferable because of frequency of allergy in these patients, especially to fruits and condiments, as well as to milk, wheat, eggs, chocolate, and other foods eliminated from our CFE diet. Lockey reported lower abdominal pain, nausea, melena, and hematuria especially from eggs in an eczematous child.

The physician's challenge is to find a diet that relieves the patient's symptoms for a definitely longer period than previous periods of relief. If such relief does not occur in two to four weeks, one of our minimal elimination diets is advisable, remembering that it is necessary in occasional patients to study possible allergy to most foods, as advised in Chapter 3. Allergens in city water as from vegetations, animal life, including chlorine in such water, may require study with pure spring water or distilled water. After a relieving diet is assured, foods individually can be added, eliminating those which definitely reproduce symptoms (Chapt. 3).

Control of Inhalant Allergy

Inhalant allergy at times is relieved by environmental control. When the causative inhalants cannot be avoided or eliminated from the air of the patient's environments, desensitization as advised in Chapter 4 is required. Definite assurance of allergy to such inhalants is important, since desensitization usually is required for months or longer periods to obtain and especially maintain good relief. Unnecessary desensitization to pollens and other inhalants too often occurs merely because of positive skin reactions to such inhalants when no evidence of clinical allergy thereto has been obtained.

Control of Drug Allergy

Drug allergy is evidenced by relief after initial elimination of all drugs, remembering that they often remain in the body for days or weeks after their discontinuance.

Medications for Relief of Symptoms

When allergy to foods, inhalants, or drugs alone is responsible for urogenital symptoms, until relief of the causes as advised above occurs, epinephrine 1:1000 in 0.2 to 0.5 cc doses hypodermically every three hours according to age is justified, especially if relief of spasm, burning, frequency of urination, itching, and pain results. For more gradual and lasting relief, corticosteroids up to 10 to 40 mg a day by mouth or when the distress and manifestations of allergy are severe given parenterally are fully justified, as advised in Chapters 6 and 8. The dose is gradually reduced and with relief omitted in five to fourteen days as the allergic causes are discovered and controlled.

When this allergy is associated with infection in the urogenital tract or cutaneous tissues, indicated and tolerated antibiotics or sulfonamides are required. Urinary retention especially in old men but even in children because of ephedrine given to relieve bronchospasm occurs.

When pathology requires urological or gynecological procedures or surgery, the control of concomitant allergic causes is important, as emphasized in Chapter 27.

SUMMARY

1. Urogenital allergy to foods and inhalants unfortunately receives little or no consideration by physicians, including most urologists, most gynecologists, and too few allergists.

2. Since Duke's epochal discussion of bladder allergy from foods, it has been confirmed by several allergists, as noted in this chapter, and most recently by Powell.

3. Case reports of such allergy in eleven of our patients from food allergy emphasizes its occurrence.

4. Renal and ureteral allergy to foods reported in the literature especially by Duke, Hansen, Vaughan, and Hawk is supported by four case reports of our relieved patients.

5. That pollen allergy can produce symptoms in the bladder is evidenced by spasm and urgency occurring during general reactions from excessive doses of pollen.

6. Allergic vulvitis and vaginitis from food are evidenced in case reports of two relieved men and three women. Urethral and prostatic allergy especially occur.

7. Enuresis especially from food allergy particularly to fruits but also to common allergenic foods was reported by Bray in 5 percent of eight hundred allergic children. Its confirmation by us in two reported cases we opine does not indicate its probable frequency.

8. Orthostatic albuminuria from food allergy as suggested by Dees in 1951 was confirmed by Matsumara in 1966.

9. Painful, frequent, even prolonged menstruation because of food allergy first reported by Duke in 1923 has been confirmed by Cooke, Vaughan, Kahn, Robinson, and Thommen and by us in the following decade and since that time.

10. Leukorrhea illustrated in two of our patients was relieved by elimination of allergenic foods determined with our elimination diets.

11. Angioneurotic edema in the Fallopian tubes has lead to exploratory surgery.

12. Cohabitation allergy from drugs, perfumes, contraceptives and rubber condoms occurs.

13. Exaggeration of allergy especially to foods during menstruation has been recognized for thirty years. Other symptoms ascribed to recurrent infection may be due to unrelieved food allergy.

14. Study and treatment of food, inhalant, and drug allergy are summarized. Medications for relief until the allergies are recognized and controlled are advised.

Chapter 22

Diagnosis and Control of the Causes of
Hematological Allergy

Food allergy as indicated in the literature and by our experience usually occurs to milk, wheat and other cereal grains, eggs, and chocolate. Other foods less frequently but significantly often cause clinical allergy.

For the initial study of food allergy, therefore, our CFE diet with no listed vegetables or fruits uncooked (as a rule) is utilized as advised in Chapter 3. If allergy to several fruits, spices, and flavors is indicated in the diet history of the patient or if relief from the strict adequate use of the above diet does not give desired relief, the FFCFE diet detailed in Chapter 3 should be prescribed, especially if a diet history of disagreements or dislikes suggests possible fruit allergy. If relief fails from strict use of these diets with necessary maintenance of nutrition for at least three weeks, a minimal elimination diet may be justified before the quest for possible food allergy is forgone.

As in other possible manifestations of food allergy, relief of symptoms usually occurs in one to three weeks with the initial diet.

Control of possible inhalant allergy indicated by history and usually by skin tests is advised in Chapter 4.

Possible drug and chemical allergies always require recognition and are controlled by elimination of the medication for two or more weeks as advised throughout this volume.

ANAPHYLACTOID PURPURA
(HENOCH-SCHONLEIN PURPURA)

This syndrome is characterized by varying degrees of red or purple skin lesions of purpura, colicky pain, vomiting and intestinal bleeding, edema and pain in and around joints, frequent hematuria, and even nephritis. It usually occurs in males between the ages of four and fourteen and also in young adults and even in old age, as reported by Stremple *et al.* (1968). The symptoms and lesions usually occur in attacks (see Chapt. 1), which suggests food allergy as a possible cause. Glomerulonephritis explained by allergic vasculitis may develop in about 30 to 50 percent of the cases (Levitt and Burbank, 1953) and is progressive in about 25 percent. Increased capillary permeability produces a) bleeding into the cutaneous and subcutaneous tissues and mucosa, or bleeding into the wall of the intestine; b) extravasation of fluid with resultant urticaria or edema into the viscera; and c) purpura especially on the buttocks, lower back, elbows, extensor surfaces of the arms and legs, ankles, and feet which blanches on pressure.

If, because of pain from visceral smooth muscle spasm, exploratory abdominal section is done, edema, inflammation, and hemorrhage in the intestinal wall and free fluid in the abdomen are found. Therefore, this syndrome should be considered and ruled out as a possible cause of abdominal pain for prevention of unnecessary surgery.

Stremple *et al.* (1968) emphasize recognition of this syndrome and conservative treatment with corticosteroids rather than surgery. We opine, however, that possible food allergy should be studied with our FFCFE diet along with the administration of large and gradually decreasing corticosteroid therapy and (possibly) epinephrine.

Though it is generally agreed that allergy causes this syndrome, food allergy has been reported and confirmed in only a limited number of cases. We opine that in the future it will be revealed more frequently. Thus the recent statement in an article on this syndrome by Gary, Mazara, and Holfelder that the cause is unknown is not justified.

Alexander and Eyermann (1937) first emphasized food allergy as a cause of the HS syndrome. Eyermann (1935) gave further information with case reports confirming food allergy as a cause. Their conclusion that food allergy was responsible was made with trial diets rather than with fallible skin testing with foods. In their patients, negative reactions to all allergens were obtained, and diet trial was necessary to determine these causative foods and give the patients the very important relief they received.

THROMBOCYTOPENIC PURPURA (WERLHOF'S DISEASE) FROM FOOD ALLERGY

Squier and Madison (1937) reported relief of this purpura with a gradual increase in the previously depressed thrombocytes by elimination of specific foods. They opined that an allergic reaction in the thrombocytes similar to that in the capillary endothelium causing HS syndrome was responsible. In discussion, Rappaport reported this disease of five years' duration causing attacks of purpura and bleeding from bullous lesions in the mouth relieved by the elimination of onions, almonds, and the cabbage group of vegetables.

The report by Squier and Madison of reduction of normal or of moderately reduced platelet counts resulting from ingested foods with relief of symptoms and an increase in the platelet count from the elimination of specific foods justifies the study of possible food allergy in other cases of this TP syndrome. Allergy to the platelets would indicate probable allergy in the megakaryocytes.

Since this syndrome has been controlled by the elimination of allergenic foods, we opine that adequate, sufficient study of such food allergy as we advise may reveal food allergy in more cases of idiopathic thrombocytopenic purpura.

Ackroyd stated that since platelets and capillary endothelium are antigenically related, the same antigen can cause allergic reactions in both of them.

DRUG ALLERGY

That drug allergy to Sedormid produces the TP syndrome was reported by Loewy (1934). Markowiez (1933) reported it to even 0.3 gm of quinidine and Peshkin and Miller (1934) to quinine and ergot. Since then its rare origin from drugs has been reported to sulfamethoxypyridazine, quinidine in 1962 by Berger, and by Thomas in 1963.

PURPURA SIMPLEX

Purpura in the skin causing tender or painful ecchymoses without bleeding in the gastrointestinal, urogenital, or other tissues occurs occasionally from food allergy. Purpura from vascular abnormalities, blood dyscrasias including coagulation defects and thrombocytopenia, infections, scurvy, effects of leukemia, myeloma, and other causes, as discussed by Wintrobe and other hematologists, must always be in mind.

Purpura simplex resulting from food allergy is caused by allergic vasculitis with increased capillary permeability. There are nearly always other manifestations of clinical allergy in the nasobronchial, cutaneous, gastrointestinal, and less frequently in other tissues.

Ancona *et al.* (1951) reported attacks of purpura with edema in the ankles, left leg, and lower back from crab and shrimp without abnormalities in the blood. A tender, slightly enlarged spleen was present. Snyder (1968) reported a woman thirty-six years of age with nonpainful bluish areas in the skin from cantaloupe.

In this category familial purpura simplex, as first reported by Davis in 1939 and again in 1941, justifies comment. He assembled information about its occurrence in twenty-seven families occurring in one generation in nine, in two generations in twelve, in three generations in five, and in four generations in one family. In the eighty-eight cases purpura simplex occurred in seventy-nine, with Schonlein's purpura in four, with Henoch's purpura in two, and from trivial bruises in two cases. Fisher *et al.* (1954) also reported inherited purpura simplex and ptoses of the eyelids in four generations. They stated that capillary fragility was the only abnormality in the blood in their cases, similar to the HS syndrome. Because of the acceptance of food allergy as the one demonstrated allergic cause of the HS syndrome, it would be justifiable to study possible food allergy as a cause of familial purpura simplex in the strict and adequate manner we advise in this volume. Inherited tendency to allergy, even to specific foods, cannot be ignored, as has been noted in Chapter 1.

EOSINOPHILES IN FOOD ALLERGY

Blood eosinophilia often occurs in the allergic individual, more often in our experience from food than from inhalant allergy. The normal percentage of eosinophiles in the blood of children varies between 1 and 6 percent. Allergy, rather than absorption of foreign protein, seems responsible for an increase. In addition to eosinophiles in the blood, they are found in the secretion from the mucosa in the nose, sinuses and bronchial, urological (Chap. 21), intestinal, and in other allergic tissues. Eosinophilia in CUC and regional enteritis indicates allergy to foods and less often to inhalants and drugs, as stated in Chapters 6 and 7. Eosinophilia from other causes than allergy includes some acute infections, digitalis therapy, intestinal parasites, and less common conditions.

Hansel, especially, has reported eosinophiles in nasal and sinal secretions resulting from allergy as contrasted with their absence when infection is present. In our experience this occurs more frequently in perennial nasal allergy from foods than in hay fever from pollens. Thorn's eosinophile depression test as a guide to ACTH or cortisone therapy, as discussed in other textbooks, must be remembered in our consideration of eosinophiles.

Eosinophiles in wheals resulting from intradermal injection of histamine have been reported for over forty years. Kline, Cohen, and Rudolph (1932) reported 25 percent of the cells were eosinophiles in fifteen minutes and that practically all of the cells were eosinophiles in twenty-five minutes.

Thus eosinophiles in blood, secretions, and tissues indicate probable allergic reactivity. In our experience a high percentage of eosinophiles often favors food allergy. The frequency of eosinophiles in the blood, nasal, and bronchial secretions in patients with nasal polyps, as stated by Sheldon, Lovell, and Matthews, is best explained, according to our experience, by perennial food allergy which we have found the usual cause of nasal polyps as well as pereninial nasal allergy and perennial bronchial asthma. The rarity of infection as a cause has been stated in Chapter 12.

The origin, mechanism, and significance of eosinophilia is not assured. Kammerer and Hansen especially have reviewed its extensive literature in their discussion of the origin and significance of eosinophiles.

EOSINOPHILIC PNEUMONOPATHY

Loffler's syndrome characterized by transient pulmonary infiltrations, blood eosinophilia, varying fever with or without cough, or malaise occurs in children and also in adults. O'Byrne reported transient areas of pneumonia in a girl five months old with fever of 101 F and moderate anemia. Eosinophiles were 8 percent with varying leukocytic counts. Relief from a milk-free diet in three weeks suggests that food allergy may be causative in other cases. Food and pollen allergies were the indicated causes in one typical case in our practice.

Tropical eosinophilia characterized by blood eosinophilia, fever, and diffuse pulmonary infiltrations may be an equivalent of Loffler's syndrome.

This is not to be confused, moreover, with the serious collagen pulmonary diseases or with the rare transient infiltrates in the lungs from allergy to para-amino-salicylic acid or other drugs or from transient infiltrations in bronchial asthma or obstructive pneumonitis at times without atelectases.

Disseminated visceral lesions associated with extreme eosinophilia were reported by Zuelzer and Apt (1949) in whose patient pulmonary infiltrations, asthma, urticaria, joint symptoms, and convulsions occured and were attributed to an allergic hyperergic tissue reaction. Study of atopic allergy especially to foods as we advise in an adequate, strict manner would have been justifiable.

BLOOD CHANGES IN ALLERGY, ESPECIALLY TO FOODS

The following changes in addition to eosinophilia in the normal blood count may occur from food and other atopic allergy.

1. When perennial nasal and bronchial allergy, especially bronchial asthma, occur in children and adolescents, the leukocytes may be increased at times up to twenty to thirty thousand. This occurs in the absence of obvious or secondary infection. Determinations of leukocyte and differential counts in 147 children with allergic dermatitis are reported according to age in Table XLIV. In a large majority of these cases food, with or without inhalant, allergy was the major cause.

2. The hemoglobin is within normal limits except for its depression in undernourished children with anorexia and at times malnutrition. In such children determination of electrolytes, carbon dioxide, blood sugar, cholesterol, and enzymes in the serum may be advisable as recommended in other texts.

3. Though the leukocytes do usually decrease in an hour or so after the ingestion of an allergenic food, the leukopenic index advised by Vaughan is not used in our practice because the necessary blood counts are time-consuming and fraught with possible errors. In our experience, moreover, information about chronic cumulative food allergy, which is not evi-

dent up to even twenty-four or more hours after the ingestion of a food, usually is misleading or absent. After the symptoms have been controlled for days or weeks, the allergenicity of a food added to those in the elimination diet is best determined by a provocation feeding test with that food (Chapt. 3).

BLEEDING AND HEMORRHAGES IN BODY TISSUES FROM ALLERGY, ESPECIALLY TO FOODS

Manwaring stressed the increased permeability of vascular endothelium with resultant bleeding arising during anaphylactic shock in animals. A reduction in the coagulability of blood, especially in canine anaphylaxis, has been long reported. In man, bleeding in Henoch-Schonlein purpura and purpura from thrombocytopenic purpura has been discussed in this chapter. Though food allergy is not the sole assured cause in all of these cases, its demonstrated occurrence makes the study of food allergy as well as of possible inhalant and drug allergies justifiable as a possible sole or associated cause of unexplained bleeding and hemorrhage. Such allergy needs consideration in unexplained, severe, recurrent nose bleeds; excessive menstruation; and gastrointestinal bleeding. That melena in children requires study of food allergy, especially to milk, has been reported by Heiner and other pediatricians. Conjunctival bleeding from food allergy and retinal hemorrhages from serum allergy have been noted in Chapter 20. Hematemesis and later bleeding from the bladder from food allergy is reported below in Case 183. Tzanck (1932) reported gastric hemorrhage from food allergy.

Rappaport, in discussing the article by Squier and Madison, reported severe hemorrhages from the nose, rectum, and vagina after the ingestion of individual foods to which skin reactions were negative. Squier reported severe menorrhagia during pollen therapy for ragweed hay fever. A gynecologist found no cause for it. This recurred during two successive pollen seasons. There was a drop in her platelets and leukocytes and a rise in her blood eosinophiles thirty minutes after an injection of a maximum dose of pollen.

HEMATURIA FROM ALLERGY, ESPECIALLY TO FOODS

Hematuria from food and less often to drug allergy with or without other manifestations of allergy has been reported for many years. This has been noted in Chapter 21. Manwaring, in 1927, reported allergic reactivity in the urinary bladder in rabbits. Hematuria may be due to food allergy alone or associated with bleeding in other tissues or with urticaria, colic and other gastrointestinal symptoms, pain and swelling of the joints, and nephritis occurring in the Henoch-Schonlein syndrome (HS) as discussed previously in this chapter. Brown reported hematuria as a major symptom in the HS syndrome resulting from tomato. Similar occurrence to foods listed in Table XLII have been reported by Kittredge and Lazarus. Gairdner reported hematuria in twelve cases of HS syndrome with entire recovery from the associated nephritis in seven cases. Glaser stated that food allergy should be studied when hematuria of unrecognized origin develops. That allergic inflammation of the bladder causes hematuria is evident in our Case 160 in Chapter 21.

DRUG ALLERGY

Hematuria from drugs, especially to Sedormid and aspirin, indicates possible hematuria from other medications. Gastric bleeding in varying degrees from ingested aspirin is increasingly reported. Local tox-

TABLE XLII

CASES OF THE HENOCH-SCHONLEIN SYNDROME RESULTING FROM
HYPERSENSITIVITY TO FOODS

Author	Case No.	Foods causing syndrome	Symptoms Produced by Administration of Causative Food						
			Purpura	*Erythema*	*Urticaria*	*Blood in stools*	*Hematuria*	*Colic*	*Joint Pains*
Galloway (1903)	1	Blackberries and nuts	+	+	.	+	+	.	.
Sachs (1916)	1	Anchovy paste	+	.	.	.	.	.	.
Alexander and Eyermann (1927)	2	Milk	+	.	.	.	.	+	.
	3	Egg	+	.	.	.	.	.	+
Alexander and Eyermann (1929)	1	Milk	+	.	.	.	.	+	.
	2	Egg, potato & wheat	+	.	.	.	.	+	.
	3	Egg, chicken & beans	+	.	.	.	.	+	.
	4	Plums	+	.	.	.	.	+	.
	5	Wheat	+	.	.	.	.	+	+
	6	Pork, onions & strawberries	+	.	.	.	.	+	.
Barthelme (1930)	1	Wheat	+	.	.	.	.	.	+
		Egg yolk	+	.	.	.	.	+	.
Eyermann (1935)	1	Egg, chicken & beans	+	.	.	.	.	+	.
		Fish and lamb	.	.	.	.	.	+	.
Diamond (1936)	1	Milk	+	.	.	.	.	.	+
	2	Tomato & chocolate	+	.	.	.	.	+	.
	3	Popcorn	+	.	.	.	.	.	.
	4	Egg	+	.	.	.	.	.	.
	6	Chocolate	+	.	.	.	.	.	.
	7	Chocolate	+	.	.	.	.	.	.
	8	Chocolate	+	.	.	.	.	.	.
	9	Rolled oats & chocolate	+	.	.	.	.	.	.
Althausen and Deamer (1937)	1	Egg, orange	+	.	.	.	.	+	.
Kempton (1940)	1	Milk	+	.	.	+	.	+	+
		Potato	+	.	.	+	.	+	.
	2	Carrot, milk, wheat, pineapple, apple, orange prune & string beans	+	.	.	.	.	+	+
Brown (1946)	1	Tomato	+	.	+	+	+	+	+
Rowe (1938)	1	Milk	+	.	.	.	.	+	+
	2	Wheat, milk, egg, rye, corn, citrus fruits	+	.	.	.	.	+	+
Lazarus (1949)	1	Rice							

icity rather than allergy seems responsible. al-Mondhiry and Spaet recently reported reduced stickiness of platelets and decreased clumping of platelets which seal off wounds from aspirin.

COLONIC BLEEDING FROM FOOD AND POLLEN ALLERGY

Bleeding from allergic inflammation and resultant tissue changes in the large bowel from food and less often pollen allergy has been reported in many contributions since 1942 and is emphasized in our discussion of chronic ulcerative colitis in Chapter 6 of this book and in our chapter on Children's Allergies.

Thus the increased permeability of the endothelium of small blood vessels and the capillary walls resulting from localized allergy requires consideration of allergy to foods, drugs, and pollens in the differential study of bleeding in body tissues. As in all study of possible food allergy, failure of relief from skin test-negative diets does not exclude it as a cause. Diet trial with our CFE diet or its modification has to be done in the adequate, informed manner we advise in this volume.

PERSONAL CASES

Case 182: Bleeding from the bronchial mucosa in four to six hours after the ingestion of even traces of milk, small amounts of butter, or cheese developed at the age of sixty-seven in a patient who had had perennial nasal allergy from milk for many years.

This and another similar case justify the study of food and possible inhalant allergy as a cause of unexplained hemoptysis. Bleeding from the lungs in Goodpasture's syndrome in our opinion also justifies the study of possible allergy, especially to foods. Our review of the literature shows that such study of food allergy with adequate, sufficient use of our CFE diet or its modifications never has been done.

The associated nephritis with death from azotemia is best explained by allergic vasculitis in the kidney or with food allergy as a possible cause. Bleeding from the gums and even the oral mucosa from allergy to various foods is at times recognized even by the allergic individual.

Case 183: A woman forty-five years of age had had severe hematemesis three times in the preceding three years. X-rays of the upper gastrointestinal tract were normal, revealing no evidence of duodenal ulcer. In addition, she had had bronchial asthma in the winter months for eight years which required study of food allergy as the cause. Skin reactions were negative to all common foods and airborne allergens in her vicinity.

Her diet history indicated possible fruit allergy. With our FFCFE diet, asthma and moderate gastric distress were controlled. No hematemesis had recurred for twelve years except eight years ago when fruits had been eaten without permission. With strict adherence to the diet since then, no hematemesis had developed. Her asthma has required the additional elimination of milk and cereal grains and their products through the years.

Bleeding from allergic inflammation and resultant tissue changes in the urinary bladder occurred three years ago after fruits had been added to the diet without permission for one month.

EASY BRUISING OF TISSUES

Easy bruising occurs in various patients suffering with the HS syndrome. Squier reports the development of "purpuric spots" when his patient with T.C.P. from food allergy attempted to get out of bed during a period of bedrest for two months because of her continued hemorrhages from nose and gums. After food allergy was controlled, this purpura and nasal hemorrhage stopped. Easy bruising, moreover, is noted by Cohen in familial purpura simplex.

If depressed platelets, increased capillary permeability, and red blood cell fragility with possible increased eosinophiles are present in patients susceptible to easy bruising, the study of possible food and less often pollen allergy as a cause is justifiable.

CLINICAL ALLERGY FROM TRANSFUSIONS

Asthma, with occasional shock and more often urticaria, has occurred after transfusions from properly matched donors who had eaten foods to which the patient was allergic just before the blood was drawn. Moreover, patients can be passively sensitized with antibodies to foods or other allergens present in the donor's blood.

Asthma from the inhalation of horse dander from antibodies in the patient after transfusion from a horse-sensitive donor was first reported by Ramirez in 1919. Fasting donors reduce the likelihood of transfusion reactions in food-sensitive patients. The elimination of specific foods to which the patient may be allergic from the donor's diet for one to two days may be necessary to prevent such post-transfusion allergy. The transfusion of washed, properly grouped red blood cells in normal saline also reduces possible allergic reactions.

Randolph, in 1945, reported enlarged peripheral lymph nodes, especially in the neck, increased lymphoid tissue in the pharynx, enlarged tonsils along with leukocytosis, and atypical large lymphocytes in the blood in adolescents and young adults in whom allergic toxemia and fatigue from food allergy were present. Negative heterophile antibody tests disproved infectious mononucleosis as the cause. Crook (1969) confirmed this pseudomononucleosis to be due to food allergy rather than to infection.

SUMMARY

1. Henoch-Schonlein's (HS) syndrome, characterized by purpura, colicky pain, vomiting, intestinal bleeding, edema and pain in joints, frequent hematuria, and at times nephritis was first attributed to food allergy by Galloway in 1903, Sachs in 1916, and especially by Alexander and Eyermann to foods in 1927.

2. Since then allergists have confirmed food allergy as the usual cause. Two case reports of allergenic foods in the causation of HS purpura and two of our cases are summarized.

3. Thrombocytopenic purpura from food allergy reported by Squier and Madison is discussed.

4. Purpura simplex from increased capillary permeability from food allergy reported by Ancona *et al.* in 1951 and Snyder in 1968 is more often due to drug than to food allergy, as to Sedormid.

5. Familial purpura simplex first reported by Davis justifies the study of food allergy as we advise in this volume as a possible activating inherited factor.

6. Eosinophilia and eosinophilic infiltration of tissues, according to our experience, occurs more frequently and to a greater degree from food allergy than inhalant allergy. Its frequency from certain parasites and some drugs must be remembered.

7. The role of possible food allergy in Loffler's syndrome of eosinophilic pneumonopathy needs consideration.

8. Because leukocytosis occurs after ingesting allergenic foods, Warren Vaughan advised the leukopenic index test. Its fallibility and the necessity of confirming positive results with trial diet disfavors its use rather than our elimination diet in our practice.

9. Permeability of capillaries from allergy causes bleeding and hemorrhages, especially from food allergy. Bleeding in oral, gastrointestinal, and colonic mucosa in RE and especially in CUC from food allergy or in the skin, as in HS purpura, is reported in this chapter.

10. Hermaturia from food as well as drug allergy is reported.

11. That bleeding from the bronchial mucosa in Goodpasture's syndrome requires study of food allergy, especially to milk, is indicated in two of our patients.

12. Easy bruising of tissues warrants study of allergy, especially to foods, as one possible cause, especially if corticosteroids are not being given.

13. Asthma, urticaria, or a generalized allergic reaction in a food-sensitive patient after transfusions with accurately matched

blood can be explained by allergens of foods in the donor's blood. This suggests giving blood from a fasting donor to a food-sensitive recipient.

Chapter 23

Food Allergy and the Arthropathies

Since our main challenge in this book is the role of food allergy in its many clinical manifestations, the joint symptoms attributed to or requiring the study of food allergy receive initial and special discussion.

That joints and synovial membranes are susceptible to allergic reactions is evidenced by the arthropathies arising from allergy, especially from parenteral foreign serum therapy, but also to many drugs and from general reactions arising during desensitization to allergens, especially pollen allergens.

ARTHRITIS FROM FOOD ALLERGY

Food allergy as a cause of arthritic pain or arthralgia and swelling occurs not infrequently. Many physicians are noting that swelling, stiffness, and pain in small and large joints of the body occur from specific foods. That it may also affect synovial sheaths and even muscles, probably through their blood vessels, is evidenced in Case 193. Allergic synovitis from walnuts every two months for six years was recorded by Lewin and Taub (1936). Low backache with radiation of pain into the lower abdomen and down the thighs also arises from food allergy. It was associated with vomiting, headache, and fatigue in one of our patients from wheat and egg allergy.

Talbot (1917) and Cooke (1918) suggested that arthritic pain in certain patients might result from food allergy. Turnbull (1924) drew attention to relief from longstanding joint pains from test-negative diets. Such allergy cannot be assumed as a cause of hypertrophic changes. Edema and exudation into joint capsules may occur in the presence of rheumatoid or hypertrophic arthritis. Criep (1946) reported recurrent arthritis in the right ankle and wrist from egg allergy to which a large skin reaction occurred. Blood eosinophilia was 10 percent.

Gudzent (1935) stressed the frequency of food allergy as a cause of chronic arthritis. He noted that unsatisfactory results frequently were obtained from removal of foci of infection and vaccine therapy. The possibility of inhalant allergy as a cause of arthritic reactivity was discussed and one case relieved of polyarthritis by the recognition and control of causative allergy from fungi was recorded. He stated that the rheumatic processes in joints, muscles and nerves are best explained by allergy.

Neck and shoulder pain, which we listed in the allergic toxemia and fatigue syndrome in 1928, 1930, and especially in 1950, was emphasized by Randolph in his article on allergic torticollis and in the posterior cervical and trapezius muscle as summarized in Chapter 19.

Of interest is the report of Epstein of Madison, Wisconsin, on page 5 of vol. 23 of *Correspondence Letters of Allergists* that severe attacks of pain in joints for several days were due to sodium nitrate as a food additive in frozen vegetables, tomato juice, sausage, and other foods.

Personal Cases

Our work for over forty years has affirmed such pain and at times swelling in joints from food allergy. One patient invariably had such symptoms in the right ankle when tomatoes, rhubarb, strawberries, or beef were eaten. Pain in the right lower back, suggestive of arthritis, with severe pain radiating down the leg in the tissues supplied by the obturator nerve arose from grapefruit, red wine, and port in another patient. One man had pain in the calves, knees, ankles, and probably tendons whenever string beans were eaten. Gay told me of tomatoes as such a cause in two patients. Citrus fruits and tomatoes were responsible in one of our cases. Apples and apricots caused pain and stiffness in the joints and soreness in the right arm of another patient. One woman fifty-five years of age had had mucous colitis, pain and stiffness in her knees (so she could not bend them to go down stairs), and in the hips and nerves of the legs which kept her awake for years. Increasing disability was entirely relieved with the use of our FFCFE diet (Chapt. 3), which demonstrated that tomatoes and wheat especially were causative.

One patient with potential food allergy had severe pain in the sacrum and buttocks attributed to an automobile accident. It was only relieved, however, with use and manipulation of our elimination diet. The injury possibly made synovial membranes or nerve structures susceptible to the food reactions.

One woman seventy-six years of age had swelling and pains in ankles, knees, shoulders, and elbows with recurrent headaches and toxemia resulting from food allergy. Traces of milk reproduced all of her complaints. The joint involvements in allergic purpura, especially Henoch-Schonlein purpura, reported in Chapter 22 also arise from food allergy. Some of our patients state that elimination diets which have controlled urticaria, asthma, gastrointestinal allergy, or migraine have also relieved pains and swellings in joints, including the lower back.

It is unlikely that deformities of joints as found in the two types of chronic arthritis ever arise from allergic reactions alone. However, repeated allergic reactions in joints may gradually lead to organization and thickening of the tissues and might produce moderate enlargement thereby. Two patients with rheumatoid arthritis of long standing were markedly relieved of joint pain when with the use of elimination diets, specific foods were found which also were apparently producing allergic edema or reactions in the deformed joints.

LITERATURE

Fletcher (1922, 1933) and Fletcher and Graham (1930) benefitted patients with chronic arthritis with diets low in carbohydrates. Pemberton (1934) also reported such help and stated that 3.6 grams of water accumulates in the body with the storage of every gram of carbohydrate. It is interesting that three of Fletcher's patients were also relieved of chronic eczema. Two were allergic to milk.

Transient, at times more persistent, pain, swelling, and limitation of motion in the joints resulting from food allergy have long been recognized. Absence of fever, increased sedimentation rates, and abnormal x-ray findings rule out infection as the cause. Other clinical manifestations of allergy are usually present. Such negative findings have encouraged the consideration of psychoneurosis as a cause.

Criep, in 1946, reported the following case reports of arthritis from food allergy.

A woman forty years of age had excruciating pain in the nuchal area radiating down the right arm for five months. Pain often occurred suddenly, at times awakening her. Tenderness was present in the trapezius and deltoid muscles and upper spinous processes as reported by Randolph (Chapt. 18). Laboratory tests and x-rays of bones were negative. Pain and inflammation and fusiform swelling occurred in the third right finger. Severe urticaria had occurred. Diet trial revealed grapes and wine as major causes.

A man thirty-seven years of age had recurrent pain and swelling of the right great toe and at times of the right knee. This kept him abed once for six weeks. Hives had occurred two times. Ingestion of peanuts, almonds, and wheat was found responsible.

A girl twelve years of age had intermittent swellings in the right ankle and wrists for several hours, painful with motion. There was no evidence of infection. Eggs, even traces thereof, caused swellings in joints.

A man sixty-five years of age had pain and swelling of several fingers and brief blindness in one eye after eating fish.

Recently Zussman (1966) reported swelling, soreness, and pain in joints suggesting rheumatoid arthritis from food allergy. Three illustrative cases were published, summaries of which follow. Food allergy was demonstrated with the use of our CFE diet. Skin tests were not helpful, being done largely "for psychological reasons."

1. A woman fifty-four years of age had intermittent pains in fingers, toes, knees, elbows, and shoulders for five years. Slight nasal allergy and recurrent headaches indicative especially of food allergy were present. Joints were not enlarged. X-rays of the joints were negative. With our CFE diet, pain disappeared in two weeks. Provocation tests then showed milk, wheat, and coffee as the causes.

2. A woman forty years of age had "arthritis" with no enlargement of many painful joints for twenty years. Migraine, hay fever, and arthritis were in the family. Elimination of foods she suspected because of disagreements gave no relief and left her "at the end of her rope."

Nasal edema, eosinophiles in the mucus, swelling, and soreness in most fingers producing fusi-

form shape as seen in rheumatoid arthritis were present. Serum latex and sedimentation rates were normal. X-rays showed no changes in the joints.

The swelling with pain in the joints and headaches were relieved with our CFE diet. Provocation tests revealed wheat, milk, eggs, and legumes as the causes. Bananas, chocolate, and nuts caused bloating and diarrhea but no arthritic pain. This arthritis had been attributed to rheumatoid arthritis for twenty years.

3. A woman forty-one years of age had had pains in muscles, joints (especially in the right shoulder, knee, and wrist) and proximal finger joints and edema in the face, hands, feet, and legs for eighteen months. Medical advice had yielded no help. She was told she was "allergic to everything." With our FFCFE diet, edema disappeared in ten days, and pains in the muscles and joints gradually lessened in degree. Provocation tests with additional foods showed that wheat, rye, milk, and pork reactivated pains in four hours.

FOOD ALLERGY IN RHEUMATOID ARTHRITIS

That food allergy may play an active or secondary role in cases of rheumatoid arthritis was also stated by Zeller in 1949. He advised study and attempted control of possible food allergy in addition to the study and control of other possible causes especially when a personal or family history of probable atopic allergy is present. In addition to indicated laboratory tests, x-ray studies, and physical examination in such patients, study of food allergy with trial diets was advised. Varying degrees of improvement with the elimination of specific foods was reported in five patients in all of whom there were other manifestations of clinical allergy.

Though my study of possible food allergy in rheumatoid arthritis has been of little or no help, its control seems to have definitely relieved pain and soreness in two patients. One patient with advancing pulmonary tuberculosis in 1938, before chemo-therapy was available, had diffuse arthritis of the rheumatoid type. Marked relief of pains and soreness in the joints occurred as she adhered to my fruit and cereal-free elimination diet with an adequate caloric intake and multiple vitamins.

REPORTS OF ARTHRITIS IN OUR PATIENTS RELIEVED BY ELIMINATION OF ALLERGENIC FOODS

Case 184: A woman twenty-five years of age had had pain in her right buttocks and thighs with pain in elbows and edema in fingers for 1½ years. Scratch tests with foods and inhalants and x-rays of painful joints were negative.

Pain decreased in one month and was absent in 1½ months with adherence to our FFCFE diet. In 2⅓ months provocation tests with additional foods revealed egg as the sole cause. It reactivated pain in buttocks, thighs, and fingers in twelve hours, disappearing in forty-eight hours after exclusion of eggs.

Case 185: A woman thirty-nine years of age had had stiff, painful, and moderately swollen joints in the neck, shoulders, and knees for six years. Recurrent "colds" and headaches from the age of twenty to thirty years suggested food allergy. Pressure and burning in the epigastrium for six years indicated the allergic epigastric syndrome (see Chap. 5). That pains in the joints disappeared in pregnancy also suggested food allergy. Her son had severe infantile eczema relieved with our CFE diet.

The joint pains and epigastric distress were controlled with our FFCFE diet in three weeks. In three months fruits and condiments reactivated symptoms in six to ten hours. This fruit allergy continued for ten years until death from cancer.

Case 186: A woman fifty-nine years of age had had pain, edema, and enlargement in fingers, knuckles, wrists, nuchal area, hips, and thighs for five years. Menstrual sick headaches had occurred. Food allergy as a possible cause of retinal detachments helped by three operations in the last four years is discussed in Chapter 20.

Milk caused nasal congestion, and fruits produced constipation.

With our FFCFE diet, pain and edema of joints disappeared in three weeks. In the last fourteen years fruits and condiments have reactivated her arthralgia.

In view of her food allergy the possibility that her retinal detachments were due to allergy in the choroid needs the above consideration.

Case 187: A woman fifty years of age had had pain and aching in the right shoulder, knees, right hip, and other joints for five years. Failure of relief from medicines and corticosteroids caused discouragement. Epigastric aching and distention persisted. Dopiness, drowsiness, and fatigue indicated allergic toxemia (Chapt. 19).

Milk caused vomiting or diarrhea. Pyrosis occurred from wheat.

Her mother had severe sick headaches.

With our FFCFE diet, she felt "wonderful" in one week, being free of distress "present for years." No medicines or corticosteroids had been taken.

In four months relief had continued. It was the first winter she was free of head colds and brochitis. Indigestion and fatigue were absent. "I can do anything."

Provocation tests with additional foods reactivated arthralgia. All fruits, corn, wheat, milk, and uncooked vegetables caused moderate indigestion. A minimum diet of rice, white potatoes, pearl tapioca (see recipe), beef, lamb, chicken, turkey, tea, sugar, rice-potato bread, and cookies relieved joint pains and other symptoms.

Case 188: A woman sixty-four years of age had had pain, aching, and stiffness "in all joints of the body" intermittently for eight years. Painful, swollen, stiff hands prevented their use five years ago. At present neck and shoulders especially were painful. All muscles ached, especially in the legs. Distress had always been worse in the late fall and winter, indicating food allergy (see Chap. 1).

Perennial postnasal mucus and blocking of Eustachian tubes (see Chap. 12) especially in the winter, suggested food allergy. Treatment by several physicians had failed.

With strict adherence to our fruit-free and cereal-free elimination diet, relief of all symptoms gradually occurred in four weeks. After assured relief in three months, provocation tests with additional foods gradually showed that all fruits, condiments, milk, and wheat produced symptoms. In fourteen years she reports that pains still recur when the above foods are eaten. Fruits and condiments especially are detrimental.

Case 189: A woman forty-nine years of age

had had pain and aching in the right shoulder, right hip, with aching in other joints most of the time for four to five years. Corticosteroids gave brief but no lasting relief. Epigastric distress, vomiting, or diarrhea occurred from milk. Pyrosis resulted from wheat. Bronchitis occurred for several weeks every two to three months, especially in the fall and winter (Chapt. 9). Dopiness, dullness, and fatigue were nearly constant, indicating allergic fatigue and toxemia (Chapt. 19). Her mother had sick headaches.

With our fruit-free and cereal-free elimination diet, she felt "100 percent better in one week." In three weeks symptoms she had had for years disappeared. No medications or corticosteroids were given.

Provocation feeding tests showed that peaches, pears, and apricots reproduced aching and pain in joints and gastrointestinal symptoms in three to five hours, lasting four to five days. In one year she reported complete relief as she maintained her strict diet.

LIFELONG PAIN IN JOINTS AND MUSCLES

The following history deserves emphasis because of lifelong invaliding joint and muscle pains associated with fatigue, toxemia, and headaches, relieved for ten years by a minimal elimination diet. Familial gastrointestinal allergy was present.

Case 190: A woman thirty-two years of age had had pains in her joints and especially the muscles particularly in arms, chest, upper and lower back, calves of legs, and thighs all her life. In adolescence and twenties pain had increased in back, arms, and chest. Walking became increasingly difficult attributed by physicians to "relaxation of ligaments in the back." For three years she had worn a lumbosacral support extending below the buttocks with a detached supporting bra "heavier and stronger than her maternity corset." Aching was worse in the winter, suggesting to us possible food allergy (Chapt. 1). "Popping sounds" occurred in back and knees.

Asthma had occurred at fifteen to twenty-eight years. Perennial nasal allergy had occurred all her lift.

Epigastric burning and aching had recurred for several years, indicating our allergic epigastric

syndrome (Chapt. 5).

Weakness and also depression because of failure of medical help existed.

Moderate headaches had been frequent for twenty years.

Diet history revealed suspicion of fruits as a major cause of pain and indigestion. Wheat and pork increased muscle pains. Milk and eggs caused asthma.

Drug and environmental histories were negative for allergy.

Family history revealed gastrointestinal symptoms and nasal allergy in the mother, hives and severe colitis in an aunt, and eczema is another aunt. Two nieces had gastrointestinal allergy, toxemia, and pains in muscles. "Popping joints" were present in her father and his brother.

Skin testing gave no scratch reactions to foods or inhalants.

Treatment: To study food allergy, a minimal elimination diet was ordered consisting of rice, pearl tapioca, lamb, chicken, turkey, carrot, squash, peas, sugar, salt, water, and Willow Run (milk-free) margarine. A multiple vitamin was given, but no corticosteroids were used.

In six weeks pain and aching in muscles and joints were less. Desensitization to tree, grass, fall, and cultivated flower pollens present in her environment (not determined by skin tests) was gradually increased into the 1:200 dilution and continued for two years. With a gradual disappearance of pain in muscles and joints, she discarded her bracing support in one year, working in the garden without pain.

She moved to the midwest, where deviations in the diet at intervals reactivated pains but without impaired activity.

She writes eight years later, "My strict diet is lamb, chicken, rice, white potato, peas, squash, cane sugar, noniodized salt, and multiple vitamins. I am teaching psychology in the university."

Pain, stiffness, soreness in the joints especially in the hands preventing piano teaching due to fruit allergy is of special interest in the following case.

Case 191: A woman fifty-one years of age had had intermittent stiffness and swelling in the joints of the left thumb for three years and during the last eight months stiffness and soreness in all the finger joints of the right hand. For one year, moreover, intermittent aching in the right hip, knee, and ankle had occurred. This arthritis in her fingers increasingly interfered with her piano teaching. Perennial nasal congestion causing blocking and coryza associated with some itching of her ears had occurred. Urticaria had been present in childhood. Canker sores had occurred at intervals throughout life, indicating probable food allergy as a cause (see Chapt. 5). For one year some intermittent wheezing and coughing had been present.

Her diet history revealed the eating of more raw fruit since being in California for the last four or five years.

Family history revealed sick headaches in the mother, perennial hay fever in the sister, and bronchial asthma in an aunt.

Scratch tests with all ingested foods and inhaled allergens and routine laboratory work were negative.

Treatment and Results: Food allergy was studied with our fruit-free and cereal-free elimination diet. In seven days there was less nasal congestion and coryza than during her life. Pains and stiffness in the finger joints had decreased. This relief increased during the next two months. Ingestion provocation tests with several fruits reactivated the pain and stiffness in her joints. Milk reproduced nasal allergy. Tomatoes produced itching of the skin. In two years her arthritis was still under good control. The ingestion of apple and orange had reproduced arthritic pain for two or three days in her fingers. Pit fruits had rapidly produced arthritis in the fingers and also in the knees and had caused stiffness in the neck.

In ten years she reported that her arthritis, nasal congestion, and nasal allergy were still under good control. The control of her arthritis in the fingers and other joints and her nasal allergy still required the elimination of the same foods. At that time she was actively engaged in piano teaching, was doing all of her housework, and was also working in the garden.

Case 192: Arthralgia. Neuralgia. A man twenty-nine years of age during the last three years had had pain in both hips and in the lumbar and sacroiliac regions. During the last three years his back had been painful, and with any change in position sharp, shooting pains in his hips had occurred. A roentgen ray picture of his back and hips had shown no abnormality. Medical treatment at the hands of specialists had been ineffectual. For seven months he had

worn a supporting brace on his back, with no relief. The pain had been so severe, especially in the early mornings, that sleep had frequently been impossible.

During the last three months he had found that the daily use of enemas had ameliorated his pain, favoring possible food allergy. He had been suspicious that milk had increased his symptoms. He had never had any definite history of allergy, and there was no history of allergy in his family. His physical examination was negative, and his laboratory tests were negative. Skin reactions to foods showed the following positive reactions:

Foods:

Wheat, glutenin	+
Wheat, leucosin	+ +
Barley	+
Turnip	+ +
Orange	+
Cabbage	+ +
Carrot	+
Cauliflower	+
Celery	+
Spinach	+ +

Because of his positive skin reactions to foods and the history of some relief from enemas, it was felt that his pain might be due to food allergy. He was therefore given our CFE diet plus rice and oats. He reported in one week that one day after starting the diet, the pain had disappeared and that he had been practically free ever since.

Since then it has been found that milk and eggs definitely reproduced the severe pain in the back and hips. After taking milk for two days the pain in his back began in the early morning. He continued the milk for four days and the pain became steadily worse. After discontinuing the milk the pain disappeared at the end of the first day. After being free from the pain for three weeks one egg was taken and that night severe pain in the back and hips occurred. A few days later another egg was taken, and the same pain resulted. Ever since then he has continued on a milk-free and egg-free diet. Wheat has been included, and he has been entirely free from all of the severe pain.

Comment: The arthralgia in this patient has been definitely shown to be due to food allergy. There was little in the history to indicate its presence. It is interesting that the skin reactions, though positive, did not indicate the true type of allergy. The patient has found that he can take all of the foods to which positive reactions occurred without any difficulty and that his pain was due to wheat and milk, to which negative cutaneous reactions occurred. The importance of the elimination method of diet trial such as we have described is therefore especially apparent.

ALLERGIC SYNOVITIS

Allergic inflammation and edema in the membranes of the joints and tendons may occur from food allergy.

When transient synovitis of the hip joint occurs in a child, allergy requires study, as it did in twenty-two children studied by Finder (1936), whose average age was 5.4 years. Spasm of the muscles about the hip holds it in an uncomfortable position. Fever from 99 to 101 F usually occurs. Serious diseases such as tuberculosis, pyogenic infection, osteomyelitis, and aseptic bone disease (Legg-Perthes disease) must be ruled out.

Possible food allergy requires study with trial diet, especially our CFE diet and later if relief fails in two to three weeks without fruits. Such study is justified by our case reports concerning food allergy and of other allergists already summarized.

Edwards (1952) reported thirteen children under the age of ten with transient synovitis in the hip causing muscle spasm and limited motion. No infection was evident. Personal history of allergy occurred in four. Atopic allergy was a suggested cause. Food allergy, we opine, should have been studied, especially with our fruit-free and cereal-free elimination diet.

SYNOVIAL MEMBRANE EDEMA RESULTING FROM FOOD ALLERGY

Tendon sheath and synovial membrane edema we reported in 1938 from food allergy justifies the following summary:

Case 193: A woman fifty years of age for three years had had swellings with pain in the tendon sheaths of the fingers, wrists, forearms, knees, thighs, and legs. In the first year they were intermittent every few months, suggestive of food allergy. In the last year they had rarely been absent more than a week, and she was constantly aware of some pain or stiffness in the extremities, hands, or feet, especially with exercise. Use of her hands as in driving, working, or knitting always increased or precipitated swellings in various tendon sheaths, joints, and at times in soft tissues. Severe generalized urticaria had occurred fifteen years ago. The severe attacks had usually appeared suddenly, lasting forty-eight to seventy-two hours and disappeared rather rapidly, again suggesting food allergy (Chapt. 1). Attacks of mucous colitis, bloating, and epigastric discomfort had recurred for five years. Marked nervousness and fatigue had been present, especially with the attacks.

Shellfish, chocolate, tomatoes, and lemonade produced indigestion. Former physicians had found no cause for her swellings. One sister had eczema. A paternal uncle had asthma. All skin reactions to allergens were negative. With elimination diets it was found that milk, eggs, wheat, spinach, and chocolate caused the swellings of her tendon sheaths. With a strict diet no difficulty has been present during five years while follow-up was maintained. Her lumbago, nervousness, indigestion, and mucous colitis remained absent. Occasional butter and other slight breaks in her diet caused a return of the symptoms, which required three weeks of strict dieting to eradicate. This relief occurred before corticoids were available. No medications were taken.

INTERMITTENT HYDRARTHROSIS AND PALINDROMIC RHEUMATISM

The intermittent swelling of joints in intermittent hydrarthrosis and palindromic rheumatism along with other characteristics of these syndromes have long suggested allergy as the probable cause. Food allergy especially must be studied because of the usual cyclid recurrence of their manifestations often with interim relief. This recurrent characteristic is especially exemplified in recurrent bronchial asthma, which is better in the summer, being exaggerated in the fall and winter, resulting from food allergy, which we have long reported in the literature (Chapt. 1). Recurrence, moreover, of sick headaches, migraine, urticaria, and angioneurotic edema and at times epilepsy also requires adequate study of food allergy as we have advised throughout this volume.

Evidence that inhalant allergy and bacterial allergy cause these regular recurrent swellings in joints is questionable or absent, as discussed in the literature.

Intermittent Hydrarthrosis

Intermittent hydrarthrosis (IH) has been attributed to possible atopic allergy for over forty years. Even in 1924 Miller and Lewin presented evidence favoring such etiology in an excellent review of this rare condition. They stated that Schlessinger (1899) first emphasized the similarity of IH to angioneurotic edema. The marked periodicity of attacks of IH was similar to that at times of migraine and as we have recorded, in bronchial asthma resulting from food allergy. They noted that Garot reported IH associated with urticaria and also with transient edema of the eyes and lips. Goix recorded IH accompanied by edema of the face. Senator also observed it in a boy seventeen years of age who had had recurrent edema in the gluteal region up to the age of twelve years. Bierring reported relief of IH in eight of nine patients during pregnancy. Miller *et al.* stated that other manifestations of food allergy, as recurrent migraine and in our experience bronchial asthma, are inactivated at times in some patients during pregnancy, as we discussed in Chapter 8. Paviot *et al.* (1932), in an article on allergic arthropathies, discussed slight swelling, stiffness, and pains in various joints because of food allergy as we have discussed in the first part of this chapter. He also stated that IH occurring usually in women in mid-life usually in the knees was best explained by allergy.

Favoring allergy is the report of temporary cessation of fluid formation after an initial injection of corticosteroid into the knee joint or other joint cavities or relief from initial large and decreasing doses by mouth. If adequate, accurate use of our elimination diets or their modifications with or without corticoid therapy suggested above relieves and prevents the recurrence of swellings, it would make surgical removal of secreting synovial membrane of the knee or less often other joint capsules unnecessary, thus preventing the time and expense incurred by surgery and hospitalization and the restricted use of the joint, especially of the leg, and the resulting inactivity for two to three months thereafter.

Palindromic Rheumatism (PR)

Hench and Rosenberg (1941) reviewed twenty-four cases of afebrile recurrent attacks of swellings in various joints, which they named palindromic rheumatism. Palindromic indicated recurrence with interim relief. Because of involvement of the joints and particularly para-articular structures, it was also named rheumatism. In contrast to the usual involvement of only one joint in IH, involvement of different joints, particularly fingers, wrists, shoulders, knees, elbows, toes (especially the great toe), necessitating the exclusion of gout, and less frequently of other joints occurs in PR. Varying degrees of pain, aching, at times agonizing and severe in degree, with varying degrees of disability occur during the attacks.

Blood tests, other routine laboratory tests, and x-rays were negative. Relief of swellings with sudden onset and disappearance of attacks with no residual tissue changes, the history of possible food allergy in sixteen of thirty-four cases reported by Hench, the occurrence of varying manifestations of probable allergy in eighteen patients, and the occurrence of arthritis, hives, and edema in relatives also suggested possible allergy.

Failure of relief of diets excluding skin-reacting foods and failure to exaggerate or reproduce swellings with large feedings of such foods indicated incorrectly to the authors that food allergy was not causative. As emphasized throughout this volume, food allergy cannot be excluded by failure to relieve symptoms with test-negative diets. This, on the contrary, necessitates for its study the use of trial diets, particularly our cereal-free elimination diet, usually without fruit, as we advise.

In the first edition of this volume in 1931, we included the report of our valued friend in years past, V. G. Alderson, M.D., which exemplifies Henoch's palindromic rheumatism rather than intermittent hydrarthrosis.

Case 194: A woman thirty years of age had had swellings of her hands, knees, and ankle joints on the same side all of her life. At first they occurred every one to three weeks. For three years they occurred every week or almost constantly. Swellings increased or occurred in four to five hours after eating. Fluctuating fluid distended the joint capsule. Moderate asthma and hives had occurred. There was seasonal asthma in the mother, hay fever in a brother, hives in two sisters, and convulsive seizures in a brother which had been relieved by the elimination of specific foods.

With history, trial diet, and partial help of skin tests, wheat, milk, and beef were found responsible for the joint swelling. Milk caused marked fatigue as well as drowsiness.

Evidence favoring bacterial allergy and angioneurosis also was lacking, according to Hench.

In our opinion, food allergy needs further study in all of these patients. Failure to relieve food allergy by test-negative diets does not justify the decision that food allergy is not operative. Such failure necessitates its study with our elimination diets as we advise with recognition and control of less possible inhalant and drug allergy if indicated.

SUMMARY

1. That food allergy produces pain and varying swellings in joints, especially in the synovial membrane, has been reported by allergists for many years, as suggested by Talbot in 1917 and Cooke in 1918.

2. This has been confirmed by Criep, in 1946, by Zussman, in 1966, with use of our elimination diets, and by us and is summarized in eight informative case reports.

3. Relief of stiffness and aching in various joints, especially in the finger joints of a piano teacher, by elimination of allergenic foods with our fruit-free and cereal-free elimination diet is of special interest.

4. Pain and edema from food allergy may be associated with bacterial allergy responsible for rheumatoid arthritis.

5. Transient synovitis in hip joints in children justifies study of food allergy as we advise.

6. Tendon sheath and synovial membrane edema causing pain and swelling because of food allergy is reported in Case 193.

7. Intermittent hydarthrosis in the knees and other large joints and of palindromic rheumatism in smaller joints require study of atopic allergy, as in Case 194. The regular intermittent reactions in the joints favor food allergy as stressed in Chapter 1 of this volume.

8. As in other manifestations of possible food allergy, its study and control, as we advise in Chapters 3 and 30 is indicated.

Chapter 24

Fever Resulting From Food Allergy

Food allergy requires recognition as one cause of "unexplained fever." Fever from drug and serum allergy is generally recognized. Very occasionally, fever also arises from allergy to pollens or other inhalants, as reported since 1931 by Rowe, Gottlieb and Urbach, Rinkel, Randolph, and others. Though fever from food allergy was first reported by Barnathan in 1911 and by Laroche, Richet, and Saint Girons in 1919 and has been reported by other observers as noted in our article Fever due to Food Allergy in 1948, since then its recognition has been too long delayed. Failure to recognize the role of allergy usually is due to not realizing its occurrence, failure of test-negative diets to evidence food allergy, and failure to study food allergy as we advise.

Cooke, in 1933, reported fever up to 104 F associated with cyclic gastrointestinal symptoms resulting from milk allergy in a girl from the age of one year to her present age of sixteen years. Similar recurrent gastrointestinal symptoms with fever of 101 F for two days in a girl fourteen years of age because of allergy to milk and beef was reported. These cases have been summarized in Chapter 5.

Periodic fever as a manifestation of periodic disease requires study of allergy especially to foods as reported especially by Reimann in 1942 and as discussed in Chapter 2 of this volume.

In 1936 Gay reported one patient with "habitual fever" from food allergy. This patient had been treated for months for tuberculosis in spite of the absence of abnormal findings. A second patient had been at rest in bed for eight years because of moderate afternoon fever attributed to unproven tuberculosis. She had purpura, nasal allergy, and a family history of nasal allergy. Food allergy was the proven cause. A third patient had fever for two years with repeated negative findings. She had had asthma, hives, and recurrent headaches. Diet trial gave relief.

Failure to recognize food allergy as one cause of fever accounts for some unjustified diagnoses of idiopathic or psychogenic fever, subclinical tuberculosis, brucellosis, or other questionable infections. It has led to unnecessary operations on tonsils, appendices, gallbladders, and pelvic organs. Needless surgery has been performed on nasal sinuses because of the association of fever with nasal congestion, blocking, or postnasal mucus, especially with swollen membranes, opacities in the antra, or other sinuses which were not due to infection but to allergy, especially to foods. Such fever often has constituted the chief reason for prolonged, unnecessary inactivity or vacations, for bedrest in hospitals or sanitaria, and for extensive clinical and laboratory investigations.

Food allergy should be considered as a cause of fever when the physical examination and laboratory studies give no explanatory clues and especially when treatment based on positive findings gives no relief. As in other possible clinical allergy from food, this study is especially necessary if the patient has a personal history of other allergic manifestations and/or a familial history of allergy. Thus in the case described below, aversion to milk and probable colonic allergy stressed study of food allergy as one cause of the fever. The absence of any familial allergy did not detract from this necessity. The most likely explanation of allergic fever is a disturbance in the temperature-regulating center of the brain by a localized or generalized allergic reaction.

Fever resulting from food allergy often occurs in the first one or two days of the typical recurrent attacks of bronchial asthma from food allergy reported by us for over thirty-five years. This history in our opinion and experience is pathognomonic of asthma resulting from food allergy. As stated in Chapters 8 and 25, fever varies from 99 to 104 F during the first one or two days of the attack and decreases to normal in one or two days without antibacterial therapy. If the fever continues for three to four days, secondary infection may be responsible. If pneumonitis or infection of tonsils is assured, antibiotics along with the accurate use of our CFE diet are important.

Periodic sore throats with nasal congestion and other upper respiratory symptoms along with fever up to 104 F for one to two days require study of food allergy with or without secondary infection as the cause, as reported in Cases 65 and 66.

Fever in recurrent attacks of serious otitis media, as stated in Chapter 13, is usually due to food allergy rather than infection. Since food allergy often produces recurrent attacks of the symptoms, as emphasized in Chapter 2, its consideration as a possible cause of cyclic fever always requires adequate study as we advise. Food allergy as a cause of periodic fever must be studied with our CFE diet and if necessary with its modifications.

Food allergy also produces persistent fever nearly always in association with other manifestations including perennial nasal, bronchial, urogenital, or gastrointestinal allergy. In CUC and RE fever may be due to food allergy alone, as evidenced by its relief with the control only of food allergy without antibiotics as reported in Chapters 6 and 7. Secondary infection in CUC and RE may also be present, requiring antibacterial treatment. The importance of recognizing and controlling fever from food allergy to prevent needless medical investigations and treatment, unnecessary operations, prescribed inactivity, and even psychological therapy has been emphasized above.

Recurrent febrile seizures or prolonged convulsions especially if Dilantin or another anticonvulsant drug is given justify this study of possible food allergy as we advise as a cause of the fever and also of possible epilepsy as discussed in Chapter 18 and also in Chapter 25 on clinical allergy in infants and children.

The following case report illustrates prolonged fever with recent colonic symptoms as a result of allergy, especially to milk. Lifelong anorexia and aversion for milk had occurred. Because of the fever, hospitalization continued for 4 ½ months, during which many laboratory and clinical investigations had given no relief. A diagnosis of psychogenic fever had been made. A summary of the history, our study and control of food allergy, and the fluctuating but persistent fever is described. This case as published in 1948 is the only published report of prolonged fever from food allergy.

CASE REPORT

Case 195: A girl eighteen years of age developed fatigue and anorexia in July of 1942 with cramping in the abdomen, night sweats, and afternoon fever of 102 F during a two-month period. Continued fever led to study and treatment in two different hospitals where she was at complete rest for 4½ months. Investigations were negative except for slight bleeding in the rectal mucosa seen by proctoscope. Laboratory studies done in these hospitals revealed normal blood counts except for an eosinophilia several times up to 23 percent, which should have suggested allergy, other causes having been excluded. This eosinophilia reduced to 7 percent in seven days and to 4 percent in twenty-one days after the fever was controlled by our CFE diet. A rapid sedimentation rate up to 25 mm in one hour was also explained by uncontrolled food allergy. This rate was 10 mm one month after the elimination of allergenic foods. Leukocytosis, which at times occurs from food allergy, was absent.

In spite of bedrest for 4½ months and sulfadiazine given for several weeks, fever persisted until her referral to us for the study of allergy.

Food allergy was immediately suggested as a cause of her long aversion to milk. She had been forced to take milk in childhood. She had been encouraged to drink it in the hospitals, especially by her mother, a trained nurse. Otherwise, her personal and family histories were negative for allergy. Scratch tests were negative to inhalants and foods except for 1 plus reactions to nuts and peanuts. Scratch reactions to milk were negative in spite of our later demonstration that milk was the major cause of her food allergy (see Chapt. 2).

Food allergy was studied with our CFE diet. As shown in the temperature chart, fever disappeared in twenty-four hours after this diet was started. In one week she left the hospital. Her appetite and energy had definitely increased. In three weeks weight had increased from 108 to 119 pounds in spite of the elimination of milk, wheat, and eggs from her diet. Provocation tests thereafter with chocolate, peanuts, walnuts, and finally milk produced fever and colonic symptoms. In six weeks she drank 1 oz and the next day 2 oz of milk. On the third day abdominal pain and fever of 99.2 F developed. With the elimination of milk, these symptoms again disappeared in seven days.

As we heard from her for seven years thereafter, milk and to a lesser degree chocolate continued to reproduce symptoms. Weight increased twenty-six pounds in six months.

Thus this fever was of the persistent type without intermittent relief which often arises from refractoriness after recurrent attacks of food allergy. Moderate refractoriness at intervals during her 4½ months' hospitalization was indicated by slight reduction in fever. The persistence of fever, however, is recorded in her chart.

Comment: Chilling, goose flesh and night sweats occurred in the patient and were relieved by the elimination of allergenic foods. Children and at times adults perspire, especially on the neck and shoulders, at night soon after retiring because of food allergy, as noted in Chapter 25. Chronic food allergy is a common cause of anorexia, especially in childhood and at times in adolescents and adults.

Her initial symptoms suggested possible chronic ulcerative colitis especially because of the friability and slight oozing of bloody mucus in the rectal mucosa. If food allergy had not been recognized, CUC might have developed.

CONCLUSIONS

1. Food allergy as one cause of "unexplained fever" must be recognized. Although any food may be responsible, milk is a common offender.

2. Failure to consider allergic fever accounts for a) needless surgical operations performed because of possible foci of infection or other lesions and also for b) the unnecessary bed rest in home, hospital, or sanitarium.

3. Other manifestations of food allergy of varying severity may accompany allergic fever.

4. Chilling and night sweats often occur. Night sweats, moreover, may result from chronic food allergy in the absence of allergic fever.

5. Leukocytosis, eosinophilia, and a rapid sedimentation rate may or may not be present.

6. Allergic fever because of food allergy may occur in recurrent attacks. Usually it is persistent and somewhat fluctuating. It needs study as a cause of the convulsions in febrile seizures.

7. One case of fever resulting from food allergy associated with allergic toxemia and colitis with the recorded temperature during hospitalization for 122 days before allergy was suggested as one possible cause is reported and discussed. This graphic record of prolonged fever from food allergy is the first of its kind in the literature.

Chapter 25

Clinical Allergy in Infancy and Childhood

Allergic symptoms are extremely common in infancy and childhood resulting from allergic reactivity especially in the gastrointestinal, nasobronchial, cutaneous, and cerebral tissues and to a lesser extent in other tissues of the body. Cow's milk in early infancy and other foods as they are gradually added to the diet are responsible for most clinical allergy during the first one to two years of life. Thereafter, inhalant allergy, especially to pollens, increases with or at times without the more dominant food allergy. Possible allergy to animal emanations and other inhalants must be recognized. Glaser stated in 1956 that approximately 60 percent of children in his practice developed some clinical allergy in the first six years. Prophylactic elimination of animals and feathers and the control of dust are advisable especially if there is a familial history indicating such possible inhalant allergy.

At times ingestant and inhalant sensitizations concomitantly affect the older infants and especially children, producing the same or different allergic symptoms. Though bacterial allergy is responsible for many symptoms in infectious diseases, it rarely if ever is a fundamental cause of allergic symptoms in infants and children. This infrequency of bacterial allergy as the cause of atopic clinical allergy has been discussed and reported by many allergists and in our books in 1931, 1937, 1944, and most recently in our book on bronchial asthma in 1963. Drug allergies arise infrequently in childhood compared with adult

life. Contact allergy occasionally occurs in infants and children, requiring the avoidance of contactant allergens.

Severe, moderate, or slight manifestations of allergy occur in varying degrees in most children. The tendency to develop clinical allergy is increased when a familial history of it occurs, especially in both parents or their relatives. Many children gradually gain tolerance to allergenic foods so that gastrointestinal, nasobronchial, or cutaneous manifestations decrease or disappear in the sixth to twelfth years, especially if the allergenic foods have been eliminated from the diet for several years. Potential allergy, especially to foods, however, persists, so that the same or another manifestation of food allergy may reappear in a few years or even at any time during adult life. Inhalant allergy once established, however, usually persists and without environmental control and desensitization therapy increases in degree. All allergists emphasize the importance of the control of the early symptoms of allergy and the justification of indicated control and treatment with continued supervision for months or years to prevent chronicity and the establishment of complications and disability.

As in other periods of life, atopic allergies as a cause of symptoms frequently are overlooked. This is especially true of food allergy because of the failure to realize its many manifestations discussed in this chapter and throughout this book, failure to remember its characteristics as discussed below and in Chapter 2, failure to remember the fallibility of routine skin testing in the determination of clinical food allergy, and failure to use trial diets, especially our CFE diet or its modifications in the strict and adequate manner required to obtain good results as emphasized through this volume, particularly in Chapter 3.

OUTGROWING FOOD ALLERGY

The opinion that food allergy usually disappears during childhood is due in part to the diminishing frequency of skin reactions during this period as reported by us and other allergists and originally by Stuart and Farnham. However, when large scratch reactions as to eggs, fish, peanuts, and other foods occur which cause immediate symptoms after their ingestion, they usually persist for years even though the foods have not been eaten. When a decrease occurs, it can be explained by the exhaustion of skin-sensitizing antibodies even though other tissues of the body may still react to such allergies. The underlying sensitizations in the shock tissues have not necessarily been eradicated. Potential allergy often persists to reappear in months or years or in other manifestations of allergy to the food.

That children usually outgrow food allergy, therefore, often is not corroborated by long follow-ups of the patient. Postponing or denying children adequate study and experienced control of their allergies too often subjects them to unfortunate suffering, incapacitation, and damage to their bodies. All allergists emphasize the importance of early control of symptoms and the advisability of indicated therapy and supervision for months or years not only of inhalant allergy but, as we have long emphasized, especially food allergy to prevent chronicity and

serious complications. Such control of food allergy has increasingly been confirmed with our continued study and control with our CFE diet and its modifications.

ESTABLISHMENT OF ALLERGY, ESPECIALLY TO FOODS, IN INFANCY AND CHILDHOOD

1. Sensitization to foods *in utero* has been demonstrated especially through the studies of Ratner. His articles (1928, 1932) pointed out that overeating by the mother during pregnancy often leads to specific allergies revealed when the foods are first eaten by the infant. He attributed this fetal sensitization to the passage of the food allergens through the placenta. With such active sensitization, the mother is not necessarily allergic to the same food, though passive sensitization from the mother to the fetus may also occur. Mayerhofer (1935) emphasized sensitization in the uterus as a cause of toxic erythema, pylorospasm, melena neonatorum, laryngeal edema, and most dyspepsias in early infancy. Volkheimer (see Chapt. 28) has shown that entire solid food granules can enter the fetus from the maternal circulation. This is particularly true of starch granules found in unboiled starch as occurs in piecrust, shortbread, cookies, popcorn, and some dry breakfast cereals.

2. The studies of Shannon, O'Keefe, and Donnolly indicated that sensitization can also be established in the nursing infant by means of food proteins in the mother's milk. Walzer (1926) demonstrated conclusively that the gastrointestinal mucosa is normally permeable to whole proteins taken into the alimentary tract even in adults, and Schloss and Worthen (1916) found this especially so in marasmic infants and in those with intestinal disorders. Lippard and Schloss (1936) showed that the gastrointestinal wall remains permeable

to minute amounts of milk proteins for several months after birth and this may lead to milk allergy. Overindulgence in specific foods during nursing therefore should be discouraged, since it undoubtedly increases such proteins in the breast milk. Of interest was the finding of Kwit and Hatcher (1935) that the taking of bromide resulted in appreciable amounts of it in the breast milk. This was not so with morphine, codeine, phthalein, barbital, and only slightly with salicylate medication. Again, Volkheimer has found starch granules from food in mother's milk.

3. Food sensitization in infancy and to a lesser extent in adult life results from overfeeding and especially from the forcing of foods which are not well tolerated. It is probable, as will be pointed out later in this chapter, that many aversions and distastes which infants and children evince for specific foods are protective in nature in order that gradual immunity may be established for such foods or in order to actually prevent the infant from taking foods which are productive of allergic reactions. Thus the desire to overnourish young children should be discouraged because of possible sensitizations which may be established as well as for other reasons well recognized by pediatricians. Feeding during digestive upsets or where digestive power is below normal should be conducted with care, and well-cooked foods with moderate amounts of the indicated fresh ones should be administered.

ESTABLISHMENT AND PREVENTION OF ALLERGY TO FOODS, INHALANTS AND DRUGS IN INFANCY AND CHILDHOOD

1. It has been stated already that food allergy is the most frequent type of sensitization in infants. This most likely is due to the fact that the foreign allergens to which the infant is most exposed *in utero* are those of foods, as emphasized by Ratner, and this holds true in large part in early infancy of other food proteins eaten by the mother which appear in her breast milk. More and more intimate and prolonged exposures to the inhalant allergens, first to special animal emanations and later when the child is taken out of doors to the pollens, occur with increasing age. These sensitizations are therefore most often established after the first year. Ingestant allergy to drugs might also occur in the fetus by passive or active sensitization from the mother. Bacterial allergy might arise, though it is rarely if ever responsible for the allergic manifestations in infancy and only occasionally in late childhood. Contact eczema may arise in infancy and childhood from continued exposures to any allergenic substance as discussed but is not common in early years.

2. Possible ways in which food allergy may be established in infancy and childhood follows:

a) Overeating by the mother during pregnancy, as suggested by Ratner, and during the nursing period, according to Shannon and O'Keefe, should be interdicted. This is especially important when there is a definite allergic inheritance in the family and particularly when food allergy has been present.

b) Overfeeding in infancy and childhood, especially during digestive upsets and particularly when there is a family history of allergy, is to be avoided. Such overnourishment in the attempt to fatten patients who are underweight has in our experience resulted at times in mild or severe sensitizations and is especially unwise where allergic tendencies exist in the patient.

c) Intermittent feeding of specific foods to infants has been warned against by various students, such as MacBride (1916), Schloss, Talbot, Unger, and others. The feeding of a food, such as egg-white or cow's milk, on one or two occasions during early infancy followed by the stopping of such feeding for more than two weeks theoretically might result in sensitization from the viewpoint of experimental anaphylaxis. If a food is to be given, small amounts should be fed at first, to be followed by gradually increasing amounts every day or two until rather large amounts have been taken every day for several weeks. Such feeding should help to establish immunity and prevent the origin of a specific allergy.

3. As stated by Stuart and Farnham (1926), certain physicians recommend that in infants, especially with an allergic family history, those foods which are known to produce especially violent or active sensitizations in infancy should not be fed during the first year or two. Thus eggs are at times withheld for about eighteen months, and fish, nuts, and fresh fruits other than orange for even a longer period. This may be advisable in children with a strong inherited tendency to allergy and especially when there is a tendency to food sensitization. As a usual procedure it is unnecessary, though intermittent feeding is not advisable. Pounders (1932) recommended in infants predisposed to allergy that cow's milk be started gradually with boiled, powdered, or evaporated products and continued for several months before a gradual change to the unboiled form.

4. Infants who have definite family histories of allergy, especially to inhalants, should be protected against unnecessary inhalation of substances which might lead to allergy. Pillows might well be covered with a thin rubberized or absolutely dust-proof slip. Sensitizations to horse hair, rabbit hair, kapok, and especially to feathers according to contents of pillows have long been recognized in infants and children. Such children should not have fuzzy woolen blankets or woolen comforters. Mattresses might be covered, and the sleeping room should be devoid of carpets, furniture, drapes, flowers, and so forth which might lead to inhalant allergy. The clothing of parents or nurses as possible sources of such allergy to wool, silk, or cosmetics or allergens of dyes or fixing agents in fabrics as causes of sensitization must be considered. Coverings and fillings of toys must also receive study. During nasobronchial infections especially, the establishment of inhalant allergy from the above named sources is possible.

5. Drug and contact allergies must be thought of in infancy and childhood. The possibility of the development of sensitizations to any medicine used in the eyes, nose, and throat, given by mouth, or applied to the skin must be kept in mind. One child had slight redness from a mercury ointment soon after birth. With a reapplication, a generalized scaling erythema developed.

6. Eczema, asthma, or other manifestations of allergy present in infancy or childhood may gradually subside or disappear, the atopic allergy being reactivated in adolescence or adult life in the same or a different manifestation.

MILK AND OTHER FOOD ALLERGIES IN INFANTS

Since cow's milk is the major or only food ingested by infants, allergy to it is the usual cause of the gastrointestinal, nasobronchial, and cutaneous clinical allergies which we will discuss and which already have received consideration in our former chapters. Since cow's milk is not the natural food for the infant, the body often tries to reject it with allergic re-activity, especially when a familial tendency to allergy exists.

In brief, Schlossman, Moro, and Finkelstein (1905) first reported marked allergic symptoms from cow's milk. Hutinel (1908), Finizio (1911), and Halberstadt (1916) reported such clinical allergy including severe dramatic symptoms, even death, in infants and young children. Such death was reported by Kerley (1936) and by Parish, Barnett, *et al.* (1960). Death from probable milk allergy was also reported by Gerrard, Heiner, *et al.* (1963), pulmonary edema and congested alveolar capillaries being found at autopsy.

In the twenties Schloss, Blackfan, Talbot, and especially Park reported symptoms in children resulting from cow's milk allergy. In the next ten years O'Keefe, Kerley, Peshkin, Duke, Vaughan, Rowe, Campbell, Andresen, Casparis, and others increasingly reported clinical allergy to cow's milk.

The frequency and importance of clinical allergy to cow's milk, especially in infancy, as a sole or major cause associated with allergy to other gradually ingested foods extending throughout life justifies extended discussion, including additional reviews of articles into the thirties in Chapter 29. Case reports of invaliding and severe symptoms from milk allergy reprinted from a translation of *Alimentary Anaphylaxis* by Laroche, Richet, and Saint Girons (1908) are of special interest and importance. Personal observations and good results from recognition and control of milk with or without allergy to other foods are informative.

In the last thirty years allergy to cow's milk has received increasing emphasis by Clein, Stoesser, Rinkel, Randolph, Dees, Glaser in his excellent book *Allergy in Childhood,* Collins-Williams, Fries, Bigler, Tudor, and especially by Gerrard *et al.*

Our study of clinical allergy to cow's milk and to wheat, other cereal grains, eggs, chocolate, fish, and other less allergenic foods, all of which are out of our CFE diet, has indicated that allergy to these foods in varying degrees and especially to cow's milk, cereal grains, and eggs is frequent in children as well as in adults.

Clein's excellent article of "Cow's Milk Allergy" needs special comment. Of 140 allergic infants sensitized to cow's milk, pylorospasm occurred in 39 percent, severe colic in 29 percent, diarrhea in 24 percent, and "a very unhappy child" in 20 percent. Allergic symptoms developed during the first four months in 82 percent and were present in the first month in 39 percent. Eczema also developed in 42 percent, croup and cough in 9 percent, nasal allergy ("one cold after another") in 8 percent, asthma in 5 percent, and allergic toxemia (see Chapt. 19) in 2 percent. Other less frequent manifestations of allergy are listed in his article.

Bigler, in 1955 in his article on clinical allergy to cow's milk, reported six typical informative case histories of a) colic and diarrhea starting ten days after cow's milk was given; b) diarrhea and colic with hypoproteinemia and anorexia at the age of three months; c) severe, frequent vomiting in an infant three months of age; d) diarrhea, colic, eczema, and fever up to 105 F (from food allergy) in a child age three months; e) vomiting after meals for two years with headaches and pain in the abdomen and knees in a boy seven years of age who had been forced to drink milk (elimination of milk, egg and banana gave relief); and f) attack of swollen joints in hands, wrists, ankles, and feet with fever of 104 F (from food allergy) associated with hives in a boy seven years of age. In five years asthma from reactivated food allergy occurred, brought under control once again by the elimination of cow's milk.

In 1956 Tudor emphasized allergy to cow's milk in causing colic, vomiting, diarrhea, nasal stuffiness, coughing, wheezing, and even shock, as exemplified in infants as follows: a) constant crying and apparent abdominal pain from canned cow's milk starting in an infant at the age of two weeks; b) constant crying and pain for three weeks after canned cow's milk had replaced breast feedings (symptoms stopped in 4 days after Mull-Soy replaced cow's milk); c) vomiting all feedings of canned milk by a boy from the age of two weeks to two months (after Mull-Soy replaced cow's milk, vomiting ceased); d) daily diarrhea requiring parenteral feedings in a premature infant fed on dried milk for four days (Mull-Soy after the 21st day gave rapid lasting relief); e) diarrhea in another infant relieved with Mull-Soy; f) a rash starting in one month and naso-bronchial symptoms in two months in a boy being fed evaporated cow's milk, cereal, and vegetables being controlled by substituting canned goat's milk for cow's milk; and g) diarrhea at the age of five days in a boy fed on evaporated cow's milk who became flaccid and "limp as a rag." Many laboratory and spinal fluid tests were negative. Symptoms were relieved with our meat-base formula and recurred with evaporated milk.

A summary of recent articles on milk allergy follows.

In 1963 and especially in 1967 Gerrard *et al.* discussed allergy to cow's milk and its various manifestations in 150 sensitized infants and children and added important confirmation of the importance and frequency of cow's milk allergy and its vari-ous manifestations, as reported in this chapter. A summary of information contained in his articles follows.

The diagnosis of food allergy including that to milk depends on relief from the elimination of milk or other allergenic foods and the reproduction of the specific manifestations of the food by its inclusion in the diet. Skin testing and serum antibodies to milk proteins were of little or no help in the diagnosis. The possible role of lactase deficiency was not demonstrated.

Important symptoms of cow's milk allergy follow: diarrhea occurred in 50 of the 150 cases, diarrhea with blood in 20, vomiting in 51, recurrent bronchitis (asthmatic) in 77, rhinorrhea in 43, colic and pain in 28, asthma in 26, and eczema in 20. After initial ingestion of milk, sensitization with resultant symptoms developed in one week in 56 percent of the cases, in two weeks in 11 percent, in three to four weeks in 8 percent, in five to six weeks in 9 percent, in thirteen to twenty-four weeks in 6 percent and in twenty-five weeks to twelve years in 5 percent.

Tolerance for milk developed in ½ to 12 ½ years, allowing the inclusion of milk in the diet without obvious resultant clinical manifestations. Sensitization to other foods occurred: to soy in 27 of the 150 cases, to egg in 11, to wheat in 11, to rice and oats in 8, to beef in 7, and to chicken in 4 cases. Possible cow's milk allergy occurred in 17 percent of mothers, 7 percent of fathers, and in 34 of the 225 siblings.

Breast milk relieved practically all allergic symptoms arising from cow's milk. Tolerance for cow's milk and not for breast milk occurred in only two babies. This suggests that there were foods secreted from the mother's diet into her milk to which the child was allergic. One child was relieved by the elimination of cow's milk from the mother's diet. Later 8 cc of milk in the mother's coffee reproduced asthma in the nursing child. This helps to confirm the secretion of cow's milk allergen and that of other ingested foods into the mother's milk. Hence allergic symptoms in a nursing infant may be relieved by the exclusion of allergenic foods in the mother's diet, best accomplished with our CFE diet as advised in Chapter 3. The importance of preventing the baby's inhalation of possible airborne food allergens from the cooking of allergenic foods not mentioned by Gerrard has been emphasized in this book, particularly in Chapter 3. The presence of foods in cow's milk from the foods eaten by the cow suggests, according to Gerrard, that clinical allergy may vary according to foods eaten by the cow. The recognition and control of allergy to cow's milk and other foods will reduce concern and frustration of parents and also decrease medical expense for the control of the child's allergic symptoms.

Gerrard advises soy milk if the baby is not breast fed. As stated in Chapter 3, we use Mull-Soy, which contains cane rather than corn sugar. He also advises our meat-base formula if soy allergy occurs.

Additional information about allergy to cow's milk was published by Goldman *et al.* in eighty-nine children in 1963 which is summarized in Chapter 29. Deaths reported by him are probably comparable to "crib deaths" reported in the literature. Hill in 1940 reported shock and collapse in nursing infants from ingestion of a trace of cow's milk.

Additional information about the literature of milk allergy which we published in 1938 is in Chapter 29.

Gryboski, in 1967, reported histological evidence of colitis from milk allergy in twenty-one infants studied in a sixteen-year period. Age varied from 2 days to 2½

years. Symptoms developed in the first six weeks of life. Vomiting and colic occurred in some infants. Relief failed with soybean formulae and only with our lamb-base formula in three infants. Melena occurred in two cases. Tolerance for milk seemed to occur in three to five years. Other manifestations of allergy occurred in ten patients.

LACTASE DEFICIENCY VERSUS MILK ALLERGY

That disaccharide intolerance resulting from deficiency of disaccharidase activity in the intestinal mucosa in celiac disease might cause diarrhea was reported by Wisgers *et al.* in 1966. Gerrard and Lubos, in 1967, emphasized usual relief from a wheat-free and rye-free diet and advised later from elimination of lactase in milk and disaccharide when the exclusion of gluten fails. It was also discussed recently by McDonagh (1969) in the causation of gastrointestinal symptoms.

That the relief from total elimination of milk can be explained by allergy rather than by lactase deficiency has been opined by several investigators, including Gerrard. In regard to milk, allergy thereto seems a more likely cause than lactase deficiency, since the amount of lactose in a minute quantity of ingested milk, which will prevent relief of celiac disease and other clinical manifestations of milk allergy such as asthma, eczema, CUC, and RE, would not appear to contain sufficient lactose to cause these diseases. Symptoms from ingested lactose also do not necessarily confirm this etiology as most lactose is contaminated by milk proteins (see also Chapt. 28 and Table XLV).

EGG ALLERGY

Allergy to eggs in infancy and young children occurs less frequently than to cow's milk. In contrast to cow's milk, it causes more severe, immediate clinical manifestations of allergy. When it is severe in degree, it gives rise to bronchial asthma, nasal allergy, eczema, or gastrointestinal symptoms in a few to thirty minutes. Large scratch reactions to eggs, four to six plus in size, occur when such severe immediate clinical allergy arises, causing erythema and edema in the lips, tongue, or mouth when egg is tasted or even when it touches the lips. Fastidious elimination of traces of egg from the diet is imperative. Localized or generalized hives or nasal allergy, varying degrees of asthma, and activation or exaggeration of eczema or of other manifestations of egg allergy may rapidly arise. When such severe allergy is present, the child should not inhale any odor from eggs when they are cooked or be in a room when eggs are even broken or being mixed in other foods. It also is often advisable to keep eggs out of the refrigerator, even out of the house when large four to six plus scratch reactions occur to eggs and particularly when obvious immediate allergy to eggs occurs.

Egg allergy was more frequent in infants before 1930 when eggs especially the yolks were often included in infant's feedings. This incorporation led to the development of clinical allergy in susceptible infants to eggs, often of a severe degree. Clein stated that 90 percent of allergic babies before 1934 fed milk formulae containing raw eggs developed a rash, pylorospasm, or gastrointestinal distress greatly reduced since the discontinuance of egg yolk in infant's formulae. The manifestations of egg allergy still develop in sensitized infants while they are in kitchens where eggs are being cooked as such or cooked with other foods.

The occurrence of large scratch reactions to eggs, fish, peanuts, or to a lesser

extent other foods which may cause the immediate severe type of clinical allergy justifies routine scratch tests with all foods eaten by older infants or children, as discussed in Chapter 2, even though most foods causing delayed or cumulative clinical allergy are not demonstrated by scratch reactions. And, as reiterated in this book, the clinical importance of most of these large reactions and especially of the smaller reactions to foods must be determined by provocation tests in the symptom-free patient. These provocative tests are unnecessary if the child's history reveals indisputable immediate clinical allergy to the large-reacting foods in whom, for example, the tasting of egg and especially the swallowing of it has been known to cause edema of the mouth, throat, or even the larynx; severe edema of the esophagus or stomach; asthma collapse; and in very rare occasions death.

ALLERGY TO OTHER FOODS AS THEY ARE ADDED TO THE INFANT'S AND CHILD'S DIET

Pediatricians for years, even up to the present time, have given orange juice along with cow's milk in the initial infant's formulae. This had led to sensitization to orange evidenced by varying degrees of erythema or eruption on the skin. This accounts in part for today's opinion that it is not advisable to include orange juice in the diets of young infants and also accounts for its omission from our CFE diet (Chapt. 3) for the study of food allergy even in those described for older children and adults.

As stated above, moreover, allergy to additional foods, especially to wheat, corn, rice and oats, chocolate, fish, and to meats, fowl, vegetables, fruits, spices, and condiments develops in a limited number of infants, children, and adults as such foods are gradually added to the diet. Though such sensitizations are not the rule, they do occur particularly when there is a familial inheritance of allergy, especially to foods, and when such inheritance occurs in the families of both parents.

Our discussion of clinical allergies to these various foods, as published in 1937 and with additional information since then, is reported in Chapter 29.

CROUP

Croup characterized by recurrent attacks of spasmodic laryngitis lasting for two to four days especially at night and by usual moderate tracheitis and pharyngitis with slight or absent fever is best explained by food allergy rather than infection. The occurrence of colic, usually to milk allergy, and the later development of nasal allergy and of bronchial asthma with its typical history because of food allergy we have long reported favor allergy in the causation of croup.

Attacks of bronchial asthma or allergic bronchitis are often misdiagnosed as croup or even pneumonia. Bronchospasm and cough with varying amounts of mucus require the study of food allergy as their cause. As emphasized in Chapter 24 fever in such attacks is usually due to food allergy rather than infection.

If secondary infection in the larynx, trachea, or nasosinal tissues occurs, antibiotics are required. Diphtheria must always be considered.

STUDY AND CONTROL OF ALLERGIC CAUSES OF CROUP

When cow's milk is in the infant's or child's diet, allergy to it should be studied by its substitution with Mull-Soy (which contains sucrose rather than corn sugar). If allergy to soy is evident, then our beef or lamb-base formulae (Gerber) will usually relieve allergy to cow's or goat's milk.

If croup occurs in breast-fed infants, sensitization to food allergens in the milk through their ingestion by the mother may be responsible. Then croup may be controlled when the mother's diet is limited to the foods in our CFE diet as advised in this chapter. Traces of milk from unclean dishes, spoons or pans, on lips from adults by kissing, or by inhalation of allergens from cooking milk products may explain clinical allergy from milk.

When croup occurs in older infants and children who are eating most foods, probable food allergy is studied and usually controlled with our CFE diet or its modifications advised in Chapter 3.

SKIN TESTS WITH FOOD

Skin tests with milk and egg allergens may be done even in the first two or three months of life. As reiterated throughout this volume, however, a negative test to milk does not rule out clinical allergy thereto. A large scratch reaction to eggs often indicates severe allergy to eggs. This makes removal of eggs from the refrigerator and at times from the home advisable, even though the baby is not eating eggs. The infant, moreover, should not be in the kitchen when foods eliminated from the diet, especially eggs, are cooked.

When other foods are being eaten, skin testing with the puncture method in infants after the age of one or two months and with the puncture or scratch test in older infants and young children is routine in our practice, as advised in Chapter 2. Though information from skin testing is limited, it is justifiable but only with those foods ingested and inhalants inhaled by the child. Interpretation of the clinical significance of positive reactions and also of negative reactions to allergenic foods as well as inhalants is advised in Chapter 2.

The gradual development of positive protein skin reactions to foods in childhood and their usual absence in the first month or two of infancy has long been reported.

POSSIBLE INHALANT ALLERGY

As a routine when croup or other nasal bronchial allergy is present, the mattress should be covered with extra sheets and a Dacron pillow or no pillow should be used. Though inhalant allergy in infancy and in older children is an unlikely cause of croup, its consideration is justifiable. Food allergy is the probable cause and requires accurate study and control as we advise.

CONTROL OF THE SYMPTOMS OF CROUP WITH DRUGS

Since allergy requires study as the major cause of severe croup, hypodermic administration of .05 to .15 cc of epinephrine 1:1000 dilution, the dose varying with age and weight of the child, is justified. If relief occurs, the dose can be repeated every one to two hours for relief.

Corticosteroids are also justified in doses advised for each commercial preparation according to the child's age to relieve the symptoms of recurrent attacks or gradually control the persistent cough between such episodes. Long-term use of corticosteroids is never allowed in our practice, nor is it necessary because of our control of allergy, especially to foods.

In older infants and children, syrup of ipecac in doses advised in pediatric textbooks to produce vomiting of mucus may be justified.

Absence of advice in textbooks on pediatrics about the study and control of allergy, especially to foods, as the major cause of croup is unfortunate, according to our experience. Nonrecognition of food allergy is due to too frequent skepticism about the major role of food allergy in bronchial asthma and other nasobronchial symptoms. Realization of the important role of food allergy in croup will occur if an open mind about the frequency of food allergy develops and especially with the accurate use of our CFE diet and its modifications for study and control of such allergy.

CASE HISTORIES

Case 196: A boy 2½ years of age first developed croup, causing a barking cough, choking, and shortness of breath associated with slight or no fever lasting two to five days, recurring every month or so at the age of one year. Its absence in the summer favored food allergy (Chapt. 1). In the fall and winter, in addition to these severe attacks, an unproductive cough occurred each night associated with irritability, crying, and crankiness. Moderate coughing during the day had occurred for four months. Allergy was not suggested in his history. His grandmother, maternal uncle, and paternal great-uncle had bronchial asthma. Moderate rhonchi and wheezing were heard throughout the lungs. Skin reactions to foods and inhalants were negative.

Treatment: With the study of food allergy with our CFE diet, all symptoms of croup disappeared in 1½ weeks' time. Rice, oats, and additional vegetables and fruits were added in the following six months, and no reactivation of his symptoms occurred. Tolerance for all foods was reported in 1½ years, during which time croup had not recurred.

Case 197: A girl eight years of age had had bronchial attacks every month except July and August diagnosed as croup for four years. Fever and vomiting were absent. For two months shortness of breath and some wheezing had indicated bronchial asthma.

She had disliked and refused milk all her life. Chocolate had caused vomiting. A great uncle had asthma. An aunt had eczema of the ears.

Edema of the nasal mucosa and wheezing were present. Scratch tests gave moderate reactions to pollens but none to foods.

Treatment: Since the history indicated food allergy, it was studied with our CFE diet. All symptoms disappeared in a month's time. "Marked increase in energy and appetite and pep" occurred. No symptoms recurred with a general diet during the summer until October, when our CFE diet was required to control reactivated bronchial symptoms.

Thus these symptoms formerly diagnosed as croup constituted the early equivalent of bronchial asthma.

BRONCHIOLITIS (CAPILLARY BRONCHITIS)

Bronchiolitis is characterized by coughing, diffuse moist rales and rhonchi throughout the lungs, shortness of breath, and nasal congestion and discharge with only moderate or no fever. The attacks usually last for three to five days, recurring every two to four weeks. At times interim moderate nasobronchial symptoms, even a croupy cough, occur.

This syndrome, according to our experience, is practically always the equivalent of recurrent bronchial asthma resulting from food allergy, as reported in this chapter and Chapter 8. These cases always require study of allergy to inhalants and especially to foods as we advise. Though wheezing and marked bronchospasm may be absent or mild in degree, the symptoms often evolve into obvious recurrent bronchial asthma resulting from food allergy. Other manifestations of atopic allergy are often present or gradually develop. A familial history of allergy is frequent.

Secondary infection in the nasopharyngeal and bronchial tissues may occur and require antibiotics best given by mouth with a preference to the mycin drugs rather than penicillin. Though pneumonitis is infrequent, it must be suspected if fever increases and persists for two or three days. Its demonstration by x-ray is important. Even if definite infection is present, accurate study of allergy, especially to foods, as advised in our discussion of bronchial asthma in this chapter and in Chapter 8 is mandatory. Along with the immediate

study of food allergy and of infrequent inhalant allergy with environmental control, relief of symptoms with Adrenalin® and corticoids, as advised in "The Treatment of Bronchial Asthma" in this chapter is important. If secondary infection is probable, antibiotics, especially with a mycin drug, is indicated.

These attacks of bronchiolitis usually are controlled in one to four days. Placing these children in mistogen or moisture-laden air is unnecessary when the control of allergy, especially to foods, is immediately established. Difficulty in breathing may be increased, causing restlessness and general discomfort in a vapor-filled atmosphere. As in bronchial asthma, sedatives are contraindicated because of impairment of respiratory efficiency. If coughing is severe, small doses of codeine in simple elixir, however, may be justifiable for a few days until food allergy is controlled.

The importance of controlling allergy in these patients is supported by the reports of Wittig, Crawford, and Glaser; of a history of respiratory allergy in 49 percent of the cases; and the development of bronchial asthma in 32 percent of children with bronchiolitis. Favoring food allergy, moreover, is the occurrence of two of the important characteristics of such allergy in histories of patients with bronchiolitis:

1. The cyclic recurrence of the attacks.
2. Their occurrence in the fall, winter, and spring, with usual absence in the summer.

These characteristics are further discussed in Chapter 1. Dennis, moreover, reported recurrent bronchiolitis in infancy in 54 percent of asthmatic children, indicating that the early bronchiolitis was probably an equivalent of the recurrent bronchial asthma resulting from food allergy which gradually developed thereafter. We opine that such allergy must be studied with our CFE diet as advised for infants and young children in this and especially in Chapter 3.

HISTORIES

Case 198: A girl six years of age had "recurrent bronchiolitis" with moderate wheezing and a fever at times up to 104 F. Attacks lasted three to four days every month from September to June, with relief in the summer. Such attacks had occurred since the age of one week. Attacks were initiated with nasal congestion and sneezing. There was some interim nasal congestion and a hacking cough in the morning and evening. Penicillin had always been given during the attacks.

Irritability, restless sleep, and frequent crying during the night evidenced probable allergic toxemia (see Chapt. 19).

The maternal grandmother had asthma. The mother had eczema.

Scratch testing gave reactions to a few pollens and to wheat and milk.

Because of a history being equivalent to the pathognomonic history of bronchial asthma resulting from food allergy, such allergy was studied with our CFE diet. During the next five years bronchiolitis and evidence of bronchial asthma did not recur except when milk, wheat, and other cereal grains were added to her diet.

RECURRENT OR CHRONIC BRONCHITIS OR HEAD COLDS

It is important to consider allergy as the cause of chronic bronchitis in children as it is in adults, as emphasized in Chapter 9. If the bronchitis is activated in the fall, winter, and early spring and especially if it is exaggerated for a few days or a week or so every three to four weeks, even though daily coughing especially during the night continues, food allergy requires definite consideration. Such recurrent attacks of coughing with varying degrees of bronchial mucus are equivalent to recurrent attacks of bronchial asthma resulting from food allergy which are decreased in the summer months. That food allergy especially to milk in children must be stud-

ied as the cause of recurrent bronchitis with or without wheezing and usually with rhinorrhea and the frequency of its familial occurrence is reported by Gerrard in an excellent article in 1966. On the contrary, bronchial cough from pollen allergy in the spring, summer, and fall is absent or definitely decreased during the winter, and it does not occur or become activated in cyclic attacks. Pollen allergy produces symptoms every day that causative pollens are in the air, decreasing on rainy days during the pollen season.

Though food allergy is the major cause of these symptoms in the fall, winter, and early spring, allergy to house dust, animal emanations, and other environmental allergens in the home or working environments also produces daily cough. Such symptoms, however, are not activated at regular recurrent intervals as are the bronchial symptoms from food allergy (see Chapt. 8). Before assuming and limiting treatment to inhalant allergies, sufficient strict study and control of food allergy is important, as we advise. This especially is indicated if treatment based on inhalant allergy has not been beneficial. Animal emanation allergy is important to recognize if animals, including birds, are in the home or have been kept in the house by previous occupants. Though skin reactions to such emanations usually occur, they may be absent. The diagnosis then depends on a well-taken history. As emphasized in our following discussion of bronchial asthma resulting from food allergy "head colds" before recurrent bronchial asthma or bronchitis are practically always due to food allergy rather than infection.

Continued coughing with or without asthma or nasal allergy may also be due to allergies to spores of fungi in the air of the home or other environments. Such spores may come from fungi in carpets or from damp areas on the floors in which fungi are growing on the grounds, girders, or foundation under the house, particularly if dampness is present. Allergy to airborne fungi out-of-doors is, according to our experience, infrequent possibly because of the low humidity which is characteristic of most of the California and adjoining mountain areas or because of our persistent and advised study and frequent recognition of food allergy. Evidence of allergy to airborne spores of fungi in our practice is less frequent in children than it is in adults (Chapt. 8).

Nasobronchial allergy to house dust alone may cause bronchitis. It is worthy of consideration if large scratch reactions occurs to stock dust or to an antigen made from the carpet or floor dust of the patient's home. It must be remembered, however, that many patients with large reactions to house dust have no clinical allergy thereto. This is also true of many patients who give reactions to pollen or other inhalant allergens.

Strict control of the house dust together with allergen-free pillow, bedding, furniture, and carpets as advised in most textbooks on asthma will relieve most house dust allergy without desensitization. Too often such desensitization is given and continued for months or longer periods when strict environmental control alone would render relief. Too often, moreover, desensitization with "conventional antigens" containing dust, fungi, and other inhalants, including pollen, is given, even for years, when unrecognized and uncontrolled food allergy is the sole cause. It must be remembered, however, that chronic bronchitis with or without asthma, which is relieved by moving into dust-free and animal emanation-free houses and recurs on return to the patient's former home, requires study of allergy to animal emana-

tion, fungi, and other environmental dusts in the home. As noted above, however, unrecognized food allergy may be the sole or an associated cause. Allergy to pollens during the winter, when they are absent from the air, can be excluded as a cause of persistent bronchial allergy unless pollens remain in house dusts. Perennial desensitization with skin-reacting pollens rarely if ever will relieve symptoms present during the winter.

As emphasized in Chapters 8 and 9, the many marked or infrequent causes of coughing, wheezing, and shortness of breath other than allergy must be remembered and ruled out by physical examination or indicated x-ray and laboratory studies in chronic bronchitis and in bronchial asthma as discussed later in this chapter.

Food allergy especially needs emphasis as a cause of bronchitis and coughing and mucoid expectoration at times associated with mild fever or exaggerated during the fall and winter and spring months. Food allergy unfortunately is overlooked by many physicians and allergists today as a cause of nasobronchial and the many other manifestations of food allergy because of the usual impossibility of demonstrating any or all food allergy by protein skin tests and because of the failure to use trial diets, especially our CFE diet, in an adequate manner as emphasized and advised throughout this volume. Allergy to other inhalants as the cause of bronchitis during the fall, winter, and early spring months must be remembered but is a less frequent cause in our experience than food allergy. As emphasized above, viral and bacterial infections as causes of bronchitis, which does not produce regular recurrent attacks and may arise during the summer months, always need recognition and proper therapy.

RECURRENT HEAD COLDS

Allergy to foods and less so to inhalants in causing "head colds" pertains only to quite regularly "recurrent colds." Colds from viral or bacterial infections are usually followed by relative immunity for more than three or four weeks and are usually associated with fever, malaise, nausea, or bodily aching.

Allergy especially to foods causes nasal and sinal colds at fairly regular intervals every month or so, particularly in the fall, winter, and early spring. Fever may or may not be present. When infectious colds occur, antibiotics are advisable. The "mycin" drugs rather than penicillin are preferred in our practice.

CASE HISTORY

Case 199: A girl nine years of age had had recurrent "colds" characterized by nasal congestion, sneezing, coughing, and no itching of eyes or nose or fever lasting one to two weeks every one to two months especially from early fall to late spring for seven years. After tonsillectomy, perennial nasal blocking had increased, and hearing diminished.

Scratch tests with protein food and inhalant allergens were negative.

A grandmother had sick headaches.

Treatment and results: Food allergy indicated by the quite regular recurrence of the colds, worse in the winter half of the year was studied with our CFE diet. After relief for three months breaks in diet caused a recurrence of the "colds." "Radium treatment" was given for three months with no benefit. Then our CFE diet was resumed, with resulting relief for five months. Provocation tests with additional foods showed milk and all cereal grains reproduced the head colds.

BRONCHIAL ASTHMA IN CHILDREN FROM FOOD AND INHALANT ALLERGIES

Food allergy in our experience is a more frequent cause of bronchial asthma in childhood, especially in infants and young children up to the age of six years, than inhalant allergy. Our increasingly excellent or good control of such asthma has affirmed our statement thirty-eight years ago in the first edition of this book that "bronchial asthma in the first two or three years of life is most frequently due to food allergy" with a gradual increase of inhalant allergy during late childhood. This importance of food allergy in bronchial asthma in childhood was emphasized by our analysis of its causes in 411 controlled patients cooperating for a minimum of six months treated during a six-year period up to and including 1947 and by good results reported in former articles. Its importance increasingly has been confirmed, moreover, in the last twenty-four years, as reported in articles on bronchial asthma resulting from food allergy in 1952, 1959, and especially in our book *Bronchial Asthma—Its Diagnosis and Treatment* in 1963. The reader is referred particularly to our article "Bronchial Asthma in Infants and Children" in 1948, in which the following statistics on 156 children, ages 0 to 5, and 255 children, ages 5 to 15, relieved of bronchial asthma in the preceding seven years were reported.

These statistics are also included in Table XVIII in Chapter 8 along with those relieved of bronchial asthma in adult life and in old age. Of great importance was the occurrence of this relief up to 1947 before corticosteroids were available. It must also be emphasized that all of these patients cooperated with us for a minimum of six months extending to six years. Cooperation for one or even two months is not adequate and unfortunately results in the conclusion that our CFE diet is of questionable value in recognizing and controlling food allergy in perennial bronchial asthma.

In infancy and early childhood, food allergy alone was adjudged causative in 50 percent. From the age of five to fifteen it was the sole cause in 25 percent. This latter percentage is to be compared to the 20 percent in adult life and with 40 percent in old age as shown in Chapter 8.

In childhood mild to severe food allergy with or without inhalant allergy required control in 82 percent as compared with inhalant allergy, especially to pollens, in 66 percent. House dust and fungus allergy probably are decreased by the low humidity and the mild winters in Northern California. In contrast to other opinions, bacterial allergy or infectant asthma was not the sole cause in any patient and was a secondary factor in only 1 percent, as stressed in Chapter 8. Tonsillectomy, nasal or sinal surgery, or irradiation of the nasal pharynx was not done in any patient to obtain these good results. Previous tonsillectomy, however, has been done in many patients without benefit. Further comments on infectant allergy are in this chapter and also Chapter 8. We agree that tonsils should be removed only because of infection, remembering however the onset of asthma after tonsillectomy, as reported by Peshkin, Piness, Tuft, and others, a result in our opinion, of uncontrolled inhalant and especially food allergy.

With control of inhalant and especially of food allergy, evidence of infectant, intrinsic, and psychogenic causes has reduced to a minimum. With cooperation of children and parents in our control of inhalant and especially of food allergy, psychological studies on children and parents, parentectomy, breathing exercises, and long-term sanitarium care or residential treatment have been unnecessary. It must be emphasized that no long-term corticoid therapy has been or is being given to control asthma in our young and older children treated and with the parents' cooperation, as we advise.

If inhalant and especially food allergy were controlled as we advise, most asthma in children being sent to sanitaria, in our opinion, would be controlled at home. Moreover, in our opinion food allergy should be so studied and controlled as we advise in all recurrently activated or persistent perennial asthma while in such sanitaria.

RETARDATION OF GROWTH AND NUTRITION FROM PERENNIAL ASTHMA RESULTING FROM FOOD ALLERGY

This has been discussed in Chapter 8.

TYPICAL HISTORY OF BRONCHIAL ASTHMA RESULTING FROM FOOD ALLERGY IN INFANTS AND CHILDREN

The typical and in our opinion pathognomonic history of bronchial asthma resulting from food allergy in childhood, at times extending into adolescence and young adult life, reported by us for over twenty-five years would not have been recognized without the accurate and strict use of our CFE diet. This deserves special emphasis. This important history, already described in Chapter 5, is summarized as follows:

A pathognomonic history of bronchial asthma (resulting from food allergy), especially in children (Fig. 6, Chapt. 8) has long been evident in our cases. Attacks usually begin in the fourteenth to the twenty-fourth month, although they may commence at any time in infancy and adult life. They recur regularly every two to eight weeks. They are often absent or less frequent or severe in the summer, recurring from the fall to the late spring, especially in the winter. Nasal allergy suggesting a cold often precedes and/or accompanies the asthma. Asthma with varying dyspnea, wheezing, tightness in the chest, or coughing then develops. This lasts for one to three days with a sudden or gradual decrease up to five days. Anorexia may precede and continue during the attacks. When severe, vomiting and fever up to 104 F (40 C) from food allergy and not from infection, as noted in Chapter 24 may occur. As the attacks recur, interim relief may be replaced by moderate wheezing, coughing, and tightness in the chest, especially with exercise and at night if food allergy is not controlled.

This history is characterized by recurrent attacks of asthma in the fall, winter, and spring, absent or infrequent in the summer, often with vomiting, usually with preceding "colds" for one to three days, often associated with fever even up to 105 F for one day because of food allergy in our opinion and not to infection. The attacks recur every two to six weeks, lasting two to five days, varying in degree. Coryza, nasal congestion, sneezing, and often fever up to 105 F rectally because food allergy rather than infectious colds may precede the asthma by four to twenty-four hours or may arise with and continue through the attack. Itching or sneezing are absent or rare compared to that from inhalant and especially pollen allergy.

This usual regularity of attacks of exaggeration of symptoms from food allergy may be altered by variables. These include temporary delay in the increase of the specific reacting antibodies sufficient to produce the severe attacks of asthma or a temporary decrease in the allergic reactivity or even a partial anergy, all of which are hypothetical and are only supported by clinical observations. These attacks and symptoms in certain patients are also favorably influenced in inland, dry areas and also in the late spring and summer months, as already discussed.

We hypothesize that during these attacks antibodies to specific foods attached to the cells of the lungs and especially the airways and nasal mucosa are inactivated by uniting with their respective blood-borne previously ingested food allergens. The exhaustion of these antibodies allows the causative foods to be eaten with no symptoms after the attack. When the antibodies reaccumulate above the hypothetical reacting threshold, attacks of asthma recur as the allergenic foods continue to be eaten. During sudden, severe attacks terminating in one to three days, all reacting antibodies seem to be exhausted, whereas during more moderate and longer attacks these assumed antibodies are inactivated more slowly. If food allergy is not controlled, the length of refractoriness after attacks is decreased and moderate coughing, wheezing, and nasal allergy persist because of failure of antibodies to decrease below the hypothetical reacting threshold. If food allergy is not controlled, especially as we advise, refractoriness after attacks decreases, and daily coughing usually with wheezing and dyspnea with exercise and especially on retiring and through the night continues and intractable asthma may result. These persistent symptoms usually are recurrently exaggerated especially in the fall and winter, such exaggeration being the equivalent of the previous cyclic attacks of bronchial asthma because of food allergy. This recurrence of bronchial allergy from food sensitization was reported by Gerrard in 1966.

We have reported this typical pathognomonic history of bronchial asthma resulting from food allergy, especially in 1948, 1959, and in 1967 and also in our book *Bronchial Asthma—Its Diagnosis and Treatment*, in 1963. In Chapter 7 of the above book there are detailed summaries of typical histories, laboratory tests, and good results from the use of our CFE diet in eighteen infants and children up to the age of fifteen years in all of whom definite, often chronic recurrent bronchial asthma was present.

These results emphasize the importance of food allergy alone and at times in association with inhalant allergy as a cause of bronchial asthma. As stated in Chapter 8, summaries of only a few cases of marked bronchial asthma resulting from pollen and other inhalant allergies alone or at times associated with food allergy were reported because of the general recognition of inhalant allergy in the causation of such asthma.

INDICATIONS OF FOOD ALLERGY IN BRONCHIAL ASTHMA

1. The pathognomonic history resulting from food allergy already summarized.

2. History of asthma from specific foods (see Chapt. 2).

a. Dislikes or disagreements suggest but do not prove clinical allergy.

b. Diet diaries rarely list all ingested foods. We feel, therefore, that time required in the preparation of such diaries and in the analyses of such diaries by the doctor usually is not warranted.

3. Former croup, recurrent bronchiolitis, nasobronchial colds, recurrent serous otitis media, fever up to 104 to 105 F and other manifestations as a result of possible allergy to foods, especially animal milk.

4. These indications of food allergy are more fully discussed in Chapter 1.

5. Large scratch reactions to foods may indicate immediate allergy. Other scratch tests often fail to reveal any or all allergenic foods. Scratch and not intradermal tests are routine.

a. Ingestion provocation tests are necessary to confirm possible allergy to foods

indicated by positive even large skin tests or to foods giving negative skin reactions.

6. Test-negative diets infrequently control food allergy.

7. Relief of at least two anticipated recurrent attacks and interim symptoms with our CFE diet or its modification with no injectant or drug therapy or corticosteroids confirms food allergy. Associated inhalant allergy must be recognized.

(These have been discussed more fully in Chapter 2.)

INHALANT ALLERGY

Inhalant allergy as evidenced in Chapter 8 has been the sole indicated cause of asthma in 10 percent and a contributing cause associated with food allergy in 39 percent. Thus asthma especially in the fall, winter, and early spring is often due to food, with symptoms in the late spring, summer, and early fall resulting from pollen allergy. Other inhalant allergy also modifies the pathognomonic or its equivalent history because of food allergy. The role of such inhalant allergies in causation of asthma is indicated by history aided by skin test results.

INDICATIONS OF INHALANT ALLERGY

1. Symptoms when airborne allergens of pollens, animal emanations, house dust, spores of fungi, and other environmental allergens are inhaled.

2. Positive skin reactions to inhalants.

a. May be negative in 10 percent to 15 percent of cases though history indicates clinical allergy.

b. All positive reactions do not indicate clinical allergy.

3. Positive provocation inhalant tests and relief from desensitization or environmental control confirm such allergy.

EVIDENCE AGAINST INFECTANT ASTHMA

1. When food allergy is controlled, recurrent "colds" at times with fever up to 104 F (from food allergy) associated or followed by bronchial asthma do not occur.

2. Removal of infected tonsils and adenoidectomy has not relieved asthma.

3. When allergy, especially to foods, is controlled, infectious colds do not cause asthma.

4. Vaccine therapy has not been used to control asthma and when given by other allergists has not yielded results comparable to ours with such therapy.

Our experience supports our statement in the first edition of this book in 1931 "that much so-called bacterial asthma in children is really due to unrecognized food allergy."

FOOD ALLERGY AS A SOLE CAUSE OF ASTHMA IN INFANTS AND CHILDREN

To emphasize food allergy as a sole cause of bronchial asthma, the statistics in Table XLIII on 130 infants and children published in 1967 follow. These corroborate the conclusions from similar statistics on fifty cases we published in the *JAMA* in 1959.

The asthma in these 130 infants and children whose statistics are in Table XLIII was controlled with the elimination of allergenic foods alone with no injections of inhalant allergens, no vaccines or gamma globulin, and with no corticosteroids or antibiotics. Many more cases resulting from food allergy alone are omitted because of brief or longer injections of antigens or vaccines even on one or two occasions which we now realize were given largely because of positive skin reactions or hoping to increase bacterial or viral immunity. Though antibiotics are not given to control

TABLE XLIII

BRONCHIAL ASTHMA IN 130 INFANTS AND CHILDREN FROM FOOD ALLERGY ALONE

(No corticoids, drugs, vaccine, or desensitization given to maintain relief)

Males	70%
Females	30%
Age, in years	3/4-13
Age, at onset (av. 1.6)	1/20-11
Years of asthma (av. 3.4)	1/4-12
Typical history from food allergy	72%
Less typical history	16%
"Cold" at onset	70%
Fever (99.6-105 F)	54%
Vomiting	22%
Attacks absent in summer	64%
Attacks less in summer	22%
Between attacks	
Nasal symptoms	52%
Coughing	20%
Former eczema	30%
Former GI symptoms	20%
History of possible food allergy	36%
Family history of possible allergy	73%
Eosinophilia (4%-37%)	60%
Skin Reactions (Scratch)	
Foods	27%
Pollens*	34%
Animal emanations*	11%
Miscellaneous inhalants*	4%
House dust*	20%
Years of cooperation (½-10 years)	
Average years	2.8

*No desensitization to inhalants. Relief a result of control of food allergy.

asthma, they were given if occasional definite infection in tonsils, nose, sinuses, or lungs as indicated by laboratory or x-ray studies or if respiratory infection occurs without asthma between the attacks.

The classic or nearly typical history of bronchial asthma resulting from food allergy occurred in 72 percent, as shown in Table XLIII. Initial "colds" from food allergy and suggesting infection occurred in 70 percent. Fever nearly always a result of food allergy occurred in 86 percent. Nasal allergy between the attacks occurred in 52 percent. Associated eczema and gastrointestinal symptoms occurred in 30 and 20 percent, respectively. The skin reactions to foods in 27 percent were of little clinical importance. Desensitization based solely on reactions to inhalants was not given in these cases. The diet history of possible or proven food allergies correlated with clinical allergies in only a few patients.

CASE REPORTS

Case 200: A boy twenty-six months of age had had bronchial asthma every month for 1½ years starting with a "nasal cold" followed by dyspnea, coughing, wheezing, and fever of 101 F for 2 days.

Recurrent "head colds" every month had recurred in infancy. Eczema on the face lasted for three to nine months. His diet history was negative for allergy. Skin tests were positive to feathers, dog hair, and fall pollens.

Because of his recurrent attacks, food allergy was studied with our CFE diet. No desensitization to inhalants or vaccine was given. In the first year asthma recurred two times after the ingestion of rice. In the second all foods were tolerated except milk.

Case 201: A boy five years of age had attacks of asthma every two weeks in the first year and every month since then, symptoms being absent in summer. All were preceded by nasal symptoms. Skin tests were positive to spring and fall pollens and negative to foods.

With the CFE diet asthma was absent in one month. Rice, corn, and oats were added in the summer. Asthma recurred in September, and the cereals were eliminated, with resultant relief. Control has continued for three years, the original diet being necessary during the fall to late spring and all foods being tolerated in June, July, and August. Former absence from school one half of the time was replaced by no absences. No desensitization to inhalants was given.

Case 202: A boy fourteen years of age, had had asthma for two to three days every ten to fourteen days preceded by "a head cold" from the age of two to fourteen years. He was better in the summer. For three years asthma continued with no severe attacks with the inhalation of epinephrine 1:100 five to seven times a day. Skin tests were positive to dust, cat hair, spring and fall pollens, corn, rice, and wheat. X-ray of the lungs revealed hyperinflation. With our CFE diet symptoms were controlled in one month. No desensitization was given. Asthma recurred from eating cereal grains. In three years milk alone caused asthma in the winter. He had gained seventeen pounds and grown three inches. No desensitization or vaccines were given.

Many more case reports of bronchial asthma from food allergy alone are in the Appendix of our book *Bronchial Asthma—Its Diagnosis and Treatment,* 1963, the reading of which is strongly advised to the physician challenged with bronchial asthma in infants and children.

Inhalant allergy with or without food allergy receives important discussion in this chapter.

CONTROL OF FOOD ALLERGY

When the above indications of food allergy occur, our CFE diet is immediately ordered in office, clinic, or hospital. Its successful use has emphasized the necessity of the initial study of allergy to all cereals including wheat along with milk and eggs and other foods causing less frequent allergy. Because of negative skin reactions and the fallibility of positive skin reactions to reveal clinical allergy, test-negative diets are rarely used. The list of prescribed foods, menus, and recipes for bakery products must be given to the parents or patients.

The CFE diet for infants with menus is detailed in Chapter 3. For successful use of this diet, directions for its cooking, maintenance, and manipulation as indicated by our continued and successful use of this diet for thirty-six years, as summarized also in Chapter 3, must be read and accurately followed. Detailed discussion of this diet and its accurate use is in Chapter 3 and also in Chapter 4 of our book *Bronchial Asthma—Its Diagnosis and Treatment.*

Strict adherence to the diet, necessary maintenance of weight and nutrition, persistence of foods in the body for more than one to even four weeks, and slow disappearance of tissue changes because of food allergy (see Fig. 16 and Plate I Part 8) must be realized for good results.

After two anticipated attacks of asthma have not occurred or persisting asthma has been relieved for three to four weeks, individual foods can be added, one every three to five days, eliminating any that reactivates the symptoms as advised in Chapter 3. Such provocation tests are best done in the fall to late spring because of the phenomenon already described, that is, frequent inactivation of food allergy in the summer.

Soy milk is accepted by most infants. Mull-Soy is used, since it contains sucrose instead of corn glucose. If it disagrees, our beef-base or lamb-base formula made at home or by Gerber is substituted.

If older children dislike soy milk, bread, and cookies, they are omitted. Muffins and hot cakes made from Cellu-Grainless Mix and water or lima-potato bakery products may be accepted. If both are refused, more white potato, tapioca, meat, and chicken are given to maintain weight and nutrition as we have advised in Chapter 3.

If additional foods are gradually added, especially in the spring and summer, with no nasal or bronchial symptoms and asthma recurs in the fall or winter, the initial CFE diet which gave relief previous to the summer should be strictly resumed. In many of these patients the CFE diet is required in the winter half of the year for several years, as stated in Chapter 3.

With elimination of allergenic foods for one to three years, tolerance may increase to most or all foods, especially in children. Such increase rarely occurs in adults. Hypodermic desensitization to proven allergenic foods is not effective according to our long experience. This is further discussed in Chapters 3 and 8.

CONTROL OF INHALANT ALLERGY

Inhalant allergy to pollens, animal emanations, fungi, dusts, and other inhalants was associated with food allergy as a major or secondary cause in approximately 40 percent and was a sole cause in about 10 percent of our asthmatic infants and children.

Strict environmental control often relieves allergy, especially to dusts, animal emanations, and miscellaneous allergens. Moving to an area in which causative pollens are absent gives relief. Electrostatic pollen filters may decrease symptoms in the home but not out-of-doors.

When inhalants causing the patient's symptoms cannot be removed from his inhaled air by environmental control and air filtration, desensitization is required. Positive skin tests without a definite history of nasobronchial allergy to the reacting inhalants and not confirmed by provocation inhalant tests, however, do not justify initiation of necessarily prolonged desensitization.

When food allergy, moreover, is probable, its control often relieves symptoms without any desensitization to inhalants which give positive reactions, as illustrated in Table XLIII.

We must emphasize that many of our patients in childhood and adult life readily relieved of asthma by the control of unrecognized food allergy had been desensitized with multiple inhalant antigens for one to six to even twenty years in extreme instances without satisfactory results.

The practice of allergy today, we feel, too often is based on a) an inadequate history taken without due considerations of characteristics of food allergy, b) skin testing often performed with an unnecessarily large number of allergens and injections given with one or more multiple antigens containing only skin-reacting allergens, allergy to which is not indicated by history and especially provocation tests (as advised in Chapter 2, our information about possible atopic allergy is obtained from scratch tests done in one to three visits and not in five to as many as sixteen), c) many physicians guided by advice in literature of commercial companies making and selling antigens containing pollens, spores of fungi, house and various other dusts, and other inhalants because of skin reactions interpreted too often by inexperienced technicians or by physicians without any indications in the patient's history of definite or even probable clinical allergy to such inhalant allergens and with no knowledge of the botanical flora in the patient's area or local environment. Too frequently, inadequate or no study is given to the most important cause of bronchial asthma in most patients—food allergy.

CONTROL OF SECONDARY INFECTION

Since infectant asthma is rare or nonexistent as emphasized in this and in Chapter 8, autogenous or stock vaccines are not given to control asthma. Small doses of immune globulin, moreover, have not proven beneficial. Antibiotics are not indicated unless complicating tonsillitis or bronchial infection usually with fever for more than two to three days occurs. Because of possible allergy to penicillin, tetracyclines are preferred. If there is a reduced resistance to bacterial or viral infections, limited use of stock, viral, or bacterial vaccines is justified to prevent or benefit respiratory infections. Fever resulting from food allergy alone is repeatedly noted in this, Chapter 8, 1, and in other chapters of this volume.

RELIEF OF SYMPTOMS WITH MEDICATIONS

Along with the immediate ordering of our CFE diet to study possible food allergy and environmental control with later desensitization to control definite or indicated inhalant allergy, the symptoms of asthma must be relieved by medications as advised in Chapter 8. Epinephrine 1:1000, 0.1 cc to 0.4 cc hypodermically every one to three hours according to the patient's age and weight and severity of asthma, is important. Unusual syncope after even 0.05 cc epinephrine 1:1000 reported by Rappaport was confirmed by Speer and Topay in 1970. Aminophyllin 1.5 to 3.5 grains by rectum every six to twelve hours is justified according to the patient's age and weight after the age of three years. It is not given to younger children. Bronchodilating drugs in suspension or tablets and epinephrine 1:100 or Isuprel 1:200 by inhalation especially with a hand atomizer may be indicated. No intermittent positive pressure therapy is used in our children. Inhalation of steam or mistogen in tents is not necessary with immediate control of inhalants and especially of food allergies and the above medications.

Relief of dehydration and electrolyte deficiency in intractable asthma is important. Because of the necessity of considering allergy to cereal grains when food allergy is indicated in the history and the frequency of allergy to corn in such patients, we give invert sugar instead of glucose solutions when intravenous fluids are advisable. This is justified by the demonstration of corn dextrin antigens in commercial glucose solutions for intravenous use by Arthur Lietze, Ph.D. as reported in Chapter 28 of this volume.

In these patients with intractable or severe asthma it is immediately necessary to limit the diets to those foods in our CFE diet for infants and children, serving them in the liquid, pureed, or soft form until regularly cooked foods are desired.

No opiates, Demerol, or sedatives except occasionally small doses of phenobarbitol have been given. Their omission especially has made possible our study of food and inhalant allergies and use of our advised medications, including corticosteroids, explaining the absence of deaths from asthma in our control of bronchial asthma in our infants and children cooperating in our antiallergic study and control.

For further discussion of control of asthma resulting from food, inhalant, and less often drug allergy, the reader is referred to Chapters 3 and 8 and especially to our book *Bronchial Asthma—Its Diagnosis and Treatment,* 1963.

CORTICOSTEROID THERAPY

Long-term corticosteroid and corticotrophin therapy has not been necessary for the continued control of bronchial asthma in our infants and children because of our continued and intensive efforts to control atopic allergy—especially from foods.

Today corticosteroids are being given too often to control perennial bronchial asthma or its recurrent, often frequent attacks without any or adequate study and control of inhalant and especially of food allergy. When atopic allergy, particularly to foods, is adequately controlled as we advise in this chapter and also in Chapters 3 and 8, corticosteroids if given previously gradually can be reduced and discontinued in children. As already stated, no long-term corticosteroid therapy has been necessary for the continued control of either intermittent or perennial bronchial asthma in infants or children.

Unfortunately many current textbooks, monographs, medical articles, and printed advertisements of pharmaceutical companies advise such long-term therapy, failing to stress the responsibility of controlling inhalant and especially food allergy before and along with its temporary use.

No long-term corticosteroid therapy every one to two days for four to six months to control perennial bronchial asthma has been required in our children or adolescents because of the important cooperation of the patients and parents in our advised control of inhalant and especially food allergy. The importance of this has been already emphasized in this chapter and in Chapter 8. This is comparable to our disuse of long-term corticosteroid therapy in adults as reported in Chapter 8. It receives added discussion and emphasis in Chapter 30.

This does not exclude corticosteroids for the initial control of asthma especially of severe attacks and status asthmaticus and of activated wheezing, dyspnea, coughing, and expectoration resulting from deviations from the necessary elimination diet or from uncontrolled inhalant allergy resulting from inadequate environmental control or desensitization to allergenic inhalants.

Such long-term corticosteroid therapy becomes unnecessary when the required control of the allergenic causes is established and maintained by adamant cooperation of the patient and parents in our advised control and treatment of allergic causes.

This control of perennial asthma without long-term corticosteroid therapy has been emphasized, especially by Fontana as achieved by his recognition and control of atopic allergy including that to foods. He decries "the promiscuous and indiscriminate use of corticosteroids in asthmatic children."

When long-term corticosteroid therapy is gradually stopped, it must be remembered that adrenocortical suppression may persist even for a year. This often necessitates temporary later readministration of these hormones when stress from accidents, illness, or operations reduces the production of these adrenal hormones. Parents and older children are informed about this necessity.

Corticosteroids in large initial doses according to age are both necessary and justified for the control of severe intractable asthma when used in conjunction with indicated sympathomimetic drugs, xanthines, antibiotics, fluid and electrolyte replacements and the necessary immediate study of food and inhalant allergies. As symptoms are relieved by control of atopic allergies, corticosteroid doses are reduced and gradually terminated.

When severe exacerbations of asthma result from diet breaks or inadequate control of inhalant allergy, resumption of short-term corticosteroid therapy in conjunction with other treatment is at times justified.

The reader is referred especially to our discussion of prevention and complications of long-term corticosteroid therapy in Chapter 8.

PERENNIAL NASAL ALLERGY RESULTING FROM FOODS

Food allergy is nearly always the cause of perennial nasal congestion, especially blocking throughout life, including infancy, childhood, and adolescence as already emphasized in Chapter 12. In comparison to inhalant allergy, particularly to pollens, food allergy produces practically no itching. Sneezing may occur in the morning on arising and at times through the day during which it is much less marked and frequent than from inhalant allergy, especially to pollens. The edema of the nasal mucosa and in varying degrees of the mucosa of the sinuses produces nasal blocking to relieve

which nostrils are pushed upward with the palm and twisting of the nostrils with movement of the face from side-to-side often occurs. This blocking from food allergy is the common cause of mouth and noisy breathing, particularly at night and at times snoring, even in infancy and early childhood. A nasal sound to the voice, concomitant blocking, or edema of the eustachian tubes with varying degrees of decreased hearing and at times serous otitis media, as reported in Chapter 13, occurs. A mucoid rather than a watery nasal discharge arises from food allergy. Eosinophiles are usually present in the mucus.

Food allergy is the usual cause of recurrent colds and coughs rather than infection, though infection at times may be a secondary complication, as already discussed in this chapter.

In infants and especially in older children postnasal mucus develops from food allergy in the back of the nose or in the pharynx, causing a hacking cough, clearing of the throat, and at times laryngeal edema, hoarseness, and as in adults, a loss of voice.

As this allergic edema continues into late adolescence and adult life in the nasal and especially sinal mucosa, polyps may develop in the sinuses, the larger ones extruding into the nasal passages from the maxillary antra and smaller ones from the ethmoids. These in our experience nearly always result from food allergy, as discussed in Chapter 12. The constant reactivity of food allergy in the mucosal tissues for years rather than the intermittent allergic reactivity of inhalant allergy explains this development of polyps from food sensitization. It is generally agreed that bacterial allergy is not responsible.

Though nasal congestion, blocking, and other symptoms arise from inhalant allergy, perennial nasal allergy is practically always due to food sensitization. Investigation and control of food allergy, as we advise, have been summarized in this chapter and fully discussed in Chapter 3.

NASAL ALLERGY FROM POLLENS (SEASONAL HAY FEVER) IN CHILDHOOD

Nasal allergy from pollens in childhood increases in frequency after infancy. It has not been recognized in infants in our practice. In the second and third years it develops along with skin reactions as shown in Table XLIV in children with eczema from the age of zero to three years. From the ages of three to eight years and more so from eight to fifteen years, hay fever from pollens increases in frequency from early March to late October in our patients in the western United States. Bronchial allergy causing allergic bronchitis or asthma with or without hay fever develops in about a half of the patients with seasonal hay fever, justifying the control of hay fever when indicated by desensitization therapy.

Thus puncture tests with a few tree, grass, and fall pollens which are in the air in the patient's environment are justified in older infants and children up to the age of three years. Scratch or puncture tests with more pollens and inhalants, as advised in Chapter 2, are advisable in older children and adolescents when seasonal hay fever is indicated in the history. Tests with a few airborne fungi, especially with *Alternaria*, may also be advisable. Allergy to the spores of fungi in childhood, especially in young children, is rare or absent in our practice. Before desensitization is started with a fungus antigen, allergy to the fungi must be assured by provocation inhalant tests which must always be done in the symptom-free patient. Desensitization to pollens that cannot be eliminated from the patient's environment is impor-

tant, as already discussed in Chapter 4.

NASAL ALLERGY FROM INHALANTS OTHER THAN POLLENS

With increasing age from infancy to mid-adolescence, nasal and sinal allergy from animal emanations, house and recreational dusts, and other miscellaneous inhalants may develop. Allergy to spores of fungi is less frequent, as discussed above. Such allergy may be indicated by sneezing and coryza and nasal congestion in environments in which these various allergens are in the air. Positive scratch reactions are usually present, though their clinical importance must always be determined by an unquestioned history or by provocation tests. Animal emanations in carpets and coverings of furniture may persist in the living environment in spite of ordinary cleaning procedures. If animals or birds are in the house or were kept in the home by former occupants, the possibility of nasal or bronchial allergy to emanations from them especially in the carpets and furnishings must be considered. They may remain in the carpets and coverings of furniture in spite of usual cleaning procedures, requiring the removal of such fabrics and carpets and substitution with new floor and furniture coverings.

When these allergens are assured causes of the patient's perennial symptoms and especially if they occur during the fall, winter, and early spring, it is also imperative to study and control possible concomitant food allergy which is usually exaggerated in the fall and winter months. Formerly assumed environmental allergy may prove to have been due to foods.

To control nasal allergy resulting from the above inhalants, environmental control as advised in Chapter 8 may suffice. Desensitization to those inhalants which cannot be eliminated from the air of the patient's environment may be required.

EMPHYSEMA IN INFANCY AND CHILDHOOD

Overinflation of the lung during acute attacks of bronchial asthma subsides after attacks. When such asthma continues with recurrent exaggeration, hyperinflation persists and the chest cage enlarges, especially in anterior-posterior diameter. Chronic cough especially increases this condition. The diaphragms become depressed and flattened.

If the causes of asthma persist and especially if the airways become obstructive with tenacious thick mucus and by edema of the mucosa, along with bronchospasm, destruction of alveoli may occur, resulting in varying degrees of destructive and obstructive emphysema, as reported in Chapter 11 on obstructive emphysema in adults. In youth, however, emphysema is usually due to overinflation without alveolar destruction, and control of the allergy, especially to foods, reverses the condition. When the chronic asthma or bronchitis with shortness of breath persists with a distended, even barrel-shaped chest with higher shoulders and widened costal angle, destructive emphysema may have developed along with other pathology of obstructive lung disease.

To relieve the shortness of breath, the rales and rhonchi, and wheezing and suppressed breath sounds, and varying degrees of bronchorrhea, adequate, sufficient study, especially of food allergy, as advised in Chapter 8 in this volume is required. This is necessary especially if symptoms are marked and recurrently intensified in the fall, winter, and early spring when food allergy so often is reactivated and severe in degree. Even when cysts or bullae are evident in the x-ray and bronchiectasis is demonstrated, such study and control of possible food allergy along with that of inhalant allergy, if present, is important, as noted in Chapter 8.

BRONCHIESTASIS IN CHILDHOOD

That allergy needs consideration as an initial or complicating cause of bronchiectasis in children is supported by its necessary consideration in adults according to our limited but challenging evidence reported in Chapter 10. That smooth muscle spasm, the mucosal edema, and mucoid secretions are best explained by allergy is stressed therein. Bronchial allergy associated with or complicating pneumonia or pertussis occurring in about one-half of the cases of bronchiectasis in childhood increases the chances of obstruction of the airways, causing increased persistent cough with resultant tubular cylindrical dilation of the bronchi. Its persistent occurrence increasingly through the years produces varying degrees of saccular lesions.

Important information about bronchiectasis in childhood in three articles by Field was published in 1949. Of 160 cases of irreversible lesions, 20 percent developed in the first year. In five years 50 percent had developed it.

Bronchial asthma occurred in over one-half of the children. The frequent origin of bronchiectasis in childhood is due to obstruction of the small bronchus with mucus, the origin of which is best explained by allergy, especially to food, with subsequent secondary infection. This can result not only in cylindrical but often in saccular bronchiectasis. Since our long experience indicated allergy to food and not to infectants as the cause of most perennial bronchial asthma in childhood, its adequate study and control along with that of less frequent causative inhalant allergy if present, as we advise, is most necessary.

In 1957 Kulczycki *et al.* discussed bronchiectasis and atelectasis in cystic fibrosis and reported four operations for it in lower lobes of the lungs.

Because of the possibility of food allergy as a sole or contributing cause of saccular and also of cylindrical bronchiectasis in infants and young children, it should be studied adequately as we advise as a possible initial cause. A history of nasal and sinal congestion, bronchial congestion, or bronchitis and especially of possible or definite bronchial asthma in infancy and childhood as well as in adult life emphasizes such study and control, as we have stated in Chapter 8. The advisability of considering food allergy in infants and young children in the possible causation of these symptoms is emphasized throughout this chapter. Concomitant antibiotic therapy, if infection rather than allergy is or seems a major possibility or if it is a possible secondary cause, is important. Moderate and decreasing doses of a corticosteroid for one to three weeks would be justified, as advised in our discussion of bronchial asthma in this chapter.

Study of possible food allergy and if definitely indicated by history (not by skin tests alone) inhalant allergy, we opine, is very important before surgical resection of lobes of the lung in older children is contemplated. This is especially important if "cylindrical bronchiectasis" is evident in bronchograms. When bronchorrhea and bronchospasm with resultant cough are present, the challenge is to recognize and control the allergic causes rather than only to encourage expectoration of the constantly forming mucus and the attempted control of bronchospasm with intermittent inhalant or positive pressure therapy and varying amounts of bronchodilator drugs and possible Adrenalin 1:1000 hypodermically. If allergy is a problem because of possible or definite nasobronchial allergy,

study and control of the allergy, especially to foods, with indicated limited corticosteroid therapy and minimal or no bronchodilator therapy are very important, often yielding definite benefit. Relief of coughing, expectoration, and bronchospasm with or without definite asthma may occur with the accurate, sufficient use of our CFE diet.

Indications of atopic allergy in cystic fibrosis as discussed later in this chapter justify its adequate study for possible or more definite atopic allergy, especially to foods, as we advise. Food allergy has never been studied as a major or associated cause not only of this serious, usually fatal disease but also as a factor in bronchiectasis or in cystic fibrosis as well as in Kartagener's syndrome, as reported in these two diseases and noted later in this chapter.

KARTAGENER'S SYNDROME

Kartagener, in 1933, reported the association of bronchiectasis, situs inversus, and sinusitis in four cases in childhood. Bergstrom *et al.*, in 1950, tabulated statistics on eighty-four published cases including two of their own who were among six siblings in one family. The association of bronchiectasis and situs inversus was found to occur in 12 to 23 percent of patients with such transposition of viscera. A hereditary predisposition has been a considered cause. Olsen (1932) reported thirteen cases in eighty-five patients with dextracardia in ten of which nasal polyps, which require study of food allergy (Chapt. 12), were present.

An error in development or lesions in the bronchial walls arising from cardiovascular anomalies were suggested explanations of the bronchiectasis. Atelectasis probably is a forerunner. Bronchiectasis according to Conway is usually tubular in these patients rather than cystic. The latter would indicate a congenital origin. Dickey (1953) reported five cases in children present at the age of six weeks and others occurring from the age of four to fourteen years in which nasal congestion and coughing had been continuous since infancy associated with attacks of asthma present all of his life in a fourteen-year-old boy which justifies the study of perennial allergy, especially to foods.

As Glaser states in his excellent discussion of this syndrome (1956), the occurrence of nasal congestion, "sinusitis," bronchial cough, and at times bronchial asthma and especially nasal polyps challenges the allergist concerning the role of allergy in the causation of this syndrome and particularly of the bronchiectasis. Failure of benefit from the study and treatment of possible food allergy up to now, we opine, could have been due to the usual dependence on positive skin tests to determine food allergy rather than trial diet as we advise.

This further study of food allergy in our opinion with the strict and adequate use of our CFE diet, as we advise throughout this volume, may evidence food allergy as the important cause in this syndrome. The frequency of food allergy as the major cause of perennial nasal allergy and of nasal polyps (Chapt. 12) and of perennial nasal and bronchial symptoms in children, including recurrent bronchial asthma, as discussed in this chapter, supports this probability.

The lesser probability of inhalant allergy also discussed in this and other chapters must be studied when atopic allergy is considered in the etiology. In regard to bronchiectasis the frequency with which it is initiated by bronchial asthma always requires the study of food allergy as the initial cause, as we have discussed in Chapter 8.

ALLERGIC DERMATITIS (ECZEMA) IN INFANTS AND CHILDREN

That eczema in infancy and childhood as well as in adult life, including old age, always requires study of atopic allergy especially to foods and to a less extent inhalants, particularly to pollens, has been emphasized in Chapter 14. Necessary recognition of drug, chemical, and contact allergy has been stressed.

In this chapter additional information about atopic eczema resulting from food and inhalant allergy garnered from our study and results of control of these causes for over forty years will be reported. This emphasizes that such allergy can be the demonstrated cause of this dermatitis when adequate cooperation of parents and children is obtained in the study and control of food and inhalant allergy as we advise in this chapter and in Chapter 14. Those physicians, especially dermatologists, who are skeptical about the role of atopic allergy both to inhalants and foods, in the causation of atopic dermatitis can confirm the role of such allergy with their study and control of inhalant and especially of food allergy as we advise. Thereby, the unsupported statements such as "Desensitization therapy is not warranted" and "Food sensitivity alone is not responsible for atopic dermatitis" will not be made. Clark, in 1948, deplored the tardiness of dermatologists to recognize and control atopic allergy to food and inhalants including atopic eczema.

As noted in this chapter, eczema in infants fed only with cow's milk requires the study of allergy to such milk as the cause. Even if milk is given for a few days after birth, replacing it entirely with breast milk, sensitization to the cow's milk may have developed and may result in eczema, nasobronchial allergy, colic, or other manifestations of allergy when cow's milk replaces breast milk several weeks later with the termination of breast feeding. Even infants on breast milk alone may develop eczema or other allergic manifestations from allergy to foods eaten by the mother and excreted in her breast milk, as reported long ago by Shannon, O'Keefe, and Ratner.

In occasional infants purchased breast milk is used to control atopic dermatitis or other manifestations of allergy in the infant, as discussed in this chapter.

When the infant has been on cow's milk alone, allergy to it must be studied with soybean milk or if it is not tolerated, with our meat-base formula manufactured by Gerber or made at home as advised in Chapter 3. If other foods in addition to cow's milk have been in the diet of older infants, our CFE diet for infants is prescribed as advised in Chapter 3.

Food allergy as a cause of atopic dermatitis as emphasized throughout this volume is indicated by:

1. Perennial symptoms which are exaggerated in the fall, winter, and early spring with decrease of it, even absence in the summer. "Winter eczema" is often due to food allergy.

2. Disagreements and dislikes for specific or many foods.

3. Large positive protein scratch tests to foods which may indicate allergy to reacting foods. The clinical significance of these large reactions must be determined by provocation tests or undoubted history of clinical allergy thereto.

The reader is referred to our further discussion of the characteristics of food allergy and about the exaggeration of food allergy in the winter half of the year in Chapter 1 and indications of clinical food allergy by the diet history in Chapter 2.

In a few patients eczema resulting from food allergy can be controlled by elimination of foods giving large protein scratch tests or of foods to which a history of food dislikes or disagreements is obtained. That eczema or other manifestations of food allergy can continue or be activated by the inhalation of the odors of foods in the raw state and especially during cooking has been emphasized in Chapter 3. Infants and children who have obvious or probable allergy to foods and especially those giving large reactions should be out of the kitchen when such foods are being cooked. At times, as already stated in this book, such foods, particularly eggs, may have to be eliminated from the house, including the refrigerator.

It is important to emphasize that food allergy, according to our experience, cannot be excluded as the cause of atopic dermatitis or other manifestations of food allergy until our CFE diet has been adhered to with no deviation and with maintenance of nutrition for one to two months, since it takes up to three or four weeks for previously ingested foods to leave the body and a longer time for the pathological changes in the shock tissues of allergy to decrease and especially to disappear (see Fig. 19 in Chapt. 14). If relief does not occur, modification of this trial diet and the possible use of minimal elimination diets (Chapt. 3) must be employed before food allergy is excluded as a cause of atopic dermatitis or other manifestations of possible food allergy. As emphasized in Chapter 14 and throughout this volume, possible inhalant allergy associated with food allergy or as a sole cause must be remembered.

Evidence of milk allergy as the cause of allergic dermatitis in infants usually is evidenced by evidence of relief which occurs in one to two weeks after Mull-Soy or our meat-base formula with indicated additional vitamins replaces cow's milk. When our CFE diet is used to study food allergy as a cause of atopic dermatitis in older infants and children, evidence of improvement may not occur for two to three weeks even with strict and adequate maintenance of the diet. It must be emphasized, however, that successful study and control of food allergy by a physician is not always possible with his first use of diet trial, especially with our CFE diet. Our discussion of the ordering of the diet must be read and reread in this volume in Chapter 3 and in our other publications. The diet must be used in more than a few patients for several months by the physician, allergist, dermatologist, or other specialist before dependable facility in its use occurs. Bakery products must be made by our recipes by a trusted baker or in the home. The true content of the commercial bakery products cannot be assumed by the printed labels on the wrapping of the products, as emphasized in our article *Hypoallergenic Breads—Wheat Content of Products Available* published in 1967.

The importance of accurate, adequate, and persisting use of our CFE diet and (if necessary) of its modifications must be emphasized to all physicians and specialists, since manifestations of food allergy are a challenge to the entire profession, as evidenced throughout this volume. The time required to recognize and study food allergy alone or in association with inhalant, and at times drug allergy is comparable to that required by physicians in other specialities than allergy to learn and master the methods of diagnosis, treatment, and control of coronary occlusion, fractured hips, removal of cataracts, gallstones, tumors of the lung, or the many other medical or surgical challenges. Thus the failure to relieve allergic symptoms with the initial use of elimination diets, at times advised on a single page of a textbook or medical article, utilized in one or even a few pa-

tients with no study of the causes of allergy, no recording of the history from the allergic viewpoint (see Chapt. 2), failure to prescribe and later manipulate the CFE diet or our advised modifications, and too often the delegation of such study to an inexperienced physician, nurse, or even a dietitian does not justify skepticism about the role of food allergy as the cause of its many manifestations such as allergic or atopic dermatitis.

Evidence of the major importance of food and to a less extent of inhalant and particularly of pollen allergy in the causation of allergic dermatitis (atopic eczema) relieved by our control of such inhalant and especially food allergy is shown in our statistics on 147 cases from the ages of one month to fifteen years in three age groups, "one to three," "three to eight," and "eight to fifteen" we report in Table XLIV. The frequency of eczema in young infants especially because of milk and less frequently egg and other foods is evidenced in these statistics.

As in bronchial asthma more boys than girls were in the unselected age groups. In the three groups of increasing age, the average age of onset remained in the first 2½ years. The duration of the uncontrolled dermatitis increased, indicating that atopic dermatitis often continues from infancy into late adolescence and as shown in Chapter 14, into adult life. These statistics, especially after the third year, show the frequency of eczema in the cubital and popliteal areas with its lesser frequency on the face, ears, neck and forearms, hands, and legs, in all of which food was found to be of major importance.

That all areas of the skin are susceptible to the spreading tendency of atopic dermatitis is shown in these statistics. It first appeared on the face in twelve cases and on the cubital areas in nineteen, compared

TABLE XLIV
STATISTICS ON 147 INFANTS AND CHILDREN WITH ALLERGIC DERMATITIS RELIEVED BY CONTROL OF FOOD AND/OR POLLEN ALLERGY

	84 Cases 0-3 yrs	34 Cases 3-8 yrs	29 Cases 8-15 yrs
Age (av.)	1.9	5	11
Males	56%	42%	58%
Females	44%	48%	42%
Duration	1/12-3	1-5	3-12
	Av. 1.4 yrs	Av. 3.5 yrs	Av. 5.7 yrs
Age of onset	Av. 1.1 yrs	Av. 1.5 yrs	Av. 2.5 yrs
Recurrently exaggerated		8%	
Generalized	9%	32%	20%
Face	24% (1st in 6)	32% (1st in 3)	60% (1st in 3)
Scalp	15% (1st in 1)	10%	6%
Ears	25% (1st in 1)	14%	40%
Neck	26% (1st in 1)	23%	29%
Chest	5% (1st in 1)	6%	4%
Arms	15%	24%	48%
Forearms	25%	20%	40%
Cubital	40% (1st in 7)	35% (1st in 6)	45% (1st in 7)
Hands	20% (1st in 1)	14%	10%
Thighs	13%	10%	14%
Legs	34%	22%	45%
Popliteal	10%	43%	60%
Feet	8%	3%	15%
Personal History of Probable Allergy			
Colds and coughs	8%	10%	14%
Nasal symptoms	7%	20%	15%
Asthma	17%	30%	34%
Colic	8%		
Worse in winter	28%	40%	49%
Family History			
Eczema	30%	23%	20%
Asthma	24%	30%	22%
Nasal allergy	11%	10%	
Hives	20%		
Diet history	20%	18%	22%
Drug history			5%
Skin Tests			
Grass	18%	15%	68%
Tree	3%	6%	8%
Fall	6%	2%	20%
Milk	19%	0	0
Egg	29% (4+ in 24)	14%	20%
Soy	2.4%	0.9%	
Wheat	1.1%	6%	
Beef	0	0	
Lamb	0		
Peanut	5% (4+ in 3)	1%	
Fish	1%	1%	
Fruits	0	0	
Animal emanations	2 only	0	2 only
House dust	3 only	0	3 only
Fungi	0	0	0
Silk	1 (4 plus)	0	0
Causes			
Foods	90%	91%	82%
Pollens	8.4% (sole cause in 1)	10%	7% (sole cause) with foods 29%
Animal emanations plus food		9%	
Dust			14%
Animal emanations			10%
Fungi			10%
Blood Count			
White	11,150	11,200	12,500
Lymphocytes	50%	41%	47%
Eosinophiles	10%	11%	8%

with five on the popliteal areas. In days or weeks thereafter it spread in varying degrees and frequency to other cutaneous areas, as indicated in the statistics. Further information about eczema on the ears and eyelids is detailed in Chapter 20 on Ocular Allergy and in Chapter 13 on Ear Allergy as well as in Chapter 14 on Allergic Dermatitis.

The relief of longstanding eczema of the scalp, including "cradle cap" in 12 to 20 percent of our patients, especially resulting from our control of food allergy, aided in the initial weeks of such therapy with decreasing use of corticosteroids is evidenced. These hormones were finally decreased and omitted as the eczema of the scalp was controlled with elimination of allergenic foods alone. Its occurrence in adults was discussed in Chapter 14.

"Diaper rash" also needs study of food allergy, as shown by its relief in five cases in our infants with our CFE diet or at times with its modifications.

In the personal histories frequency of colds and coughs at times associated with asthma, particularly during the fall and winter months, indicated food allergy as the major cause. This was confirmed by its control with our CFE diet. The usual relief of colic by the replacement of cow's milk with soybean milk, or especially Mull-Soy or by meat-base formula in seven patients in infancy are more fully discussed in this chapter. The occurrence of eczema and asthma in the family history of these patients with atopic eczema correlated with such findings in our statistics on bronchial asthma in children in this chapter and in Chapter 8. There also was a definite tendency to develop the same manifestations of allergy in successive generations of the family.

The increased frequency of exaggeration of eczema in the fall and winter with ad-

vancing age through childhood up to 62 percent of patients in the eight-year to fifteen-year group is explained by the exaggeration of food allergy during these months as reiterated in this volume, especially in Chapter 2.

Scratch skin reactions with foods gave large positive reactions, especially to eggs, in 12 of these 147 patients. In ten of these patients rapid exaggeration of eczema and in three patients, of bronchial asthma occurred after ingestion of slight amounts of egg and usually with inhalation of its airborne odor, especially when the child was in the kitchen when eggs were being cooked. Thus, when eczema is severe or definite asthma is present in patients giving these large scratch reactions to eggs or other foods, the patients are excluded from the kitchen when possible allergenic foods, especially eggs or fish, are being cooked. When allergy is severe, large scratch-reacting foods are excluded from the house, including the refrigerator. One baby of three months developed severe asthma sitting in the highchair in the kitchen immediately after an egg was broken.

In contrast to the questionable clinical significance of large scratch reactions to eggs and other foods in the opinion of allergists and dermatologists twenty to forty years ago, our experience indicates that such large reactions usually indicate the immediate severe type of food allergy. Former skepticism, we believe, was due to failure to eliminate any trace of large skin-reacting foods, especially eggs, peanuts, and fish, from the diet, even preventing the inhalation of odors of such foods. Moreover, the frequency of negative or questionable skin reactions to foods causing clinical atopic allergy was not known in these years. This requires the use of trial diets, particularly our CFE diet, for three or more weeks before evidence of relief from the elimination of allergenic foods occurs.

Though milk allergy was studied in all patients with our CFE diet, revealing its major clinical importance by good results, a definite scratch reaction occurred in only one case. Large reactions to peanuts occurred in three cases in whom marked immediate clinical allergy to them was present. Negative skin reactions to foods causing severe clinical allergy, however, do occur.

The skin reactions to grass pollens in thirty-six cases were large in three and moderate in the others. Moderate reactions to fall pollens occurred in seventeen cases. One very large reaction occurred to *Hormodendron,* which proved of no clinical significance. There were slight or indefinite reactions to other fungi in children which caused no clinical allergy.

Pollen allergy was the sole cause of atopic eczema in five cases in our children three to fifteen years of age. Pollen allergy, on the contrary, was not the cause of clinical allergy in the infants and children up to three years of age. Allergy to pollens, animal emanations, and other inhalants was associated with food allergy in eight cases in the three to fifteen year age group.

Thus preponderance of food allergy over inhalant allergy in the causation of atopic dermatitis is supported by these statistics.

Of interest was the blood eosinophilia (3%-20%) in these infants and children. Leukocytes varied from 7,000 to 21,000. Lymphocytes varied from 15 to 65 percent.

Control of the eczema occurred in sixty-seven patients before corticosteroids were available. In our other eighty-seven cases small doses of corticoids were given by mouth to only forty-six patients. In no patient was long-term corticoid therapy continued to maintain control of the eczema after the first one to four weeks of our antiallergic therapy.

Our evaluation of the causes of this allergic dermatitis in these 147 cases is as follows:

Food allergy was the indicated sole cause of 85 percent of the group zero to three years of age, in 70 percent in the three- to eight-year group and in 70 percent of the eight- to fifteen-year-old group. As age increased, food and pollen allergies were associated causes in approximately 10 percent in each group. Whereas pollen allergy alone was not evident in the zero- to three-year group in contrast to its sole role in 8 percent of the three to fifteen group, control of pollen and other inhalant allergy when necessary with desensitization therapy at times with minute doses is advised in Chapter 4. Allergy to animal emanations and other inhalants with or without allergy to pollens and usually in association with food allergy were indicated causes in 2 to 10 percent in different groups. Thus food allergy and less frequent pollen allergy were the evident major causes of this allergic dermatitis in infants and children in our practice. Failure of relief of atopic eczema from desensitization to inhalants for two to six years has been reversed by the control of food allergy alone as we advise, which had previously not been recognized.

Case 203: A boy ten months of age had scattered areas of dermatitis under the diaper and on the scrotum. This had started as a generalized rash at the age of six weeks when fruits were first given. The dermatitis had coalesced into a brown granular 2-by-6 inch area on the left thigh at the lower border of the diaper. The exaggeration of cubital, popliteal, and nuchal eczema being exaggerated every two weeks suggested food allergy. Colic had occurred two to three times a week for the first five months, suggesting milk allergy.

Nasal congestion exaggerated every few weeks especially in winters suggested food allergy.

Diet history revealed increased eczema from eggs and oranges.

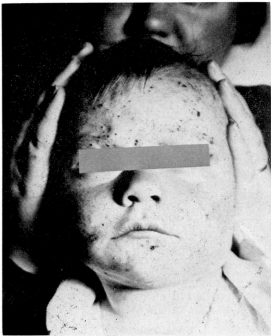

Figure 40. Facial eczema with flexural involvement resulting from allergy to cereal grains, milk, wheat, and chocolate. Thickened lichenified moderately erythematous diffusely papular, slightly excoriated areas 2 by 4 inches in the cubital and popliteal areas; a diffuse papular, dry, moderately excoriated dermatitis over buttocks and lower back; a diffuse papular dry eruption on the left neck; roughness of the skin of the cheeks; and a fine, sandy, papular dry character of the skin of the anterior upper chest had been present for four years during the winter and definitely decreased in the summer.

Family history revealed asthma and hay fever in the mother and her mother.

Scratch tests were negative to foods and inhalants. Hemoglobin 71 percent, leukocytes 16,450, and eosinophiles 5 percent.

Treatment and results: Because of the perennial dermatitis and especially because of its recurrent exaggeration and increased symptoms in the winter and the great frequency of allergy to milk in colic, our CFE diet was ordered. Since soy milk had caused abdominal cramps, our meat-base formula (Gerber) was prescribed. No corticosteroids were given.

In four weeks the dermatitis had cleared except for slight residual dermatitis on the flexures. After continued relief for three more weeks, one

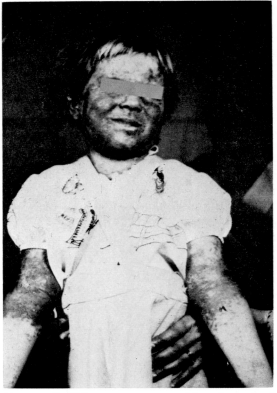

Figure 41. Winter eczema resulting from food allergy controlled with our CFE diet.

ounce of milk reactivated the eczema, relieved with return to our CFE diet.

In four years the dermatitis still recurs when milk, eggs, chocolate, citrus fruits, spices, and condiments are included in the diet.

Case 204: A girl fifteen years of age at the age of five months developed eczema on the face involving the scalp, the upper back, and neck. She had been fed with canned cow's milk, goat's milk, and finally Mull-Soy and later Gerber's meat formula without improvement. These changes in diet were made rather rapidly.

A cousin had eczema from eggs. Her father had hay fever. There was a large reaction to eggs and also to chicken. Eosinophiles were 16 percent in 23,000 lymphocytes.

An initial diet contained meat-base formula, white potatoes, peas, carrots, squash, salt, water, sugar, pears, peaches, plums, and tapioca pudding. Eggs were excluded from the house. There was definite improvement in a month. At the end of three years all foods were tolerated except eggs.

Case 205: A girl developed eczema at the age of ten months. It was exaggerated in the spring until this year, clearing in the winter. It was exaggerated especially in the cubital and popliteal areas in May for two years. It was generalized in May a year prior to the first visit. There was a dry, diffuse, minute, excoriated scaling dermatitis on the upper and lower extremities, buttocks, and back. Cortisone ointment was used freely and gave no relief. In addition she had some wheezing and coughing when playing in the last two months.

Skin tests gave large reactions to grasses and to lamb, codfish, and milk. She had 10 percent eosinophiles. She was desensitized to pollens beginning with a 10^{-14} dilution with a gradual increase into the 10^{-6}. Of interest was the mother's statement that the pollen therapy with the #14 and then the #13 dilutions had been of great help.

Case 206: A boy 8½ years of age developed eczema first on the cubital and popliteal areas, gradually spreading to all areas of the body except the scalp in the winter of 1947. In the winter of 1948 he was hospitalized and placed on a diet of peas, Ry Krisp, soy, bananas, Knox gelatin, corn, and carrots, which cleared his skin entirely. It was again exaggerated in the spring months. Since then it had been better in the summer and exaggerated during the fall, winter, and spring. He had had perennial nasal allergy with moderate blocking of the nose for three years, especially around alfalfa, and exaggerated in the spring months. He had been constipated since infancy.

The parents did not actually know any foods which exaggerated or activated his eczema. Prunes, however, seemed detrimental.

The father had eczema in childhood, remaining on the hands in the preceding seven years. He also had asthma from the age of eleven to sixteen years. The mother had hay fever.

Skin testing gave large reactions to the grass pollens, one to two plus reactions to the fall and tree pollens, and three plus reactions to *Cladosporium, Hormodendrum,* and *Chaetomium.*

Brief desensitization to pollens in June gave no lasting relief. In one year in April eczema was all over the body except the hands and face. Because eczema continued in the winter months, he was placed on our FFCFE diet. Desensitization was resumed with a 1:5000 multiple pollen antigen. Gradually eczema de-

creased and disappeared. During the summer of 1955 he had no eczema. Desensitization had been increased into the #1 dilution. Pollen desensitization was continued for two more years, with no return of the eczema. After the first six months continued relief did not require elimination of foods from his diet.

URICARIA IN INFANCY AND CHILDHOOD

Urticaria, infrequent in infancy, increases in childhood and into adolescence. As stated in Chapter 15 on urticaria, the three common causes of urticaria must always be remembered, namely allergy to drugs or chemicals, to foods, and to inhalant allergens, especially pollens. In children as in adults, drugs are readily eliminated as a cause by their total discontinuance, remembering that it requires one or two weeks and even a longer period for them to leave the body. In young and older infants food allergy is the most frequent cause of hives. As age increases through childhood into adolescence, inhalant allergy to animal emanations, environmental allergens and dusts, and especially to pollens increases in frequency, though food or drug allergy alone or associated with inhalant allergy may be the dominant cause.

CONTROL OF ATOPIC ALLERGY IN URTICARIA TO FOODS, INHALANTS (ESPECIALLY TO POLLENS), AND TO DRUGS AND SERA

Since it is generally agreed that food allergy is difficult and often impossible to demonstrate with present methods of testing with available allergens, particularly in urticaria, diet trial especially with our fruit-free and cereal-free elimination diet (FFCFE) is usually important to study possible food allergy as advised in Chapter 3. At times the parents suspect specific foods, especially fruits, nuts, chocolate, or fish, the sole elimination of which may relieve the urticaria.

The importance of allergy to fruits, condiments, and flavors as well as to other foods which commonly cause clinical allergy which are excluded from our FFCFE diet must be remembered for the study of food allergy in urticaria.

In spite of the fallibility of skin testing in demonstrating foods that cause urticaria, scratch tests with all foods eaten by the child are routine in our practice. When large scratch or puncture tests to foods, especially to milk, eggs, peanuts, fish, and occasionally to meat, soy, or rarely other foods occur, the possibility of urticaria to them may be studied only by their elimination. Practically all of these, however, are eliminated from our FFCFE diet. With the preparation and adequate use and manipulation of this diet as advised in Chapter 3 the frequency of food allergy in urticaria and important relief will occur in many patients. Confirmation of the allergenic effect of any individual food must be made by provocation feeding tests (read Chapt. 3).

The history of urticaria arising from allergy to inhalants, especially to pollens, which cause urticaria only during the pollen seasons is necessary to recognize and record in the patient's history.

Further discussion of urticaria and advice about the use of the elimination diets to reveal and control food allergy and the use of skin tests, environmental control, and desensitization to inhalants, especially to pollens in infants, children, and adolescents, are discussed more fully in Chapter 15.

Since corticosteroids and epinephrine 1:1000 rarely cause clinical allergy, they can be given to control urticaria until its causes can be found.

Contact allergy to feathers, wool, silk, and other environmental allergens at times causes localized urticarial wheals and are discussed in other textbooks on allergy including our own. Urticaria and localized edemas from insect bites also discussed in most books in clinical allergy must be remembered.

ANGIONEUROTIC EDEMA

This condition resulting from food allergy is very rare in infancy. Its frequency increases through childhood and early adolescence, though it is less common than in later life. Lyon, in 1928, did describe varying and extensive swellings of the body especially of the labia in a breast-fed infant six weeks of age because of corn and beans ingested by the mother and excreted in her milk.

The occurrence of localized swellings in young and old adults from allergy to animal sera, drugs, food, and other ingestant and inhalants, especially pollens, is discussed in Chapter 16 on localized swellings.

Though these edemas can occur in any part of the skin they do arise at times in the gastrointestinal, genitourinary, central nervous system, ocular, and other tissues, as reported throughout this volume. They are especially prone to occur in the eyelids, face, and particularly around the mouth, on the lips, in the nasal mucosa, and on the tongue. With such localization in the oral tissues, possible laryngeal and pharyngeal edema must be anticipated, which has at times caused death by suffocation.

Treatment

Thus when such swellings may develop in the face and especially in the lips and mouth, the patient, spouse, or parent must be provided with and be taught to administer epinephrine 1:1000 with a dispensable, sterile, 1 cc syringe in a dose of 0.1 to

0.20 cc to children according to age and weight and 0.4 to 0.5 cc hypodermically to adults, repeating the injection every five to fifteen minutes until free breathing occurs and until a physician is consulted for further advice. Suffocation resulting from such swellings can occur before the patient can be so treated by a physician.

GASTROINTESTINAL ALLERGY

Gastrointestinal allergy is very common in infancy, decreasing in frequency in early childhood. Such allergy, especially to cow's milk, causes nearly all infantile colic, pylorospasm, cyclic vomiting, and best explains most hypertrophic pyloric stenosis, all of which will be discussed individually in this chapter.

Food allergy usually to cow's milk and less often to soy milk and to other foods as they are added to the diet also causes most vomiting, abdominal pain, cramping, diarrhea, or other gastrointestinal symptoms in infants and children.

That cow's milk is by far the major cause of gastrointestinal symptoms in childhood and especially in infancy has been noted in the first section of this chapter and also in Chapter 24 where studies and observations of pediatricians and allergists since 1905 have been reviewed. The development of allergy to cow's milk in ten to thirty days after its initial ingestion by the infant is comparable to the development of allergy after ten to fourteen days in an experimental animal after parenteral injection of the allergen. Ratner, moreover, sensitized many rabbits by oral feedings of cow's milk as occurs in infants after the initial ingestion of such milk.

That gastrointestinal, nasobronchial, cutaneous, and other manifestations of clinical allergy develop to other foods after they are added to the diet has been pointed out. Information about the gastrointestinal symptoms resulting especially from cow's milk in the excellent articles by Clein, Collins-Williams, Bigler, Tudor, and recently by Gerrard, and some of their case reports of allergy to cow's milk have already been summarized. Gastrointestinal allergy to eggs, oranges, cereal grains, and other foods after their addition to the diet of infants and children as already discussed must be remembered.

The frequency of clinical allergy to milk and its common origin in the first month of life with the gradual onset of allergy to other ingested foods has been reported above.

COLIC

Food allergy to cow's milk increasingly has become recognized during the last fifty years as the cause of most infantile colic. Starting at the age of two to three weeks, it usually lasts for two to four months. However, unrelieved colic may continue through infancy into early childhood. Colic associated at times with regurgitation, diarrhea, melena, nasobronchial symptoms, and especially eczema has been reported by Richet in 1911, Laroche, Richet, and Saint Girons in 1919, Schloss in 1920, Shannon in 1921, especially by White in 1929, Rowe in 1931, Greer in 1933, and by other allergists, especially Glaser (1933) and Speer (1958) since then. As Glaser stated in his discussion of colic in his excellent book on *Pediatric Allergy*, crying indicative of pain is a major symptom which causes great concern and distraction in parents and doctors.

Glaser especially discussed evidence that allergy to milk is the major cause of colic. The development of colic ten to twenty days after birth can be explained by allergy to cow's milk if it is given during the first two or three days of life, after which allergy develops. Eosinophiles in mucus of stools suggest atopic allergy. Transient blood eosinophilia as new foods are eaten suggests allergy may occur.

The familial history suggesting food allergy especially to milk and other foods or of gastrointestinal allergy justifies the study of possible allergic colic in the child. Martin, in 1956, reported colic in 60.1 percent of 611 infants with a family history of allergy and in 25 percent of 296 infants from nonallergic families. Of 841 infants 36.1 percent were colicky babies. Speer, in 1958, reported that 6.3 percent of 152 infants with colic were relieved by the end of the second month by food substitution.

As we advised in croup, if cow's milk is the only ingested food, its substitution with soy milk, especially with Mull-Soy, which contains no corn sugar, is recommended. If diarrhea occurs, particularly if additional digestive symptoms arise indicating allergy to soy, then our meat (beef)-base or lamb-base formula advised in Chapter 3 should be given. Though required calcium, other minerals, and vitamins are in both formulae, small doses of synthetic liquid vitamins may also be ordered. If allergy to cow's milk is mild, the use of condensed or dry cow's milk may relieve the colic. The occasional relief with goat's milk is explained by allergy to lactalbumin in cow's milk and not to casein, which is identical in both milks. In our practice we replace animal milks with Mull-Soy or my meat-base formulae. After assured relief, possible tolerance for goat's milk may be determined.

If such substitutes for cow's milk fail to relieve colic, breast milk from another mother or from a breast milk bank, if it is available, may give relief. If colic continues when other foods in addition to cow's milk are ingested, then our CFE diet as advised for infants in Chapter 3 should be prescribed.

After relief, individual foods in our CFE diet are added, one daily every three to five days, eliminating any which reactivates the clinical allergy (Chapt. 3). That other causes produce abdominal cramping, intestinal obstruction, peritoneal infection, hunger, air swallowing, and emotional disturbances must be remembered. Crying may also be due to unrecognized otitis media.

If colic occurs in infants who have been entirely breast-fed, the possibility that the child is allergic to the foods eaten by the mother being excreted in her breast milk justifies placing the mother on our CFE diet, as suggested in our discussion of diet control in croup. Speer, in 1958, reported that one or more foods in the mother's diet were responsible for colic in twenty-three of thirty-three breast-fed infants. In the infant Mull-Soy or our beef-base or lamb-base formula also are advised instead of cow's milk or goat's milk.

Skin testing only with ingested foods by the puncture method on the back is our routine in infancy after the first month. In older infants and young children, scratch tests with all ingested foods and limited inhalants are advised. As reiterated throughout this volume, negative reactions, however, do not rule out food allergy, and positive skin reactions do not necessarily indicate clinical allergy.

OTHER POSSIBLE CAUSES OF INFANTILE COLIC

Some physicians have attributed infantile colic characterized by constant crying, abdominal distention, regurgitation, at times vomiting, flexing of legs on abdomen, passing of flatus, and abdominal pain to tension and unexplained unhappiness in the infant who usually is well nourished. Such tension is suggested by the temporary or more lasting relief from patting, rocking, burping, or continued holding and walking of the child by parents or nurses. Relief from a mouth-held pacifier supports this assumed cause.

Moreover, the transmission of the mother's tension, concern, and emotional turmoil to the infant caused by its continued crying and apparent abdominal distress and pain, her loss of sleep, and frequent use of sedatives have been blamed for the colic.

However, allergy to foods, especially to cow's milk, or to food allergy in the mother's milk is the logical explanation.

According to our experience and that of other physicians, the tension, pain, and unhappiness in the infant and the nervousness and emotional disturbance in the mother disappear when the relief of food allergy results in a happy, comfortable child and happy parents.

The usual decrease of colic in three to five months can be explained by varying degrees of refractoriness to allergy to milk or other food in the intestine, often, however, with the development of cutaneous, nasobronchial, or other tissue allergy.

Other suggested causes of infantile colic according to Breslow are poor feeding technique (2%), organic causes including intestinal obstruction (13%), hunger (11%), carbohydrate intolerance (31%), and butter fat intolerance (31%). In our experience the last two possibilities are eliminated with our advised control of food allergy.

PYLOROSPASM AND HYPERTROPHIC PYLORIC STENOSIS

That food allergy, especially to milk, requires study as the cause of pylorospasm and stenosis was well stated by Glaser in his *Treatis on Allergy in Childhood* in 1956. He noted that allergy as the cause of pylorospasm was suggested by Halberstadt even in 1911 and by Lesne and Dreyfus in 1913, as reported in our translation of *Ali-*

mentary Anaphylaxis (1919) published in 1930. To Cohen and Brietbart belongs the credit, however, of emphasizing allergy in the etiology of pylorospasm with or without stenosis. Other manifestations of infantile allergy were noted. McCarthy and Wiseman (1937) reported pylorospasm in 0.8 percent of five hundred infants, projectile vomiting being the important sign of stenosis and allergy to milk usually being responsible.

Pounders (1933) reported two operations at four weeks and three years for pyloric stenosis before it was relieved by the elimination of eggs and milk, preventing continued abdominal symptoms. Atopic eczema was also relieved. At a second operation in their patient and in an infant reported by Rosenblum, there was no evidence of the first surgery.

In adults we reported gastric retention after ingestion of allergenic foods, as shown in several x-ray studies (1933).

Barrie and Anderson reported concentric hypertrophy and eosinophilia of the musculature of the stomach, pylorus, and duodenum in a food-sensitive patient with constant blood eosinophilia.

When hypertrophic pyloric stenosis soon after birth requires surgery, Glaser states that allergy in the pyloric muscles to milk could be explained by sensitization *in utero* to such allergens in the mother's blood, passing the placental barrier, as discussed in Chapter 1.

Gastric retention in adults with resultant symptoms because of milk and other foods revealed by roentgen ray studies were reported by us in the *JAMA* in 1933.

CASE REPORTS

Case 207: A child 1½ years of age had cried nearly continuously because of apparent intermittent abdominal cramping and pain since the age of six weeks. Evidencing the pain and abdominal distress was the flexing of her legs on her abdomen intermittently. Milk curds and other undigested foods were passed in the stools. Severe attacks had lasted for three or four days and had recurred every two to three weeks. Enemas had given some relief to the pain.

Breast feedings had been supplemented with cow's milk during the first four months. Weight was maintained.

Skin reactions were negative.

The mother had hay fever. Milk had disagreed and caused nausea in the mother and in her sister. The patient's brother had had pyloric spasm in childhood.

Treatment: To study probable food allergy, our CFE diet, modified for a young child, was prescribed. Mull-Soy supplanted cow's milk. In two weeks the mother reported 90 percent relief, a marked improvement in disposition, and a disappearance of symptoms with increased appetite. Gradually other foods were added in the next six months, with no recurrence of symptoms.

Comment: That food allergy was responsible for the pylorospasm, colic, persistent abdominal distress, and the passing of undigested milk curds and other foods in the stools in this patient was indicated by the relief from the elimination of cow's milk and other common allergenic foods. The record emphasizes the importance of considering food allergy in gastrointestinal disturbances in infancy and childhood.

Comment: The persistence of symptoms of a similar nature in the patient's older brother, up to the age of five years, illustrates familial occurrence of food allergy. A definite history of milk sensitization in three generations in this family also illustrates the frequent tendency for specific food allergies to be inherited. These gastrointestinal symptoms resulting from food allergy in older children are shown in the following record:

Case 208: A boy nine years of age had had transient cramping and abdominal pain occurring one to two hours after meals and associated with nausea, vomiting, and at times with diarrhea. These attacks had occurred every two to three months from the age of three to seven years. They usually lasted one day and were associated with fever with no associated infection. Eczema on the face and head developed from the age of six months to two years and had been very severe, resisting all treatment. The eczema

had been replaced by recurrent vomiting. He had frequent attacks of bronchitis and colds. As an infant he had been difficult to feed. Cream of wheat and eggs had caused nausea and "indigestion." He had been constipated. Hay fever and asthma were present in the mother and her family. The boy's examinations were all negative. There were no positive scratch reactions.

Treatment: By the use of our CFE diet the symptoms proved to be due to eggs and wheat.

RECURRENT GASTROINTESTINAL SYMPTOMS WITH FEVER FROM ALLERGY TO FOODS, ESPECIALLY TO MILK

Cooke's report in 1933 of cyclic attacks of gastrointestinal symptoms with fever up to 104 F from infancy to the age of sixteen years because of allergy to cow's milk supported the frequency of the periodicity of symptoms from food allergy first reported by Schloss; by Barnethan in 1910; by Laroche, Richet, and Saint Girons in 1919; and confirmed by us in 1926 and in the first edition of this book in 1931. Supporting our emphasis of negative skin tests to allergens of foods causing clinical allergy was Cooke's report of negative skin tests to cow's milk. Fever resulting from food and other allergens receives our special discussion in Chapter 24.

In 1967 Deraney reported attacks of similar symptoms including abdominal pain, nausea, weakness, listlessness, and fever of 101 F (recurring every month for 3 years and with her periods for the last 2 years) in a girl fourteen years of age. Physical examination with over twenty-five indicated laboratory tests and gynecological consultation were negative.

The similarity of this history to that of Cooke's summarized above indicated the study of food allergy. With trial diet, cow's milk and beef proved responsible.

He excluded the possibility of lactase deficiency because of interim relief which occurred when cow's milk was being ingested and because of the occurrence of symptoms in one to two hours after ingestion of milk when lactase deficiency is not responsible.

The history of regularly recurring symptoms with interim relief and of associated fever resulting from food allergy is the equivalent of the pathognomonic history of bronchial asthma from food allergy we have long emphasized. The activation of food allergy during menstruation receives further discussion in Chapter 21.

Supporting our emphasis of negative skin tests to allergens causing clinical allergy is the report of Cooke of negative tests to ingested foods, especially to the causative milk.

This report of Derancy's is worthy of additional study.

DISTENTION, BELCHING, EPIGASTRIC PAIN, RECURRENT HEADACHES, URTICARIA, AND BRONCHIAL ASTHMA

Case 209: A boy twelve years of age had had irregular attacks of distention and belching after eating lasting for two or three days every two to four weeks for two years. Between attacks belching had occurred. He had acute pain in the epigastrium, with vomiting of undigested food and intermittent headaches lasting two to three days, recurring every one to two weeks for five years. Occasional canker sores from grapes had occurred. His bowels had always been constipated.

Family history revealed constipation in the mother and headaches in her family. Laboratory tests, physical examination, and the skin reactions to all important foods were negative.

Treatment: The patient was placed on our CFE diet, and relief occurred in seven days. Provocation tests with other foods revealed cow's milk as the sole cause.

Comment: The occurrence of intermittent headaches, urticaria, and absence of physical as well as laboratory findings in explaining the cause of the boy's distress justified the study of food allergy as a cause of his symptoms. His mother stated that the boy could never drink milk "since he knew anything" and that it had

been forced on him against his desire all of his life and often in a disguised form! The mother herself had never been able to drink milk even as a child.

CYCLIC RECURRENT VOMITING

Cyclic recurrent vomiting develops in childhood and it also occurs in adolescence and adult life. The vomiting often lasts two to six days with intervening relief until the subsequent attack in two to six weeks or even longer. Years ago these attacks were called bilious attacks because of which calomel was usually advised. They may be preceded by fatigue, irritability and drowsiness, and other symptoms of allergic fatigue and toxemia we reported in the first edition of this book and discussed in Chapter 19 of this volume. Headache may be severe, mild, or absent. Diarrhea, weakness, and frequent acidosis occur. If they continue for more than a year or even after the initial attacks, interim, mild daily headaches or gastrointestinal symptoms may occur. They may evolve during adolescence or later years into recurrent migraine from food allergy as reported in Chapter 17.

Fries and Jennings, in 1940, assembled evidence from the literature and their own experience that food allergy is the usual cause of cyclic vomiting. They referred to articles by Kerley (1914), Tileston (1918), Schers (1929), Balyeat and Rinkel (1931), Efron (1932), Smith, Dutton, and Tallerman (1934), Ott (1936), Rowe (1937), Smith (1937), and Glaser (1937) reporting food allergy as a possible cause. Hinnant and Halpin (1936) published more evidence of food allergy in cyclic vomiting in twenty children. Tallerman (1934) reported increased frequency of the family history of allergy in children with this malady. Tuft (1937), Clausen (1938), and Vaughan (1939) favored food allergy as the cause. Brown and Brown (1942), in discussing such cyclical vomiting, included confirmatory articles by Casparis (1933), Fries and Jennings (1940), Tallerman (1934) and Hinnant and Halpin (1936) in their Bibliography. Fries and Jennings stated that the recurrence of symptoms with interim relief favors allergy. This is supported by our opinion emphasized in this book that such recurrent attacks of symptoms with interim relief are usually due to food allergy, as is recurrent bronchial asthma from food allergy in this and also in Chapters 2 and 8. The failure of vomiting soon after the eating of the assured allergenic food can be explained by its ingestion in the refractory period between attacks when specific antibodies are absent or by eating the allergenic food in the summer when food allergy often is inactivated. Cyclic vomiting in young girls may occur before or during menstruation and associated with sick headaches or migraine especially from food allergy in adult women. Other manifestations of food allergy, especially bronchial asthma, may also be activated or intensified during menstruation (Chapt. 21).

For many years some pediatricians who have not recognized and controlled food allergy have attributed cyclic vomiting to nervousness. In our patients relief of tension and nervousness which has occurred with the control of causative food allergies has disproved such a psychological cause.

Recurrent vomiting in childhood may be supplanted by recurrent migraine with or without gastrointestinal allergy or by allergic toxemia and fatigue in adult life.

During the study of food allergy as a cause of recurrent vomiting in children and young adults, other causes must be considered. Intussusception, appendicitis, pyloric stenosis, brain tumor or abscess, hydrocephalus, acute infections, and other accepted causes must be remembered. The recurrent nature of cyclic vomiting and the absence of obvious pathological causes and the usual occurrence of a family, personal, or diet history of allergy emphasize the probable allergic origin of the symptoms. Acidosis which may accompany the vomiting is the result rather than the cause of the headaches and other symptoms arising from inability to ingest and assimilate the carbohydrates.

Accurate and adequate diet trial is imperative in every case of cyclic vomiting if the patient is to receive the advantage of our present knowledge of allergy. Several young girls with prolonged invalidism and restriction of social, educational, and recreational activities in spite of former study and treatment by physicians have been entirely relieved by the elimination of allergenic foods as we advise.

CASE REPORTS

We have observed cyclic vomiting associated with bronchial asthma both being relieved with the elimination of allergenic foods.

Case 210: One child eight years of age had diabetes and cyclic vomiting. Another child twelve years of age had the same combination of symptoms. Both were relieved of vomiting and nausea with diets which eliminated their allergenic foods and also have been adjusted to their requirements as advised for diabetics suffering from food allergy in Chapter 30.

Case 211: Another girl had recurrent attacks of vomiting, fever, prostration, and diarrhea with moderate acidosis every two to three months, lasting three to eleven days from the age of twenty-two months until we saw her at the age of six years. Appendectomy was ineffective. Relief occurred with our CFE diet. Thereafter, the gradual addition of foods revealed that wheat was the only cause of her vomiting. No attacks have occurred for eight years except when wheat on rare occasions has been eaten.

VOMITING (NONCYCLIC) BECAUSE OF FOOD ALLERGY

Vomiting or regurgitation of cow's milk in various formulae always requires consideration of allergy to cow's milk or occasionally to other foods added to the formulae or given separately to the infant or child. Formerly when egg yolk was a frequent addition to such formulae, allergy at times developed to it in ten to twenty days after its first ingestion, causing vomiting and other allergic symptoms. If this vomiting continues into childhood and adolescence, it may gradually evolve into cyclic vomiting previously discussed.

When allergy to soy develops in two to three weeks after its initial use, vomiting may arise but less frequently than distention and diarrhea. As already stated in our discussion of infantile colic and gastrointestinal allergy, vomiting is a common occurrence in such symptoms. Vomiting with varying degrees of abdominal pain has been emphasized in our discussion of pylorospasm from cow's milk allergy and also in our discussion of hypertrophic pyloric stenosis in which allergy to cow's milk always requires definite study. Such vomiting may be projectile in type. Gastric retention, demonstrated especially by Fries in children with pylorospasm from milk, has been noted in our discussion of such spasm.

After other foods are added to the infants' and especially to the diet of children, adolescents, and adults, allergy to foods in addition to milk may cause vomiting, especially when sick headaches or classical migraine occur.

DIARRHEA

Diarrhea alone or associated with the other manifestations of food allergy discussed in this chapter deserves additional comment. Kunstadter and Schultz (1953) emphasized the frequency of diarrhea from cow's milk. Clein's report of diarrhea in 24 percent of 140 infants from allergy to cow's milk and Garrod's report of diarrhea in 50 of his 150 infants and children and diarrhea with melena in another 20 cases because of food allergy have already been noted in the discussions of the manifestations of cow's milk allergy. Tudor's report of constant daily diarrhea from allergy to evaporated cow's milk is illustrative of diarrhea alone or associated with other gastrointestinal manifestations of milk and other food allergy.

It is also important to remember that diarrhea and to a less extent other abdominal manifestations of allergy can arise quite frequently from sensitization to soy in soybean milks. As in cow's milk, such symptoms usually develop in ten to twenty days after soy milk is first given, during which time allergy gradually develops.

It is because of this diarrhea and other gastrointestinal symptoms arising from soy milk in children and especially in infants that we proposed in the first edition of this book in 1931 a substitute formula containing meat juice as its protein. Since meat juice only contains 5 percent protein, large amounts of it were necessary to furnish the protein required for a child's nutrition and growth. We therefore asked various processors of meat to make a strained or liquified meat which was first prepared by Clapp and Company in Rochester, New York, in 1939. With this meat we published a meat-base formula, the successful use of which was reported by Glaser in 1956. Then Armour and Swift placed strained meat on the market, which made it unnecessary for mothers to scrape meat for the feeding of infants and children. And since 1942 Gerber has manufactured our meat-base formula containing beef and our lamb-base formula which are in wide use by allergists, pediatricians, and other physicians caring for or directing the feeding of infants and children in this country. As we have used this formula, not only made by Gerber but also by mothers in their homes according to our published directions, the gastrointestinal symptoms, especially diarrhea, colic, abdominal pain, and vomiting because of cow's or goat's milk and soy milk have been relieved in practically every case.

When the beef-base formula does not give desired relief in one to two weeks, the lamb-base formula in practically all cases has produced satisfactory results. As foods other than cow's milk or its substitute are added individually to the infant's diet, diarrhea or other gastrointestinal symptoms may develop from allergy to such foods.

Sudden occurrence of diarrhea with increasing blood and mucus in the stools not only in infancy but at any time during childhood and adult life requires the consideration of chronic ulcerative colitis (CUC) and less frequently regional enteritis as a possible cause. In both of these conditions we have emphasized an eczematouslike allergic inflammation in the mucosa extending into the rest of the tissues in the walls of the bowel resulting especially from food and less frequently to pollens. This important role of allergy in CUC and regional enteritis in adults has been discussed in Chapters 6 and 7. Because of the great importance of its recognition in infants and children, CUC is discussed and emphasized in Chapter 6.

Other causes of diarrhea, especially in children, adolescents, and adults, such as parasites, infection, and from other colonic pathology, always must be considered in the determination of the causes.

Advice of colectomy in young children and even infants because of severe intractable diarrhea from nonspecific enterocolitis

by Avery *et al.* (1968) is in our opinion unjustifiable, especially because of reported deaths in six of twenty infants, unless all other possible causes including food allergy, especially to milk as advised in our discussion of CUC and in this chapter, have received expertized study.

The occurrence of a pathogen in the stools or an ingested food does not obviate the possibility of food allergy, especially if diarrhea continues after the pathogen has been eliminated by drug therapy. The reader is advised to read and study our discussion of allergy to foods and also to pollens and at times drugs as the cause of diarrhea in Chapters 5, 6, and 7. Other causes of diarrhea, including parasites and viral infections, must be in mind. Grampositive bacterial flora resulting from repeated antibiotic therapy must be considered.

Case 212: Thus a child five years of age developed diarrhea attributed to bacteria cultivated from egg yolk. Diarrhea continued, though repeated stool cultures were negative. Our study of food allergy gave large scratch reactions to eggs, the exclusion of which eliminated the diarrhea; thus a recent journey to a midwestern clinic with no benefit was unnecessary.

ABDOMINAL PAIN IN CHILDREN

Abdominal pain requires consideration of possible appendicitis, peritonitis, diverticulitis, intestinal obstruction, intussusception, herniation, and (in older children) cholecystitis or occasional pancreatitis.

If such pathology can be ruled out and vomiting from viral infections can be excluded, pain from abdominal allergy, nearly always to foods, requires adequate and experienced consideration and study. This was recognized and discussed by Ratner (1945). The pain in infantile colic and pylorospasm and pyloric hypertrophic stenosis from allergic reactivity in the muscles of the pylorus have been noted in our previous discussion of these symptoms. Pain may occur in a localized area of the abdomen as a result of food allergy, especially to cow's milk, eggs, fruits, wheat, corn, and other common allergenic foods. Failure to recognize allergy as a cause of such abdominal pain has resulted in too many unnecessary exploratory operations. Pain in the anal canal may arise from allergy, especially to foods.

Seasonal recurrence of pain in the spring to winter months may be due to pollen allergy, as discussed in Chapter 4. Other manifestations of allergy to pollens may or may not occur. Scratch reactions likewise may or may not be present.

Appendiceal type of pain from allergic inflammation in the appendix and/or cecum because of atopic allergy, especially to foods, is discussed in Chapter 5. Since secondary infection may occur, operation is required if rigidity and leukocytosis indicating infection are present.

CELIAC SYNDROME

The celiac syndrome (CS) described by Andersen and di Sant'Agnese (1952) is characterized by indigestion causing bulky, foul stools containing undigested starch, fat, and particles of food with varying degrees of steatorrhea. Intermittent diarrhea and constipation occur. There may be a protuberant abdomen and flabby and even wasting and weak muscles. Deficiency in vitamins and minerals occurs.

Andersen discussed different forms of the syndrome arising from a) an idiopathic possible metabolic familial defect, b) congenital mucoviscidosis, c) severe dietary deficiency, d) chronic impaired absorption, e) chronic enteric or parasitic infection, or f) gastrointestinal allergy.

Kundstadter (1942) and especially McKhann et al. (1943) first attributed the celiac syndrome to gastrointestinal allergy, especially to cow's milk. McKhann noted the similarity of the symptoms in some cases of gastrointestinal allergy and in the CS. McCreary (1951) confirmed cow's milk as a common cause and advised its elimination for several weeks in every case of CS to ascertain possible relief. This was also Kundstadter's advise in 1953. Of thirty-six cases of allergic diarrhea in infants and children, 30.5 percent were typical of the CS. Of these 23.5 percent started in the first three months of life, arising from allergy to cow's milk. Other manifestations of allergy were present in 50 percent of these infants. Tolerance for cow's milk occurred by itself after its elimination in eleven to forty-two months.

Dicke, in 1950, confirmed by Andersen and di Sant'Agnese opined that gluten of wheat and other cereals was the major cause of CS. Weijers and Van de Kamer reported the gliadin fraction of gluten as the major offender in wheat. Taylor, Thomsen, Truelove and Wright (1961) reported serum antibodies to a proteolysed fraction of wheat gluten and to casein, alpha-lactalbumin and beta-lactoglobulin in a higher incidence and titre in these patients than in the sera of normal subjects.

The control of CS with the elimination of gluten, especially in wheat, reported by Andersen and with the elimination of milk by Kundstadter, McKhann, and others indicates allergy as the probable cause of CS. Allergy to other foods also has been suggested in cases of CS which have not been satisfactorily relieved by the elimination of wheat and milk. Davidson (1957) reported diarrhea from beta-lactalbumin and not alpha-lactalbumin in whey which caused steatorrhea. Johnstone opined that the gluten celiac syndrome may be due to allergy. Spector favored food allergy as the cause as Holt noted evidence that allergy to milk as well as to wheat require consideration as the cause of CS. That allergy to other foods also needs consideration was stated by Davidson. Though allergy to milk rather than disacchardide intolerance best explains the control of symptoms by elimination of milk, deficiency in lactase must be in mind, as discussed especially by Arthur, Clayton, *et al.* in 1966.

Because of the advised elimination of wheat and other gluten-containing cereals, of animal milks, and of other possible allergenic foods, we suggest that this challenge of food allergy in CS may best be studied with our FFCFE diet modified for infants and children (Chapt. 3). Because of the acknowledged inaccuracy of protein skin testing in the determination of clinical food allergy, the exclusion of food allergy because of the failure of relief from test-negative diets is not justifiable.

The similarity of idiopathic sprue to the celiac syndrome as noted by other students would also justify the study of possible causative food allergy with our FFCFE diet modified in adolescents and adults as advised in Chapter 3. In 1956 Roberts reported control of sprue and its associated symptoms with a wheat-free diet. Johnstone, in 1970, stated that vitamin A absorption curve returns to normal when allergenic foods are eliminated.

Davidson and Burnstein (1957) reported gastrointestinal symptoms with steatorrhea simulating sprue in a child three months of age with diarrhea from cow's milk. Feeding tests showed allergy to alpha-lactalbumin and not to beta-lactalbumin of the whey protein which even in 1/100 of the normal amount in a quart of whole cow's milk caused considerable steatorrhea. Malabsorption with vomiting, diarrhea, and steatorrhea controlled by elimination of milk in infancy recurred in 1½ years from gradually acquired allergy to gluten, as re-ported by Fallstrom *et al.* in 1965.

FIBROCYSTIC DISEASE OF THE PANCREAS MUCOVISCIDOSIS

Andersen, in 1938, first reported cases of fibrocystic disease of the pancreas associated with recurrent and gradually persisting changes and resultant symptoms in the bronchial tissues. Because it is a disease of the mucus-secreting glands of the pancreatic, nasal, sinal, bronchial, and hepatic mucosae, Farber in 1945 named it mucoviscidosis. Today cystic fibrosis (CF) is the preferred name for this disease, especially affecting the exocrine glands of the body secreting mucus and sweat. Of great importance was the report of Darling, Andersen, *et al.* in 1953 of heightened sodium and chloride excretion from the sweat-producing gland. This was confirmed by di Sant'Agnese, Darling, *et al.* in 1953.

The frequency of CF in the United States is estimated between 0.7 and 1.7 per 1000 neonates. Deaths in twenty-five patients between 6 and 14½ years of age because of purulent bronchitis, bronchiectasis, and pneumonia were reported by Fisher, Van Metre, and Winkerwerder in 1960.

Indigestion and irritable colon with hypoglycemic attacks, weakness, and varying evidence of our clinical allergy resulting from probable gluten allergy causing roentgen ray changes in the small bowel were reported by Pack-Steen and Lorenzen in an informative article in 1968.

Of informative interest are the following statistics of Van Metre, Jr., *et al.* (1960) indicative of CF in nineteen patients in whom allergy also was present.

	19 Patients With CF and Allergy %	135 Patients With CF %
Family history of cystic fibrosis	32	30
Abnormal stools	90	96
Pancreatin enzyme deficiency	79	73

Rectal prolapse	11	10
Meconium ileus	11	7
Respiratory disease symptoms	100	96
Emphysema	100	91
Pulmonary infiltrates	100	
Wheezing	63	38
Clubbing of fingers	79	45
Rhinitis	95	79
Failure to thrive	95	96
Death from CF	32	41

Concern from the allergic viewpoint has encouraged continued reports of recurrent and later persistent respiratory symptoms and especially of evident bronchial asthma as by Abbott *et al.* in 1957 in 10 percent of 102 patients, by Van Metre *et al.* (1960) in 11 percent of 116 patients, and by Derbes *et al.* (1957) in 33 percent of 68 patients. Bodian (1953) reported incidence of allergy in 11 percent of 116 such patients.

Kulczychi *et al.* (1957) reported allergy in 36.6 percent of 266 patients and respiratory allergy in 16.6 percent.

Evidence of possible allergy in CF reported by Kulczychi *et al.* included the following:

1. Familial history indicating allergy.

2. Hay fever or nasal or ocular symptoms of probable allergy.

3. Nasal polyps with chronic sinusitis.

4. Asthmatic symptoms.

5. Cutaneous allergy.

6. Indications of food allergy, especially colic, vomiting, and diarrhea in infants and children.

That the changes in the bronchial tissues in cystic fibrosis and in bronchial asthma are similar has been reported by Andersen, Farber, and Atkins. Atkins, in 1948, stated that bronchoscopy in CF showed similar findings to those in bronchial asthma. The dramatic response of bronchospasm when present in CF to epinephrine also favors allergy as the cause, as stated by Derbes *et al.*

The necessary occurrence of a high content of sodium and chlorides in the sweat in the diagnosis of cystic fibrosis must be emphasized.

As Fisher, Van Metre, and Winkerwerder (1960) warn, the evidence of allergy must not divert attention from the recognition of concomitant and major CF. Derbes also advises recognition of CF in young patients in whom persisting cough, shortness of breath, and wheezing indicate bronchial asthma.

COMMENT

Allergy to inhalants has been studied and treated in a limited number of patients with confirmed CF with no benefit. Because of failure of relief with diets excluding positive skin-reacting foods along with negative reactions to foods and negative diet histories indicating possible food allergy, food allergy also has been excluded on insufficient evidence as a major or associated cause of CF. Because of this absence of evidence of inhalant and food allergy, therefore, the slight or more definite asthma in these patients has been attributed, unjustifiably in our opinion, to intrinsic or possible infectant causes.

According to our experience, however, unrecognized atopic allergy, especially to foods, with or without inhalant allergy is responsible for most perennial asthma and much chronic bronchitis often ascribed to intrinsic or infectant causes.

As we peruse the articles on CF in which there has been consideration of allergy, especially in the nasobronchial tissues, there is no evidence that food allergy has been studied with trial diets, especially with our CFE diet or its modifications as we advise in Chapter 3 and throughout this volume in the adequate strict and sufficient manner we recommend. Existent or probable inhalant allergy also must be recognized and controlled.

Though patients with CF have not been

referred to us for the study of atopic allergy, we opine that our advised study of allergy, especially to foods, should be made in a large number of cases of CF. Such study by us and many other physicians has confirmed food allergy with or without inhalant allergy as the sole or major cause of most cyclic recurrent asthma in children and young adults as reported in this chapter, of much perennial bronchial asthma throughout life (Chapt. 8), much chronic bronchitis (Chapt. 9), and of most bronchospasm and bronchorrhea in obstructive emphysema (Chapt. 11).

Adequate study of food allergy is especially important moreover when nasal polyps, which are frequent in CF, are present which usually are due to chronic food allergy according to our experience (Chapt. 12).

With such study and control of possible food and of indicated inhalant allergy, food allergy especially may prove a frequent associated or major cause of CF. It is the common cause of thick, often inspissated, mucus in bronchial asthma and obstructive emphysema as confirmed by us for many years.

Moreover, because of the increasing evidence that all tissues of the body are subject to food and other allergy, it is also possible that it may play a major or adjunctive role in the secretion of thick inspissated mucus and tissue changes in the pancreatic ducts, as we state in Chapter 27. If so, the heightened sodium and chlorides would need explanation.

Thus with the control of such possible allergy and the judicious use of corticosteroids, the symptoms and tissue changes of CF in the respiratory tissues and in the pancreas might gradually subside and result in increased longevity in these presently unfortunate children.

ALLERGIC GASTROENTEROPATHY CAUSING PROTEIN LOSS BECAUSE OF FOOD ALLERGY

Waldman *et al.*, in 1967, reported allergic gastroenteropathy causing marked protein loss from the gastrointestinal tract associated with generalized edema (especially periorbital edema), retarded growth, hypoalbuminemia, hypogammaglobulinemia, anemia with eosinophilia, and other manifestations of allergy including asthma, eczema, and allergic rhinitis. There was eosinophilic infiltration of the lamina propria in the mucosa of the small bowel in six reported cases. Five had definite evidence of milk allergy. After marked relief in three from elimination of allergenic foods, especially of milk, the symptoms recurred from the ingestion of milk. Symptoms had started from the age of 4 months to 2.5 years (average 1.5 years). A history of milk intolerance was usual.

Low serum albumins are reported in regional enteritis and ulcerative colitis in which gastric neoplasm and other malabsorption states are present.

Other nutritional deficiencies reported from an exclusive milk diet also suggest milk allergy as the cause.

Intestinal permeability to milk and other food proteins, as evidenced by a positive Prausnitz-Kustner reaction, is paralleled by the passage of starch particles through the mucosa of the gastrointestinal tract into various body tissues, as reported by Volkheimer and by Dr. Lietze in Chapter 28 of this volume.

Varying degrees of intestinal food allergy therefore are suggested causes of malabsorption, malnutrition, and retarded growth in children.

That food allergy and to a lesser degree pollen and at times drug allergy cause the eczematouslike inflammation in the mucosa of the colon and small bowel, causing chronic ulcerative colitis and regional enteritis, has long been reported by us as discussed in Chapters 6 and 7 of this volume.

These reports of Waldman's and of other physicians referred to by him are worthy of special study when symptoms in this syndrome challenge the physician.

ALLERGIC FATIGUE AND TOXEMIA

Allergic toxemia and fatigue from food allergy which we first reported in 1930 and in the first edition of this book in 1931 occurs in children as well as adults, as has been discussed in Chapter 19. Lack of energy, lifelessness, unwillingness to play, drowsiness, nervousness, irritability, frequent whining, and crying often result. Restlessness and nightmares and at times insomnia may arise from food allergy. Fever up to 104 F from food allergy and not infection (as reported in Chapt. 24), chilling, gooseflesh, and sweating with slight exertion may be present. Other manifestations of food allergy (especially in the gastrointestinal tract), perennial nasal allergy, headaches, and less often cutaneous and bronchial allergy along with a familial history of the allergy are the rule. These manifestations of allergic toxemia and fatigue in children are fully discussed in Chapter 19, in which case histories are included and the use of our elimination diets to study and control the causative food allergies are advised. Reports of a change in the child's personality "from a little devil to a little saint" or of a little girl who formerly "just sat" and "was climbing trees and wearing out her shoes in a few months" or the history of a rebellious, militant boy who became quiet and corrigible when food allergies were controlled with additional comments on these manifestations in children are included in the aforementioned chapter.

The frequency and importance of recognition of allergic fatigue and toxemia which we reported in the first volume of this book in 1931 have been confirmed and emphasized by Randolph, Speer, and by ourselves and other allergists, including Davison, through the intervening years. The reader is again referred to Chapter 19 on allergic fatigue and toxemia.

MALNUTRITION AND CACHEXIA

When gastrointestinal allergy, especially to milk, causes nausea, cramping, diarrhea, and at times vomiting, especially when it is associated with atopic eczema, anemia, malnutrition, underweight, weakness, and fatigue may arise. When these results of food allergy are severe, exudative diathesis described by Czerny many years ago and confirmed by Abt and subsequent pediatricians may result. Food allergy, especially to milk, may cause slight colonic bleeding. Actual melena has been reported especially by Rubin in 1940. Protein losing allergic gastroenteropathy reported by Waldman in 1967 has received previous discussion in this chapter. With the use of soy milk or our infant's meat-base formula as the substitute for milk and the use of our CFE diet in older infants and children together with indicated vitamins, these manifestations of food allergy often are controlled.

ANOREXIA AND FOOD AVERSIONS

Dislikes or aversions to specific foods often are due to food allergy. Finicky eating, moreover, often arises from allergy to some but not all ingested foods. Allergy to one or to two foods may decrease appetite for other important foods to which allergy is absent. If food allergy is a challenge, a child should not be forced to eat suspected allergenic foods. Freeman, in 1920, opined that dislikes for food were frequently due to food allergy and not to fancies or whims. Ratner, in 1922, emphasized distaste for foods as presumptive evidence of allergy. Fenwick warned against forcing children to eat probable or definite allergy-producing foods. Articles by our former distinguished confrere and friend, Clifford Sweet, on poor appetites considered allergy as one important cause. The selection of a balanced, nourishing diet by the unaided infant was beautifully demonstrated by Davis (1928) and also by Sweet. It is probable that during the first months or years of life, tolerance for allergic foods gradually develops. Delayed tolerance may account for the slowness with which new foods are usually accepted by many children and for aversions to various foods which may persist for many years. Food allergy, therefore, as a common cause of anorexia needs constant consideration.

NERVOUS AND PSYCHIC DISTURBANCES IN CHILDHOOD FROM ALLERGY

Food allergy in childhood can produce localized or general reactions in the brain and in other nervous tissues which may result in various mental and psychic disturbances, including restlessness, incorrigibility, irritability, bursts of temper, drowsiness, sullenness, depression, somnolence, and marked changes in disposition.

Disturbed sleep and nightmares often occur in children with nasal allergy because in large measure of the irritation, fullness, and occlusion in the nose and throat with extension of the allergy into the meninges, vascular, and possibly other cerebral tissues, especially in the frontal lobe.

These results of food allergy were especially stressed by Shannon in 1922, who reported many interesting case records in his article on nervous manifestations of food allergy in childhood. It is well recognized that migraine begins in the teens in many cases and as Tileston has reported, it may begin in childhood. Such migraine, as stated in Chapter 17 requires adequate study of food allergy. It may be preceded or accompanied by cyclic vomiting as noted in this chapter. I have several records of recurrent headaches in young children associated with other types of allergy, all of which were due to food sensitization.

Marked restlessness in sleep and "jumping" or "leaping" during the night which might have been due to food allergy occurred, as in two children recently relieved with elimination of causative foods. Pounding of the head in early childhood also can result from allergy, especially to foods. Somnolence, mental sluggishness and recurrent convulsive seizures were due to food allergy in another young patient. This latter child also had a pollen allergy which was necessary to control.

These symptoms have been more fully discussed in Chapter 19 on Allergic Fatigue and Toxemia and in Chapter 18 on Cerebral and Neural Allergy.

The probability that epilepsy, especially in children, may be due to food and pollen and other inhalant allergy has been discussed in Chapter 18. Such etiology must be seriously considered in all cases of idiopathic epilepsy.

The reader is referred to the above chapter on the nervous manifestations of allergy for a further consideration of this subject. It is realized that some pediatricians will opine that many of these symptoms are due to lack of rest or to nervous strain or poorly controlled daily routines in the affected children. Such possibilities had been thought of and therapy based on such likelihoods had been carried out without benefit in many patients suffering with such symptoms from allergy, especially to foods. Of interest was the study of Piness and Miller (1937), showing that the intelligence rating of allergic children is the same as that of normals.

FEVER

Allergic fever in childhood as well as in adult life may be due to food allergy. Low-grade fevers from allergy may wrongly be assumed to result from possible undemonstrated pyelitis, bronchitis, tonsillitis, sinusitis, or other possible foci of infection. Prolonged bed rest for assumed tuberculosis, impossible however to demonstrate, occurred especially before its present control with drugs. Zybells' case of fever from milk in a child three years of age was reported by Laroche, Richet, and Saint Girons, and other similar cases in the literature are referred to in Chapter 29. The reader is referred to our further discussion of fever from food allergy in Chapter 24.

Atopic allergy, especially to foods, must be adequately studied as advised in this chapter as a conjoint cause of recurrent convulsive seizures and of fever when febrile seizures recur, especially if Dilantin or other anticonvulsive drug has been suggested or given. All other possible causes also must be considered (see Chapt. 22).

ENURESIS

The possibility that bed wetting may arise from allergy with our illustrated case has been discussed in Chapter 21. Bray (1931) reported relief in a number of children from the elimination of causative foods. He stated that because of similar enervation of the lungs and bladder, stimulating of the parasympathetic system may lead to spasm in the bronchi or bladder.

Enuresis from food and at times inhalant allergy has occurred, and additional discussion is in Chapter 21.

ORTHOSTATIC ALBUMINURIA FROM FOOD ALLERGY

This has been discussed in Chapter 21.

NEPHROTIC SYNDROME

Evidence that inhalant allergy to pollens is one cause of the nephrotic syndrome was reported by Hardwick in 1959. It was confirmed by Wittig and Goldman in 1970 to airborne spores of fungi in one case and to pollens in two cases. Their report with a discussion of the possible immunological pathogenesis and references is important.

Because of this probable role of inhalant allergy, the study of possible food allergy as advised in this volume with our cereal-free elimination diet as a cause of the nephrotic syndrome is a definite challenge, remembering however its rarity in about 7 in 100,000 children under the age of five years as stated in the article by Wittig and Goldman.

FINAL COMMENT

It is very evident that food, inhalant, and other types of allergy must be in the minds of all physicians treating or supervising infants and children. In infancy food allergy is the first type of sensitization that nearly always develops. It often persists throughout childhood even into adult life. It also must be emphasized that food allergy can develop at any time of life, however, even in old age.

SUMMARY

1. Allergy, especially to foods, in infancy and childhood causes symptoms in gastrointestinal, nasobronchial, cutaneous, ocular, cerebral, urogenital, and other body tissues. Cow's milk is the sole or most common cause of allergy in infancy.

2. As other foods are added, allergy to them must be suspected. This can be stud-

ied with modifications of our CFE diet as advised in Chapter 3.

3. Inhalant allergy increases during later years. The manifestations of food allergy often decrease through childhood. However, it may persist or be reactivated through life, including old age.

4. Establishment and prevention of food, inhalant, and drug allergies are discussed. Allergy to cow's milk is the usual cause of croup, bronchiolitis, bronchitis in the first five to twelve months, as emphasized by Cline, Bigler, Tudor, and recently by Gerrard. Illustrative histories are summarized.

5. Perennial nasal allergy and "recurrent head colds" at times with fever are usually due to food allergy, especially to milk, cereal grains, eggs, chocolate, and other foods.

6. Recognition of our pathognomonic history of bronchial asthma from food allergy is emphasized, as evidenced in statistics in Table XVIII on such asthma in infants and children.

7. In our experience bacterial allergy is rare or absent.

8. Control of food and inhalant allergy and initial control of asthma with drugs are advised.

9. Though corticosteroids are justified for initial control of symptoms, no long-term corticosteroid therapy is required when our advised control of food and inhalant allergy is strictly maintained.

10. Perennial nasal allergy from foods, with or without inhalant (especially pollen) allergy is emphasized.

11. Bronchiectasis usually starting in childhood, especially after attacks of bronchial asthma, receives special discussion in Chapter 10. Kartagener's syndrome and its allergic possibilities must be recognized.

12. Allergic dermatitis in infancy and childhood is usually due to cow's milk and

to other foods as they are added to the diet. Pollen and other inhalants become active in late childhood.

13. Statistics on 147 cases of allergic dermatitis in infancy and childhood relieved by control of allergy are tabulated. Advised treatment is discussed.

14. Urticaria and angioneurotic edema are usually due to food and less often to drug and inhalants than in adults.

15. Gastrointestinal allergy, especially to milk, is the usual cause of colic, pylorospasm, and hypertrophic pyloric stenosis in infancy.

16. Recurrent gastrointestinal symptoms with fever from food allergy, as reported by Cooke in 1933, we opine is the equivalent of our pathognomonic history of bronchial asthma from food allergy.

17. Food allergy causing cyclic vomiting and noninfectious diarrhea is best investigated with our CFE diet or its modifications advised in Chapter 3.

18. That allergy to milk rather than deficiency in lactase explains most symptoms resulting from milk is emphasized.

19. Food allergy as a common cause of diarrhea, abdominal pain, and also of celiac syndrome and its abdominal symptoms is best studied as we advise.

20. Because of indications of personal and familial allergy in patients with cystic fibrosis, the challenge of food allergy requires study as we recommend.

21. Our advised study of food allergy in protein losing allergic gastroenteropathy and especially in allergic toxemia and fatigue and as an important cause of anorexia, malnutrition, cachexia and food aversions, allergic fever, and enuresis is discussed in this chapter.

22. The role of atopic allergy in orthostatic albuminuria and the nephrotic syndrome is discussed.

The study and control of food allergy

and of inhalant allergy are outlined and discussed *in extenso* in Chapters 3 and 4.

23. Thus the various manifestations of allergy as encountered in childhood have been discussed in this chapter. The reader is referred, moreover, to previous chapters in this book in which a more complete consideration of many of these manifestations of allergy, especially to foods, has been reported. The negative skin reactions and the importance of trial diet, especially our elimination diets, to study and control food allergy in childhood as well as in adult life have been emphasized.

Chapter 26

Cardiovascular, Glandular, Renal, Hepatic, and Constitutional Effects With Blood Changes From Allergy

The many manifestations of allergy already described emphasize the fact that practically any tissue of the body is likely to have such disturbances. It also illustrates the localized nature of allergic reactivity—the predilection that food allergy, for instance, has to produce evident symptoms in the gastrointestinal tract in one patient, the nasobronchial tissues in another, or the skin in another with or without major clinical allergy in other tissues. Potential sensitization probably exists, however, in practically all tissues in such patients.

Our previous discussion, moreover, has shown the localization of the allergic manifestations circumscribed in special areas of one tissue of the body best illustrated by eczema from food on one or more fingers or only in the aural canals, with no other obvious involvement of the rest of the integument. As we have stated many times, allergy produces three main types of reactions, namely smooth muscle spasm, edema, and hypersecretion of the mucosal glands arising with varying evidence and degrees from vascular allergy. Increasing evidence shows that these reactions may occur in any tissue of the body, especially in their vascular tissues. Clinical experience also directs attention to its special frequency in the skin, nasobronchial, and gastrointestinal tract. We have also discussed

its manifestations in the meninges, brain, nerve sheaths and other nervous tissues, synovial membranes of joints and tendons, and in the ocular and other tissues.

Pearson, according to Bray (1935), observed recurrent edema from allergy in the parotids similar to a case we report in this chapter. This of course indicates that other glands may be intermittently or chronically affected by allergy, as in the lymphatic glands. The cardiovascular tissues, including the capillaries, moreover, are not exempt. Sulzberger (1934) stated that vascular allergy is the fundamental reaction in allergy, leading to changes in vascular permeability and surrounding tissue edema. Such edema would result in disturbances in cellular metabolism with resultant increased or prolonged symptomatology. As yet, clinical evidence of allergic reactions from vascular allergy in the osseous tissues is questionable, though interference with function of the bone marrow and other blood-forming organs may be evidenced by leukopenia, thrombopenia, and decrease in blood coagulability arising from allergy, impairing bone development and growth, as reported by Cohen. It is possible that allergic reactions arise in the localized areas of the vascular structure of the bone itself, producing transient or severe pain of varying degrees, as in "leg pains" in childhood. Thus it is likely that no structure of the body is exempt from allergic reactivity.

Definite or hypothetical evidence of other manifestations of clinical allergy other than those previously discussed will now be presented. The following information and discussions including hypothetical considerations will be mainly concerned with food allergy, the chief challenge in this volume, and less inhalant allergy.

MISCELLANEOUS DISEASED STATES IN WHICH ATOPIC ALLERGY HAS BEEN STUDIED OR DESERVES STUDY

That atopic allergy to foods and inhalants, especially to the most common cause of the latter, namely pollens, produces allergic reactivity in vascular and other tissues of the heart, kidney, liver, and other vital organs with resultant acute or chronic symptoms is supported by the following:

Acute and chronic anaphylaxis in the above tissues of animals arise from the union of antibodies resulting from the parenteral injection of eggs, milk, and other food allergens or of inhalant allergens with the same antigen injected into or even ingested by the animal. a) In man similar pathological lesions in blood vessels and other tissues in the lungs, liver, pancreas, heart, vascular tissues, kidneys, and adrenals from anaphylaxis to foods and inhalant allergens have been recorded in the literature for seventy years. b) That anaphylaxis to drugs also causes similar tissue reactions in varying degrees in the above tissues in man is also recorded in the literature.

Since atopic allergy to foods in association with allergy to inhalants is the main challenge in this volume, evidence and probability of its occurrence in the vital organs and blood in man will be discussed.

Those diseases of unknown etiology in which immunological factors exert a defi-

nite, secondary, or possible poorly understood influence in their pathogenesis will not be our challenge. The reader is referred to the many excellent articles published in the last forty years on the immunological aspects of the following diseases as summarized recently by Neal A. Vanselow, M.D., in *Clinical Allergy,* published by Sheldon, Lovell, and Matthew (1967) and discussed under the editorship of John H. Vaughan, M.D., in *Immunological Diseases,* edited by Max Samter in 1965.

Though in all of these diseases the possible role of atopic allergy, especially to foods, has not been demonstrated, its possibility in our opinion has not been adequately investigated and excluded.

These diseases include rheumatoid arthritis, systemic lupus erythematosis, polyarteritis nodosa, polymyositis, dermatomysitis, progressive systemic sclerosis, scleroderma, and Sjogren's Syndrome. Neither have the immunological aspects of specific organ diseases authoritatively discussed in the above books been demonstrated, including demyelenating diseases, endogenous uveitis, thyroiditis, acquired hemolytic diseases, pernicious anemia and gastritis, diseases of the liver, adrenalitis, aspermatogenesis, orchitis, infertility, and myasthenia gravis.

The role of allergy to drugs as to iodine in periarteritis nodosum reported by Rasmusson in 1955 must be realized.

That atopic allergy especially to foods and less frequently to pollens and rarely to drugs is the major and often sole confirmed cause of chronic ulcerative colitis (CUC) and regional enteritis (RE) has been reported by Andresen and us in many articles during the last twenty-seven years. As we have stated in the *JAMA* in 1954 and recently in 1968, with the adequate study and strict control of such allergies as we advise, gastroenterologists and other physicians can duplicate our results. Thereby, the possible role of antibodies to foods, inhalants, and rarely to drugs which we have long reported rather than autotissue antibodies as hypothesized especially by Kirsner in 1960 will receive confirmation of great importance to the unfortunate victims of these allergic diseases.

The role of atopic allergy in CUC and RE and our methods of its adequate study and control have received extended discussion in Chapters 6 and 7. Case 62 reported in Chapter 6 is that of an infant with CUC which developed in the first week of life but which continues to be relieved with the control of atopic allergy for the last five years.

The demonstrated and probable role of allergy to foods, inhalants, and drugs in ocular allergy receives extended discussion in Chapter 20. With adequate study of food and pollen allergies as we advise, more evidence of atopic allergy in most ocular tissues will occur with a decrease in the possibilities of autoimmunity, especially in endogenous uveitis.

PAROTID SWELLINGS FROM FOOD ALLERGY

Swellings of the parotids from food allergy reported in 1947 and confirmed by us in the following case summary indicates that other glandular tissues may harbor allergy to foods as well as inhalants, drugs, or chemicals as we hypothesize in this chapter.

Waldbolt and Shea, in 1947, reported recurrent edema of the parotid to cottonseed allergen in its oil one-half hour after its ingestion. "The throat closes up," and "the chest becomes tight." A slight skin reaction was obtained. Swellings in a second patient were relieved with the elimination of sauerkraut, onion, and iodized salt. Swellings in a third patient were re-

produced by tuna, lettuce, and bread. Asthma was present in all three.

Johnston, in 1947, also reported relief of edemas in the parotid with elimination of wheat, cheese, tomato, and chocolate. Previously Meyer, in 1934, reported "probable benefit" from elimination of several foods. According to Bray (1935) Pearson studied recurrent parotitis similar to our case below.

The periodicity of unilateral or bilateral swellings, which is a definite important characteristic of food allergy occurred in Hansel's, Waldbott's, and our patient. Such periodicity suggesting food allergy was first reported by Burton-Fanning in 1925, McKaskey in 1942, Reason in 1935 and 1936, Sier in 1937, Hansel in 1941 with plugging of Stensen's duct with eosinophiles, Zindler and Frazer in 1948, and in an excellent report by Bookman in 1950 in patients in all of whom specific foods were not identified. Study of atopic allergy to inhalants and especially to foods because of the periodic attacks, we opine, probably would have revealed allergenic foods with or without less likely inhalant allergy.

References to pertinent articles are in those of Waldbott, Johnstone, and Bookman and are also included in the Bibliography of this volume.

Case Summary

Case 213: A girl nineteen years of age (D.G.) was first seen in 1960 because of swellings of the parotids for five years which had developed suddenly, lasting for five to seven days associated with slight pain, with a gradual recovery in three to twenty days. Salivation was not increased. Swellings recurred every one to two months, more frequently in the winter and early spring than in the summer. Fatigue, drowsiness, and difficulty in concentration accompanied the attacks. Between the attacks, moderate fatigue and drowiness and tension continued.

Hay fever had been present all of her life characterized by coryza, congestion in the nose, and edema in the lids exaggerated in the spring and summer. Treatment for one year four years previously had been ineffectual. Asthma never occurred. Susceptibility to head colds without fever had occurred in the last ten years, especially from November to May, suggesting food allergy. Hives had occurred from strawberries. A rash had occurred from contact with Bermuda grass.

She had had pyrosis and epigastric distention for two years up to four years previously and at intervals since then. Canker sores had occurred at times. She had had headaches two to three times a week for one to two years.

Diet history revealed no apparent idiosyncrasies or dislikes for food.

She had slept on a feather pillow. There were many trees in the vicinity of her home.

Family history of allergy was absent.

Skin testing revealed large reactions to Rye and Bermuda grass pollens and lesser ones to other grass pollens. She gave large reactions to fruit tree pollens, to sycamore, and one and two plus reactions to several of the fall and other tree pollens.

Blood and urine analyses were negative except for 11 percent eosinophiles.

Food allergy was studied with our CFE diet. In two months no parotid swellings had occurred. Desensitization to a multiple pollen antigen was started with a 1:50 million dilution (See Appendix for notation).

In four months there had been no swellings. Cereal grains and extra vegetables did not cause swellings. Pollen therapy had been continued into the #5 dilution. In January, 1961, she reported that she had deviated from the diet for two months, with resultant swellings of her parotids.

During the last nine years control of the swellings has required elimination of milk, eggs, and wheat from the diet. Desensitization with her pollen antigen has continued every three to four weeks. She reported seven years later she had had no swellings except when milk, eggs, and wheat were eaten, especially in the winter months. Control of her pollen allergy had been dependent on her cooperation in the self-administration of required multiple pollen antigens under our intermittent supervision.

In March of 1969 she reported failure to adhere to her diet for over a year. Swellings of the parotids had been recurring every one to two months. She was taking the #4 dilution of her antigen of which she could tolerate only 0.10 cc. Her blood and urine analyses were negative.

CARDIOVASCULAR DISTURBANCES FROM ATOPIC ALLERGY

The smooth muscle spasm already discussed in the arterioles, larger arteries, and probably the capillaries which leads to edema and disturbed cellular metabolism can explain many symptoms which are due to allergy. Food allergy especially seems to cause such disturbances of sufficient degree to demand relief. Evidence presented below also shows that pollen and other inhalant allergy produces vascular allergy as evidenced in anaphylactic shock from excessive doses of pollen. The probable role of tobacco allergy is also discussed. It must be remembered that allergic shock is a primarily cardiovascular disturbance. Vallery-Radot, Ledoux-Lebard, Hamburger, Hugo, and Calderon (1935) demonstrated by arteriography with thorium dioxide vasoconstriction in the femoral arteries of rabbits in anaphylactic shock. Harkavy even in 1934 stated that the possibility of allergy in arterial and coronary disease had been too little considered.

The emphasis on the recognition of allergy to tobacco in the systemic and cardiac vasculature by Harkavy during the last thirty years is of great importance. His recent review of his admirable studies and conclusions in 1968 and in his important book on *Vascular Allergy* in 1963 are mandatory reading for physicians treating adults and especially for cardiologists, heart and vascular surgeons, and allergists.

Kline and Young (1935) suggested that the necrotic intimal lesions in the arterioles in nephrosclerosis may be due to allergy. Hyperergic arteritis as studied by Rossle and others and its relation to disease in man is of great importance and receives further discussion later in this chapter.

That the heart muscle may be subject to allergy is evident from the fact that it is a modified type of smooth muscle from the vascular tube in the embryo, every muscle cell being liberally supplied with blood. Duke, in 1925, saw no reason why cardiac muscle should be exempt from localized allergy. Mild cardiovascular allergy may be very common but too slight to cause evident symptoms. Patients occasionally know that certain foods produce palpitation, flushing, cardiac irregularity, or discomfort in the chest. Patients with marked extrasystoles from food sensitizations have come to our attention. Werley (1932) also reported extrasystoles from probable food allergy. Criep (1931) noted that anaphylaxis may produce in experimental animals changes in rate, arrhythmias, auricular and ventricular asystole, and even cardiac standstill. The extrasystoles, tachycardia, and slight or definite anginal pain or discomfort are experienced by some individuals from the slightest whiff of tobacco smoke. Melli (1930) determined feather allergy as a cause of gallop rhythm with duplication of the P_2 sound and a transient A-V block.

Healey, Gallison, and Brudno (1934) found intraventricular block from food allergy as shown by the electrocardiograph. The patient had cramping, mid- and low abdominal pain, tenesmus, and diarrhea from wheat allergy. A white count of 34,000 with seventy percent eosinophiles and eosinophiles in the urine were present in the absence of infection. Thus rhythm and conduction in the heart may be affected by allergic reactions in the tissues concerned. Food allergy as a possible cause can be studied with our CFE diet and its modifications, as advised in Chapter 3.

Paroxysmal tachycardia has apparently arisen from allergy in many cases. We have studied three patients whose attacks were greatly decreased in frequency and severity by "elimination diets." One woman was freed from attacks when wheat was excluded from her diet. She also had hay fever from grass pollens. One had gastrointestinal allergy and the other recurrent corneal ulcers from food allergy. Several other patients were prone to transient spells of tachycardia when allergenic foods were ingested. Coffee was the cause in two patients. Thomas and Post (1925) and Bassoe (1933) stated that paroxysmal tachycardia may often replace or accompany migraine (Chapt. 17). Critchley and Ferguson (1933) called such tachycardia a migrainous equivalent. Hoffman (1910) observed that migraine, epilepsy, and paroxysmal tachycardia were at times associated. A patient of Vallery-Radot's (1925) had alternating attacks of migraine and tachycardia from food allergy. As reported by Shookhoff (1933), Luria and Wilensky, Weill (1932), and Mussio-Fournier (1932) stressed food allergy in the etiology of paroxysmal tachycardia. Kern (1932) reported one woman with recurrent attacks since the age of five years. Specific foods were causative to which skin reactions were negative. L.P. Gay reported several cases of tachycardia controlled with food eliminations. The intermittent nature of this malady, its frequent association with other allergic manifestations, a marked history of allergy in the family, the lack of definite pathology in the heart muscle, and the absence of changes in the electrocardiographic tracings between attacks favor an allergic origin. Hyperirritability of the heart muscle from various causes may be present, and allergy might be the added factor to initiate the attack. However, allergy alone, especially to foods, must be studied as a cause of this condition. Vascular spasm with possible edema in the cardiac muscle would well explain a "functional upset."

Anginal pain may arise at times from vascular spasm and surrounding tissue edema in the heart muscle from allergy. Liveing and Osler commented on the relation of angina to migraine, asthma, angiospasm, and transient paralyses. Osler even suggested anaphylaxis as a cause of angina, with resulting spasm of arteries and ischemia of the myocardium. In our book on food allergy in 1931 we pointed out the possibility of food allergy as one cause of angina. Since then Gay told us of a patient with angina pectoris and even syncope apparently from food allergy. Werley (1932), in a study of sixty-two cases of angina and infarction, concluded that food allergy needed frequent consideration. Recurrent angina pectoris in two patients were definitely controlled by our elimination diets. Migraine in 55 percent, urticaria in 32 percent, asthma in 17 percent, hay fever in 11 percent, and angioneurotic edema in 11 percent of his patients pointed to an allergic status in many of these individuals. He felt that allergy established in the cardiac muscle and possibly the autonomic nerves is a trigger mechanism so that spasm suddenly occurs or is initiated even by psychoneurotic influences, cold or other nonspecific factors. He felt also that spasm from allergy may arise in partly sclerosed arteries and may even precipitate patients with angina pectoris. These patients should be studied from the allergic viewpoint, especially with our elimination diets.

Werley (1935) again reported food allergy as a factor in many cases of angina pectoris. In discussion Herrmann commended Werley's contribution and stated that "elimination diets" were logical means for study of possible food allergies. Lichtwitz (1925), Finch (1930), Dattner (1931), and Jones (1932) discussed angina pectoris from the allergic viewpoint, and Eiselsberg (1934) reported two cases apparently arising from food sensitizations. Shookhoff and Lieberman (1933) presented a case with angina, hypertension, and arteriosclerosis benefited greatly by pollen therapy and with pollen-free air. In discussion the writer told of a patient whose anginal attacks were greatly diminished by similar treatment. She had been afflicted with coronary spasm for several years, especially in the spring and summer months. Shookhoff also reported three patients with angina attributed to aspirin allergy. Two of them had urticaria. Thus food allergy and less frequently pollen and drug allergy may play a more or less important role in producing anginal pain and even occlusion. This is especially true in middle age or the early sixties. While possible allergy is being considered, however, it is most necessary to utilize other recognized diagnostic and therapeutic measures and study other more common possible causes.

PERIPHERAL VASCULAR ALLERGY

Cardiovascular manifestations of hypersensitivity with associated and resultant tissue changes and pathology arising from tobacco, antibiotics, other drugs, inhalants, foods, and infection, as reported by Harkavy in his prestigious book, are summarized in his recent article in November of 1969, which will be of special interest to the reader. That arthralgia, edema, purpura, loss of weight, subcutaneous nodules, pneumonitis, dermatitis, tender muscles, weakness, neuritis, gastrointestinal edema, erythema, bleeding, and vasculitis and even failure in kidney occur is stated by Harkavy. Periarteritis nodosa, dermatomyositis, lupus erythematosus, and scleroderma result from such vasculitis.

Harkavy especially stresses allergy in the

peripheral blood vessels and in the heart. Allergy needs study as a cause of vasculitis and thrombosis of some migrating phlebitis and thromboangitis obliterans of angina pectoris and cardiac arrythmias.

Harkavy reaffirms food allergy to fish and citrus fruits in migrating phlebitis as reported by him in 1963 and Conner even in 1920. His emphasis since 1932 of tobacco as the common cause of this allergy and of coronary artery disease must be remembered. Recurrent coronary arteritis, he states, causes fibrin deposits on the intima, gradually resulting in stenosing arteritis which is similar to primary arteriosclerosis causing occlusion from superimposed thrombosis.

Of importance in this volume is Harkavy's opinion that atopic allergy, especially to foods, requires study as a cause of cardiac arrhythmias in patients with previously normal hearts rather than emotional and digestive disturbances, fatigue, alcohol, tobacco, and other suggested causes. This is especially possible when other clinical allergies are present. The electrocardiographic abnormalities reported by several investigators from anaphylaxis in experimental animals are summarized in Harkavy's article. Of added importance are the electrocardiographic changes in man during anaphylaxis in one case arising from ingestion of cereal grains as reported by Booth and Patterson in 1970.

Illustrative of arrhythmias arising from food reported by Harkavy are the following cases:

1. Supraventricular tachycardia after ingestion of milk, chocolate, and orange by a boy nine years of age.

2. Daily ventricular extrasystoles for nine years with recurrent paroxysmal tachycardia from milk, rye, corn, and soybean in a woman thirty-two years of age.

3 and 4. Paroxysmal tachycardia from chocolate in two children.

5. Paroxysmal tachycardia had occurred twenty-four hours after beer, whiskey, and cognac for several years in a man thirty-three years of age. During a severe attack after coffee, paroxysmal tachycardia, right bundle branch block, and coronary insufficiency occurred, being relieved by an injection of Benadryl as seen in the published ECG records.

6. Paroxysmal tachycardia after chocolate, milk, oranges, and after inhalation of cat hair in a woman forty years of age.

7. Attacks of atrial fibrillation for eight years, especially in the summer, from shellfish, spices, tobacco, and allergy to trees, grasses, and ragweed which had never caused nasobronchial symptoms in a man forty-eight years of age.

8. Daily attacks of fibrillation for two years controlled for four years without quinidine by eliminating oranges, tomatoes, milk, and coffee in a woman fifty-nine years of age. Angioneurotic edema of the tongue was due to shellfish.

9. Atrial fibrillation from tobacco occurred in a man twenty-six years of age.

Harkavy cites reports of paroxysmal tachycardia by Weil, Lavbry and Mussio-Fournier, Luria, and Wilensky; Davidson, Thoroughan, and Bowcock which are included in his five important references. Kern opined that 25 percent of cases of tachycardia were due to food allergy.

Allergic reactions in the blood vessels beyond the heart probably cause more manifestations than we now realize. Animal experimentation especially by Rossle and by Gerlach, Klinge, Masugi and Sato, and many others has demonstrated allergic inflammation in and around the walls of blood vessels, especially the arteries and capillaries. Periarteritis nodosa and diffuse glomerular nephritis are probable results of such hyperergic arteritis, as noted later in this chapter. Knepper and Waaler (1935) reported such arteritis in the lungs and hearts of animals injected intravenously with an antigen.

Sulzberger (1933) and Harkavy (1934) reported the likelihood that thromboangiitis obliterans is most frequently due to vascular allergy with increasing occlusion from tobacco and possibly from ingestant and other allergy. Their studies have shown that smokers give positive reactions to the intradermal injection of specially prepared extracts from various kinds of tobacco much more often than do nonsmokers and that such allergy affects particularly the smooth muscle of the arterial system. This might explain the dizziness, nervousness, headache, neuralgia, cardiac discomfort, and even pain experienced by certain smokers.

Transient pareses, paralyses, paraesthesias, and loss of function in the cranial nerves resulting especially in disturbances in eyesight and hearing might arise from temporary smooth muscle spasm and edema in the cerebral or spinal cord arteries. Vascular crises in the extremities, heart, brain, abdomen, eyes, and other parts of the body have long been described by Riesman (1933) and might arise from such allergy in the arteries supplying such tissues. However, sclerosis with impaired elasticity and reduced lumen in the arteries and associated disturbances in the blood supply to adjacent tissues in elderly people must receive primary consideration. Kline and Young (1935) presented evidence in favor of allergy as a cause of periarteritis nodosa, a disease of the medium-sized arteries as discussed below. In an article on allergy in hypertension, Funck (1926) suggested that food allergy might cause proliferation of the intima in the artery and encourage sclerotic changes. Fishberg (1925) noted

that sclerosis only occurred in one percent of patients with hypertension. This emphasizes spasm as a sole cause itself, as discussed on page 503.

Localized flushing of the skin, especially of the face, relieved by the elimination of specific foods may occur in patients with other manifestations of food allergy. This also may be due to a localized vascular allergy or possibly to an interference with the function of the sympathetic nervous system as a result of allergy.

Duke (1932) has maintained that heat and cold allergy or abnormal reactions thereto may produce cardiac irregularities, tachycardia, angina, and other vascular spasm. Whether such agents activate an underlying ingestant, inhalant, or possibly a bacterial allergy or act as stimulating or irritating factors as such or create a changed body protein to which the vascular tissues may be sensitized has already been discussed on page 302.

Feingen and Prager have reviewed the effects of immune reactions in the isolated heart. For these reactions to occur, either the antigen or the antibody must be fixed to suspectible cells in the cardiac tissue. Reaginic skin-sensitizing antibody is of course capable of attaching to any living cells, and thus any atopic allergy to foods or other allergens can affect the heart. Feingen and Prager state that fibrillation, decreased polarization rate of the intracellular potential, increased rate and amplitude of contraction, coronary constriction, and atrioventricular block can result from antigen-antibody reactions in the heart.

ATOPIC ALLERGY IN THE LIVER, GALLBLADDER, AND BILE DUCTS

That these tissues are susceptible to allergic reactivity has been long reported in experimental animals from anaphylactic shock. In the dog the liver is the main shock tissue. Because of spasmodic contraction of the hepatic vein, the liver may enlarge to two to three times its normal size. Smooth muscles in any part of the biliary tract can contract from an allergic reaction which causes pain, colic associated with soreness, enlargement of the liver, and slight jaundice. Hepatic allergy to drugs may also produce slight jaundice and liver enlargement.

As in other tissues of the body, sensitization to the products of hepatic and biliary tissues after injury, surgery, invasion by new growths, or infection may theoretically produce autoantibodies. These could cause immunological reactions in the tissues similar to that arising from proteins of the thyroid or of the ocular lens of uveal pigment discussed in Chapter 20. These possible autoimmune reactions are discussed in *Immunological Diseases,* edited by John H. Vaughan, M.D., referred to in the first section of this chapter.

Apparent allergic reactions in the hepatic and biliary tissues from food allergy have been noted in Chapter 5, along with symptoms suggesting gallbladder and hepatic disease from gastrointestinal allergy to foods. In the statistics in Chapter 5 on 270 patients with indicated gastrointestinal allergy, pain and distress in the upper right quadrant relieved by the control of food allergy occurred in 60 percent of the cases.

ATOPIC ALLERGY LOCALIZED IN THE KIDNEY

Evidence of atopic allergy in the urogenital tract has been presented in Chapter 21.

That allergic reactivity occurs in the kidney in experimental anaphylaxis as in other vital organs and all tissues of the body already has been emphasized in this chapter. That such reactions can arise from milk, egg, wheat, or other food allergens

justifies the study of possible acute or chronic allergy in the kidneys arising especially from ingested foods.

Our review of important articles reporting inflammatory or degenerated lesions in the kidney from experimental anaphylaxis published in *Clinical Allergy* in 1937 is reprinted in Chapter 26. Masugi's use of egg albumin as well as of horse serum in establishing diffuse glomerular nephritis and the allergic reactions in the kidney from allergy to ingested horse meat along with the albumin casts, red and white blood cells, and hematuria often occurring in Henoch's purpura which requires the consideration of food allergy as a cause, as stated in Chapter 21, justifies more study of such atopic allergy as a cause of nephritis. Glomerulonephritis as a complication of Schonlein-Henoch's syndrome was reported by Levitt and Burbank in 1953 and by many others in the literature.

Possible food allergy as a cause of nephrosis is suggested by the benefit from corticosteroid therapy. This, in our opinion, justifies adequate and sufficient study of food allergy as we advise, which has never been done in nephrosis.

DELAYED HEALING OF WOUNDS BECAUSE OF FOOD ALLERGY

With our FFCFE diet in a boy seventeen years of age, abdominal cramping, right-sided abdominal soreness and pain, and distention present since childhood were relieved, and a nonhealing wound from a futile appendectomy two years previously with a recurrent serosanguineous discharge healed in one month. With the gradual addition of other foods, milk only reproduced the cramping, distention, and soreness in the wound and the right abdomen. Indicative of milk allergy, moreover, was the history of colic in infancy which practically always is due to such allergy to cow's milk, as emphasized in Chapter 25. Negative scratch tests to all foods along with those to inhalants did not rule out atopic allergy, especially to foods.

Since no residual sutures or necrotic tissues were removed before our elimination diet was ordered and since there was no reaction to implantation of Nylon, catgut, or kangaroo sutures in the cutaneous or subcutaneous tissues, control of food allergy rather than possible allergy to sutures explained the nonhealing of this wound.

The experiments of Hopps (1944) reported that inflammation and necrosis occur in the ears of rabbits previously sensitized to horse serum after irritation of the ears with xylol followed by intravenous injection of such serum. Concentration of antibodies in the inflamed tissues of the ear probably occurs, according to Hopps, followed by necrosis after the injection of the horse serum. He stated, moreover, that hemolysins, agglutins, and antitoxins accumulated in the areas of acute inflammation, including tissues in operative wounds. Nonhealing wounds occurred in eleven rabbits previously sensitized to egg or horse serum after the allergen was given intravenously subsequent to the establishment of the wounds by surgery.

According to the literature Hopps reported that 1.5 to 2 percent of abdominal wounds disrupted with death occurring in 35 percent.

Since allergy to milk best explained the nonhealing of the wound in our patient, the study of atopic allergy, especially to foods, would seem justified as a cause of the nonhealing of other wounds. Moreover, since allergy to inhalants, especially pollens, also produces manifestations of allergy in most tissues of the body, including the skin, the gastrointestinal tract and other abdominal tissues (Chapts. 5 and 21),

sensitization in the tissues of cutaneous wounds to ingested foods and less often to inhaled and even to bacterial allergens is a challenge as a possible cause of disruptive, slow healing or discharging wounds or even as a cause of progressive gangrene in operative wounds.

Tenderness and pain in abdominal wounds may also be due to localized allergy, especially to foods. Even after healing, antibodies and allergens of foods to which a patient is allergic according to Hopps can be assumed to be attracted to the tissues in and around the wound, causing persistent allergic reactions and resulting in continued localized soreness and sensitivity in the wound or its adjacent tissues, as in the following patient:

Case 214: One patient with longstanding gastrointestinal allergy to foods had continued right-sided abdominal distress and soreness in the wound after a futile appendectomy. Suspected adhesions as a cause of this distress were not found, however, six years later during a second abdominal exploratory operation for possible but nonpresent intestinal obstruction. Engorgement of the peritoneum over the intestines and omentum and free fluid in the abdomen were found. Peritonitis was suspected. The wound was loosely closed because of possible peritonitis and large cigarette drains were placed down into the pelvis. With no ingestion of foods for five days, distress ceased, and the wound healed in a month's time during which suspected food allergy was studied with our FFCFE diet. The former gastrointestinal symptoms, tenderness, and soreness in the wound in the right lower quadrant have remained absent during the last forty years except when even small amounts of allergenic foods, especially fruits, condiments, spices, coffee, wheat, and corn excluded from the prescribed diet have been ingested.

These results suggest the study of allergy especially to foods and to inhalants when a history indicative of such allergy is obtained with or without positive skin tests as one possible cause of nonhealing or tender wounds, especially when other manifestations of atopic allergy are evident in the patient's history. The interested reader is also referred to a careful perusal of the articles of Hopps as well as of our own article on allergy as a cause of non-healing of abdominal wounds.

Starch on surgeon's gloves is an allergen and can produce granulomas. Ruth S. Davis, M.D., has reported a case to me.

The patient had numerous granulomas remaining after previous surgery. Removal of these granulomas by a surgeon wearing starch-free gloves was successful. Examination of the granulomas revealed numerous starch grains still remaining from the previous surgery (Plate I Part 7). Serum from this patient tested negative for antibodies to starch, so this granuloma is probably a result of cellular-type hypersensitivity to starch.

SUMMARY

1. Since atopic allergy involves vascular and secondarily adjunctive tissues of all types, including mucosa, smooth muscle, cutaneous, and glandular tissues, it is evident that all types of body tissues in varying degrees are susceptible.

2. This susceptibility depends partly on predisposition through inheritance and on varying degrees of excessive inhalation and ingestion and exposure to the allergens.

3. Though many diseases including lupus erythematosis, systemic sclerosis, scleroderma, and others, as discussed by many investigators, are attributed to auto-immunity, immunological aspects of which are not understood, the study of possible adjunctive role of atopic allergy, as we advise, may be considered.

4. Because autoimmune allergy is especially evident in thyroid disease, it has been investigated as a cause of disease in other glands and vital organs.

5. In chronic ulcerative colitis and regional enteritis in which it has been studied, our experience shows that atopic allergy, especially to foods and less to pollens, is the major cause rather than auto-tissue immunity. This suggests that atopic allergy may be an unrecognized cause in other assumed possible autoimmune disease.

6. That atopic allergy may involve glandular tissues is indicated by its localization, especially to foods, in the parotids, as first reported by Waldbott and illustrated in one of our cases from food and pollen allergy in this chapter.

7. Enlargement of cervical and abdominal lymph glands in our patients has been relieved along with the control of other concomitant manifestations of allergy from foods.

8. Such involvement of glandular tissues justifies study of possible allergy in relapsing pancreatitis and even in genital glands, as already suggested.

9. Atopic allergy to foods, drugs, and possibly to inhalants in cardiovascular tissues has been reported by many allergists and clinical investigators for many years, as summarized by us in 1931 and 1938 and discussed *in extenso* by Hansen in 1956.

10. Duke, in 1925, opined that the cardiovascular tissues and muscle are susceptible to reactions from atopic allergy. Criep commented on abnormal cardiac arrhythmias and asystoles occurring in experimental anaphylaxis.

11. Other reports of cardiac arrhythmia, tachycardia, increased blood pressure, paroxysmal tachycardia, and anginal pain attributed to food allergy are noted, discussed, and summarized in this chapter.

12. That vascular allergy to tobacco, causing pain, vascular crises, thromboses, and resultant symptoms has long been emphasized, especially by Harkavy.

13. That unrecognized atopic allergy

especially to foods may influence the apparent autoimmune tissue reaction, causing the recurrent postpericardiotomy syndrome, is suggested.

14. The possible role of atopic allergy in nephrosis, as indicated in the literature, and by the reported benefit of corticosteroids is considered.

15. Our report of the delayed healing of an abdominal wound by the control of allergy to milk along with the experimental evidence of delayed healing of wounds in animals resulting from allergic reactions by Hopps is of special interest. That painful postoperative wounds may also be due to uncontrolled food allergy is opined.

Chapter 27

Prevention of Elective, Exploratory and Emergency Surgery by the Recognition and Control of Atopic Allergy, Especially to Foods

NOSE, THROAT AND EAR ALLERGY

Possible surgery in the tissues in the upper respiratory tract is increasingly being prevented by control of allergy to foods and less often to environmental allergens and especially to pollens if symptoms are exaggerated or only present during the spring to late fall.

Thus control of atopic allergy to inhalants and especially to foods minimizes or eliminates:

1. Removal of moderate deviation of nasal septums.

2. Removal of allergically enlarged turbinates, irrigation of antra, especially through surgically established antral windows, or the Luc-Caldwell operation with removal of edematous mucosa in the antra. Demonstrated secondary infection persisting after antibiotics may require surgery if allergy is not controlled.

3. Tonsillectomies because of recurrent head colds from allergy, especially to foods, without demonstrated infection.

4. Myringotomies for recurrent serous otitis with or without fever from food allergy and not infection, the history being equivalent to that of recurrent bronchial asthma from food allergy (Chaps. 8 and 25). With the control of foods usually in absence of inhalant allergy, insertion of tubes into the middle ear can be prevented and terminated.

5. Repeated insufflations of Eustachian tubes because of edema in the nasal mucosa from allergy, especially to foods, and not infection.

SURGERY IN BRONCHIAL ASTHMA, CHRONIC BRONCHITIS, AND OBSTRUCTIVE LUNG DISEASE

With the study and control of atopic allergy, especially to foods, and of indicated inhalant allergy in perennial bronchial asthma along with the use of corticosteroids in initial large and gradually reducing doses to a minimum and their entire elimination and adjunctive drug therapy as advised in Chapter 8, the following surgery or operative procedures requiring the advice and experience of surgical specialists are rarely necessary and usually are contraindicated.

1. Benefit from glomectomy advised by Nakayama in 1961 has not been confirmed by us and other allergists.

2. Operations on sympathetic ganglia of the vagus nerve suggested twenty to thirty years ago are no longer justifiable.

Thus we agree with Prigal and with practically all allergists that formerly suggested surgical procedures by thoracic and neurosurgeons for relief of bronchial asthma are to be definitely avoided. This does not exclude their necessary advice and skill when pneumothorax, empyema, or new growths or possible foreign bodies in the airways or other complications requiring their help develop.

Whenever such investigations or procedures are considered, continued or immediate control of possible food and/or inhalant and drug allergy with adjunctive therapy as advised in Chapters 3 and 8 is mandatory.

3. Bronchoscopies to remove "mucus plugs" and "relax bronchi" are no longer advised, being relegated into disuse as is induced artificial fever which was utilized before our presently successful relief of severe asthma and status asthmaticus as advised in Chapter 8, which has occurred in the last twenty years, with our adequate study and control of atopic allergy especially to foods and of course to inhalants and the fortunate initial availability of corticosteroids with their gradual decrease and usual discontinuance, as advised in Chapter 8. Moreover, artificial fever therapy with drugs and psychotherapy as discussed in our book on *Bronchial Asthma* in 1963 very rarely requires consideration. When foreign bodies are present or possible bronchoscopy of course is important and may be mandatory. With adequate and strict control of inhalant and especially food allergies as advised in Chapter 3 possible intrinsic causes of asthma have steadily decreased or disappeared.

Since pulmonary complications causing morbidity and even death often occur in surgery patients with early or established obstructive lung disease indicated by simple pulmonary function tests, atopic allergy to inhalants and especially to foods requires definite consideration as the cause complicated at times with secondary infection.

As in chronic bronchitis, bronchial asthma, and obstructive emphysema, perennial symptoms especially exaggerated in the fall and winter always require study of food allergy, especially with our CFE diet or

its modifications as we advise in Chapters 8, 9, and 11. In addition, indicated medications including antibiotics are required to control possible infection.

With such study of allergy in our surgery patients inhalation adrenergic therapy, postural drainage, and bronchodilator drugs usually advised as by Stein and Cassara in 1970 and by others referred to in their article have been reduced to a minimum or eliminated, and IPP therapy has infrequently been advised. This has changed the patient from a poor into a risk category.

Therefore, we urge the routine use of our CFE diet in such surgery patients rather than a general soft or regularly cooked diet which includes foods which most commonly cause bronchospasm and mucoid expectoration from food allergy.

EYE ALLERGY

The recognition and control of atopic allergy to foods and less often to inhalants and at times to drugs may prevent much local or oral treatment with drugs and may also prevent some eye surgery and hasten healing after indicated necessary surgery, as noted later in this chapter.

1. Control of eczema, especially on the face and eyelids, particularly when perennial because of foods and at times to inhalants a) may prevent development of incipient cataracts with or without keratitis, and b) is required by most ophthalmologists before removal of mature cataracts and after surgery to improve and hasten healing.

2. Increasing realization that atopic allergy requires consideration as a cause of the exudative type of detachment of retina is illustrated in Case 148, in which the control of such detachments first by ACTH injections and thereafter by the control of food allergy with our CFE diet has pre-

vented initial or subsequent surgery or repeated retinal detachments. Such good results from the use of our CFE diet have continued for the last two years in the above patient.

This benefit justifies study and control of allergy, especially to foods, when symptoms occur through the year, especially in the winter months (see Chapt. 1) and to pollens if symptoms increase or originate during the pollen seasons.

3. Paresis of muscles with or without other manifestations of ocular allergy require study and indicated control of allergy, especially to foods, by ophthalmologists, allergists, and other physicians, as evidenced in our discussion of the literature and also in Case 148.

4. Though surgery has not been recorded in patients with tunnel vision from food allergy (Case 65) and in patients with hemianopsia occurring with migraine headaches, as discussed in Chapter 18 and especially in Case 149, realization of the important role of food allergy and its study and control as advised in this volume is most important to remember. This will often prevent unnecessary and unrewarding investigative procedures in many patients.

NEUROLOGICAL AND CEREBRAL SURGERY

The challenge of adequate study and control of atopic allergy, especially to foods, exists in trigeminal neuralgia if the pain is perennial and especially if it is recurrently intensified, particularly in the fall to late spring months, and to pollens or to other inhalants if pain occurs or is exaggerated when those allergens are in the air, as advised in Chapter 18. The possibility of avoiding operations on the Gasserian ganglion justifies such study, as noted in Chapter 18.

The control of severe pain in the arms

and forearms during the spring, summer, and fall from pollen allergy with desensitization to causative pollens prevented a scheduled exploratory surgery of the brachial plexus as reported in Chapter 18.

The challenge of studying pollen and especially food and chemical allergies as a possible cause of peripheral neuritis receives further discussion in Chapter 18.

Brain and Spinal Cord Surgery

Angioneurotic edema in the brain or spinal cord discovered at exploratory surgery for possible tumors reported in Chapter 16 emphasizes the thorough consideration of allergy, particularly to foods, other manifestations of which are usually present in the history.

Moreover, since allergy, especially to foods, must be a considered cause of idiopathic epilepsy or its equivalents, as reported in Chapter 18, the study of such possible allergy as we advise is important for relief of the disease before surgery for removal of a possible cerebral focus of irritation is undertaken.

ABDOMINAL SURGERY

That adequate and expertised study and control of food allergy and less often of drug and inhalant allergy, especially to pollens, as the possible cause of various symptoms in the gastrointestinal tract and of other abdominal symptoms will prevent some abdominal (including intestinal) surgery needs special discussion and emphasis in addition to that in Chapters 5, 6, and 7.

Such study and control, especially as described in Chapter 5, will relieve various symptoms in the upper right quadrant, thus preventing gallbladder, gastric, duodenal, or exploratory surgery. The various manifestations of food allergy causing such symptoms are listed in our discussion of the allergic epigastric syndrome and upper right quadrant in Chapter 5. Control of additional symptoms in the allergic epigastric syndrome by the recognition and control of food allergy as advised in Chapters 2 and 3 to relieve recurrence of persistent symptoms justifying previous surgery often explains symptoms which might indicate further surgery.

That control of food allergy may prevent or relieve pyloric hypertrophy and surgery in children, as noted in Chapter 25 and in adults, was reported by us in 1931, followed by similar reports in children by Fries. Before surgery is done in cardiospasm (achalazia of the esophagus) and because of the "failure of surgery to relieve symptoms in prolapse of the gastric mucosa into the duodenum" reported by Rappaport *et al.* in 1953, study of possible food allergy as advised in Chapter 5 is in our opinion important.

As discussed in Chapter 5, increasing clinical and experimental studies evidence that duodenal inflammation and ulcer are usually due to a canker sorelike lesion usually from food and at times to other allergens has been supported by our control of such allergy, especially to fruits, condiments, and spices, as reported in Chapters 3 and 5. With our advised study and control such allergy will be increasingly confirmed, and surgical relief of symptoms of duodenal ulcer we opine, including postoperative symptoms requiring subsequent surgery, will be decreased.

Gudmand-Höyer, in 1969, reported that 37 percent of ninety-five patients developed abdominal symptoms from milk after surgery for peptic ulcer.

Though lactose intolerance was the suggested cause, food allergy opined by us in Chapters 5 and 29 is the usual cause.

The necessity of studying food allergy and less frequent drug and inhalant allergy as the cause of epigastric symptoms with x-rays of the upper gastrointestinal tract often reveals a diaphragmatic hernia which too often is blamed for the symptoms. Surgical correction of such herniae, it must be emphasized, should not be done until study of allergy, especially to foods and also to drugs, has been done for two to three months as advised in this volume to reveal or rule out allergy to foods or drugs as the cause. Persistent symptoms after such operations without previous study of gastric allergy also requires the study of such allergy, which should have been done before the surgery.

RECURRENT CHRONIC PANCREATITIS

Since food allergy is one recognized cause of inflammation and edema of the parotid (Chapt. 26), it is justifiable to consider its occurrence in other exocrine glands, including the pancreas, especially when pancreatitis of unknown etiology is recurrent. We opine that this possibility justifies study, especially because of the severe pain and discomfort that often result in increasing use of drugs and alcohol and the possibility of preventing surgery which is of questionable value.

CUC AND RE FROM ATOPIC ALLERGY, ESPECIALLY TO FOODS AND INHALANTS

Our continued confirmation of atopic allergy, as reported by Andresen in 1925 to foods and less often to pollens reported by us in 1941 and occasionally to drugs as the main cause of chronic ulcerative colitis and regional enteritis during the last thirty years justifies the adequate and accurate study as advised in this volume and especially in Chapters 6 and 7 before surgery is done. With such study and continued necessary cooperation of the patient, initial ileostomies and colectomies and subsequent complications after surgery because of failure of cooperation has been minimal.

This important acceptance of atopic allergy as the cause cannot be overemphasized, as we have stressed for three decades. The partial control of symptoms with continued administration of corticosteroids does not excuse the patient's physician from the responsibility of controlling the causative allergies, as was necessary in our cases before corticoids were available and as our continued good results with little or no corticoids continues.

SORENESS AND PAIN IN THE RIGHT LOWER QUADRANT

Soreness and pain in the right lower abdomen, especially without rigidity or fever, require study and control of possible food allergy, as we advise in Chapter 5.

1. Allergic inflammation may be in the cecum alone and also in the appendix. If other manifestations of food allergy and dislikes or idiosyncrasies to specific foods are recognized in the diet history, study of allergy for one to three weeks often confirms such allergy. However, if rigidity and rebound tenderness, fever and blood counts, indicate infection, appendectomy is important to prevent possible rupture and peritonitis, even though atopic allergy may be the underlying cause. If allergic inflammation to foods with secondary bacterial infection was responsible, continued pain and postoperative soreness will require study and control of such allergy as we advise. Allergic reactions occurring in the peritoneal glands or the cecum, especially in children, would need consideration. Unrelieved soreness in the wound as noted below may be due to food allergy.

2. Allergic edema including angioneurotic edema in the Fallopian tube has been reported, requiring consideration especially if urticaria and other tissue edemas require study of allergy as advised in Chapters 16 and 21 which may prevent unnecessary surgery. If edema is found, such antiallergic therapy rather than surgical resection is important.

HEMORRHOIDS AND PRURITUS ANI

That allergy in the lower rectum and anal canal, especially to foods and at times from inhalants, especially to pollens, during the spring, summer, and/or fall causes hemorrhoids as discussed in Chapter 5 has long been evident in our practice. Usually other manifestations of gastrointestinal allergy such as CUC or RE (Chapts. 6 and 7) or allergic proctitis, clinical allergy in other body tissues, a history of familial allergy, or of allergy to foods or drugs is easily obtained.

With control of probable or definite causes of allergy and corticosteroid therapy as advised in our discussion of hemorrhoids from allergy in Chapter 5, initial surgery gradually can be prevented. And if surgical removal is done without such control of allergy, our advised study and control of existent or even probable atopic or drug allergy during and after surgery is advisable to hasten healing and prevent future localized allergic inflammation.

Pruritus ani with or without hemorrhoids as stated in Chapter 5 also requires such control of atopic allergy which may be complicated with localized allergy to medicaments in antipruritic lotions or ointments as to mercury and especially to caine drugs. Failure to recognize allergy to foods complicated with allergy to a caine ointment causing long-continued excoriation had been responsible for surgical excision of perianal skin with no relief until longstanding food allergies were controlled with our FFCFE diet.

HENOCH-SCHONLEIN PURPURA AND POSSIBLE SURGERY

In addition to the cutaneous purpura and urticaria, nausea, and vomiting, melena, arthritis and varying degrees of fever, abdominal pain, and soreness from purpura in the walls in the intestine may indicate possible surgery. Though exploratory surgery may be indicated or required, hemorrhagically involved acres of the small bowel, as illustrated in Chapter 22, rarely if ever require resection. This is especially emphasized by Stremple *et al.*, in 1968, in their article "The Acute Nonsurgical Abdomen of Henoch-Schonlein Purpura in the Elderly Patient."

Since food allergy is a common cause of Henoch-Schonlein purpura, its study as advised in this volume is required.

Though control of food allergy with adjunctive help of corticosteroids usually controls the symptoms, such control is also indicated after exploratory surgery to control postoperative symptoms. That food allergy is the major and probable sole cause of such purpura must be realized by all physicians, including surgeons. The futility of surgery in these patients was stated by Althausen, Deamer, and Kerr in 1937. Fitzsimmons, in 1968, reported testicular pain and scrotal swelling and stated that surgery is contraindicated. Doubtful benefit from initial steroid therapy we opine would have been reversed if probable food allergy had been studied and controlled as we advise.

GENITOURINARY ALLERGY

The importance of recognizing and controlling atopic allergy, especially to foods, in the genitourinary tissues has been emphasized in Chapter 21.

1. With the control of food allergy, ureteral, bladder, and urethral inflammation and pain can prevent many diagnostic studies and unrelieving surgery, as evidenced in case records in Chapter 21. Prevention of scheduled "intrabladder surgery" by relief of pain and improved emptying of urine by control of unrecognized food allergy is reported in Case 161.

2. Hysterectomies because of severe menstrual headaches and other symptoms occurring during periods are contraindicated until adequate sufficient study of the most usual cause, namely food allergy, has been done as advised in Chapters 3 and 17. Termination of periods by x-ray also should be preceded by such study of possible allergy.

3. Angioneurotic edema in the Fallopian tube requiring control of allergy rather than surgery has been discussed above.

JOINT ALLERGY

Recognition and control of allergy, especially to foods, may eliminate surgery and injectant therapy in some allergically involved joints.

Recognition and control of food allergy as a cause of intermittent hydrarthrosis and palindromic rheumatism can prevent surgery which has been advised (Chapt. 23).

Moreover, since relief of atopic allergy is one explanation for relief of pain, swelling, and impaired activity in joints by intracapsular injections of corticoids or by parenteral administration of corticosteroids, the possibility of continued relief without steroids resulting from the study and control of allergy, especially to foods alone, may control symptoms without corticosteroids (Chapt. 23). Food allergy may be recognized as a complicating cause in swellings of joints in rheumatoid arthritis, thus preventing synovectomies, especially of the knee, advised by Todd and Tkach (1969) and others.

HEALING OF WOUNDS

That tenderness or delayed healing and even necrosis of wounds can result from uncontrolled food allergy, as evidenced in experimental animals and illustrated in our patient reported in Chapter 26 justifies its frequent consideration by surgeons. Such allergy can cause otherwise unexplained abdominal evisceration. Reading of our article on the delayed healing of wounds is strongly advised.

TRANSFUSIONS

That manifestations of allergy to foods may be activated by their allergens in transfused blood of donors who have eaten such foods a few hours before their blood is drawn and given to the patient has favored previous fasting for twelve hours by the donor.

Though allergens of foods therefore are reduced by such fasting, protein allergens and also carbohydrate allergens according to our clinical evidence and as reported by Arthur Lietze, Ph.D., in Chapter 28 remain in the blood and body tissues for several days. Fasting for twelve hours may decrease but not prevent activation of severe allergy to foods in the patient who is markedly sensitive to foods last eaten by the donor. Unless marked allergy to specific foods exist in the patient, fasting of donors thus might not be necessary.

FEVER AS AN INDICATION FOR SURGERY

Realization that food allergy produces fever nearly always with activation or persistence of major manifestations of clinical allergy, especially bronchial asthma, serous otitis media, gastrointestinal allergy, and especially in CUC and RE, as emphasized throughout this volume and initially in Chapter 1 requires the adequate study and control of possible food allergy as a cause

of fever when surgery in the nose, throat, ears, gastrointestinal tract, urogenital, ocular, or other tissues is being considered, as discussed in this chapter and throughout this volume. Reading Chapter 24 on allergic fever especially is suggested.

Removal of noninfected tonsils because of recurrent asthma or "colds" with no fever without consideration of atopic allergy especially to foods is illustrative of the necessary discernment by the surgeon in regard to possible food allergy as the major cause.

CARDIAC AND VASCULAR ALLERGY

Finally, because of the frequency of clinical food allergy in most tissues of the body, originating as it usually does in vascular tissues, and because of its demonstration or probability as a cause of various symptoms in the vascular and cardiac tissues as noted in Chapter 26, its possible influence on the results of cardiac and vascular allergy needs consideration. If postoperative feeding of foods to which there are many antibodies in the patient's blood were prevented, then antibodies to transplanted heart tissue as reported by Kaplan and Frengley would be less likely to delay postoperative healing and the recipient's acceptance of the donor's tissues might be improved. This also needs consideration in transplants of kidney, liver, or other organs in present and future surgery.

Comment

This cognition and control of atopic allergy as the cause of allergic vasculitis and resultant tissue changes in most body tissues as reported through this volume because of which surgery is considered and too often done without expertized and adequate study of allergy, especially to foods, will aid in decreasing the frequency of unnecessary surgery which has been commented on by Bunker in 1970.

SUMMARY

The important recognition and control of atopic allergy to inhalants and especially to foods for the prevention of unnecessary diagnostic procedures and surgery are discussed for the following:

1. Ear, nose, sinuses, and throat.

2. Bronchial asthma, chronic bronchitis, and obstructive lung disease.

3. Eye, especially in cataracts, at times in detached retinae, tunnel vision, and especially in ocular migraine.

4. Cerebral and neural tissues as in idiopathic epilepsy, trigeminal and peripheral neuralgia, and in other manifestations of allergy discussed in Chapters 17 and 18.

5. Abdominal tissues including the gallbladder, stomach, and duodenum, especially gastritis and duodenal ulcer, cardiospasm, recurrent pancreatitis, chronic ulcerative colitis and regional enteritis, appendiceal and cecal pain, and hemorrhoids.

6. Abdominal symptoms from Henoch-Schonlein purpura resulting from food allergy.

7. Genitourinary tissues.

8. Joints.

In addition delayed healing of wounds, fever and transfusion reactions, and cardiac and vascular allergy as discussed in Chapter 26 from food allergy are discussed.

Finally, if emergency or planned surgery is done on a patient for a condition unrelated to allergy but in whom clinical allergy, especially to foods, has been controlled, the required elimination diet must be maintained, if necessary, in a liquid or soft or pureed form until regularly cooked foods are tolerated.

Chapter 28

Immunological Aspects of Food Allergy

ARTHUR LIETZE

ALLERGENS

The great majority of food substances are insoluble in water. When an extract of a food is made for skin testing, therefore, most of the chemical species present are simply not taken up in the extract, and there is no possibility of detecting allergy to them with the skin tests. Seinfeld and McCombs have proposed a modified skin test which may be able to detect allergy to insoluble foods. Bryan and Bryan (1960) have developed an *in vitro* test involving leukocytes which also is a potential means of testing for allergy to insolubles.

Soluble Food Allergens

There are many food allergens, of course, which are water soluble. Thus in addition to the gluten and starch of wheat, which are insoluble, there is at least one allergen in the soluble proteins of wheat flour responsible for the positive skin tests given by some wheat-sensitive patients. In a study of the antigens of wheat giving passive hemagglutination reactions with sera of wheat allergy patients, we found that the soluble globulins of wheat extract reacted with sera from those wheat allergy patients most easily identified by skin tests or history. Sera of patients who were benefitted by the Cereal-Free Elimination Diet (Rowe) but whose sensitivity to wheat was unknown, however, did not react with the globulins but did react with the gluten or starch of wheat. We concluded that persons allergic to insoluble food substances who are not identifiable by skin tests are not identifiable by history either, since an insoluble allergen must take time to diffuse to the target organ and when once there must be highly persistent.

All allergens of milk would appear to be soluble, but casein micelles are actually large enough to be filtered out by a bacterial filter, and thus casein is less likely to elicit a skin reaction in patients allergic to it. The principal soluble allergen of milk appears to be beta-lactoglobulin, a protein which is not present in human milk but is present in all others commonly used in the diet. Thus a patient allergic to cow's milk is also likely to be allergic to goat milk, sheep milk, water buffalo milk, and so on.

Beta-lactoglobulin is only partially stable to heat and as a whey protein is present in considerably reduced amounts in most cheeses. Thus some milk-sensitive patients may be able to tolerate moderate amounts of heated milk products or cheese. Bleumink and Berrens, on the other hand, have found that the allergenicity of beta-lactoglobulin is enhanced by heating with reducing sugars such as lactose.

Much gastrointestinal illness is ascribed to lactose intolerance. Persons with a deficiency of disaccharidase cannot hydrolyze the lactose, and illness of such patients is attributed to osmotic flow of water into the intestines because of persisting high concentration of lactose. Lobos *et al.*, however, believe the disaccharidase deficiency can be an *effect* of destruction tissue. They reported that feeding disaccharides does not precipitate the illness. Flatz, Saengudom, and Sanguanbhokhai also report that although substantially all the people of Thailand are lactose intolerant not all Thai by far suffer from diseases associated with lactose intolerance, not even Thai dairymen who drink milk habitually. In this connection we have found that lactose contains a residue after dialysis and lyophilization. This residue is as active as casein, weight-for-weight, at inhibiting the hemagglutination reaction between erythrocytes coupled to casein and rabbit anticasein antibody (Sylvana Co.) (Table XLV). Percent residues found in food quality and chemical grade lactose (Nutritional Biochemical Corp.) are 0.059 percent and 0.098 percent, respectively. Therefore, lactose can never be considered free of milk allergens unless their absence is proved rigorously for each batch of lactose. This is because lactose is prepared from whey, a by-product of cheese-making. Caplin and Haynes have also reported sufficient milk allergen to precipitate symptoms in lactose used in an asthma inhalor.

It has been reported (Fällström *et al.*, Gryboski *et al.*) that gluten intolerance is a sequel to cow's milk sensitivity. Infants with a history of cow's milk sensitivity should not, therefore, be given any wheat food without being carefully observed.

The cause of infant cot deaths are still obscure. There is evidence, however, that a form of allergy to milk resulting from a diminished ability to develop immunity is a principal factor in these deaths. Underdeveloped parathyroid glands also appear to be involved. Thus the pathogenesis of cot deaths appears to be first excess maternal parathyroid hormone inhibiting formation

TABLE XLV

CASEIN PASSIVE HEMAGGLUTINATION TITERS

Antibody Dilution	No Inhibitor	Casein Inhibitor 10 μg/well	Lactose Residue 10 μg/well
1/25	++++	++++	++++
1/50	++++	+++	+++
1/100	++++	++	+++
1/200	+++	−	−
1/400	+++	−	−
1/800	+++	−	−
1/1000	−	−	−

Note: BDB-erythrocytes (equal to 0.05 ml packed) sensitized with 2¼ mg casein. Cells brought to 2.5 ml and 0.05 ml placed in each well with ½ ml antibody dilution.

of the fetal parathyroid gland, then exposure of the baby to nonhuman (cow's) milk, even one feeding, and finally an allergic reaction to ingested milk resulting in sudden death of the infant.

It would appear to be highly advisable to give an infant *no opportunity* to become sensitized to nonhuman milk because of the danger of atopic allergy as well as cot deaths. The risk is simply not worth the nutritional benefit.

In contrast to cot deaths, allergic reactions seem to be associated with increased parathyroid activity, as suggested by our recent review article in the *Journal of Asthma Research*. To test this hypothesis, supplemental calcium and magnesium in the form of dolomite, and vitamin D in the absence of binding anions such as phosphate or sulfate was given to one food allergy patient. After two months of treatment, there was no longer any evidence of this patient being allergic to food. Nevertheless, one meal with two slices of bread eaten *without* dolomite being taken first was enough to produce asthma.

There are three substances in egg whites implicated in egg allergy: ovalbumin, conalbumin, and ovomucoid. Antibodies to milk and egg proteins can be detected (Matsumura *et al.*) in sera of young children with allergy to these foods, but these antibodies seem to disappear (at least in serum) in later life though the allergy persists. On the basis of BDB-hemagglutination Frick reports that the antigens of importance in egg allergy are the ovalbumin and the conalbumin. To ovomucoid he assigns a lesser importance. On the other hand, Bleumink and Young (1969) state on the basis of skin tests that the atopic allergen of egg whites is ovomucoid.

Antibody secreted into the intestine is known as "copro-antibody." This antibody is apparently secretory IgA produced in the cells in the mucosa. Such precipitating coproantibodies have been found to milk and to eggs when the serum contained no such antibodies. We have found that soy hemagglutinin shares the immunosuppressive properties of jack bean hemagglutinin. Thus the large amount of soybean products in the Rowe elimination diets may act to suppress coproantibody formation.

Aas has studied the crystalline allergen from codfish. It is a heat-stable myogen of a group of muscle proteins occurring in fish but not in mammals. The allergen of salmon has different specificity to that of cod, so it is possible for a patient to be allergic to one fish and not to another. Aas does not mention any brown color for this allergen. Such a color would be expected if it contained Maillard complexes (*vide infra*).

Berrens' group has prepared an allergen from tomatoes whose spectrum indicates that it contains Maillard complexes formed by reaction between lysine amino groups of the protein and a reducing sugar such as glucose of lactose. They suggest that these Maillard complexes are what makes allergens allergenic. It would seem, therefore, to be important to make a determined effort to detect them in codfish allergen. They have shown that lactoglobulin becomes more reactive in skin tests if it is

warmed with lactose and point out that this implies that pasteurized milk may be allergenic to patients who could tolerate raw milk.

The allergen in tomatoes does not occur in ripe fruit but only appears on ripening. Thus a person allergic to tomatoes might well be able to eat pickled green tomatoes with safety.

Insoluble Food Allergens

Some of the potentially allergenic insoluble food components are: muscle fibers, collagen fibers, keratin, wheat gluten, corn zein, pectin, cellulose fibers (particularly with adhering protein), and the starches.

Gluten

Of the insoluble antigens listed, the best known as an allergen is gluten. Since gluten is the protein which enables bread to rise, it turns up in foods not containing wheat flour as such. Even bread labeled as "wheat-free" may actually contain gluten undeclared on the label. A good rule of thumb is to assume that any bread which has risen well is gluten-containing, regardless of *what* may be on the label.

The reactions of gluten with soluble antibody can be studied in three or more ways. Frazer has found that gluten can be hydrolyzed with proteases to form a soluble peptide with similar antigenic properties. Malik *et al.* have shown the presence of gluten derivative in the intestinal epithelium with fluorescent antibody. We have coated erythrocytes with gluten for hemagglutination studies by slowly adding an aluminum lactate solution of gluten into erythrocytes being stirred rapidly. These methods have shown a connection with antibodies to gluten in celiac disease and in allergy of various kinds relieved by Rowe elimination diets but without any definite implication of wheat by skin tests or histories.

Starch

We have found that BDB-erythrocytes treated with wheat or corn starches will hemagglutinate in sera of some food allergy patients, particularly those whose allergies are not detectable by skin tests or histories. We believe that this phenomenon and the similar findings with gluten are both the result of the insoluble nature of the allergens. Skin tests do not work with insoluble allergens, and insoluble allergens take longer to get to the target organs and stay at the target organs for longer periods of time.

In contrast to the results with wheat and corn starch, we find very little evidence of antibody to potato and tapioca starches. The Cereal-Free Elimination diets (Rowe) have long stressed these foods as hypoallergenic sources of starches.

We have since found further evidence of antibodies to starch in sera of food allergy patients by a mixed hemadsorption technique and by radial immunodiffusion. The radial immunodiffusion technique, particularly, shows great promise as a means of detecting allergy to starch. The specific starches to which a patient may be sensitive are not as yet discernible by this method, but we have found differences between the reactions of sera of patients with different starch allergies and the corresponding amylopectins when the parameter measured is the shrinkage in ring size after the serum is heated to 56 C. By the radial immunodiffusion criterion, the most allergenic kind of starch is corn, followed in decreasing order by wheat, potato, tapioca, arrowroot, and sego. Rice and oats seem to be the least allergenic starches, but their rings are of atypical appearance.

Dextrins—Corn Syrup and Intravenous Dextrose

We have found antigenic dextrins (starch derivatives) in corn syrup by a passive hemagglutination technique. Dextrose prepared for intravenous feeding also contains small amounts of these dextrins, as shown by specific hemagglutination inhibition. Thus we feel that intravenous feeding with dextrose is unnecessarily hazardous. We recommend that invert sugar be used instead as Rowe and Randolph have advised in papers on cereal-free diets. We also recommend that dextrose be made from nonallergenic starches.

PERSORPTION

Volkheimer has reported that insoluble food components, such as unboiled starch, pass directly from the intestinal tract into the lymphatic circulation. For this to take place, the particles must be small and sharp as well as hard. Many of the starch granules then become filtered out in the pulmonary capillaries (and other tissues later), where they remain until they are eliminated into the pulmonary lumen, dissolved by enzymes, or phagocytized. If a patient allergic to starch has these particles in his pulmonary capillaries, inflammation can surely be expected to persist until all starch has gone. It is for this reason that the Rowe elimination diet should be strictly maintained in each patient for over three weeks before any firm conclusions are drawn.

Starch which has been cooked in the presence of adequate amounts of water cannot be persorbed, but persorbable starch is eaten in the form of piecrust, shortbread, cookies, popcorn, tortillas, and some dry breakfast cereals. The persorbability of the starch in a food can be found by examining it in a microscope with crossed polaroids. Persorbable starch will show a black cross on a white background (Plate I).

EMPHYSEMA

Major complications of pulmonary emphysema are bronchorrhea and bronchospasm. Satisfactory treatment must remove all sources of this bronchorrhea and bronchospasm and this must include removing all food allergens. We have found a high incidence of allergy to starch, as judged by radial immunodiffusion tests, among emphysema patients. A portion of our data are given in Table XLVI. These emphysema patients, however, do not seem to include any with emphysema associated with antitrypsin deficiency, since the antitrypsin emphysema typically does not involve any bronchitis.

Fagerhol and Hauge report that only 8 patients of 503 with all pulmonary diseases (1 out of 14 emphysema) had this deficiency.

ANTIBODIES

Antibodies are common to all immunology and not just food allergy. Hence ex-

cellent reviews of antibodies are available elsewhere, and we will provide only a discussion of those points of greatest interest to us. A summary of the major immunoglobulins is shown in Table XLVII.

Dysgammaglobulinemia

When IgA is deficient, patients will frequently suffer from recurrent upper respiratory tract infections which can be confused with allergy. Analyses of their sera for IgA can identify such patients.

SKIN TEST FAILURES

Experience has shown that skin tests are not usually reliable for diagnosis of food allergy. There are at least ten reasons why this is so:

1. Dilution of allergens by inert protein in the same food can suppress skin reactions.

2. Insoluble food allergens exist. Extracts of insoluble allergen cannot, by definition, contain any allergen and thus cannot give positive skin tests.

3. Some allergens may not exist in the native food but only appear as a result of digestive processes.

TABLE XLVI

PERCENT OF SERA OF GROUPS OF PATIENTS WITH ANTIBODY TO STARCH

Patient Type	Antibody to Amylose Fraction of Corn Starch % Sera	Antibody to Whole Corn Starch % Sera	Number of Sera Tested
Cord Blood (C)	0	0	33
Normal (N)	13.9	20.2	101
Asthma (AS)	58.3	22.0	24
Normal old people (AGE)	23.1	42.3	26
G.I. problems, allergic (GA)	25.0	44.3	60
Emphysema (E)	41.5	45.7	50
G.I. problems, allergy suspected (GO)	30.4	45.7	46
Known allergy to starch foods (ST)	45.7	47.3	35
Chronic ulcerative colitis (CUC)	18.2	56.8	44

Significant Differences, p < 0.05 (Wilcoxon Method)
Corn Starch   CUC, GO, GA > E, AS, ST > AGE > N > C
Amylose   AS, ST, E, > CUC, GO, GA, AGE > N > C

Acknowledgment: We are most grateful to Priv.-Doz. Dr. med. G. Volkheimer for sending us sera from his gastroenterological diagnostic practice in Berlin.

TABLE XLVII

IMMUNOGLOBULINS AND THEIR ANTIBODY
ACTIVITIES

	IgM	IgG	IgE	IgA	IgD	Cellular
Time of formation in the immune response	early	late	early, late in atopy	late	?	early
Molecular weight	850,000	161,000	200,000	173,000 (serum) 370,000 (secretions)	184,000	—
Places of function	serum	serum	secretions & tissues	secretions & serum	?	bloodstream
Normal adult serum concentration mg%	100	1200 1600	3μg%	200	3	—

4. Many antigens must undergo a Maillard reaction with reducing sugars (glucose, lactose) before becoming allergenic.

5. Fruit extracts lose much of their allergens after about twenty-four hours.

6. Food allergen preparations from different manufacturers vary widely in potency.

7. Some food allergens exist as haptenes, not becoming allergenic until they have combined with body proteins.

8. There may be a high endogenous titer of blocking antibody. Even if blocking antibody does not protect against allergen, the usual exposure to a food is many orders of magnitude higher than the usual exposure to inhalant allergen.

9. Previously eaten food allergen may have combined with all the circulating reagin, leaving only that on the target organ. Indeed, it may have used up the reagin on the target organ also, leaving the patient in a temporary tolerant state (anergy).

10. Only certain organs may be able to react with a particular allergen. Thus the skin may not be a target organ for allergens which cause inflammation in other tissues. On the other hand, the skin may react to an allergen which no other organ reacts with and thus give a false positive skin reaction.

"Atopic Allergens"

Bleumink and Young (*Int Arch Allerg,* 34:521, 35:1, 1968) classify certain allergens as "atopic allergens" according to whether or not they give positive skin tests. In the light of the previous section we simply cannot see that this is a useful concept. If anything, atopic illness from insoluble nonskin-reactive allergens is surely more severe and long-lasting than from soluble allergens.

RADIAL IMMUNODIFFUSION

In radial immunodiffusion one reactant, usually the antibody, is dissolved in an agar plate and solutions of the other reactant placed in wells in the plate. Rings of precipitate form, and the area of the rings after equilibration is a measure of the concentration of antigen placed in the wells. For a given concentration of antigen in the wells, the area of the rings increases with *decreasing* antibody concentrations.

We have shown that valid results can be obtained when polyvalent antibody is dissolved in the gel and a mixture of antigens placed in the wells. Such multiple radial immunodiffusion can be used to measure adulterants in food, as wheat in "wheat-free" hypoallergenic bread.

Radial immunodiffusion can be used to detect starch allergy. A solution of starch in agar is prepared for the plates and patients' sera placed in the wells. There is a naturally occurring substance precipitating with starch in human sera, but if atopic reaginlike antibody is present, the rings formed with this substance become much larger. This is believed to be the result of competitive inhibition between the reagin and the precipitating substance for the same starch molecules.

In principle there can be many variations on this method. If, for example, a gel is used containing antibody to soluble wheat proteins and the wells are filled with patient sera, allowed to dry, and refilled with wheat protein the rings can be expected to be *smaller* when reagin is present. If the gel contains the allergen and patient serum mixed with precipitating antibodies to the allergen is placed in the wells, *larger* rings will be formed if the patient serum contains antibody. When human serum and a precipitating antibody are used together, the human serum should have all of any antibody present against the animal from which the precipitating antibody was drawn removed by adsorption. In all these experiments one must avoid too high a ratio of reaginic to precipitating antibody because if the ratio is too high only soluble complexes will form.

Cereal Cross Reactions

Quantitative multiple radial immunodiffusion has been used to measure antigens common to different grains. We have found that there are five well-defined groups. Wheat, rye, and barley belong together, as do corn and sorghum. Millet is slightly related to corn, and rice and wild rice form groups in themselves. Antibody to oats, however, reacts with a number of grains of many different botanical tribes. The inference is that patients allergic to oats may have a generalized allergy to all cereals.

CLIMATE

It has been reported, especially by Rowe, that climate has a bearing on the severity of food allergy. Patients have more trouble with food allergy during the winter than summer in the San Francisco Bay Area and at any time of the year they do better in inland areas than at the coast. These findings have been confirmed by Kantor *et al.*, who showed that inland areas in Israel make good health resorts for asthmatics, even though the mold and pollen counts are about the same as on the coast. This phenomenon may be the result of mineralization (Ca, Mg) in the inland drinking water, see the parathyroid discussion above. Tromp has shown that when an asthma patient is subjected to abrupt temperature changes, his asthma gets worse. In the San Francisco Bay Area there are frequent changes in temperature during the winter but not during the summer.

REFERENCES

A review article by me has recently appeared (*J Asthma Res*, September 1969 and March 1970). References for this chapter, when not explicitly given in the text, and a more complete exposition of the subject matter can be found there.

SUMMARY

Food allergens may be soluble or may be insoluble. Those food constituents which are insoluble (the great majority of them) cannot be expected to give positive skin tests. More soluble food allergens than insoluble, however, have been studied in the laboratory. These include wheat, milk, eggs, fish, potatoes, tomatoes, and so on. Those insoluble food allergens which occur as crystalline solids, for example, starch, can be shown to enter the circulation unchanged by the persorption process, be phagocytized, and stimulate an immune response. When a patient is allergic to starch, his serum will form an enlarged ring in a radial immunodiffusion plate containing starch. By this criterion we have found that more obstructive emphysema patients have starch allergy than do other food allergy patients. The relationships of food allergy to other parameters such as parathyroid function, climate, and geographic location are not as yet closely defined.

Plate I. Most of these color slides have been photographed in crossed polaroid optics. Under these conditions starch granules appear as white objects divided into four sectors by dark lines. In some cases, for even more unequivocal identification of starch, R I and $\lambda/4$ phase plates have also been placed in the light path. With these plates alternate segments of the starch granules appear in contrasting colors, as red and green.

We are indebted to Priv.-Doz. Dr. med. G. Volkheimer for permission to reproduce Parts 1 through 6 and to Ruth S. Davis, M. D., for the specimens in Parts 7 and 8.

Part 1: Persorbed starch granule entering a villus (rat).

Part 2: Starch granule in a lymph vessel of the intestinal wall, jejunum (rat).

Part 3: Starch granule in the alveolar tissue.

Part 4: Starch granule in the alveolar tissue (pig).

Part 5: Starch granule in the alveolar tissue (pig).

Part 6: Phagocytized starch granules.

Part 7: Granuloma which appeared after surgery in which the surgeon used gloves dusted with starch. No excess of humoral starch precipitating substance was found in this patient's blood serum.

Part 8: Autopsy specimen. Lung from a female seventy-two years of age who died from a blood clot in the middle artery of the left side of the brain. History gave no indication of emphysema during life, but the lung slide did give some evidence of this disease. Intravenous feeding and clear liquids only for the last eleven days of life.

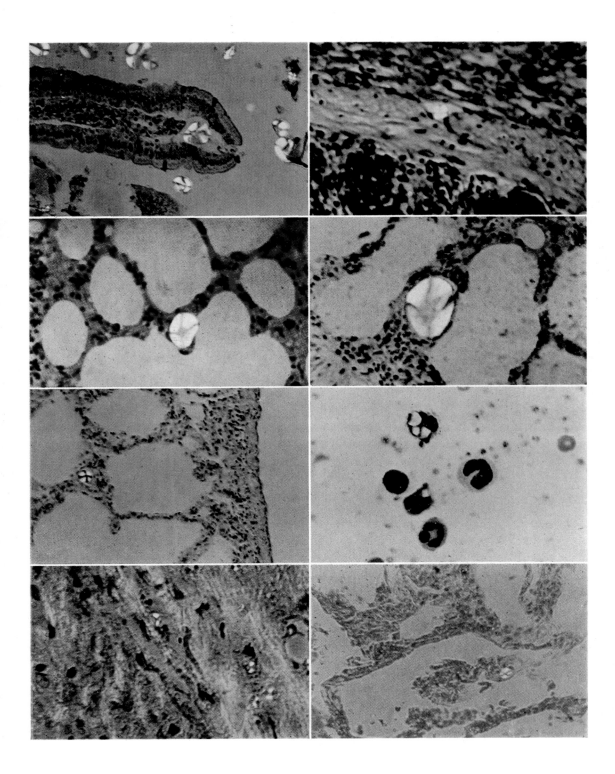

Chapter 29

Individual Food and Drug Allergies and
Their Control

Information in this chapter and literature about clinical allergy to specific foods in our practice was reported in our book on *Food Allergy* in 1931 and in *Clinical Allergy* in 1937. In the last thirty years our study of food allergy has affirmed such symptoms from specific foods, making additional reports unnecessary. Moreover, reports in the literature of allergic symptoms from individual foods have been replaced by results of immunological research in many laboratories, as in our food allergy research laboratory in the Merritt Hospital in Oakland.

FREQUENCY OF VARIOUS FOOD ALLERGIES
Determined by Skin Reactions

Positive skin reactions obtained by the cutaneous as well as the intradermal method do not necessarily indicate clinical sensitization. All through the literature there is evidence that positive reactions must be checked with diet trial to determine their real allergic role. Many patients have come under our observation who give some large reactions to foods which can be eaten without any clinical evidence of allergy. In such patients a generalized immunity is undoubtedly present to the specific foods in question. The interesting record of a man who gave negative reactions to fruits which produced marked specific gastric distress and who gave positive reactions to vegetables which were eaten without any symptoms illustrates the necessity of diet trial to determine clinical food sensitizations in all cases. The following skin reactions to foods occurred without any evidence of clinical disturbances whatsoever in a patient suffering with hay fever from pollen allergy evidenced by many large pollen reactions:

However, positive scratch reactions are

Wheat glutenin	+
Wheat leucosin	++
Cabbage	+
Cucumber	++
Garlic	+
Lima bean	+
Olive	+
Onion	++
Spinach	+
String bean	+
Tomato	+
Turnip	+
Cocoanut	++
Sage	+
Camel hair	+
Orris root	+++++
Cottonseed	+

Artemisia biennis	+
A Californica	+
A dracunculus	+++
A pycnocephala	++
A tridentata	++
A vulgaris	++++
Xanthium canadense	+
Festuca elatior	+
Poa pratensis	+
Elymus condensatus	+
Lolium perenne	+
Phleum pratense	+
Olea europea	+
Eucalyptus	+
Chrysanthemum	+++
Marigold	+

of varying or no value and may indicate potential, mild, or severe hypersensitiveness. Some patients know that the large-reacting foods cause definite disagreements or are distasteful. This emphasizes the fact that many children inherently refuse or dislike food to which allergic tolerance is lacking and therefore should not be forced to eat such foods. This is especially so if large scratch reactions occur. For example, a child who gave large positive reactions to milk and eggs, giving our typical history of recurrent bronchial asthma from food allergy as we report in Chapters 8 and 25, had been forced to eat both of these foods against his strenuous objection.

The negative skin reaction in food allergy has been stressed throughout this volume, especially in Chapters 1 and 2. The frequency of its occurrence as reported by various students and the significance of the delayed reaction to food allergens have been fully discussed.

Statistics on the frequency of reactions to various food allergens have been published by MacBride and Schorer in 1916; Cooke in 1917; Walker in 1918; Talbot in 1917; Abt in 1918; O'Keefe in 1920; Baker in 1920; Longcope in 1921; Caulfeild in 1921; Piness in 1921; Hermann in 1922; Rowe in 1922, 1925, and in other articles since then; Cooper in 1925; Campbell in 1926; Menagh in 1927; Eyermann in 1930; Vaughan in 1934; Feinberg in 1934; and Hansel in 1936. The fact that skin reactions to food and other allergens occur in apparently normal individuals has been discussed.

Determined by History and Diet Trial

From the foregoing considerations it is evident that all food allergy must be determined finally by diet trial, at times by previous trials by the patient, and usually by provocation feeding tests always in the symptom-free patient for at least two to four weeks (see Chapt. 2).

The patient's history of food dislikes or disagreements is also of great help, and such a history should indicate the advisability of diet trial to determine their possible allergic action. It is important to emphasize, however, that few patients are aware of any or all of the foods to which they are sensitive.

If a symptom which is known to be due to allergy in certain patients is relieved by the elimination of specific foods and can be reproduced and again relieved by the further addition or withdrawal of the foods, it can safely be assumed that such foods are the cause of the allergic symptoms. This is the method by which the allergic role of food has been determined in our work for over forty years and in most cases reported in this volume, being called "the provocation test" in the last twenty or more years.

Use of the Leukopenic Index

As reported by Vaughan, this often gives helpful information about food allergies. As discussed in Chapter 2, it is not used in our study of food allergy with our elimination diets.

STATISTICS ON FOOD SENSITIZATIONS

A careful tabulation of the records of five hundred patients who had been tested completely with food allergens with the scratch method and in most instances intradermally with from three to fifteen common food extracts to which negative cutaneous reactions had occurred with the scratch tests was published in Table 30 in our book on *Clinical Allergy* in 1937.

The number of one, two, three, and four plus scratch reactions to 124 foods and condiments occurring in five hundred patients were reported in this table. The largest number occurred to wheat, spinach, eggs, milk, and celery and a decreased number, finally down to one plus, to the other foods.

Because of the fallibility of skin tests in determination of clinical food allergy, the necessity of doing provocation feeding tests in the symptom-free patient is advised in Chapter 2 to confirm clinical allergy to a skin-reacting food and the long realization that much food allergy occurs with positive skin tests. These positive skin reactions are not reprinted in this volume. As stated in Chapter 2, scratch testing with most common foods, however, is routine in our practice because of large reactions, three to five plus, which may occur, which often indicate severe immediate allergy, the clinical importance of which must always be determined by provocation feeding tests with the reacting food and necessarily in the symptom-free patient.

It must be emphasized, therefore, that the real frequency of food reactions cannot be determined through an analysis of the frequency and size of food reactions alone but must be made through diet trial with those foods to which positive reactions or a history of food disagreements occur with the elimination of which allergic symptoms are relieved and with the important provocation feeding tests we have advised for over forty-five years. Such a list of foods was published in our article Food Allergy in the *Journal of the American Medical Association* and formed the basis of the "elimination diets" which we proposed for the diagnosis and treatment of food allergy. The importance of these diets has been described in Chapter 3 and has been increasingly confirmed by us during the last forty years.

RELATIONSHIP OF SPECIFIC CLINICAL ALLERGY AND BOTANICAL CLASSIFICATIONS OF INGESTED FOODS, INCLUDING VEGETABLES, SPICES, CONDIMENTS AND FLAVORS OF VEGETABLE ORIGIN

Clinical allergy to foods may exist in varying degrees to all or several foods in the same botanical family, or it may only occur to those in the same genus or even in other individual species. For example, our long study of clinical allergy to cereals has increasingly emphasized the challenge of clinical allergy to all of them in the Graminacae family, requiring their necessary total exclusion in our CFE diet in the initial study of perennial clinical allergy, as advised in this volume.

The frequency of allergy to milk and eggs, moreover, has justified the initial elimination of all of them from all animals.

On the contrary, specific allergy indicated by marked symptoms and often a large scratch reaction to peanuts or celery does not necessarily indicate total elimination of all foods in the Leguminosae (Legume) family or Umbelliacae (parsley) family in the initial trial diet.

When the physician's challenge to determine an elimination diet which relieves the patient's symptoms for at least three to six weeks has been accomplished in the cooperating patient, as we advise, provocation feeding tests with individual desired additional foods are required, eliminating any which reproduce symptoms, as advised in Chapter 3. The tolerance of additional foods depends on the patient's own realization of reactivation of previous symptoms by feeding tests and not on skin testing.

Since a food in a different genus of the botanical family could be less allergenic compared with a food in the same genus or to similar species, the printing of the genera and the species in the important families of foods follows.

Botanical relationships of vegetable spices, condiments, flavors, and gums are made available to physicians challenged with food allergy, especially to fruits.

Since our elimination diet contains none of the aforementioned foods, possible clinical allergy to a desired spice or condiment must be determined by a provocation feeding test, necessarily in the patient symptom-free for two to four weeks. Tolerance for an individual desired condiment such as pepper, ginger, cinnamon, nutmeg, mustard, onion, garlic, sage, peppermint, wintergreen, or any of the many others used especially by "good cooks," chefs, and many bakers in commercially prepared foods is determined only by provocation feeding tests with the specified condiment in which the symptom-free patient has found no exaggeration of clinical allergy.

When allergy to fruits is evidenced by diet history and later by relief of symptoms from strict adherence to our FFCFE diet, allergy to spices, condiments, and flavors always must be suspected. Some patients are allergic to all fruits, spices, condiments, and flavors in varying degrees, requiring a minimal elimination diet. If tolerance for one spice, however, is demonstrated by diet trial, other closely related spices, as recorded in Table LI may be tried rather than those in other genera or families in this table—but provocation tests in the symptom-free patient remains the final arbiter.

If large reactions occur or if a history of probable allergy is obtained to a desired food, spice, condiment, or flavor in this group, its addition must be contraindicated, or if added, its allergenic effect must be carefully evaluated. If it is tolerated, provocation tests are justified to other closely related spices and flavors with preference to those in the same botanical genus.

Information about the above relationships of spices, condiments, and flavors in Table LI was assembled by Shirley L. Willcox, B.S., and is published below. Their more detailed review of the plants, spices, and other flavoring materials is available in the library of our food allergy research institute in the Samuel Merritt Hospital, Oakland, California. Information about this subject from the American Spice Trade Association, 82 Wall Street, New York City, New York, also contains interesting information.

There is possible allergy to vegetable gums used in the manufacture and cooking of food products. In addition to this information about the sources of allergenic gums and their common use in commercial foods, pharmaceutical, industrial, and household products by Nilsson in 1960 will be important in some patients of allergists and other physicians. Similar information has been published by Gelfand, in 1943, in his article on Allergenic Properties of Vegetable Gums.

Adulteration with coloring, flavoring, and preservative agents must also be remembered because of their possible detrimental (not necessarily allergenic) reactions, as emphasized by S. D. Lockey, M.D., in Lancaster, Pennsylvania, and long reported by Theron Randolph, M.D., as referred to in many publications as in his Diagnosis and Control of Detrimental Ecological Influences on Health.

When allergenic symptoms have been relieved with one of our elimination diets or its modification and especially when allergy to fruits has been demonstrated, allergy to additional spices, condiments, flavors, and gums which are not necessary for nutrition must be adjudged necessarily with individual provocation tests and always in the symptom-free patient. When relief of serious and often invaliding clinical food allergy results from the elimination of allergenic foods, continued relief requires accurate maintenance of necessary elimination thereof not only at home and at work but also in restaurants or friends' homes. The relief may be so important and gratifying that the continued endeavor to add additional foods, unnecessary for nutrition, may be unrewarding. The patient's philosophy must be to "eat to live," and not to "live to eat."

Clinical Allergy to Botanically Related Foods

Several case reports were summarized by Vaughan, some of which will be mentioned. Thus a man had enterocolitis from peaches and almonds, both of which belong to the Drupaceae. The following case record illustrates the diversity of clinical effects of botanically related foods. A woman had indigestion, mucous colitis, and urticaria. She knew "cherry, prune, plum, apricot, and peach produced attacks of colitis, urticaria, angioneurotic edema, swelling of the gums with bleeding of the mucous membranes of the mouth, and itching in the mouth." Almonds gave no trouble. Positive tests occurred to cherries, apricots, and peaches as well as to almonds. Other nuts gave negative reactions. Apples caused indigestion, and uncooked pears made her mouth itch and swell. A positive

TABLE XLVIII

CEREAL GRAIN TAXONOMY—FAMILY GRAMINEAE (ROWE)

Subfamily	Tribe	Genus	Species	Common Names
1. Festucoideae	Triticeae	*Triticum*	*aestivum et al.*	Wheat
Festucoideae	Triticeae	*Secale*	*cereale*	Rye
Festucoideae	Triticeae	*Hordeum*	*vulgare*	Barley
Festucoideae	Aveneae	*Avena*	*fatua* var. *sativa*	Oat
2. Panicoideae	Panicaeae	*Pennisetum*	*glaucum*	Pearl millet; Indian & African millet
Panicoideae	Panicaeae	*Panicum*	*miliaceum*	Hog millet, Proso
Panicoideae	Panicaeae	*Panicum*	*texanum*	Texas millet
Panicoideae	Panicaeae	*Setaria*	*italica*	Foxtail millet; German, Siberian, & Turkestan millet
3. Panicoideae	Panicaeae	*Echinochloa*	*crus-galli* var. *frumentacea*	Japanese barnyard millet
Panicoideae	Andropogoneae	*Zea*	*mays*	Corn
Panicoideae	Andropogoneae	*Saccharum*	*officinarum*	Sugar cane
Panicoideae	Andropogoneae	*Sorghum*	*vulgare*	Sorghum, milo, Jerusalem corn
4. Bambusoideae	Bambusae	various		Bamboo, used mainly for food as shoots, but also the seeds are eaten
5. Oryzoideae	Oryzeae	*Oryza*	*sativa*	Rice
Oryzoideae	Oryzeae	*Zizania*	*aguatica*	Wild rice
6. Eragrostoideae	Chlorideae	*Eleusine*	*coracana*	African millet, Ragi

Sources:
Gould, Frank W.: *Grass Systematics*. New York, McGraw-Hill, 1968.
Bailey, L. H.: *Manual of Cultivated Plants*. New York, Macmillan, Revised edition, 1949, Tenth Printing, 1968.

Wheat Species

T monococcum—	Einkorn
T dicoccum	Emmer
T spelta	Spelt
T polonicum	Polish wheat
T aestivum	Common wheat
T durum	Durum wheat
T turgidum	English wheat

TABLE XLIX

BOTANICAL CLASSIFICATION OF EDIBLE PLANTS (VAUGHAN)

Family	Genus	Species	Common Name
		Monocotyledons	
Palmaceae	*Cocos*	*nucifera*	Coconut
	Phoenix	*dactylifera*	Date
Bromeliaceae	*Ananus*	*sativus*	Pineapple
Liliaceae	*Allium*	*cepa*	Onion
		sativum	English garlic
Musaceae	*Musa*	*sapientum*	Banana
Zinziberaceae	*Zinziber*	*officinale*	Ginger
		Dicotyledons	
Moraceae	*Morus*	*nigra*	Black mulberry
	Ficus	*carica*	Fig
Polygonaceae	*Fagopyrum*	*vulgare*	Buckwheat
	Pheum	*rhaponticum*	Rhubarb
Juglandaceae	*Juglans*	*nigra*	Black walnut
		regia	English walnut
	Carya	*olivaeformis*	Pecan
		alba	Hickory
Betulaceae	*Corylus*	*avellana*	Hazelnut, filbert
	Castanea	*dentata*	Chestnut
Chenopodiaceae	*Spinacia*	*oleracea*	Spinach
	Beta	*vulgaris*	Beet
		cycla	Swiss chard
Grossulariaceae	*Ribes*	*vulgare*	Currant
		ocyancanthoides	Gooseberry
Cruciferae	*Raphanus*	*sativus*	Radish
	Radicula	*armoracia*	Horseradish
		nasturtium-aquaticum	Watercress
	Brassica	*rapa*	Turnip
		campestris	Rutabaga
		alba	White mustard
		nigra	Brown mustard
		oleracea capita	Cabbage
		oleracea acephala	Kale
		oleracea gemmifera	Brussels sprouts
		oleracea caulo-rapa	Kohlrabi
		oleracea botrytis	Cauliflower (Broccoli)
Rosaceae	*Rubus*	*nigrobaccus*	Blackberry
		occidentalis	Black raspberry
		strigosus	Red raspberry
	Fragaria	*chiloensis*	Strawberry
Pomaceae	*Malus*	*sulvestris*	Apple
	Pyrus	*communis*	Pear
Drupaceae	*Prunus*	*amygdalus*	Almond
		domestica	Plum, prune
		avium	Cherry
		armeniaca	Apricot
		persica	Peach
Leguminosae	*Pisum*	*sativum*	Pea
	Phaseolus	*vulgaris*	Kidney bean
		lunatus	Lima bean
	Lens	*esculenta*	Lentil
	Acharis	*hypogaea*	Peanut
Rutaceae	*Citrus*	*limonia*	Lemon
		grandis	Grapefruit
		sinensis	Common orange
Anacardiaceae	*Pistacia*	*vera*	Pistachio nut
Vitaceae	*Vitis*	*vinifera*	Grape, raisin

Table XLIX (Cont'd)

Family	Genus	Species	Common Name
Malvaceae	Gossypium	hirsutum	Cottonseed
		barbadense	
	Hibiscus	esculentus	Okra, gumbo
Sterculiaceae	Theobroma	cacao	Cocoa
Theaceae	Thea	sinensis	Tea
Umbelliferae	Daucus	carota	Carrot
	Pastinaca	sativa	Parsnip
	Apium	petroselinum	Parsley
		graveolens	Celery
Vacciniaceae	Gaylussacia	resinosa	Huckleberry
	Vaccinium	macrocarpon	Cranberry
Oleaceae	Olea	europoea	Olive
Convolvulaceae	Ipomoea	batatas	Sweet potato
Solanaceae	Solanum	tuberosum	Potato
		melongena	Eggplant
	Lycopersicon	esculentum	Tomato
Rubiaceae	Coffea	arabica	Coffee
Cucurbitaceae	Cucurbita	pepo	Pumpkin
		moschata	Winter squash
		maxima	Hubbard squash
	Cucumis	melo	Cantaloupe
		sativus	Cucumber
	Citrullus	vulgaris	Watermelon
Compositae (Chichoriaceae)	Lactuca	sativa	Lettuce
	Tragopogon	porrifolius	Salsify, oyster plant
	Chicorium	intybus	Chicory
		endiva	Endive
Compositae (Asteraceae)	Helianthus	tuberosus	Jerusalem artichoke
	Cynara	scolymus	Artichoke

TABLE L

Ellis (1931) published the following supplement to Vaughan's genetic classification of food allergens:

Plants

Common Name	Family	Genus	Species
	Monocotyledones		
Sorghum	Graminae	Holcus	sorghum
Leek	Liliaceae	Allium	parrum
Chive	Liliaceae	Allium	schoenoprosum
	Dicotyledones		
Hops	Moraceae	Humulus	lupulus
Hazelnut	Betulaceae	Corylus	americana
Blueberry	Ericaceae	Vaccinium	corymbosum
Dewberry	Rosaceae	Rubus	flagellaris
Tangerine	Rutaceae	Citrus	nobilis
Maple sugar	Aceraceae	Acer	saccharum
Green and red pepper	Solonaceae	Capsicum	frutescens
Ground cherry	Solonaceae	Physalis	pubescens
Yam	Dioscoreaceae	Dioscorea	batatas
Dill	Umbelliferae	Anethum	graveolens

Edible Animals

Invertebrata
Phyllum Mullusca

Common Name	Class	Family	Genus	Species
Abalone (red)	Gastropoda	Haliotidae	Haliotis	rufescens
Abalone (green)	Gastropoda	Haliotidae	Haliotis	fulgens

Table L (Cont'd)

Common Name	Class	Family	Genus	Species
Snail (edible)	Gastropoda	Helicidae	*Helix*	*pomatia*
Mussel, salt water	Pelecypoda	Mytilidae	*Mytilus*	*edulis*
Mussel, fresh	Pelecypoda	Unionidae	*Unio*	(several sp.)
Mussel, fresh	Pelecypoda	Unionidae	*Anodonta*	(several sp.)
Oysters	Pelecypoda	Ostreidae	*Ostrea*	*virginica*
Oysters	Pelecypoda	Ostreidae	*Ostrea*	*lurida*
Scallops (common)	Pelecypoda	Pectinidae	*Pecten*	*irradians*
Scallops	Pelecypoda	Pectinidae	*Pecten*	*islandicus*
Scallops (giant)	Pelecypoda	Pectinidae	*Pecten*	*magellanicus*
Clams (soft shell)	Pelecypoda	Myidae	*Mya*	*arenaria*
Clams, razor	Pelecypoda	Solenidae	*Eusis*	*viredis*
Clams, round	Pelecypoda	Veneridae	*Venus*	*mercenaria*
Squid	Cephalopoda	Loliginidae	*Loligo*	*pealei*

Phylum Arthropoda
Class—Crustacea

Common Name	Family	Genus	Species
Lobster	Nephropidae	*Homarus*	*americanus*
Lobster (European)	Nephropidae	*Homarus*	*homarus*
Lobster (Norwegian)	Nephropidae	*Nephrops*	*norwegini*
Lobster (Spanish)	Nephropidae	*Scyllarides*	*sculptus*
Crayfish	Astacidae	*Astacus*	*nigrescens*
Crayfish	Astacidae	*Cambarus*	*limosus*
Shrimp	Crangonidae	*Crangon*	*vulgaris*
Shrimp, California	Crangonidae	*Crangon*	*franciscorum*
Prawn	Palaemonidae	*Palaemon*	*vulgaris*
Prawn	Palaemonidae	*Palaemon*	*serratis*
Southern shrimp and prawn	Peneidae	*Peneus*	*setiferus*
Spiny lobster (Florida crayfish)	Palinuridae	*Palinurus*	*argus*
Crabs, rock	Cancridae	*Cancer*	*irroratus*
Crabs, Jonah	Cancridae	*Cancer*	*borealis*
Crabs, California	Cancridae	*Cancer*	*magister*
Crabs, blue	Portunidae	*Callinectes*	*sapidus*
Crabs, lady	Portunidae	*Ovalipes*	*ocellatus*

Vertebrata
Class—Pisces

Common Name	Synonym	Family	Genus	Species
Anchovy, western		Engraulidae	*Anchovia*	*delicatissima*
Anchovy, California		Engraulidae	*Engraulis*	*mordax*
Bass, black, small mouth		Centrarchidae	*Micropterus*	*dolomieu*
Bass, black, large mouth		Centrarchidae	*Micropterus*	*salmoides*
Crappie		Centrarchidae	*Pomoxis*	*annularis*
Calico bass	Strawberry bass	Centrarchidae	*Pomoxis*	*sparoides*
Rock bass	Goggle eye	Centrarchidae	*Ambloplites*	*rupestris*
Bluegill	Blue sunfish	Centrarchidae	*Lepomis*	*pallidus*
Butterfish	Harvestfish	Stromateidae	*Pronotus*	*triacanthus*
Harvestfish	Whiting	Stromateidae	*Peprilus*	*paru*
Buffalo, common		Catostomidae	*Ictiobus*	*cyprinella*
Buffalo, white		Catostomidae	*Ictiobus*	*bubolus*
Drum	Lake carp	Catostomidae	*Carpoides*	*thompsoni*
Sucker, common	White sucker	Catostomidae	*Catostomas*	*commersoni*
Catfish, blue	Mississippi cat	Siluridae	*Ictalurus*	*furcatus*
Channel cat	Spotted cat	Siluridae	*Ictalurus*	*punctatus*
Codfish		Gadidae	*Gadus*	*callarias*
Haddock		Gadidae	*Melanogrammus*	*aeglefinus*
Flounder (Atlantic)		Pleuonectidae	*Glyptocephalus*	*cyanoglussus*
Flounder (Atlantic)		Pleuonectidae	*Pleuronectes*	*americanus*
Flounder (Pacific)		Pleuonectidae	*Platichthys*	*stellatus*

TABLE L (Cont'd.)

Common Name	Synonym	Family	Genus	Species
Halibut (Atlantic or Pacific)		Pleuonectidae	*Hippoglossus*	*hippoglossus*
Halibut (Pacific)		Pleuonectidae	*Paralichthys*	*californicus*
Pike, wall eye	Jack salmon	Percidae	*Stizostedion*	*vitreum*
Pike, sand	Sauger	Percidae	*Stizostedion*	*canadense*
Perch, yellow	Ringed perch	Percidae	*Perca*	*flavescens*
Pickerel	Common pike	Esoscidae	*Esox*	*lucius*
Muskellunge		Esoscidae	*Esox*	*masquinongy*
Herring, common		Clupeidae	*Clupeus*	*larengus*
Herring	California herring	Clupeidae	*Clupeus*	*pallasii*
Shad, common		Clupeidae	*Alosa*	*sapidissima*
Sardines	Spanish sardine	Clupeidae	*Clupandon*	*pseudohispanicus*
Sardines	California sardine	Clupeidae	*Clupandon*	*ceruleus*
Smelts, American		Argentidinidae	*Osmerus*	*mordaxchthys*
Smelts, California		Argentidinidae	*Osmerus*	*thaleichthys*
Sturgeon, common		Acipenseridae	*Acipenser*	*sturio*
Salmon, pink		Salmonidae	*Oncorhynchus*	*gorbuscha*

TABLE LI

BOTANICAL RELATIONS OF VEGETABLE SPICES, CONDIMENTS, AND FLAVORS

Gymnosperms

Family	Genus, Species, Variety	Common Name
Pinaceae (Pine)	*Juniperus communis*	Juniper berries

Angiosperms

Monocotyledons

Araceae (Arum or Aroid)	*Acorus calamus*	Calamus, Sweet flag
Liliaceae (Lily)	*Allium cepa*	Onion
	A sativum	Garlic
	A schoenoprasum	Chives
	Smilax aristolochifolia	Sarsaparilla (Mexican)
	S officinalis	Sarsaparilla
	S regeli	Jamaica sarsaparilla
Iridaceae (Iris)	*Crocus sativus*	Saffron
Zingiberaceae (Ginger)	*Alpina galanga*	Galangal
	Aramonum melegueta	Grains of paradise
	Curcuma longa	Turmeric
	C zedaria	Zedoary
	Elettaria cardamomum	Cardamon
	Zingiber officinale	Ginger
Orchidaceae (Orchid)	*Vanilla planifolia*	Vanilla

Dicotyledons

Piperaceae (Pepper)	*Piper longum*	Long pepper
	P nigrum	Black pepper
	P retrofractum (also see more detailed materials on *Piper* and *Capsicum*)	Long pepper
Ranunculaceae (Buttercup)	*Nigella damascena*	Garden nigella and
	N sativa	Love-in-a-mist
Magnoliaceae (Magnolia)	*Illicium verum*	Star anise
Lauraceae (Laurel)	*Cinnamomum burmani*	Padang, Malay, and Batavia cinnamon
	C cassia	Cassia
	C loureiri	Saigon cinnamon
	C massoia	Massoia
	C tamale	India, Himalya cinnamon

TABLE LI (Cont'd)

Family	Genus, Species, Variety	Common Name
	C zeylanicum	Ceylon cinnamon
	Laurus nobilis	Bay
	Sassafras albidum	Sassafras
Myristicaceae (Nutmeg)	*Myristica fragrans*	Nutmeg, mace
Papaveraceae (Poppy)	*Papaver somniferum*	Poppy seeds
Cruciferae (Mustard)	*Armoracia lapathifolia*	Horseradish
	Brassica hirta	White mustard
	B juncea	India mustard
	B nigra	Black mustard
Capparidaceae (Capers)	*Capparis spinosa*	Capers
Rosaceae (Rose)	*Prunus amygdalus*	Almond
Leguminosae (Pea)	*Dipteryx odorata*	Dutch tonka bean
	D oppositifolia	British tonka bean
	Glycyrrhiza glabra	Licorice
	Trigonella foenum-graecum	Fenugreek
Rutaceae (Rue)	*Citrus aurantifolia*	Lime
	C limon	Lemon
	C medica	Citron
	C sinensis	Orange
	Ruta graveolens	Rue
Euphorbiaceae (Spurge)	*Manihot esculenta*	Cassava
Anacardiaceae (Sumac)	*Pistacia vera*	Pistachio
Canellaceae	*Canella winterana*	Canella
Myrtaceae (Myrtle)	*Pimenta officinalis*	Allspice
	Syzygium aromaticum	Cloves
Umbelliferae (carrot)	*Anethum graveolens*	Dill
	Angelica archangelica	Angelica
	Anthriscus cerefolium	Chervil
	Apium garveolens dulce	Celery
	Carum carvi	Caraway
	Coriandrum sativum	Coriander
	Cuminum cyminum	Cumin
	Foeniculum vulgare	Fennel
	Levisticum officinale	Lovage
	Petroselinum crispum latifolium	Parsley
	Pimpinella anisum	Anise
Ericaceae (Heath)	*Gaultheria procumbens*	Checkerberry, wintergreen
Sapotaceae (Sapodilla)	*Lucuma nervosa*	Canistel
Boraginaceae (Borage)	*Borago officinalis*	Borage
Solanaceae (Nightshade)	*Capsicum frutescens*	Pimiento, paprika
	C frutescens longum	Chilis, cayenne, capsicum
Pedaliaceae	*Sesamum indicum*	Sesame seeds
Labiatae (Mint)	*Hyssopus officinalis*	Hyssop
	Marjorana hortensis	Sweet marjoram
	Marrubium vulgare	Hoarhound
	Melissa officinalis	Balm
	Mentha arvensis piperascens	Japanese field mint
	M piperita	Peppermint
	M pulegium	Pennyroyal mint
	M spicata	Spearmint
	Nepeta cataria	Catnip
	Ocimum basilicum	Sweet basil
	O minimum	Bush basil
	Origanum vulgare	Marjoram, oregano
	Rosmarinus officinalis	Rosemary

TABLE LI (Cont'd)

Family	Genus, Species, Variety	Common Name
	Salvia sclarea	Clary
	S officinalis	Sage
	Sautereia hortensis	Summer savory
	S montana	Winter savory
	Thymus vulgaris	Thyme
Compositae (Composite or "sunflower")	*Artemesia dracunculus*	Tarragon
	Calendula officinalis	Pot marigold
	Tanacetum vulgare	Tansy

reaction occurred to apples but not to pears. Slight reactions to onions and asparagus were present, and she had vomiting from eating onions.

Several patients who reacted to various groups and gave few if any individual reactions to foods in those groups were reported. Their symptoms were found by diet trial to be due to foods belonging to the reacting groups. Other patients gave negative group reactions, a few or no reactions to individual foods in the groups, and clinical reactions to nearly all the foods in the groups. Vaughan, however, reported many positive group reactions as well as individual food reactions with no clinical evidence of allergy to the indicated foods.

He concluded that "there is not infrequent evidence of multiple reactivity to members of individual groups, that given a positive reactor in a group, other members of the same group may sometimes produce symptoms, even though their skin reactions have been negative; that the use of mixed allergens from the same group for intradermal food testing is logical and enhances diagnostic accuracy. This group testing should be adjunct to and should not supplant individual testing."

It is evident that these group tests and the botanical classification proposed by Vaughan may help in the determination of food allergy by the positive skin reaction and diet history. However, many food families are so large that group reactions are probably not the rule. The demonstration of Walker, in 1917, that sensitization to a specific protein like serum or milk of an animal did not necessarily mean that sensitizations to the meat or the hair of the same animal were present must be kept in mind in the consideration of this contribution by Vaughan. Thus his work emphasizes the negative reactions to individual foods as well as the nonspecific positive reactions. Diet trial must still be carried out, and our "elimination diet" with our advised manipulation offer a method for such trial which has proven of increasingly great value in the last forty-five years. The botanical relationship of foods, however, should be kept in mind in the analysis of the patient's history of food disagreements and his skin reactions. As Vaughan suggests, our elimination diet for the patient may well be modified on the basis of such data. If skin reactions cannot be executed by the physician, these group relationships may help in his modification of our initial "elimination diet" if a history of definite food idiosyncrasies is obtained.

WHEAT ALLERGY

Wheat sensitization, especially in adults, along with milk allergy, especially in infants and children, are more frequently encountered here in America than any other food allergies. This allergy to wheat is due undoubtedly to the large amount of bread and other wheat products which are eaten. This great frequency of wheat allergy probably is present in other countries, such as

England, France, and Italy, where this food is consumed so freely. The studies of the Food Research Institute of Stanford University have shown that wheat constitutes about one-fourth of the calories of the American diet. In the southern European countries wheat is more extensively used than in this country. Many wheat-sensitive patients, moreover, are allergic to other cereal allergens, such as rice, rye, corn, barley, and oats, because of which our CFE diet excluding all cereal grains as well as milk, eggs, chocolate, fish, condiments, and other less common allergenic foods has been our major elimination diet since 1930 (see Chapt. 3). In infancy and early childhood, as will be pointed out later, milk is more often the cause of allergy than wheat because of its greater consumption during those years. In the last thirty years, moreover, the necessity of studying milk allergy in practically all adults including old age when perennial symptoms of possible food allergy has become apparent has been increasingly evident.

This frequency of wheat as a cause of all types of allergic manifestations, especially in older children and adults, was first emphasized by the statistics of Walker, which were published during 1917 to 1920, and of Talbot in 1917. Walker discussed nine patients with bronchial asthma who were benefitted by wheat elimination or by hypodermic desensitization with wheat protein. He also, in 1918, reported the histories of three bakers who developed asthma from wheat at the ages of thirty-five, thirty-seven, and forty years. The importance of obtaining pure cereal flours unadulterated with wheat in the control of these cases was stressed. This has been emphasized in our publications for forty years. The necessity of using wheat-free bakery products has been illustrated by failure of improvement with products containing unlisted wheat,

the presence of which has been demonstrated by Arthur Lietze, Ph.D., in our Merrill Research Laboratory at the Merritt Hospital by immunological techniques (see Chapt. 28). This unlisted wheat gets in because of the baker's distress at his wheat-free bread not rising. In order to put out a product meeting his esthetic criteria, he sneaks in a little wheat gluten. Thus any bread which has risen well should be assumed to contain wheat.* Blackfan and Sanford (1920) also pointed out its common occurrence. Engman and Wander (1921), Rackemann (1918), Unger (1923), Wynn (1927), Balyeat (1929), Alexander and Eyermann (1927) (1929), Vallery-Radot (1930), Rowe (1930), and many others have published interesting case reports exemplifying the various conditions from wheat sensitization and illustrating its frequency. Baage (1933) reported seventeen cases of vasomotor rhinitis in bakers. Colmes, Guild, and Rackemann (1935) found 47 percent of thirty-two bakers were skin-positive to wheat but only one with clinical symptoms. The significance of this was noted. Coke (1932) observed a woman who had her head pushed into wheat flour in a game. Soon after, swelling of the face, lips, throat, violent sneezing, and congested eyes occurred usually at periods from wheat ingestion. Roberts, in 1956, reported two patients with gastrointestinal allergy to wheat, causing severe primary sprue in one case and diarrhea, eosinophilia, and abdominal pain in the other.

It is interesting that Gould and Pyle commented on an article by Overton in 1855 in which marked itching, colic, nausea, and vomiting were reported from wheat. This

---

*It should be pointed out that addition of gluten to "wheat-free" bread is a result of traditional ethics of bakers, who feel that it is almost unethical to sell bread which has not risen. Some bakers cannot recognize that care for their customers' health takes priority.

persisted throughout life. During infancy the ingestion of wheat pap resulted in such collapse that the child appeared dead.

Since 1931 we have in many publications, including four books that have been printed, stated that wheat allergy is more common than other types of food allergy, occurring in about 30 to 50 percent of our patients suffering with various types of sensitizations.

Wheat reactions occurred in 162 of the 500 patients who reacted to foods. These patients gave a total of 211 skin reactions to the various proteins of wheat. The occurrence of cutaneous reactions to separate protein extracts in these patients was as follows:

Wheat	+	++	+++	++++
Whole	60	15	4	
Gliadin	32	4		
Globulin	38	10	2	2
Glutenin	23	1	1	
Leucosin	39	10	1	2
Proteose	40	13	3	2

The following clinical observations in our practice have been of special interest because of the great frequency of wheat sensitization. It is futile to detail the large number of patients with cutaneous, bronchial, nasal, gastrointestinal, nervous, and bladder allergies resulting whole or in part from wheat allergy. In general many patients find that wheat and other starches produce mucus in the nose, bronchial tract, or bowels and that indigestion and especially constipation result from them. In 1938 I (Albert Rowe, Sr.) wrote:

I think that this opinion is largely due to the frequency of wheat allergy as a cause of allergic reactions in these various tissues. I have many patients with constipation frequently associated with mucous colitis due in whole or in part to wheat sensitization. It may be that so-called starch indigestion is due to specific allergens in the various cereals and other carbohydrate foods. A man had had a continuous dysentery for over a year, which had been treated with strenuous anti-

amebic therapy for six months. He had marked pollen allergy, and his diarrhea was due to wheat, to which he gave positive reactions. A young woman had severe fatigue and generalized aching whenever she ate the slightest bit of wheat. A baby had had repeated attacks of vomiting, abdominal pain, and shock which had threatened its life. The attacks were due to wheat and eggs. A crumb of bread precipitated the symptoms. Recently an attack occurred when she ate the breast meat of a chicken which had been stuffed with bread! A woman had had persistent swelling of the tissues around both eyes associated with marked dysentery for several years due to wheat to which no reaction occurred. A baby had sneezing and coughing when first fed cream of wheat at the age of three months. The mother had severe hay fever and asthma and gave among other reactions a large one to wheat. Two men with pernicious anemia who had no acid in the stomach secretions had generalized eczema due to wheat alone, to which no definite skin reactions occurred. The taking of dilute HCl and pancreatin in enteric coated granules as well as trypsin in large doses over two weeks or more gave no relief and the elimination of wheat was necessary. Wheat produced soreness of the gums within one-half hour after its ingestion in a female patient. A woman had had recurrent sore throat, nasal congestion, and headache from wheat allergy alone. Another woman with migraine due to wheat allergy had generalized chilly sensation whenever she ate any of this food. A man had had a recurrent upper right abdominal pain due to wheat allergy. The pain simulated that due to ulcer and led to an emergency exploratory operation as occurred in one of my patients. A woman had recurrent epilepsy from wheat.

Treatment

1. The complete elimination of wheat from the diet along with the exclusion of other foods to which allergy exists will relieve its symptoms. There is a definite tendency toward desensitization to and increasing tolerance for wheat as it is excluded from the diet. Such desensitization may occur in a few weeks or months, or it may never occur. When such allergy is marked, either with or without skin reac-

tions, it is best to delay the addition of wheat to the diet for three or four months.

As in all types of food allergy it may require ten to fourteen or more days before the wheat proteins are out of the tissues and blood and the resulting symptoms are relieved. The elimination of food residues from the bowel by enemas, colonic flushings, mineral oil, or physics seems to be of no lasting help, though it is advised in severe cases. In like manner, after the addition of wheat to the diet, immunity resulting from abstinence may vary so that no wheat at all is tolerated or wheat may be taken several weeks or even months before any symptoms result. The increase of food allergy from October to May (Chapt. 1) is very important to remember.

Case 215: A man with severe allergic toxemia had continued to have marked wheat allergy in addition to milk and egg allergies. His symptoms, being entirely relieved by the elimination of these foods, returned immediately after their ingestion if he had broken his diet a few days before. He has found, however, that if he has been strict with his diet for two or more weeks that he can take wheat at one meal without any marked symptoms but that its continued ingestion gives violent symptoms on the following day. This justifies a rotating diet suggested by Rinkel in some patients.

2. The denaturizing of wheat products preferably by dry heat has been known for many years to probably change the protein molecules in such a way that certain sensitive patients can tolerate this food. Thus Melba toast, especially when it is very dry, is not deleterious to some sensitized individuals. Many patients, however, with moderate or severe degree of wheat sensitization cannot tolerate the driest Melba toast when combined with digestants.

Case 216: Thus a patient with a gastric distress, sour stomach, severe constipation, and sleeplessness from food allergy, especially to wheat, after omitting wheat for six months was given Melba toast. Constipation immediately returned, and in one week her gastric symptoms recurred. Ten days of strict exclusion of wheat from the diet were required to relieve her of the gastric and intestinal trouble. During the first two days the spastic constipation was so obstinate that repeated enemas were ineffective. A repetition of the taking of Melba toast along with the administration of 2 gm doses of trypsin, as suggested by Caulfeild, apparently delayed the appearance of the symptoms for only a few days.

3. *Oral Desensitization.* The gradual feeding of increasing amounts of wheat, beginning with minute amounts, theoretically should result in desensitization in the same way that was reported in egg allergy, as described below. However, Walker (1917) stated that he had had no results from such therapy, and we can find no definite records in the literature of success with this method. In the various trials we have carried out in our own clinic, no definite assurance of help has been certain, and we have continued to depend on the total elimination of wheat from the diet itself for desired results. One must keep in mind that desensitization protects against microgram amounts of pollen, not necessarily gram amounts of food.

4. *Hypodermic Desensitization.* Walker (1917) also stated that the hypodermic desensitization to wheat proteins gave no results. Unger (1923), however, reported help from such therapy supplemented with gradual feeding in a woman forty-three years of age. We have used this method in a number of patients, especially bakers, who rather frequently become sensitized to wheat flour. Two types of extracts for therapy have been used: a) An extract of whole wheat flour prepared by Coca's method has been used, the initial dose being 0.1 cc of the dilution, which failed to give a skin reaction, and the therapy being carried out in a like manner to that outlined for pollen desensitization. b) The other extract has been prepared from the dry al-

lergens as furnished by the Arlington Chemical Company. Those split-protein extracts of wheat which give reactions in the patient are added to Coca's extracting fluid in the proportion of one to fifty and in relative amounts corresponding to their degrees of reaction. The treatment has been carried out as outlined for pollen. Results have been disappointing, symptoms often being activated by increasing strengths of even a weak antigen.

ALLERGY TO OTHER CEREALS

Allergy to other cereals than wheat occurs less frequently, as shown in our statistics published in various articles in the past few years.

Next to wheat, corn and rice have given the greatest number of reactions, oats, barley, and rye following in order with fewer reactions. Such reactions do not necessarily indicate clinical sensitiveness, but they do indicate in a general way the frequency of allergy to the various cereal grains among the patients studied here in America.

As we have stated before, sensitization probably occurs most frequently to the cereals and other foods eaten in the largest amounts by a given people as to wheat and corn in the United States. Hence, one would expect rice allergy most often in the Orientals, rye allergy in the Scandinavians and Germans, and oat sensitization especially in the Scots. But our statistics of clinical allergy indicate that reactions to any of the various cereals may occur in patients and that a general reactivity to nearly all the cereal grains usually must be assumed. That similarity of chemical structure may account for some of these reactions is suggested by the experimental studies of Wells and Osborne in which wheat and rye were shown to interact as did corn and barley.

These comments indicate the importance of studying all patients suspected of food allergy with all types of cereal allergens and to keep in mind the fact that even with negative scratch reactions, allergy to specific cereals or to all of them in varying degrees may be present. It is because of this that our CFE diet has replaced Diets 1 and 2 containing rice, corn, and rye increasingly in the last forty years in our practice.

1. Rice gives fewer clinical reactions than does wheat and so is the first starch added to the CFE diet when relief of symptoms is assured for three to six weeks. Feinberg, Johnstone, and many other allergists have confirmed our conclusion in 1931, supported in our practice since then, that rice and other cereals require initial study of possible food allergy. Thus its routine use must be accompanied by the realization that the sensitization to it occurs, though less often than to wheat. Talbot reported a case of eczema from allergy to eggs, milk, and rice. Duke (1921) reported a patient with rice sensitization. Several clinical symptoms to rice were recorded by Ramirez, Baker, Rowe, Campbell, and individual cases by other writers. Definite nasal congestion and sneezing occurred in a young woman whenever she took rice. Other foods including milk had a like effect. Years ago when she had a Chinese cook she remembers that she had continuous nasal congestion because of the daily serving of rice. A physician with migraine who gave no skin reactions was placed on an elimination diet containing rice which immediately intensified his headache. It was found that such allergy had been acquired during the World War when rice bread was eaten generally. Another physician found that his longstanding migraine was due to rice and other cereals. A woman had definite asthma and ocular congestion whenever she ate rice. Such allergy was

apparently acquired *in utero* when the mother overate rice.

When rice is used in a test diet, it can be taken in many forms and cooked in many interesting ways, as advised on page 73. Rice flour can be used alone or combined with soy flour or (if tolerated) corn meal or rye flour in the making of wheat-free bread, cake, or pastry, as described in Chapter 3. It is best to have freshly ground rice flour, since weevils are prone to grow in any rice flour which stands very long. Wild rice differs botanically from regular rice.

2. Corn also is a common cause of allergy, especially in the United States, as shown by the statistics in Table 30 of our book on *Clinical Allergy* in 1937 and increasingly confirmed by clinical experience through the years. This justified the major importance of our CFE diet first advised in 1933 and stressed increasingly in the last thirty-five years. It is found in many commercial breads, muffins, gravies, and many cereals, especially Corn Flakes and Post Toasties. It is used especially in Mexican breads, cakes, and other foods; making beer and whiskey; corn starch, glucose, laundry starch, and sizing textiles. Corn oil is used in mayonnaise and salad dressings, for frying foods, as shortening, and as a vehicle in certain viosterols and in various emulsions.

Sensitization to corn has occurred clinically with and often without skin reactions in our practice. Its frequency was emphasized correctly by Rinkel and especially by Randolph and increasingly confirmed in our practice for forty years. Articles by Randolph in 1949 and 1950 are of special importance. A most instructive and interesting example has already been recounted, a brief summary of which follows:

Case 217: A girl fifteen years of age had had continuous asthma since birth. No skin reactions were present, and no relief was obtained with "Elimination Diets" Nos. 1 and 2 until corn was excluded. After its elimination for two months it was gradually added, and no asthma resulted until corn had been used for four months in October, when asthma again occurred to be promptly relieved by corn elimination. The girl was also sensitive to wheat, milk, and eggs. The tolerance for corn established after two months' elimination and the gradual disappearance of such immunity during the ingestion of corn for a period of four months are most instructive, and as we review this reactivation of allergy, it is readily explained by increase of food allergy in October to December, as stated in Chapter 1.

This frequency of allergy to corn justifies the initial use of our CFE diet as advised throughout this volume. It also requires elimination of corn oil and especially corn sugar and glucose included in canned products, as advised in Chapter 3. It especially stresses the use of invert sugar instead of glucose in intravenous solution to prevent serious and even fatal asthma or other manifestations of clinical allergy as stressed on page 205. Since the importance of giving 5 percent invert sugar rather than 5 percent glucose by vein to patients who have known allergy to corn or when allergy to corn and other cereals is being studied with our CFE diet was first advised by Randolph in his report of marked and serious clinical allergy from intravenous glucose are recommended for careful study.

3. Barley and oats are fed rather frequently in infancy, making it possible that allergies to these cereals may arise in childhood. Schloss (1912) reported urticaria and asthma from oatmeal. Walker (1920) noted nasal allergy from it. Barley is used to thicken soups and broths. When roasted, it is used for a substitute for coffee. It is used to make certain malted milks and syrups, beer, whiskey, Mellins' Food, and is found in Grapenuts. Moreover, reactions to these may be explained

by the group reactions to cereals already mentioned. When skin reactions are present or any indications through dietary trial indicates allergy to either one, they should be excluded from the diet. This is accomplished with our CFE diet. One case of marked barley sensitization comes to mind in which malt extract gave severe clinical reactions. Ratner and Gruehl (1935) found barley malt highly ana- phylactogenic: thus a boy twelve years of age, sensitive to barley, had asthma from drinking a malted brew. Coke (1932) recorded a nettle rash on the face and in- side the mouth with asthma in one hour when oats were eaten. Barley and oats when added to the diet can be used in their various forms and incorporated in various formulas or recipes.

4. Rye being closely related to wheat causes allergic symptoms in many patients sensitive to wheat and other cereals. Before the frequency of allergy to many or all cereals was realized in the late twenties, rye bread and especially Ry Krisp was used by us and other allergists as a sub- stitute for wheat. This is now supplanted by noncereal soy-potato bakery products, though allergy to soy and legumes as stated in Chapter 3 and on page 574 must be remembered. After relief, if rye is added, it must not be adulterated with wheat, and honest bakers must make bakery products according to our recipes in Chapter 3.

5. Buckwheat is not a cereal. It belongs to the Polygonacae rather than the Grami- nae. As such it is related to rhubarb. Sheard, Caylor, and Schlotthauer (1928) fed white-haired animals buckwheat for a long time. A rash developed, and sensiti- zation was indicated by agitation, itching, scratching of ears, weakness, urticaria, and conjunctivitis. Petechial hemorrhages were in all viscera. Phyloporphyrin and chole-

hematin but not hematophorphyrin were the causes.

Buckwheat produces violent clinical re- actions in certain patients and has given positive reactions in thirty-two patients in our series of five hundred. Wyman (1872) reported hay fever and ocular congestion from its ingestion. Dunlop and Lemon (1929) encountered angioneurotic edema from buckwheat. Blumstein (1935) stated that the hulls of buckwheat are used as fuel, packing for bottled goods, and feeding stock. The middlings are used for cattle feed and for fertilizers. The whole grain is used for poultry, the straw for stock, and the flour for griddle cakes and is one of several flours in Aunt Jemima's flour, in H.O. Buckwheat Pancake flour, and Uncle Jerry's New England Self-Rising Flour. Of five hundred cases of allergy nineteen gave positive reactions and eight were clini- cally sensitive. Sugahara (1968) reported asthma from buckwheat from its frequent ingestion or inhalation of its powder in the chaff or from pillows stuffed with the vegetation.

Case 218: One of the first skin reactions to foods reported in the literature deserving special comment was that by Smith (1909) to buck- wheat. The patient, at the age of nine years, when he first ate buckwheat had immediate retching; bloodshot eyes; red, swollen features; and large hives on his lip. Later, corn ground with stones, which had previously ground buck- wheat, or corn cakes cooked on a griddle where buckwheat cakes had been cooked caused mild attacks. Eating buckwheat by mistake later in life caused terrible burning of the skin. The face, eyes, tongue, neck, shoulders, and hands were hot, inflamed, and swollen and the lips thick with hives. Terrible itching of the skin and se- vere asthma occurred, causing the patient to roll on the floor in agony. He was comfortable in six hours after an emetic, but the irritation and shedding of the skin lasted for two or three days. The application of buckwheat to a skin abrasion by Cole in Thayer's office gave a severe constitutional reaction with the other symptoms previously mentioned. Highman (1920) reported swelling of the eyelids in a man sixty-six years of age from eating of buckwheat cakes once a week. Other examples of buckwheat sensitizations have appeared in the literature, but no such graphic descriptions as that by Smith are to be found. Thus the effect of buckwheat must be carefully watched if it is included in the diet of an allergic patient.

6. Flaxseed is incorporated in some mixed cereals and may produce marked gastrointestinal, nasobronchial, or cutaneous manifestations. One patient sensitized formerly by flaxseed poultices had burning of the tongue and stomach whenever such cereal was eaten. Another patient of Dr. Hill's, after eating Roman Meal containing flaxseed, had immediate puckering of the mouth; rapid swelling of the eyes, ears, lips, and tongue; and dizziness, faintness, and vasomotor collapse with unconsciousness. Black (1930) recorded flaxseed allergy from poultices in two patients. One had tingling and burning of lips and tongue immediately with ocular, nasal congestion, and swelling, with diarrhea soon afterwards. The other man had rapid nausea, vomiting, throat and laryngeal edema, dyspnea, and asthma. Grant (1932) reviewed the literature on flaxseed allergy and reported six cases from hair stay which contained flaxseed, from inhalation of feed dusts, and from ingestion of Roman Meal. Vaughan (1927) and Barnes (1931) discussed linseed meal and oil dermatitis. Brown (1930) also reported clinical allergies to flaxseed, including severe cutaneous allergy from it.

Flaxseed is found in Roman Meal and Uncle Sam's Breakfast Food. Flaxolyn is a laxative. Flaxseed tea is used medicinally, and flaxseed is also used as a demulcent and emollient.

7. Tapioca is a carbohydrate obtained from the roots of the tropical plant called cassava, which belongs to the same botanical family as the castor bean. Sago is a carbohydrate that comes from the pith of a certain East Indian as well as a South American palm, especially the *Metroxylon laeve* or the *M rumphii*.

In our experience, as far as we can ascertain from the literature, no definite clinical allergy has been observed to either of these starches. We have obtained a few moderate reactions to them, as seen in Table 30 (1938), but no clinical allergy apparently accompanied these positive tests. Therefore, where there has been a need for carbohydrate, we have used these foods in our elimination diets for diet trial. Special recipes have been given in Chapter 3 for their use, without the inclusion of milk or eggs.

ALLERGY TO STARCHES

Allergy and antibodies to starch and derivatives of starch have all been reported.

In our research laboratory's first efforts at studying antibodies to soluble wheat antigens in sera of wheat-sensitive patients, we found erratic results which we finally traced down to a variable amount of wheat starch in the antigen preparations. Accordingly we performed the reactions (BDB-hemagglutination titers) with the pure starch and found many wheat-sensitive patients with a high titer. Three other starches were then studied also with the result that corn starch was found to give high titers also, potato starch lower titers, and tapioca starch very low titers. With the use of eighty sera (patients and normals) tested with each starch, coefficients of rank correlation could be calculated. The results indicated high correlation between antibody to one starch and antibody to another except between potato and tapioca starches. The interpretation was that potato starch and tapioca starch have different antigenic determinants ("P" and "T," respectively) but that corn and wheat starches bear both these groupings.

We used a mixed hemadsorption technique to show that at least some of the antibody to starch was IgA, with heat labile "IgA" in allergy patients.

We later solubilized corn starch in agar by boiling to make reverse radial immunodiffusion plates. Sera from a normal population (blood bank donors) produced small rings in these plates. Sera from patients known to be allergic to corn produced large rings. This suggests that most corn allergy is really allergy to the starch. Patients whose allergy to corn was unknown separated clearly into two, approximately equally sized, populations corresponding to the normal population and the corn allergy population. This indicates that about half of the patients in our allergy practice are sensitive to starch.

Another method of solubilizing starch is to boil it in sodium hydroxide and then neutralize. The previous method dissolves only the amylose but the sodium hydroxide method dissolves both the amylose and the amylopectin, thus preserving the full antigenic capability of the starch. Using plates made up in this way we found evidence for three antigens, which we call "C," "P," and "T." Large amounts of all three were found in wheat and corn starches. A large amount of P only was found in potato, a large amount of T only in tapioca, large amounts of P and T only in arrowroot, small amounts of P, T, and C in oats and rice, and a large amount of P with small amounts of C and T in a commercial starch tentatively identified as palm sago.

We are most encouraged by the fact that the results for antigenic specificity of starches by the passive hemagglutination and the radial immunodiffusion techniques are in such good agreement.

The route of sensitization to starch appears to depend on the phenomenon of "persorption" described by our friend and colleague G. Volkheimer in Berlin. Hard, ungelatinized, starch granules (found in cookies, piecrust, shortbread, popcorn, corn chips, and some dry breakfast foods) pass unchanged from the digestive tract into the lymphatic circulation. From there they go to the venous circulation, the heart, and the lungs, where many of them are filtered out. These particles are most readily phagocytized, and induction of antibody production can be expected as a result of this phagocytosis.

We are beginning to discover why starch granules are not affected by the serum amylase. There is a substance in serum which precipitates starch. This substance does not stain with Amidoschwarz and is not precipitated completely by boiling or by saturating with ammonium sulfate. Amylase *in vitro* does not dissolve starch precipitated by this substance. Thus it coats the starch granules in serum and protects them from attack by hydrolytic enzymes. Its presence in serum also explains the bimodality of frequency distribution curves of allergy patients' sera ring size on reverse radial immunodiffusion. The lower peak is the result of rings formed by this precipitating substance only and the upper peak of rings formed by the precipitating substance *plus* antibody to starch. Thus a small ring size indicates no antibody to starch and a large ring size indicates the presence of antibody to starch in the patient's serum.

ALLERGY TO EGGS

Egg holds third place to wheat and cereals and cow's milk as a cause of food allergy. Our statistics based on skin reactions and experience indicate that egg and milk sensitizations are about equal in frequency, whereas those in Table LII based on skin reactions alone show that egg allergy is more frequent than milk allergy. Our studies, however, have been made chiefly on adults, though many children are included.

The studies of Moro, Woringer, Hill, and many others have shown that egg sensitization is relatively more frequent in childhood than is wheat sensitization and that infants seem to have a predilection for developing such allergy. This may be due to the frequency of adding eggs before wheat in the infant's diet thirty to forty years ago. Since this has become infrequent, the early development of possible skin reactions and clinical allergy to eggs in infants has decreased in our experience. In fact, its severe manifestations made it one of the first foods to be reported in literature as causing allergic reactions as well as the so-called idiosyncrasies before anaphylaxis was discovered. Egg solutions are also used in the fur, photographic, and textile industries. Egg white occurs in water color prints called "tempera." Spain (1933) found them as a cause of eczema. He also studied a patient reacting to chicken eggs, meat, and feathers. Jadassohn and Schaaf (1933) found two antigens in chicken egg white. One was present in duck egg white, and they felt that both were nonprotein. Burchard (1934) found a common allergen in all fowl eggs, very little being in parrot and none in dove eggs.

The reactions to the individual proteins in eggs as they occurred in the five hundred patients in our book in 1938 were as follows:

	+	++	+++	++++
Eggs—Whole	36	10	4	
White	32	5	5	
Albumen	18	3		
Yolk	27	5		
Mucoid	19	6	1	2

The number of the five hundred patients who reacted to the various numbers of the individual egg proteins is as follows:

No. of patients reacting to 1 protein 57
No. of patients reacting to 2 proteins 20
No. of patients reacting to 3 proteins 10
No. of patients reacting to 4 proteins 4
No. of patients reacting to 5 proteins 7

Egg allergy may produce all types of clinical allergy, especially in infancy, often without skin reactions. Thus eczema, urticaria, colic, abdominal symptoms, bronchitis, and bronchial asthma are frequently due to this sensitization and as stated previously, one such manifestation may gradually change into another. Egg allergy in infancy produces very violent and rapid reactions in certain patients. Such conditions have been described, especially by Laroche, Richet, and Saint Girons, whose case reports are of striking interest. Blackfan, Schloss, Talbot, and all other students of allergy in infancy have stressed the frequent severity of egg allergy. Severe and violent reactions to eggs at times persist throughout life, as illustrated by the following history, which we published in "Allergy in the Etiology of Disease," in 1927.

Case 219: A man forty-five years of age complained of asthma and hay fever. An egg idiosyncrasy had been present since birth, and it had steadily increased in severity, so that the smallest bit of egg gave indigestion. Marshmallows, ice cream, cake, or cookies made with eggs produced marked symptoms. Eggs first produced itching of the back of the tongue and pharynx followed by swelling and burning of the buccal membranes. Forced vomiting resulted in immediate relief. If his stomach was not emptied, indigestion, consisting of fullness, burning, and distention, lasted for several days. Eggs on the skin caused urticaria. Egg shampoo on one occasion produced itching edema all over his scalp and forehead. The eating of eggs resulted in a dry cough which persisted for several days.

Egg allergy seems to be inherited by certain patients. This was reported by Laroche, Richet, Saint Girons, in another by Gould and Pyle, and in several of our own personal cases. There is a definite tendency for egg allergy to gradually decrease during childhood. As such immunity increases, the skin reaction disappears. However, allergic disturbances not infrequently persist in the teens and even in adult life because of the fact that in spite of a known egg idiosyncrasy, small amounts of eggs are given to the child or taken by the adult in various ways. Such patients may give no skin reaction by the scratch test and may even be negative to the intradermal one. We think that where an allergic condition is present, especially one which is resistant to control, eggs should be eliminated for a trial period when there is any history of a previous allergy. Because of the frequency of egg allergy, all of our elimination diets for the study of patients suspected of food sensitization exclude eggs.

The literature contains many statistics on egg allergy and case reports of its effects, especially when eggs were given early in infancy. In the last thirty years more recognition of allergy to cow's milk has occurred, as discussed next in this chapter and especially in Chapter 25. A few of the articles which have interested us especially will be mentioned: Magendie, in 1839, first described death in dogs from the injection of egg albumen. Hutchinson (1884) mentioned vomiting, faintness, and dizziness from eggs and in 1886 described severe egg poisoning in two sisters. Orton (1886) reported egg allergy in three generations. The patient herself had intense flatulence, spasms, suffocation, vomiting, and severe pain in the bowels, followed by diarrhea, bilious headache, and prostration. Nausea, coated tongue, and anorexia lasted for two days with the attacks. Gould and Pyle reported egg idiosyncrasies in four generations. In one of the girls convulsions resulted from egg.

Schofield (1908) recorded the following observations:

Case 220: A boy thirteen years of age was egg-sensitive. As a baby he spat up any food containing even the slightest bit of egg, and such food continued to produce a free flow of saliva; burning of lips; generalized itching, swelling, and an urticarial eruption of the entire skin; swelling of lips and eyelids; and asthma when taken in any amount. A bun brushed with egg for glazing, soups cleared with egg, or the slightest bit in applesauce caused the symptoms. Raw eggs blistered the tongue. Pills containing 1/10,000 of a raw egg, daily for one month, followed by 1/500 for the next month, and then the giving of 1/250, 1/75, 1/35, 1/6 for succeeding months produced immunity. Further follow-up was not established.

Landmann (1908) reported a lifelong egg allergy in a man thirty years of age. A minute quantity of egg in a few seconds produced "a sensation of severe burning in his mouth and on his skin. His eyes watered. His ears buzzed. Violent vomiting occurred, and at the end of fifteen minutes severe diarrhea developed, accompanied by a sensation of burning throughout the length of his digestive tract. The diarrhea was uncontrollable for many hours." Horwitz (1908) published the record of a man sixty years of age whose egg allergy had persisted since the age of five. The smallest bit of egg produced in one-quarter to three-quarters hour severe gastric cramps comparable to renal or hepatic colic and extremely severe localized pain, which the patient called "eierbauchweh." Lesne also reported severe abdominal symptoms, prostration, and shock from eggs, which threatened the life of a girl eight years of age. These four contributions are summarized in the monograph of Laroche, Richet, and Saint Girons. The monograph also stated that mild symptoms are more frequent than severe ones. An interesting record of chronic egg allergy in a woman, as reported by Brazis, was included. The intensity of her symptoms gradually increased over a period of years, producing itching, nausea, vomiting, abdominal pain, and general intoxication as well as an immediate tingling in the throat and ears which spread all over the body and even throughout her digestive tract. The authors also summarized their experiments in which egg allergy was established in guinea pigs by feeding large amounts of egg for a few meals. Prolonged feeding for thirty to forty-five days, on the contrary, produced immunity! Wells, in his work in 1929, stated: "With crystallized egg albumen I have succeeded in sensitizing guinea pigs with a single dose as small as 1/20,000,000 gm, and fatal sensitization has resulted from 1/1,000,000 gm." This emphasizes the very minute amount of an allergen which may sensitize or produce allergic reactions. The article of Schloss, as published in 1920, emphasized the frequency of egg allergy as a cause of cutaneous, respiratory, and gastrointestinal symptoms. His first article in 1912 contained the first detailed description of skin reactions to egg allergens. A summary of the effects of egg allergy on his patient, as described by Schloss, is as follows:

Case 221: An infant ten days old was given eggs because of a slight diarrhea. It was given the next time at the age of fourteen months. The child upon first tasting a soft-boiled egg refused it and immediately began to claw at his tongue and mouth. The buccal tissues swelled to many times their normal size, and urticarial wheals developed on the face around the mouth. At the end of the second year it was noticed that egg shells produced an urticarial rash on the arms and hands. At the age of twenty-two months egg was given for the third time, about one-eighth of an egg-white in milk. The child immediately vomited; the lips, tongue, and inner surfaces of the cheeks became swollen; and a general urticarial rash appeared. At the age of two years

egg white was again given in a sandwich. Upon swallowing a small amount, vomiting and gagging immediately occurred. The child became very ill, his lips, tongue, and mucous membranes became enormously swollen, and urticarial wheals appeared around his mouth. His face was flushed, his respirations were rapid, his mentality was dull, and he fell into a restless sleep. In two hours he was quite well. At the age of thirty-two months he ate a few small cakes and at the age of six years he took the glazing on a cake, with the immediate onset of vomiting and swellings of his lips and tongue.

The demonstration by Schloss, in 1912, of the absence of skin reactions, except on the day of the urticarial attacks, as well as the cyclic recurrence of allergic disturbances in childhood are shown in Table LII. This recurrence of clinical food allergy as a main characteristic has been emphasized by us as stated in Chapter 1 and through this volume.

Schultz and Larsen (1918), Talbot (1918) (since then in other articles), Blackfan (1916), Grulee (1921), Ratner (1922), Stuart (1926), and Campbell (1926) reported the frequency of egg allergy in childhood in those years when eggs were often given early in infancy. That egg proteins are readily absorbed into the blood has been noted by many students. Wilson and Walzer (1935) found that in 72 percent of children, egg proteins were demonstrable in the blood in from 25 to 105 minutes after ingestion.

Duke called attention to chicken sensitization in certain patients with egg allergy. This may be due to contamination of the chicken meat with unlaid eggs in hens or to common allergens in eggs and chicken meat. Coke (1923) cited the case of a lad who became ill from the glazing on a bun and later from a soup cleared with eggs. Sterling (1929) reported a child who was nursed until nine months of age. Milk and egg sensitization developed after these foods were given and resulted in generalized urticaria and eczema. A mere taste of eggs or milk would produce wheals all over the body followed in a day or two by severe papular eczema. Shock with marked dyspnea at times resulted. Acute allergy was still present at the age of 2½ years.

Walker (1918), in a study of 400 cases of asthma, found 68 patients who reacted to foods, 25 of whom gave reactions to wheat and 13 of whom reacted to egg. The following reactions he obtained are of interest (*Clinical Allergy*, Rowe, 1938, page 560).

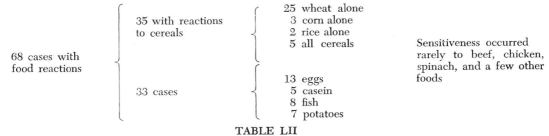

TABLE LII

POSITIVE CUTANEOUS REACTIONS TO EGGS* (SCHLOSS)

Date	Cutaneous Reaction	Symptoms	Date	Cutaneous Reaction	Symptoms
1/5	++	Urticaria	3/8	....	
1/6	....		3/10	....	
1/7	....	None	3/12	....	
1/8	....		3/14	....	None
1/10	....		3/16	....	
1/12	....	None	3/18	....	
1/14	....		3/20	....	
1/16	....	None	3/22	....	None
1/18	....		3/24	+	
1/20	....	None	3/26	++	Moderate urticaria
1/22	....				
1/24	....	None	3/28	....	
1/26	....		3/30	....	
1/28	....	None	4/1	....	
1/30	....		4/3	....	
2/1	....		4/5	....	
2/3	....		4/7	....	None
2/5	....	None	4/9	....	
2/7	....	None	4/11	....	
2/9	++	Severe urticaria	4/12	....	
			4/15	....	
2/10	....	None	4/17	....	
2/12	....		4/19	....	
2/14	....		4/21	....	None
2/16	....	None	4/23	....	
2/18	....		4/25	....	
2/20	....		4/27	....	
2/22	....	None	4/29	....	
2/24	....		5/1	....	None
2/26	....		5/3	....	
2/28	....	None	5/5	....	
3/2	....		5/7	....	
3/4	....		5/9	....	
3/6	....	None	5/11	++	Severe urticaria

*Baby, G.A., 5 months of age. Eczema; seen first on January 5, 1912. Ingestion of ¼ of an egg white caused severe generalized urticaria 15 minutes after ingestion on 4 occasions. The egg white was given on the days on which notations are made under "symptoms."

As emphasized above, provocation feeding tests to determine clinical allergy to eggs in the symptom-free patient is necessary to confirm such allergy.

Duke (1923) emphasized eggs as a cause of symptoms in adult life, and since then reported eczema on the face of an egg-sensitive child from the kissing of the child by the parents who had minute traces of eggs on their lips. Ratner (1928) reported the case of a Harvard student who committed suicide because he could not tolerate eggs! Stokes, in his discussion of the paper of Highman and Michael (1920), reported that his son had cyanosis, swelling of the face, giant urticaria, and marked swelling of the lower lip from raw but not from hard-boiled egg. Sutton (1927) stated that one patient was so sensitive to eggs that the presence of an egg in the room would provoke an attack! Urbach (1932) confirmed the reports of Joltrain and Brabant that dermatitis develops on hands of sensitive patients after handling eggs. He also cited the case of a boy who had edema of the oral mucosa, vomiting, and diarrhea if he ate bread cut with a knife that had broken an egg. He also recorded a case of anaphylactic shock in a woman twenty-seven years of age from eggs stroked on the mucous membrane of the nose. Lunsford informed us of a girl so sensitive to eggs that vesicular dermatitis developed immediately on the skin touched with egg, followed by projectile vomiting in a few minutes thereafter!

It is unnecessary to cite further case reports or examples of the various clinical manifestations of egg allergy from the articles in the literature contributed by the various writers mentioned above and by other students of the subject, such as Cooke, Alexander, Vaughan, Balyeat, Piness, and Eyermann.

PERSONAL EXPERIENCE

We have encountered all types of allergic manifestations from egg allergy. Since allergy to eggs alone is rare, the initial study of allergy to foods most frequently productive of clinical allergy, excluded from our CFE diet or its indicated modifications, is nearly always advisable. A few outstanding experiences and interesting records will be mentioned.

A child with urticaria from eggs termed her lesions "egg bites."

A girl fourteen years of age had a marked intolerance to eggs all her life. Severe vomiting and abdominal pain resulted from eating any amount of eggs. When the mother told a physician of this intolerance, he stated it was due to perverseness on the child's part and ordered large amounts of egg in the diet. This immediately produced severe acute symptoms and collapse. Recently headaches recurred, which were relieved on an egg-free diet.

A physician had chronic urticaria for fifteen years, which he finally discovered was due to egg alone. Ulcerlike epigastric pain arose from egg allergy in another patient. Herpes on the right side of the glans penis occurred forty-eight hours after egg ingestion in still another one. Headache five to six days after egg ingestion occurred in a woman. A confrere has aching epigastric pain and fatigue within one hour after eating eggs, lasting about eighteen hours. The egg in two chocolate creams will cause distress, and a whole egg gives gallbladderlike pain (see Chapt. 5). Egg sensitization occurring in two of three generations has been observed in several family records. In one family severe colic was the result of egg allergy in both mother and daughter. One mother of a child who had marked urticaria and eczema from eggs to which large reactions occurred found that her food could not be cooked in utensils in which eggs had been cooked because of the introduction of minute traces of egg into the other food. A child recently gave reactions to eggs and milk to which clinical allergy occurred. The child had been forced to eat these foods against its desire, and its eczema had steadily decreased in degree. Several cases of asthma from eggs in childhood and many more in which other foods as well as eggs were the cause have been encountered. A bronchial cough of three years' duration in a girl four years of age who gave positive reactions to eggs was immediately controlled by egg elimination alone.

Treatment

1. Elimination of eggs from the diet, as in the case of wheat, will control symptoms, providing other foods to which sensitization exists in the patient are also removed. To study most possible food allergies, our CFE diet or its modifications as advised in Chapter 3 are advised. The time required for relief of such symptoms has already been discussed and varies from ten to even thirty days. With such elimination tolerance to eggs gradually establishes itself in some patients. Schloss, Blackfan, and Ratner, in particular, have reported a gradual increase in tolerance with the elimination of eggs from the diet of infants. It is not unusual to have parents state that a child has outgrown an egg intolerance which may have been acute and absolute in infancy. It is our opinion, however, that such allergy is likely to persist or remain potentially active and that parents often fail to realize that the feeding of small amounts of egg or other allergenic foods to a child who has gradually acquired partial tolerance will produce mild obscure symptoms which impair the child's well-being and comfort, even though sometimes

in an indefinite manner. We therefore think that eggs or any other food to which marked allergy has existed in the past should be entirely excluded as long as either mild or severe symptoms are present, which might be a result of food allergy, especially if a large positive scratch test to the food is still present. It must be remembered, however, that the skin reaction may disappear or may never have been present in the food-sensitive individual. The general comments on the elimination of wheat apply to that of eggs and are important to remember.

2. Denaturization of eggs by heat has been recommended by Lesne, as reported by Laroche, Richet, and Saint Girons; Talbot; Ratner; and others. Talbot (1917, 1918) reported instances in which hard-boiled eggs were not tolerated. Our experience indicates that eggs boiled even for half an hour rarely can be tolerated by an egg-sensitive patient.

It should not be tried until eggs have been excluded for many weeks or even months. Moreover, it should be preceded by gradual oral desensitization, which is described below. Thus Talbot (1918) reported a patient who gave positive reactions to eggs and milk. Eggs were left out of the diet, and milk was reduced to 1 pint and boiled. In five days the eczema had entirely disappeared. Two weeks later a hard-boiled egg was given, and in eighteen hours an urticarial eruption appeared. When such feeding of hard-boiled eggs is without definite results in patients suspected of such allergy, it is possible that the assumed sensitization is not present. Ratner (1931) stated that boiling for thirty minutes permitted toleration in many patients.

The fear that many physicians seem to have that children are going to suffer from malnutrition if eggs, milk, or other specific foods are excluded from the diet is hard to understand. Health certainly does not depend on eating occasional bits of egg, and we feel that if there is definite evidence that egg sensitization is present and that it produces even mild symptoms, it should be excluded from the diet for a long enough period to bring about possible natural and complete desensitization or until oral desensitization aided, if desired, by hypodermic therapy, has been effective. It, however, may never occur.

3. Oral desensitization was first recommended by Schofield (1908). His case record has already been described in this discussion of egg allergy. Schloss (1912) described the following successful oral desensitization to eggs. Ovomucoid was given to a child in capsules for a period of 2½ months in doses of 2 mg daily, which were increased to 6, 12, 24, 48, 78, 190, and finally 380 mg, so that he was finally given 7 gm a day. Then gradually increasing amounts of whole egg as such or in foods were administered, though stinging and itching of the mouth occurred if too large amounts were taken. The skin reaction, moreover, gradually disappeared. As Talbot has pointed out, such oral desensitization may be retarded by reproducing symptoms with a fairly small dose. Such symptoms indicate the reduction of the dose and a more gradual increase. Casparis (1933) obtained desensitization to eggs by mouth, starting with a 1:1,000,000 dilution. It often failed, however, as it has in our experience for over forty years. Bray (1934) began with one drop of egg in a pepsin and hydrochloric mixture. A gradual increase up to one teaspoonful of egg a day then made it possible to include increasing amounts in the diet. In contrast to this work, Burchard (1934) was unable to destroy egg albumen with trypsin digestion.

Schloss (1920) stated that immunization to eggs or milk could be accomplished by the oral administration of these dried foods in capsules three times a day. At first the suggested dose was 2 to 5 mg. In small children and infants watery dilutions of milk were advised, beginning with 1/20 drop. It has been our experience that much weaker dilutions are at times advisable from the start, such as a 1:1,000 or even 1:10,000 dilution of a single drop, as was suggested in the discussion "Immunizing Against Eggs" published in the *Journal of the American Medical Association* (86: 1308, 1926). Gradual increases to 6 to 8 gm or cc a day over a period of two or even four months at times produce such tolerance that increasing amounts of the actual foods can then be taken. Schloss reported twelve patients who had been desensitized from three to seven years and were able to eat the specific foods without any discomfort. These results of Schloss have never been completely confirmed. The use of egg albumen as an inunction was noted by Burchard (1934). Urbach (1932) also used such percutaneous desensitization, with apparent help. Indifferent results were obtained.

4. *Hypodermic Desensitization.* The literature contains little confirmatory evidence that this type of therapy is successful. The failure to produce desensitization by this method, as reported by Little in the article in the *Journal of the American Medical Association* referred to in the foregoing paragraph is the experience of others as well. Cooke (1918) reported complete desensitization by egg-white injections in a boy three years of age. Ratner (1931) obtained increased tolerance to eggs by hypodermic desensitization in an infant

4½ months old. Good results, however, have not been confirmed. Urbach (1932) reported favorable results in dermatoses from egg allergy. Urbach (1932) recorded results obtained by intradermal technique suggested by Urbach and Fasal (1931) for desensitization with food allergens. Initial injections of 0.05 to 0.1 cc of a dilution of 1:100,000,000 of egg albumen with gradual increase up to a maximum of 1:10 were advised. Cooke (1922) published the following interesting case report:

Case 222: Age two years when seen in 1917. Even the first time egg was given, about one year previously, his face, lips, and tongue became swollen almost at once. He choked, coughed, and became dyspneic and cyanotic; vomited several times; and complained of abdominal pains. The father has early hay fever and the mother attacks of urticaria. On skin test the boy reacted markedly to the proteins of egg white but not to egg yolk. He was given injections of egg protein. After seven injections he could eat egg in pudding in small amounts without trouble. Four more injections were given in this year, and he could then eat one egg every other day without trouble until April, 1919, when he developed cough and hoarseness. Eight more injections were given. After this it was noted that he could eat an egg every day without symptoms. When he was put on two eggs a day, he developed edema of the face about eight hours later—again a delayed constitutional reaction. All symptoms of cough and edema disappeared forty-eight hours after egg was discontinued.

Rackemann (1928) obtained a good result from twenty-seven hypodermic injections of increasing quantities of egg white in a water solution in a young man twenty-two years of age who had had asthma all his life from eggs. Campbell (1926) reported such desensitization in a child four years of age, where the slightest trace of egg produced vomiting and where lacrimations and swelling of the eyes resulted when the patient went where eggs were being cooked. A skin reaction occurred to a 1:100,000 dilution, and treatment was begun with a 1:1,000,000 dilution. Seven months were required to complete the necessarily tedious therapy. Even then only small amounts of egg were tolerated! It would seem that in such a patient oral desensitization might have been better or that it should have been used in a gradual manner after hypodermic therapy was completed.

Personally we have not tried hypodermic desensitization to eggs or other food proteins for over thirty years, having preferred the effect of the elimination of eggs for a varying period of time. Marked skin reactions to egg proteins may disappear with the continued elimination of eggs. This has occurred in a child after the exclusion of eggs from its diet for four years. This has been followed by the gradually increased feeding of eggs.

MILK ALLERGY

In 1931 when the first edition of this book was written, the importance of allergy to milk seemed about equal to that of eggs. Since eggs have been discontinued in infants' diets and with realization of the infrequency of large or any skin reactions to milk, the greater frequency of milk allergy has occurred. This receives extended discussion in Chapter 25. Because of the frequency of clinical allergy to milk with no skin reactions and the necessity of confirmed clinical allergy to reacting foods by provocation tests, these statistics greatly minimize clinical food allergy to milk.

The reactions to the individual proteins in milk as they occurred in five hundred patients were as follows:

	+	++	+++
Milk—Whole	37	6	1
Albumen	19	6	1
Casein	16	2	

The number of the five hundred patients who reacted to the various numbers of the individual milk proteins were as follows:

No. of patients reacting to 1 protein 43
No. of patients reacting to 2 proteins 17
No. of patients reacting to 3 proteins 3

In infancy milk allergy is more frequent than at other times of life and should always be suspected. Porter and Carter, in 1927, stated that 10 percent of the well infants and 2 to 3 percent of all sick infants tolerate milk with great difficulty and that a few cannot take it at all, and they opine that such patients are probably milk-sensitive. As already stated in this chapter, the excessive drinking of milk by the mother during pregnancy may produce allergy in the fetus, and during the nursing period sensitization may arise from proteins of cow's milk which are excreted in the mother's milk. Supplemental feedings of diluted milk during the first few days of life with subsequent discontinuance of it upon the appearance of the mother's milk may also result in allergy to cow's milk in the infant as noted by Gerrard in Chapter 25. As Gerrard reported in Chapter 25 many milk-sensitive babies have milk-sensitive fathers or mothers. The overfeeding of milk, the giving of too concentrated dilutions, or the feeding of milk during severe digestive upsets are also likely to result in milk allergy, as emphasized by Laroche, Richet, and Saint Girons and especially by Schloss. The latter writer has shown that in marasmic infants especially, the feeding of milk is associated with the passage of milk proteins into the bloodstream. Such overfeeding of milk as well as of any other food at any time during life is likely to result in sensitization. Of interest was Duke's report (1932) of eczema and asthma in a woman apparently from allergy to a persisting milk secretion from her own breast. Desensitization with her own milk produced results.

It is difficult to determine what percentage of the population is milk-sensitive. In 1938 we stated that among children it may be between 0.5 to 1 percent and in adults possibly about 2 percent. In the last thirty years our continued study of milk and other food allergies indicates this estimate is too conservative. Even more people may have slight, mild, or marked clinical manifestations of some sort from milk allergy. The feeding of school children with milk should not be routine especially if evidence of perennial clinical allergy is present. If a child has cutaneous, nasobronchial, or gastrointestinal symptoms, milk or other foods should not be given in school without the sanction of a physician who appreciates the principles of allergic investigation and treatment and decides that milk is not a likely cause of allergy in the child.

Milk allergy may arise occasionally from the ingestion of beef or the inhalation of cattle dander. Simon (1934) showed experimentally that a common antigen probably exists in the hair, meat, serum, and milk proteins. Ratner and Gruehl (1935) found that animals sensitized with bovine serum reacted to raw milk, lactoglobulin, occasionally to lactalbumin, but not to casein, indicating a homologous globulin in serum and milk. These findings extended those of Crowther and Raistreck (1916) on the relation of milk colostrum and serum proteins. Wells and Osborne (1921) moreover, found the globulin of milk and beef identical. The origin of milk allergy through ingestion of meat or inhalation of dander probably is not common. Bovine serum albumin also occurs both in milk and in beef.

Milk allergy may produce any of the manifestations which have already been described in the various chapters of this volume. This is especially true in infancy and childhood and has already been pointed out in Chapter 25. As we have already stressed, gastrointestinal disturbances and symptoms are more commonly due to food allergy than is appreciated, and milk is a frequent cause of such allergy, especially in infancy and childhood. As Laroche, Richet, and Saint Girons, as well as others, have stated, it is more important to realize that such abdominal symptoms may be due to impaired digestion rather than to allergy. At times such decision is difficult to make, since it is apparently true in some patients, as emphasized by Brown, that impaired digestion in the stomach or intestine is responsible for the origin of allergic symptoms. This makes it imperative, as we have stated in our discussion of the diagnosis of food allergy, to carry out complete laboratory investigations and especially stomach analyses so that all existing pathology may be discovered. However, in the absence of such abnormal findings, the too ready dismissal of the possibility of food allergy as a cause of gastrointestinal symptoms in infancy, childhood, and adult life is unwise. The fact that meats, eggs, or other protein foods can be digested without symptoms, whereas milk or other specific foods repeatedly cause identical disturbances, is excellent evidence in favor of the presence of food sensitization rather than of indigestion.

Prophylaxis of Milk Allergy

To prevent the establishment of milk allergy, the excessive taking of milk during pregnancy and the nursing period by the mother, the taking of supplement feedings of milk by the baby for a brief period of time before the arrival of the mother's milk, the forced feeding of milk during digestive upsets, and the overfeeding of milk at any time during infancy and in certain patients during adult life are all to be avoided. This is especially true in patients and particularly in infants who have positive family histories of allergy particularly to foods. All these comments on prevention apply to eggs and wheat as well as to other foods. In infancy it is especially true in regard to milk. The frequency of wheat allergy after infancy, however, can be explained by the increasing amount of wheat consumed by the average individual as age advances.

Food Proteins Transmitted Through Milk

Sensitization to milk itself not only occurs but milk may carry other proteins from the cow's food to which the patient is sensitive. Moreover, allergy to human milk may explain intolerance of infants to one breast milk and not another, though allergy to food proteins secreted in the milk is more likely. The demonstration by Schloss of milk protein in the blood and urine of marasmic children and of egg proteins in the urine, which were reported by many investigators whose studies were summarized by Grulee and Bonar, as well as evidence reported by Shannon and O'Keefe and Donnolly that food proteins from the intestinal tract can pass into the mother's milk by way of the blood make it necessary to consider allergy not only from milk but from other foods whose proteins may be contained in cow's milk. Hermann (1922) stated that milk from cows that had fed on ragweed tops gave positive skin reactions in ragweed-sensitive patients, produced anaphylactic shock in guinea pigs sensitized to ragweed, and produced hay fever symptoms when ingested by patients who were sensitized to that pollen. Rohrbach (1925) reported seven patients who were relieved of allergic disturbances when cow's feed was changed. Thus an infant five months of age had severe alimentary intoxication, high temperature, rapid pulse, vomiting, frequent stools, and collapse resulting from the milk of certain cows. It was found that the milk obtained from those cows that fed on the weeds and grass of the hillside gave symptoms, whereas that from cows that fed on different vegetation in the meadow gave no trouble. Walzer and Bowman (1931) commented on flaxseed allergens in milk of cows fed on such fodder. G. F. Brown reported garlic and other allergens from various feeds in the milk. Balyeat, moreover, reported that milk from cows fed on bran produced severe symptoms in a wheat-sensitive patient and Black found the passage of peanut allergens through the milk of cows fed on peanut hay.

Literature on Milk Allergy

As reported by Laroche, Richet, and Saint Girons, one of the earliest clinical reports of milk allergy was made in nurslings by Hutinel (1908). The description of a few of his cases in the excellent translation by Mildred Rowe is as follows:

I have observed many patients suffering from severe colitis (dry cholera) who, when improved by treatment and rigid diet, developed severe symptoms of toxemia following one or two spoonfuls of milk. The eyes became sunken with dark brown circles, the nose became pinched, the face took on a pale or livid appearance, the extremities became cyanotic, and erythematous and urticarial eruptions appeared on the face, the arms, the limbs, and the buttocks. The stomach became scaphoid, the large intestine contracted and was cordlike to palpation; the stools soon became glairy or bloody, and nervous reactions frequently developed.

I recall particularly one of these children. I had talked to the mother about giving him milk. The attending physician believed it necessary to give some of it to him by injecting it into the bowel. Some acute symptoms resulted from this unfortunate intervention.

I have been taking care of a beautiful little girl, age eight, who has had a serious enterocolitis since her birth and has become, because of this fact, absolutely intolerant to milk. One day her mother risked giving her a spoonful of coffee with cream. Almost immediately afterward the child vomited, and in the night she had seventeen glairy stools. Later she had an extremely long and serious attack of typhoid fever; it was impossible to make her tolerate cow's milk, but fortunately she could digest goat's milk.

I have seen a beautiful little girl, age eleven months, in whom digestive symptoms occurred when at the age of nine months she was given boiled cow's milk in two nursing bottles containing 50 gm each. After this unfortunate experiment the child was nourished exclusively at the breast and throve until her nurse suddenly left her. She was given 100 gm of cow's milk. Almost immediately she was taken with vomiting, diarrhea, and prostration, and it was advised that she have another nurse immediately. My advice was heeded, and the symptoms disappeared.

These French writers also report other cases. Finkelstein, in 1905, had the following experience:

This case is that of a nursling who gave reactions every time that he received cow's milk. At each trial (5, 9, and 18 weeks) the symptoms were more severe, when at the twenty-sixth week a last trial, as a result of an unwise persistence, was attempted, and death resulted from collapse.

Finizio (1911) had a similar patient, whose record in the English translation by Mildred P. Rowe is as follows:

The following case is similar to the above. A sickly child, rachitic, tubercular, and breast-fed, took some animal milk during a previous stay at the hospital. At one year of age he was given a bottle containing 120 gm of milk. Two to three hours after serious symptoms appeared—intestinal vomiting, followed by frequent mucous and fetid diarrhea with tenesmus, dyspnea, uncountable pulse, and marked depression. Eight days later a second trial was followed by similar reactions. Trials with buttermilk, canned milk, and milk with farina still brought on reactions though less serious. Two months after the child was given 100 gm of milk; the symptoms appeared immediately—vomiting, bloody diarrhea, dyspnea, cyanosis, convulsions, and death. No autopsy was performed. It is interesting to note that the younger brother of this child likewise exhibited alimentary anaphylactic reactions to milk which were nearly fatal.

Halberstadt (1911) reported the case of a premature infant who was given supplementary feedings of buttermilk. Three months later buttermilk was again given, and collapse resulted, followed by death on the following day. Some of these patients had vomiting, glairy or bloody diarrhea, rectal tenesmus, high or low temperature, collapse, convulsions, tetany, or albuminuria. Other deaths from milk ingested were noted. Zybell reported vomiting, collapse, fever, and diarrhea in a child three years of age from milk, and Finizio had three cases afflicted with vomiting, prostration, diarrhea, tetany, or convulsions from milk allergy. Brazis reported burning and eruption on the lips of a woman from cream. The French writers recognized mild or chronic symptoms, such as urticaria, eczema, erythema, vomiting, diarrhea, asthma, migraine, emaciation, and malnutrition as results of food allergy, and especially to milk allergy, in infancy as well as in adult life.

Barnathan, a student of Richet in his pioneer treatise on food allergy in 1911, also summarized some of these same reports on milk allergy. Of definite interest Schloss, in his first article in 1912, did not mention milk allergy but gave it marked emphasis in 1915. One patient was reported with urticaria angioneurotic edema and gastrointestinal symptoms from milk, and the use of a mixture of soybean flour, washed butter, potato flour, and milk sugar was suggested as a milk substitute. He also stated that a mixture of beef protein, olive oil, dextromaltose, and rice flour gave a good result in another infant. Schloss (1920) found that lactalbumin produced more allergy than casein and reported negative skin reactions in five infants sensitized to cow's milk and suffering with gastrointestinal symptoms. Moderate amounts of thoroughly boiled milk apparently were tolerated. He reported Berger's findings of eosinophilia from seven to ten days after the first administration of cow's milk in some infants. The frequency of milk reactions, especially in eczema, was noted, and he felt that its etiological effect was difficult to prove because of the feeding problem arising with a milk-free diet. Soybean milk had not been advised. The use of milk denaturized by heat or through peptonizing or by the use of lactic acid was of value. Dried, boiled, or evaporated milk was tolerated in certain allergic infants. The passage of milk protein into the blood of marasmic infants as reported by Schloss and Anderson has already been mentioned. Talbot (1916) reported two cases of severe idiosyncrasy to cow's milk (which produced vomiting, diarrhea, high fever or subnormal temperature, weak pulse, and shock), and in 1918 he warned against giving new foods in infancy, such as milk, until the infant is able to take them steadily. Milk allergy was being recognized as frequently as egg allergy. The frequency of reactions to milk and other foods in cases of eczema reported by Blackfan, Schloss, and Talbot was reported in the first edition of this book in 1931. Talbot reported success with superheated, boiled milk and lactic acid milk, which has not been generally confirmed since then. Cooke, Walker, and Rackemann found comparatively few reactions to milk. Thus Walker, in 1918, in four hundred cases of asthma, recognized milk as an active cause in only two patients. Kerley reported near death in a baby by placing five drops of cow's milk on his tongue. Rackemann (1926), in a study of 1074 cases of asthma, found food allergy in only 30 patients!

Failure to realize the great frequency of food allergy, especially to milk, cereal grains, eggs, and less often to other foods excluded from our elimination diets, we opine, was due to failure to realize the frequency of negative scratch tests to allergenic foods and failure to use trial diagnostic diets and especially our CFE diet or its indicated modifications. This especially accounts for his conclusion that milk was active in only one child, age six, who had developed asthma and urticaria from cow's milk as well as goats! Davis *et al.* (1970) also, by failing to use our CFE diet, have actually been led to the conclusion that coproantibody to milk is clinically nonspecific. Most of their control patients were diarrhea patients not *thought* (italics ours) to be allergic to milk.

Schultz and Larsen (1918) stated that milk allergy was first described by Schloss, Moro, and Finkelstein (1905), reference to which are to be found in the trans-

lation by Mildred P. Rowe of the French monograph by Laroche, Richet, and Saint Girons. They reported pallor, at times cyanosis, vomiting, diarrhea, fever, apathy, dullness of sensoral activity, restlessness, and tremor in infants occurring immediately or within one-quarter hour after the ingestion of milk. Schultz and Larsen also cite Lust's report of two cases of laryngospasm recurring with cow's milk. They felt that the exudative diathesis of Czerny and that marasumus in infants were often due to milk allergy. Abt (1918) also felt that Czerny's exudative diathesis was probably due to allergy partly because successful therapy entailed the diminution of milk and the elimination of eggs.

Park (1920) reported a most instructive case of milk allergy in a child. The mother had had no intolerance to milk and had not drunk it excessively during pregnancy. The symptoms resulting from the ingestion of milk in Park's case are reprinted from

TABLE LIII

IMPORTANT DATA ON SEQUENTIAL REACTIONS OF PATIENT TO COW'S MILK (PARK)

Date	Age	Quantity of Milk	Mode of Administration	Interval Between Entrance of Milk Into Body and Full Development of Symptoms	Symptoms
4-13-16	6 weeks	⅔ oz	Mouth	3½-4 hr	Pallor, drowsiness, vomiting
5-11-16	10 weeks	½ tsp	Mouth	4 hr, 55 min	Drowsiness, flushed face, yawning, prostration, diarrhea
5-26-16	12 weeks	1 drop of a 1:100 solution	Skin*	4 hr	Drowsiness, vomiting, diarrhea
5-28-16	12½ weeks	0.01 cc	Skin†	3½ hr	Local induration of skin at site of test; drowsiness, flushing of face, later pallor, vomiting, yawning, prostration, diarrhea
6-1-16	13 weeks	2-3 drops sweetened	Mouth	2 hr, 50 min	Drowsiness, repeated vomiting, pallor, dyspnea, cyanosis of lips, great prostration, diarrhea
11-6-17	20 mos	4 drops	Mouth	1 hr, 10 min	Pallor, drowsiness, faintness, no vomiting
11-7-17	20 mos	5 drops	Mouth	1 hr, 15 min	Pallor, drowsiness, faintness, no vomiting
11-12-17	20 mos	7.5 drops	Mouth	1 hr, 35 min	Pallor, drowsiness, faintness

*Scarification †Intradermal injection

In 1928 he reported an infant with acute swelling of mouth, vomiting, and urticaria from milk. More food allergy would have been recognized if diet trial had been used as we advise.

his article in Table LIII and are of great interest.

The reaction at thirteen weeks resulted from the accidental administration of 2 to 3 drops of milk and was most severe in degree, being accompanied by respirations of 48 and pulse rate of 150. Desensitization was carried out as follows: November 4, 1 drop; November 5, 2 drops; November 6, 4 drops (became pale and weak); November 7, 5 drops; November 8, 10 drops; November 9, 15 drops; November 10, 30 drops; November 11, 60 drops; November 12, 7.5 cc; November 13, 10 cc; and then daily increases so that 250 cc were taken on December 10. At the age of three 1 pint of milk was being taken. Park made the important statement that milk allergy in this case was of a mild type, evidenced by the delayed clinical reaction. The possibility that natural desensitization would have arisen in this patient without attempted therapy must be considered.

Freeman (1920) reported a case of milk allergy in a man which had necessitated the use of ass's milk in infancy and stated that persistent vomiting in infancy was frequently due to milk sensitization. In discussing the article of Highman and Michael (1920), Carmichael cited the case of an infant, six months of age, who had urticaria and convulsions and nearly died after taking cow's milk. Goat's milk gave relief for eighteen months. Then 1 teaspoonful of milk gave urticaria. Reactions to milk were negative.

The studies of O'Keefe in 1920, 1922, 1923, and 1929, emphasize the frequent occurrence of milk allergy as a cause of eczema, especially in children, and the occurrence of negative skin reactions to foods. In 1929 the use of trial diets excluding milk, eggs, and wheat was recommended by O'Keefe and Rackemann.

During the last thirty years the literature has contained continued evidence of milk sensitization. The frequency of the negative skin reactions, however, has not been recognized sufficiently, especially in adult life, except by Alexander and Eyermann and O'Keefe and Rackemann. In our work "elimination diets" have been used for the last thirty years and have revealed much allergy not indicated by skin tests or even history. A few other reports of milk allergy will be added. Clearkin (1923) reported diarrhea from milk. Kerley, Ratner, Peshkin, Duke, Vaughan, Andresen, Brown, Balyeat, Piness, and others have added varying types of reports of milk sensitization to the literature. Duke (1923) reported a severe reaction in a patient who was milk-sensitive after he had received a transfusion of blood from a patient who had just drunk a large amount of milk. This would indicate the advisability of considering possible food sensitizations in recipients and of controlling the diet before the giving of blood by donors. Carr (1926) reported the interesting case of milk allergy in a patient with duodenal ulcer. Kennedy reported a case of epilepsy controlled by the elimination of milk from the diet. Campbell (1927) reported various cases of milk as well as other food allergies. In one patient severe toxemia was present. McClure and Huntsinger (1928) reported one case of typical migraine from milk. Hazen (1928) relieved neurodermatitis of nineteen years' standing in a girl by the elimination of milk. A small amount of cream reinstated the lesions. Bassoe (1926), Robinson (1927), and Joltrain (1930) recorded dermatoses from milk allergy. Sterling (1929) reported two severe cases with gastrointestinal symptoms, one simulating ulcer from milk allergy, and the other of severe urticaria, eczema, and asthma in a child. Cohen and Breitbart (1929) reported pylorospasm from milk allergy in three infants. Ashby (1929) described a case of severe eczema in an infant from the allergens in cow's milk which passed through the breast milk. Oral desensitization was carried out. In addition to the above our case reports and statistics in *Clinical Allergy* (1937), in the literature since then, and especially in Chapter 25 of this volume contain ample evidence of the importance of milk allergy.

The increasing realization of the frequency of milk allergy in infancy when milk may be the sole food at the time of onset after its initial ingestion and its manifestations including croup, colic, weakness, eczema, fatigue, tension, toxic symptoms, fever, collapse, and even death has increased in the last thirty years. This was summarized in our discussion of milk allergy in Chapter 25.

In addition, Goldman, Anderson, Sellers, *et al.*, in 1963, reported the frequency of clinical allergy to isolated milk proteins by oral provocation tests with BSA, beta-lactoglobulin, alphalactoglobulin, and casein. In 8.9 percent of seven hundred children with suspected milk allergy from the age of zero to one to ten years, the following symptoms occurred:

	%
Vomiting	33
Diarrhea	37
Colic and abdominal pain	28
Rhinitis	35
Asthma	27
Atopic dermatitis	16
Anaphylaxis during their challenge with near death in 2 patients*	9
CNS symptoms	18

*Lethargy, weakness, irritability, crying, restlessness, pallor, and darkness around eyes.

Personal Observations of Milk Allergy

It is impossible to cite the many individual cases of milk allergy with their many types of manifestations which have come under our observation. Our experience confirms the great frequency of such sensitization in infancy, its common occurrence in childhood, and its increasing recognition in adult life and old age. As has been stated before, negative skin reactions commonly occur to the scratch test and frequently to the intradermal one in all ages but especially in adult years.

Milk allergy, as has already been stated, tends to occur in families, and a history of distaste or definite disagreement for milk in such patients is frequent.* Finizio's Cases 1 and 2 showed familial milk allergy. Milk sensitization has been found to vary in degree and time of reaction. Certain patients have been found who are so sensitive that the minute amount of milk present in butter has caused severe symptoms. Milk or its products have been found to be cumulative in their allergic effects. A small amount may be tolerated on one day without difficulty, but when it is taken over a period of several days an allergic disturbance has resulted. Mildly sensitive patients have been observed who can tolerate dried, boiled, superheated, lactic acid, or buttermilk but not fresh milk. Such patients at times can take a little cream or butter. Tolerance to milk has been increased by its elimination in many individuals, and oral desensitization has been successful in a few. However, in most patients milk allergy persists in spite of elimination and attempts at desensitization. Milk sensitization as a cause of symptoms in the naso-bronchial tissues and especially in perennial nasal allergy, bronchial asthma, and obstructive emphysema has occurred often in adult life as well as in childhood. Two women in their forties with asthma were especially susceptible. In one patient cumulative effects of milk allergy produced

---

*This was emphasized by Kerley (1936). He also reported collapse and shock in infants.

asthma after it had been taken again for two or three weeks. In the other case the inclusion of a little milk in biscuits was enough to produce severe asthma again.

The following striking clinical effects of milk allergy, some of which have already been noted, will be briefly alluded to. Fever had in 1938 been observed in three adults and in several children as a result of milk allergy. A chronic excoration of the vulva was present in two small girls from milk, as well as certain other foods as determined by my trial method of "elimination diets." Pruritus ani associated with urticaria from milk occurred in a man. Several cases of chronic urticaria from food and from milk especially have been relieved. One case was a tubercular patient who had severe coughing from urticaria in the bronchial tubes from milk taken in excess for several years. Milk allergy as a cause of constipation has occurred in several instances and may explain the reputation that milk has as a cause of this symptom. In one girl longstanding constipation associated with pain in the lower right quadrant suggestive of appendicitis, together with severe menstrual cramping and vomiting, was due to milk allergy, which was also present in her sister and mother. Another girl, fourteen years of age, with a well-controlled diabetes of four years' standing, had recurrent abdominal pain with vomiting from milk allergy. A girl eight years of age developed severe asthma with temperature of 104 F and delirium a few hours after butter was taken. Milk was the chief cause of a longstanding chronic asthma. A woman had severe abdominal pain with diarrhea and joint pains especially in the lower back twenty hours after the taking of butter by mistake. A child abstained from all milk products for one year without asthma. One biscuit made

with milk was given, and asthma began in a few hours and persisted for five days.

Persistent diarrhea, associated at times with mucus and cramping pain in infants, children, and even adults, has been found a result of milk allergy, discovered with the initial use of our CFE diet, often being associated with other food sensitizations. Marked nervousness, irritability, restlessness in sleep, and nasal congestion were present in a boy four years of age from milk sensitization, and a severe case of recurrent convulsions in a child three years of age was due to a like cause. One patient among others had upper abdominal pain and soreness, suggesting ulcer or gallbladder disease, and another had persistent sour stomach and constipation from milk allergy. A coated tongue and heavy breath have been definitely due to milk sensitization in several instances, in one of which the sensation of globus hystericus resulted from this cause. A woman fifty-two years of age who had had cramping abdominal pain associated with gastric distress and constipation from this type of allergy was treating herself with cream enemas! A man sixty-four years of age developed bronchial asthma from milk without foregoing evidence of clinical allergies.

As a cause of migraine and the allergic toxemia and fatigue which we have described in Chapter 19, milk is an outstanding cause. A physician has picket fence staggers, weakness, and trembling in the arms and legs diagnostic of an epileptic equivalent (see Chapt. 18) when she takes butter. It comes in two days. She can take cream in coffee for two days but not for three days without the symptoms. Insomnia from milk allergy arose in another patient. Individual records have been cited in the respective discussions of these symptom-complexes. The tingling and chilly sensations throughout the body associated with the taking of milk, as described by Laroche, Richet, and Saint Girons, have been noted in several patients. A case of severe abdominal pain suggested kinked ureter, for which an operation was done, and another with severe abdominal pain, for which an appendectomy and cholecystectomy has been done without relief, were both found to have milk allergy as a cause, illustrating the necessary consideration of allergy especially to foods by the surgeon as emphasized in Chapter 27.

Treatment

Many of the points discussed in the previous considerations of the treatment of wheat and egg allergies apply to the control of that resulting from milk and will not be fully discussed again. The reader is also referred to the consideration of the milk-free diet and its administration especially in infancy with the aid of milk substitutes as described in Chapter 3.

1. The elimination of milk and all of its products is necessary to control allergic symptoms resulting from it. This exclusion must be complete as discussed in detail in Chapter 3. The degree of allergy and possible reestablished tolerance must be determined in the symptom-free patient by feeding tests, as advised in Chapter 3. As with the elimination of wheat and eggs, desensitization to milk frequently occurs as a result of its omission, and different degrees of tolerance in varying periods of time develop. In severe and especially longstanding cases of milk allergy, elimination alone never results in immunity, and frequently an apparent desensitization is not complete or permanent or is present only in the summer months (see Chapt. 1). The gradual addition of milk to the diet breaks down the acquired tolerance in these patients in the course of weeks or

months after such milk sensitization may remain potentially active, only to appear in the same or some other manifestation several years later.

It also must be remembered, as is true with other foods, that natural immunity establishes itself in certain patients as age increases. At times such desensitization may occur very suddenly. However, it is often only partial or is only apparent. The local manifestations of a generalized potential allergy may disappear or in another person may develop in other tissues.

The previous comments on the fear of the laity occasioned by the elimination of eggs apply even more to the exclusion of all milk. As stated, the complete elimination of all milk products, even butter, is often necessary for years or during life in sensitive patients. Many parents and physicians cannot understand that milk is not necessary for health. This was stressed by Kerley (1914) in an article already referred to, and since then various pediatricians have emphasized it. Kerley stated: "I could present dozens of records showing surprising gain in weight and marked improvement in the general well-being of the patient after a considerable withdrawal of milk, cream, and butter from the diet. A period of lactation in the human being is at most a year, and then the child is ready for other food than milk." He commented on the "unknown millions who have lived their span without it," which recalls those studies which showed the well-nourished children in Hawaii who received no milk whatsoever after being weaned. If milk produces mild or severe symptoms, it should be eliminated completely, hoping that until natural desensitization immunity by feeding or hypodermic therapy is gradually established. As already described, various substitutes for milk are available even for infants. When milk or its products are added, the patient's tolerance may be such that no symptoms arise for several weeks, especially in the summer. This delay in the reappearance of symptoms may occur in patients who retain mild or potential milk allergies.

2. The tolerance of certain milk-sensitive patients for milk denaturized by boiling, drying, evaporating, or superheating has been reported by many students such as Schloss, Blackfan, Talbot, Ratner, Porter and Carter, Kerley, and others. Kerley (1927) recommended the boiling of skimmed milk for three to six hours. The boiling of milk with cereals for long periods seems to denaturize the proteins in both. Talbot advised the removal of the coagulated scum because of the allergenicity of the contained lactalbumin. Lewis and Hayden (1932) reported increasing denaturization with increasing temperature, and Ratner (1934) concluded that evaporated milk is less allergenic than raw, pasteurized, or dried milks. This was in contrast to Cutler's findings (1929). Usually such modifications of cow's milk continue to cause symptoms, necessitating its complete elimination for weeks, months, or even longer, as advised in Chapters 3 and 25.

The use of lactic acid and predigestion only aids in the digestion and produces no denaturization of the proteins. Ratner showed that acidification of evaporated milk did not decrease its allergenicity. Wallen-Lawrence and Koch (1930) showed that trypsin digestion was more rapid and complete in evaporated and boiled milk than in raw milk and that heating destroys not only bacteria but their toxins in the milk. Therefore, the use of lactic acid as recommended by Marriott or of peptonized milk as suggested by Schloss in the twenties rarely was of help and is no longer advised. Spies *et al.* have more recently shown that predigestion produces

new milk antigens, which are possibly allergenic.

3. Oral desensitization may be carried out in the same manner as described for eggs. The dried milk or dilutions of the fluid milk may be used. Schloss described the problem of an infant who was able to be desensitized with diluted milk, the initial dose being 1/20 drop three times a day. He stated that oral desensitization usually took from three to six months. After desensitization it is important for the milk to be taken every day to prevent the reestablishment of sensitization. Schloss reported twelve patients who had been desensitized thus for three to seven years and were able to take milk without discomfort. This has not been used successfully in our practice.

FRUIT ALLERGY

The importance of recognizing allergy to individual fruits and (as stated below) to many or even all fruits, condiments, flavors, and spices and in a similar manner to vegetables became increasingly evident as we pursued the challenge of clinical food allergy from 1916 to 1928. This led to the formulation of our Elimination Diets first published in 1928 which were advised for the study and control of food allergy not only to wheat, milk and eggs, the elimination of which usually had been advised for the study of such allergy, but also to chocolate, coffee, spices and condiments, and individual fruits and vegetables, allergy to which had been recognized in our patients and reported in the literature as frequent causes of clinical allergy.

During the thirties the frequency of allergy to many or occasionally to all fruits in addition to the fallibility of skin tests to determine such possible allergy increasingly emphasized the importance of excluding all fruits and spices from the initial elimination diet for the study of allergy, especially in urticaria; localized edemas; possible gastrointestinal, urogenital, and joint tissue dysfunctions; and in other tissues as advised in Chapter 2 and other chapters throughout this volume. The importance of our FFCFE diet or its modifications has been increasingly demonstrated with its indicated routine use during the last twenty years. In addition to such routine use, this FFCFE diet has been utilized to study other possible manifestations of food allergy when a carefully recorded diet history indicates several or many definite allergies to fruits, spices, or condiments. As advised in Chapter 3, if and after the clinical allergies are controlled for more than two to four weeks, provocation tests with individual fruits to gradually determine those which can be tolerated without symptoms by the patient may be effected. Dependable information and continued relief from a nonallergenic diet, as repeatedly emphasized throughout this volume, require strict, accurate cooperation of the patient supervised by the informed, open-minded physician who is aware of the frequency and importance of clinical food allergy.

The study and control of allergy to individual fruits, condiments, and to other foods which are most common causes of clinical allergy can be achieved with our CFE diet modified with the eliminations of individual fruits or vegetables to which possible allergy is indicated by a well-taken diet history or by large scratch reactions as advised in Chapter 2. If, however, evidence of a broad-based type of fruit allergy increases, our FFCFE diet or in rare cases a minimal elimination diet, as advised in Chapter 3, may be required.

Evidence of clinical allergy to individual or botanically related fruits has been generally recognized for many years and has long been published in the medical literature. Allergy to the following fruits as reported by us in the first edition of this book in 1931 and in its revision in 1937 and which has continued and occurred in our patients in the last thirty years evidences the various symptoms arising from fruit allergy and our increasing realization of such allergy to specific fruits which justified the exclusion of frequently incriminated fruits from our CFE diet. The important recognition and control of fruit allergy first emphasized in our elimination diets in the first edition of this book and the use of our FFCFE diets, as published in 1944, as discussed above, therefore are of great importance. The important consideration of broad-based fruit (including condiments, spices, and flavors) allergy justifying our FFCFE diet and its modifications, as emphasized in Chapter 3, is necessary when manifestations of food allergy incriminate such foods.

Usually specific allergies exist to individual fruits, though closely related ones produce trouble, as discussed in Chapter 21 in certain patients. At times practically all fruits give allergic reactions in patients, as exemplified in Cases 151, 153, and 154. One physician who has many types of severe allergies has a natural aversion to all fruits. Avocado and melons produce burning in his mouth, and bananas always make him ill. Another confrere has drawing in his tongue, nausea, and vomiting in one hour after eating avocado.

Vaughan's excellent botanical study of foods, which has been summarized in Chapter 30, suggests that patients may frequently have allergic reactions to foods belonging to the same botanical group, as evidenced by mild or severe symptoms and at times positive skin reactions. The fact that patients are at times allergic to all citrus fruits or to apples and pears, or to so-called pit fruits, is an example of this group allergy. However, as will be pointed out below, quite definite specificity to fruits does occur. This also occurs in pollen allergy, where patients may be sensitized to certain grass pollens and not to others or to one atriplex or ambrosia pollen and not to another.

Allergy to fruits frequently exists without any skin reactions, and positive skin reactions less frequently exist without any ascertainable symptoms or disturbances. It has been our experience that definite dislikes or disagreements for certain fruits may be accompanied by two plus or three plus scratch reactions in some cases.

Symptoms from fruit allergy, as with other types of food sensitizations, often persist even for seven to fourteen days after the fruit has been discontinued. This also is true in certain patients even after thorough colonic cleansing has been carried out, illustrating the fact that the reactions result from blood-borne allergens which require days for final exhaustion. Thus a patient sensitized to loganberries had generalized severe urticaria for nine days after eating a few such berries for the first time in several years.

The fact that heat destroys the reacting power of fruit especially has been known by the laity probably for centuries. Tuft and Blumstein, in 1942, confirmed this in their report of large scratch reactions to fresh juice and not to dried extracts of fruits. As a general rule, fresh fruit will produce symptoms much more frequently than cooked or canned fruit, and therefore it should not be used in trial diets, especially if symptoms are not readily controlled. Quite rarely, patients can tolerate fresh and not cooked fruit. At times the skin of the fruit and not its actual edible portion causes allergy.

Separate mention will now be made of our experience in regard to the frequency of allergy to specific fruits, though we do not intend to cover the whole list. In general, allergy occurs most frequently to those fruits which are most commonly eaten in large amounts. This may vary in different individuals, though there is a tendency to take certain fruits rather than others. Thus oranges, apples, bananas, and strawberry sensitizations have been more definite and frequent in our own cases than allergies to other fruits. Severe abdominal allergy existed to the first three in a man forty years of age who had eaten excessively of these three in his boyhood. Bananas produce many allergic disturbances. Canker sores, vomiting, abdominal pain, soreness, and colonic spasm are some of its manifestations. Ramirez (1920) reported eczema on the backs of the hands from ingested fruit. Lindsay (1926), Goodale (1916), and Ratner (1928) also reported allergic symptoms from bananas. Eczema from food allergy, especially to fruits, is reported in Case 82.

Our clinical experience singles out the above-mentioned fruits as those which most frequently produce marked allergy. Along with these, melons and other berries also seem to be productive of many marked reactions. Our elimination diets, therefore, have excluded such fruits. Since sensitization to the remaining fruits occurs in apparently about the same degree of frequency in each one, three such fruits are included in each diet, and any that gives positive histories of disagreement or positive skin reactions are excluded when the diet is prescribed. Thus the effect of each fruit and of other individual foods in the prescribed elimination diets can be observed by the patient and doctor. In general, the overindulgence in any fruit should be guarded against, especially in patients predisposed to allergy. The history of the eating of a fruit such as strawberries in excess for two or three weeks to be followed by urticaria or an itching rash all over the body is not unusual.

Apple sensitization is mentioned frequently in the literature, especially by Freeman (1920), DeBesche (1923), Lindsay (1926), Goodale (1916), and Rich (1922). The latter writer stated that his patient was also sensitive to pears, which belong to the same botanical group, as described by Vaughan. Apple allergy was found to be in part responsible for severe abdominal symptoms in a man who lived on an apple ranch. A woman and her mother were so allergic to apples that even their odor made them nauseated. One child can eat red apples, but green ones give hives. Rackemann (1928) reported asthma in a boy from apples and eggs, with negative reactions to both. Apple sensitization seems to have been specifically transmitted in several families in our experience. Apples and pears produce diarrhea in one patient. Sensitization to pears, however, in our work has never been very definite except in certain patients who have a general intolerance for all fruits. One boy, however, was studied who had severe hives eight to ten hours after each ingestion of pears. Sticker (1912) encountered skin lesions from allergy to pears.

Oranges produce allergy not infrequently, especially in childhood, because of their frequent use. Patients who have allergic propensities may become sensitized or have an old potential allergy aroused by the excessive drinking of this juice. One patient has eczema on the fingers and hands when citrus fruits are eaten, and a man has eczema only on the inner side of the left fourth finger if oranges are eaten for three or four days. In one patient oranges produced a right-sided abdominal pain which

was also known to be due to other foods. This patient had been taking two or three glasses of orange juice a day for several months. Citrus fruits give pylorospasm, gastric retention, headaches, and upper right quadrant pain in a physician. A child recently was found tolerant to the juice and not to the pulp of orange. Karrenberg (1932) reported localized flushing and sweating in the head in a boy twenty months old from oranges. Another patient had puckering of her mouth and a "setting on edge" of all her teeth from all fruits. However, orange juice taken through a straw gave no disturbance. Stroud (1931) noted dermatitis from lemons. They produced migraine in one of our patients. A woman sixty-five years of age had had loose bowels all of her life. With the increased taking of orange juice, she had severe dysentery, and she found that oranges were the only fruit which produced such looseness of her bowels. Lemons and grapefruit produce equal or milder symptoms in some patients who are orange-sensitive. They may be tolerated perfectly, however. On the other hand, grapefruit produced marked allergy in a girl who was not sensitive to oranges. This patient had symptoms of hay fever from the ingestion of grapefruit and was also affected by its odor, which she could detect on first entering the house! It is interesting that peaches and pears produced the same symptoms. A young woman had marked canker sores from oranges. Another woman had diarrhea from oranges as well as from all other fruits except lemon and grapefruit. Bladder allergy especially to lemon occurred in a girl. A woman fifty-six years of age developed generalized aching from citrus fruits. The use of oil of oranges and lemons in foods and drinks must be remembered.

Peaches and apricots produce allergy less often than the above discussed fruits, though they must always be suspected. Peaches produce immediate vomiting in one man. Peaches and melons produce sores on the lips (but no canker sores) and an eruption on the arms and legs in a woman. Peaches and melons result in edema of the eyes, cheeks, lips, and penis in a boy. Recently a patient knew that all "pit fruits" caused marked indigestion, whereas citrus fruits could be taken in large amounts. Blisters on the mouth and tongue from peaches as well as fish and not from other pit fruits afflicted a girl. Lindsay (1926) noted asthma, nasal allergy, and skin edema from peaches. Vaughan has reported several sensitizations to the fruits in the Drupaceae family, including almonds, cherries, apricots, plums, and peaches. One woman can eat one variety of peach though another type produces an itching rash and giant hives in twenty minutes. It is interesting that one of our patients has severe asthma from cherries but can eat all other fruits without any trouble. Cherries and no other fruit produce marked burning in the mouth of another patient. Pineapple sensitization producing hay fever symptoms established itself in a woman who had eaten it excessively for several weeks. Such allergy in our experience is not common, however, in this country, though it may be frequent where the fruit is abundant. Many patients have gastrointestinal and cutaneous allergy to melons. At times watermelon or cantaloupe can be tolerated when honeydew, Persian, or casaba cannot. One woman has immediate asthma from watermelon. Another develops immediate hay fever from watermelon, cantaloupe, and fresh berries, especially strawberries and loganberries. Rich (1922) and Eyermann (1928) reported nasal allergy from cantaloupe. (A patient had severe intestinal cramping from all melons except watermelon. Their

close relative, squash, however, could be eaten without any discomfort.) A young woman has found that constipation occurs whenever she eats fresh fruits. "The more she eats, the worse she gets." It is not due to roughness of food, since she can eat all the lettuce, spinach, and other fibrous vegetables she desires without consequent constipation. Other mention of specific fruit allergies will not be made. The literature as well as our records give evidence of varying sensitization to all types of fruits, and in studying the allergic response of patients to trial diets, all fruits as well as other foods must be suspected, even though they may be relatively rare causes of allergy, justifying use of our FFCFE diet formulated in the late thirties.

Wyman (1872) first recorded the production of hay fever from fruits and other foods. At times such symptoms arise during eating. One of his patients had sneezing, watering of the eyes and nose, and irritation of the throat after eating or even touching peach, pear or melon. These allergies were not active in the mountains. Pears produced itching of the throat and hoarseness in another patient. Soreness of the mouth and swelling of the lips from tomatoes and peaches occurred in yet another one. One other patient had an inflamed throat and mouth from uncooked fruits except strawberries! Sliced melons and tomatoes could not be on the table. Handling apples and oranges produced immediate eye and nasal symptoms. Such observations have been duplicated in many experiences.

ALLERGY TO VEGETABLES

Allergy to specific vegetables exists in many patients, and reactions to various vegetables are not infrequent. It has been our experience, however, that many one plus reactions occur to vegetables without any ascertainable clinical disturbances. It thus becomes necessary to determine vegetable sensitiveness with actual clinical trial, as has been done in our cases. Clinical experience shows that cabbage, cauliflower, legumes, white potato, celery, tomato, and mushroom allergy most frequently exists and that carrots, squash, and lettuce are of secondary importance. There occurs a comparatively large number of two plus and three plus reactions to celery, potatoes, cauliflower, asparagus, and turnips, and these reactions in many instances checked with clinical experiences of patients. As emphasized in Chapter 3 and throughout this volume and continuously by us since 1927, clinical allergy to these reacting and nonreacting vegetables and other foods must be determined by provocation testing always in the symptom-free patient. The effect of the vegetables used in the prescribed diets must be observed by the patient and physician, and if definite evidence of disagreement or distress occurs as a result of their ingestion, they must be held under suspicion and eliminated from the diet if necessary. The incorporation of various vegetables in sauces, soups, and other foods must be remembered. Tomatoes are included in sauces, catsups, dressings, flavorings, and onion, likewise, and also in meat sauces, soups, and as flavor in cooking. Contact as well as inhalation may be instrumental in giving rise to allergic reactions to vegetables. Thus a patient sensitive to carrots could not be in the kitchen where they were cooking without getting asthma. A patient sensitive to celery and another sensitive to potatoes could not peel them without suffering allergic reactions. Dermatitis from the handling of vegetables and of fruits according to the individual specificity is not uncommon.

Most of the points brought out in regard

to fruit sensitizations apply to those resulting from vegetables. This is particularly true of the group allergy that exists to large numbers of vegetables in a few individuals. This wide variety of sensitizations may depend upon the group relations described by Vaughan, who cites records of patients with clinical sensitizations to various beans, including peanuts, as well as cabbage, carrots, cucumbers, celery, onions, garlic, and asparagus. However, specificity within food groups do occur. One of our patients had marked bladder distress from string beans and no other legumes, and Vallery-Radot and Heimann (1930) reported urticaria in a child eight years of age, from dwarf kidney and not from white kidney beans. Cauliflower and cabbage result in belching and distention and asparagus in diarrhea and cramping in ten minutes in a young woman. One patient had indigestion from radishes, turnips, cabbage, Brussel sprouts, and cauliflower, which belong to the Cruciferae family. Tomatoes produced urticaria when eaten, handled, or even touched in one individual. Another had violent nausea and vomiting from tomatoes but not from their close relatives, the potatoes. Vesicular keratitis from tomatoes arose from its ingestion in a child. A case of migraine from various types of beans was also reported. Severe grippelike aching, especially in the legs, in two men arose from eating string beans. We think, however, that markedly specific allergies to vegetables frequently exist, as have also been shown in the case of fruit allergies. In such patients the elimination diets must be modified by the exclusion of nearly all vegetables or fruits as the indications dictate, according to the suggestions for the minimal elimination diets as described in Chapter 3. It must be emphasized that sweet corn is a cereal and not a vegetable.

Evidence in the literature as well as in

our own clinical experience illustrates the frequency of allergic reactions to cabbage and its close relatives, cauliflower and sprouts, as well as to white potatoes, tomatoes, and celery. Hazen (1928) reported dermatitis, Alexander and Eyermann (1929) purpura, Rose (1928) migraine, Highman and Michael (1920) urticaria and edema, and Eyermann (1928) nasal allergy from white potatoes. It also produced abdominal pain in one patient. Raw potatoes yielded hives and slight asthma and swelling of the uvula in another. Cooked potatoes were tolerated. Potato allergy was reported by Vallery-Radot and Heimann (1930) and Joltrain (1930). Roch and Schiff (1921) recorded asthma arising from potatoes. These foods not infrequently produce rapid and acute reactions which are easily recognized by the patient. Thus one patient was so sensitive to cabbage that generalized urticaria and diffuse angioneurotic edema came on invariably about two hours after its ingestion. The peeling as well as the eating of asparagus by one patient invariably produced sneezing. Another woman was so allergic to celery that the mere taste caused marked, immediate swelling of her lips and tongue and uncontrollable vomiting followed in about fifteen minutes with generalized urticaria and asthma. A girl with pollen hay fever had stinging and burning of the mouth from celery, and her mother had angioneurotic edema of the larynx from celery, which on one occasion threatened her life. A lad sensitive to celery, to which a three plus reaction occurred, had immediate itching and swelling of the lips from it but suffered no gastrointestinal symptoms after swallowing it. This illustrates a marked degree of localized allergy. A man had severe weakness and marked pain in the neck, shoulders, and arms, with pain in the eyes and nasal passages whenever he ate raw celery. Cooked celery, however, could be eaten with impunity. Skin reactions were negative to celery. It is to be remembered that celery salt is used frequently to season foods and that celery flavor enters into cooking in many ways. Celery produced a rash on the neck and parsley and carrots caused headache in one woman. Spain (1933) reported asthma in a patient on entering a dining room where celery was on the table or driving past celery fields. Henry (1933) reported celery causing itching in 4 percent of those canning this food. Sweet potatoes occasionally give clinical reactions. They are botanically separate from white potatoes. It is interesting that sweet potatoes have been used in the glue on postage stamps. Spinach rarely produces clinical allergy in spite of its rather frequent skin reactions which are often nonspecific in origin. However, Brown, in 1929, described unconsciousness coming on two hours after eating it. A young patient of mine had allergic rhinitis from food allergy, and spinach produced a rash on the skin around his mouth. A child had colic from a specific allergy to spinach. Spinach only when eaten alone gave hives in the child. Handling spinach produced swelling and running of the eyes and asthma in a woman. Volk (1931) reported radish and horseradish, Urbach (1932) noted cucumbers, and Ellis (1931) recorded beets as causes of dermatitis.

Onion and garlic sensitizations caused marked allergic symptoms which are outstanding and may serve to emphasize their apparent frequent occurrence, which is not shown in our experience in skin tests. A physician and his brother, as well as another patient, have been sensitized to both of these vegetables since boyhood, when they frequently ate onions as they would eat apples or oranges. Such excessive ingestion probably accounted for the establishment of the allergies. One of these patients had severe bilious headaches and psychic disturbances. Another severe allergy to both of these foods, especially to onions, resulted in allergic toxemia. The remarkable sensitivity to a minute amount of onion sauce or flavor in this case is illustrative of the delicacy of many reactions in food allergy. A woman forty years of age had recurrent appendiceal pain definitely from onions. Frost, in his discussion of Talbot's paper (1917), described an onion allergy which occurred in many members of successive generations of the same family. Ratner (1925) described a garlic allergy which evidenced itself upon the taking of a little bologna. Kern (1927) also described an interesting case of onion sensitization. Walker also described allergic disturbances from its ingestion (1920), as did Highman and Michael (1920), Kahn (1929), and Beecher (1929). The wide use of onions as a flavor in cooking makes it almost impossible for patients who are thus afflicted to eat away from their own tables. In one of our patients we are now trying hypodermic desensitization.

Various beans give skin reactions in certain patients. Negative reactions do not rule out allergy. In 1938 we reported positive scratch reactions with the use of whole food extracts of several species of beans in some patients.

As has been emphasized in various contributions, peanuts belong to the bean family and should be thought of as a vegetable. Large scratch reactions may occur without reactions to other legumes usually associated with marked clinical allergy.

The fact that certain olive oils, especially imported ones, are diluted with peanut oil must be remembered, and the passage of the peanut allergen through cow's milk is of interest. A few peas in the mouth of one child always produced a tickling sensation, causing her to work her tongue back and forth for relief. Peaches produced the same effect. A physician has migraine only from peanuts or cucumbers. Death from the ingestion of peas was reported by Starck (1926). Feinberg and Avies, in 1932, reported severe asthma from peas even when their cooking odor was inhaled. Intradermal tests were positive with a 1:10,000,000 dilution. Coca and Grove, in 1925, reported serum antibodies to the protein in a patient markedly sensitive to peas. Edwards and Helming, in 1942, reported anaphylactic shock with involuntary urination and collapse several times in fifteen years from ingestion especially of peas to which a four plus scratch skin reaction occurred. Ingestion of slight amounts caused tightness in the chest and throat. Engman and Wander (1921) reported urticaria from beans. Vallery-Radot (1930) noted several reports of urticaria from legumes. A child had a specific idiosyncrasy only to kidney beans.

The frequent use of soybean flour and oil of the beans not only in food but in the industries was noted by Duke (1934). Soybean allergy causes gastrointestinal symptoms, particularly diarrhea. Because of this we asked the meat industry to make strained meat which is valuable to patients sensitive to soy as well as milk and was used in a formula which is important in infant feeding. Such a product is sold by Gerber and Company and can be used by the mother with our formula as advised in Chapter 3. Soy allergy also causes intestinal symptoms, reported by Peters in 1965, as in Case 6 in this volume and asthma or other clinical allergy in adults. One man had asthma from the dust in a soybean mill. Olsen and Prickman (1936) also reported such a case and listed the various products made from soybean flour, meal, or oil.

Peshkin (1924) noted asthma from soybean dust.

Tomatoes give a burning sensation in the mouths of patients of ours who are definitely sensitized to this vegetable.

As with fruits, allergy can exist to any vegetable, established according to the causes already discussed in various sections of this book. Squash sensitization occurs at times, usually causing mild reactions. An interesting localized sensitization exists in a friend who has a marked erythmatous swelling of the sclera of the eye if the slightest bit of juice from squash is introduced into the eye by rubbing the lids with the fingers during the peeling or handling of this vegetable. Avocados, which had been eaten rather freely by a fruit dealer, produced localized allergy in his mouth and stomach. Mushroom sensitization has been recorded in four different individuals, and it is interesting that abdominal pain and distress as well as nausea and vomiting were complained of by all patients.

The frequency of allergy to the cabbage group of vegetables and to celery and legumes, except peas, justified their elimination from our CFE diet (Chapt. 3).

ALLERGY TO MEATS AND FOWL

Sensitizations to these foods are rather infrequent. General impressions and clinical data obtained from the literature and our own experience will be presented. Some patients are sensitive to all mammalian meat proteins, probably because of a common allergen such as Simon (1934) showed exists in all mammalian sera. Pork probably produces allergic reactions more frequently and of a more acute nature than other meats. It may be that some of these reactions are due to indigestion, as is probably true with veal. If the veal is "milk-fed," however, caution in feeding it to milk allergy patients is obvious. For trial purposes, our "elimination diets" have excluded these meats, except for bacon in Diet No. 2. A remarkable record of pork sensitivity will be briefly presented on page 577. A patient with generalized eczema and anal pruritus could detect the presence of any product of pork, such as bacon grease used in frying hot cakes, by the recurrence of anal itching. Vaughan (1933) found pork causative of severe migraine, blurred vision, and blind spells. A physician sensitive to pork could not take gelatin made from hog skin. Gelatin, like glue, is made from hides, horns, connective tissue, and cartilage of various animals. It is used in cooking, capsules, bouillon tablets, and in the industries. Isinglass is discussed by Coca *et al.* Duke told of a man so sensitive to pork that his allergic symptoms persisted because of the use of lard in his biscuits. Abt (1918) reported the record of a boy with the specific inheritance of pork allergy from his father who had always disliked it. A woman developed herpes on her lips and face from pork in any form, such as pigs' feet or even mince meat. The mixed ingredients of sausages, bologna, and similar smoked and pickled meat products must be remembered. Flours, cereals, spreads, vegetables, all kinds of meat, even horse meat, are incorporated. Lesions from horse meat are encountered in Europe, as recorded by Urbach (1932). Mitra (1926) recorded allergy to various meats in India. Beef seems to produce more allergy than lamb. This may be due to the possibility that certain milk-sensitive patients may also be sensitized to beef. Eyermann (1927) described sensitization to beef, and a patient of ours has a flushed feeling followed by coryza during the eating of this meat. One doctor gets eczema on the hands when mutton or lamb are eaten. Another patient has increasing asthma, and one has urticaria when beef is taken day after day. Duke (1921) reported alimentary distress, and Blackfan (1916) noted eczema from beef ingestion. Duke (1921) reported three patients sensitized to beef, milk, and one or two other foods. Ratner (1928) described eczema in a child eighteen months of age from beef and milk. He also reported the case of a boy who was sensitized to meats. The asthma did not clear satisfactorily, and eczema persisted on the face because of the touching of his face by his father's mustache. His father's occupation was that of a butcher, which explained the reaction. Another case of nasal blocking from beef was described by Eyermann (1927). One of our patients as well as her mother had recurrent back pain from beef, which produced insomnia and a purple band across her nose and face. These symptoms even resulted from beef broth. Wells has shown that the globulin of beef is identical with that of milk, which suggests that certain patients who are sensitive to one food may also be sensitive to the other. Lamb sensitization is infrequent, though occasional reactions occur which are accompanied by clinical symptoms. Southworth, in discussing a paper by Talbot (1917), reported such allergy. One physician has nausea, cramping, dizziness, diarrhea, prolonged vomiting, and joint pains, especially in the big toe, from any kind of liver. The fact that horse serum allergy may arise from eating horse meat or inhaling its dander must be realized. Horse meat is eaten even in America, at times unwittingly. Mitra (1926) reported asthma from ingested goat meat and again from venison.

Goldman *et al.* (1963) have shown that twenty-one out of eighty-five milk allergy children react by skin test to Bovine Serum Albumin (BSA). They have also shown that twenty-three out of forty-four milk allergy children react to pure BSA taken orally. BSA is a normal constituent of beef. Thus it can be expected that about one-fourth to one-half of milk allergy patients may also be allergic to beef.

Chicken sensitization occurs at times. It is probable that unlaid eggs are frequently broken in the cleaning of hens. The eating of such hen meat which has traces of egg on it may be responsible for some symptoms. An interesting reaction was also described by Duke (1923) in a patient who could not eat ordinary chicken but could eat capon. It must also be remembered that chicken is usually allowed to stand in an egg and flour mixture before frying and that wheat flour is usually sprinkled over roasting chicken to produce a proper brown. Patients sensitized to wheat or eggs or other foods used in gravies or stuffing cooked with meats or fowl may have symptoms which are due to such added foods and not to the meats or fowl themselves. Thus a child sensitive to wheat had severe vomiting and collapse after eating the breast of a chicken which had been stuffed with bread. Another patient invariably had an acute attack of asthma within one-half hour after eating chicken. Chicken as well as rice allergy produced severe abdominal pain and distress in a lady who could eat every other food. Group sensitizations to the meats of all fowl probably exist as they do to all eggs as noted on page 550. Other sensitizations to tame or wild fowl must be suspected, especially if they have ever been eaten in excess.

In general, it is probable that sensitization exists to nearly all meats and all fowl in rare patients in a similar way that they do to fruits as a whole. This must be appreciated in the control of an occasional individual. Such a problem demands supplemental minimal diets (Chapt. 3) or elimination of all mammalian meats.

ALLERGY TO DUCTLESS GLAND PRODUCTS

In consideration of allergy from meats, mention must be made of the allergic reactions which may arise from the meat allergens contained in various glandular products which are so important in our present-day therapy. It will be evident from the following case records that the source of the glandular products, whether from beef, lamb, or pork, should be plainly printed on each product.

Case 223: A woman physician was given thyroid in doses of one grain daily for reduction purposes. After taking this small dose for two days, she broke out with a generalized erythematous itching rash which she immediately diagnosed as her previously recognized "pork rash," which had recurred since childhood whenever any product of pork, even lard, had been taken in the smallest amount. An attempt to obtain thyroid from beef was not successful on the first trial, since the taking of new tablets, supposedly from beef, was again followed by her "pork rash." It was found later that a mistake had been made. Finally, beef thyroid was obtained, and no cutaneous reactions resulted from its use.

We have used powdered pancreatin and trypsin by mouth in many cases and have obtained gastrointestinal reactions and migraine in a few patients who were sensitized to pork. One patient had a marked swelling of her body and especially on her face when she took pancreatin as well as pork. The sources of such digestant should be kept in mind in dealing with patients who may be sensitive to meats.

There is an interesting example of allergy to liver which was prescribed because of anemia to a patient who had definite food allergies.

Case 224: The woman forty years of age suddenly developed severe asthma and determined it was due to the liver which was being taken by mouth. It has since been found that she cannot take dried or fresh beef or lamb liver but that she can eat chicken liver. Apparently, however, she can tolerate the meat of beef and lamb without any allergic disturbances. Matzger reported a similar case of allergy to liver. Grun also discussed allergy to liver products and reported desensitization. The use of horse liver extracts might be possible in some patients sensitive to beef or hog liver. Heed and Goldbloom (1931) also recorded allergiclike symptoms to liver extract, which they attributed to uric acid. Allergy to liver and not to muscle may exist, as indicated by Allan and Scherer's finding of sensitization to beef pancreas and not to the muscle.

HORMONAL ALLERGY

Insulin allergy frequently arises during the first two or three weeks of therapy as itching, erythematous reactions around the site of injection or in diffuse erythematous or urticarial lesions. Tuft (1928) noted such evidences of allergy, and Collens, Lerner, and Fialka (1934) found such lesions present in 7.3 percent of 408 insulin-treated patients. Such cutaneous sensitization gradually disappears with the continued injections in varying periods of time. Local desensitization may be present. If the disappearance of such allergy is slow, desensitization with small and increasing doses as noted below may be advisable. Williams (1930) first reported a severe allergic manifestation, which fortunately is very rare. A boy twelve years of age developed vomiting, pyloric, and colonic spasms which prevented retention of rectal fluids and resulted in marked dehydration and acidosis. A leukocytosis of twenty thousand suggested surgical exploration, which was not deemed advisable. Finally, symptoms were relieved in forty-eight hours by the substitution of beef for the pork insulin. He (1932) reported a second case in a woman fifty-two years of age, who after six years of insulin therapy developed cramps and four to five stools a day with edema of the eyelids continuing for nine months. Roentgen rays showed marked hyperperistalsis and rapid emptying of the entire gastrointestinal tract. Substitution of beef for pork insulin gave relief. An intradermal test with the pork insulin was positive and reproduced the symptoms. Bayer (1934) reported severe allergy which arose on the reinjection of insulin after its discontinuance for two or three months. Five units were then injected, and in twenty minutes abdominal cramps, a macular itching generalized rash, diarrhea, choking, and spontaneous recovery occurred. Skin tests to all insulins were positive. Desensitization beginning with 1:1000 unit which just failed to react cutaneously with increasing doses every half hour was successful, so that in eight to ten hours five units were tolerated.

Davidson (1932) observed urticaria in one patient to all brands of insulin. He (1934) found that the purest insulin shows definite allergenic qualities, and he concluded that the active principle is protein in nature or bound to a haptenlike protein. Rudy (1931) and Karr, Scull and Petty (1933) described insulin resistance associated with urticaria thereto. Grishaw (1931) and Fielding-Reid (1932) reported cutaneous allergy to one brand of insulin and not to another. Cade, Barral, and Roux (1931) relieved cutaneous manifestations by a change in insulin or by desensitization with the causative type. Grieff (1931) found allergy to the insulin molecule. Allan and Scherer (1932) reported additional cases of insulin allergy.

We have observed extreme sensitization to pituitary extract associated with collapse and gastrointestinal allergy in one patient. Another patient developed generalized urticaria when pituitary extract was injected after a period of abstinence from its use for eight months. A man developed severe asthma and collapse after the eighth injection of a pituitarylike hormone. Thus allergy may arise to the protein of the animal from which glandular products are obtained or to the actual hormone recovered from such glands. Such allergy to these and probably other hormones may counteract their action or modify it in usual ways which will need study in the future. Sulzberger suggested that a new field of the immunology of hormones is opening for research.

It is also interesting that manufacturers use hog thyroids almost entirely because of the greater uniformity of their iodine content as compared with the thyroids of beef or sheep. Trypsin and pancreatin must be obtained from the pancreas of the hog, since the pancreatic glands of the herbivorous animals, such as the cow or sheep, contain very little trypsin.

ALLERGY TO FISH

Sensitization to fish and especially to shellfish are more common than to meats and are quite generally recognized by the laity because of their frequent violence, especially to crab, shrimp, and lobster. Mussels are prone to produce allergic symptoms in addition to the serious poisonous characteristics of them in certain regions. As with all food groups definite specificities to individual fish are frequent, though a tendency to a generalized allergy to all members at times occurs. One of our patients has asthma from the ingestion of any fish and cannot stand the smell of any type of fish as it cooks, though he gives a positive reaction only to crab. Strickler and Goldberg (1916) described eczema arising from ingested crab, and we found crab productive of symptoms leading to operation for assumed intestinal obstruction. Conlin (1919) found conjunctivitis from ingested flounder. Feinberg reported asthma from the odor of fish and from the odor of shrimp in another patient. Spain (1933) reported one man who had asthma if he passed a fish market. Such sensitization was reported by Rackemann (1918). A man fifty-five years of age in our practice suddenly developed an allergy to crab and shrimp evidenced by immediate smarting of the tongue and vomiting. A woman and her daughter have immediate soreness of the throat on eating crab. Another woman has vomiting twelve hours after eating any food that even touches shrimp. A man has pruritus three-quarters of an hour after eating crab. Another has severe generalized urticaria, facial edema, and bronchial asthma after oysters. A physician develops itching red dermatitis in an area six inches in diameter on the right thigh and in an area three inches in diameter on the left breast two days after eating trout. A young man twenty-four years of age had immediate swelling of his lips and tongue, generalized urticaria, and in ten or fifteen minutes sneezing and asthma from any shellfish or fish. The mother also had gastrointestinal upsets, nausea, vomiting, and diarrhea from eating fish. A confrere has twitching and blinking of the eyes from fish and mucous colitis from eggs. This man is a conservative accurate observer. Acute abdominal pain is not infrequent in patients allergic to shellfish. In one such patient an exploratory operation was performed for possible intestinal obstruction. Similar attacks have since occurred after the eating of crab. This possibility was considered when fish as a whole was excluded from our original "elimination diets." Highman (1920) described a definite specific allergy only to salmon which caused urticaria in a boy nine years of age. Another markedly specific fish allergy producing epigastric pain, nausea, and vomiting was found by Duke (1921) to be due to shad roe. Of great interest was the observation of Prausnitz and Kustner (1921) in their

classic article on passive transfer that boiled fish and not uncooked fish produced marked allergic disturbances. Sachs (1916) has reported four cases of purpura from anchovies. The odor of fish produced swelling of the eyelids and even of the entire body as noted by Kammerer (1934), Lewis and Grant (1924), and Boss (1930). This food had been eaten excessively some years before. Vallery-Radot (1930) recorded violent hives from one shrimp in a man who could eat large amounts of lobster.

Le Page's glue, which is made from fish,[*] produces severe sensitization, as has been described by Cooke in a fatal case resulting from intradermal testing (1922), by Duke (1924), and by Eyermann (1927). Duke's patient, after licking a postage stamp, had swelling of the tongue, lips, generalized erythema, itching, urticaria and angioneurotic edema of the skin, and collapse, which lasted one hour. Such a reaction occurred after putting on shoes in which inner soles were glued. The scratch test with glue produced such a general reaction that his life was in danger. Rackemann (1926) described a case of a young surgeon with asthma from fish who had swelling of his tongue and mouth even if he licked a postage stamp. Andrews and McNitt (1931) in an article on glue sensitivity reported a girl eighteen years of age who had had swelling of lips, tongue, throat, coryza, and mild asthma in five minutes after eating codfish cakes. Licking labels and postage stamps except those of the United States did the same. Asthmatic attacks arose if she remained in a drafting room for fifteen minutes. Skin reactions as large as the hand occurred in the scratch test with fish glue. Moderate benefit was received from hypodermic therapy. One of our patients with allergic dermatitis who gave tremen-

[*]Sensitive patients usually give large reactions to glue and fin fish.

dous reactions in the scratch test with glue and reactions to many pollens and animal emanations and foods was desensitized with glue and other inhalant substances. Initial therapy with a dilution of 1: 500,000,000 was necessary. Dr. Langhorst reported a patient so sensitive to glue that she could detect it in a room. Cooke reported such allergy to glue in which asthma and nasal symptoms occurred in forty-five minutes when its odor was inhaled by the patient in a small room. A tremendous scratch reaction to fish was obtained. Fish when eaten gave burning and itching of the mucous membranes of the nose, throat, and digestive tract; severe itching of the genitalia; asthma; flushing of the face and trunk; abdominal pain, nausea; vomiting; and diffuse large purple hives. Such acute symptoms lasted two days and were followed by great exhaustion for two more days.

Some of the most severe and acute cutaneous, gastrointestinal, and (less frequently) bronchial allergies result from shellfish, as described in the monograph by Laroche, Richet, and Saint Girons (1919). Hazen (1914) described sensitization to oysters. Such shellfish reactions are so frequent that they have not been described to any extent in the literature. An interesting local reaction called crabhand in fishermen was mentioned by Hirschberg similar to the localized dermatitis which arises after the handling of other foods, such as vegetables or fruits. J. A. Clarke (1927) studied a patient who had severe vomiting and diarrhea three hours after eating clams on three different occasions. Skin reactions were negative. A similar reaction on the hands to trout was described by us (1927). This sensitization was transmitted through three generations, and it was so specific that it supports the theory of occasional

tendency to specific food inheritance which probably occurs. Fordyce, in discussing Highman's paper (1920), reported sensitization to shellfish which resulted in generalized urticaria even when the patient used a form which had merely touched fish. Another asthmatic was sensitive to fish and eggs, and two others were sensitized to fish. Stoesser (1932) reported asthma from cod fish.

These patients who give positive reactions to a specific fish should probably have all fish excluded from their diets until the symptoms are well controlled, after which those fish giving negative or questionable reactions can be tried. If the "elimination diets" are used without skin reactions for diagnosis, when relief is obtained, fish such as sole, white fish, or salmon may be tried after a few weeks. Fish sensitization is usually acquired after childhood, as it is gradually included in the regular diet. Its intermittent ingestion and its excessive intake by certain patients may explain the origin of some of the sensitizations. Rolleston (1927) described the sudden acquisition of an allergy to oysters in a physician fifty years of age. It is important to mention the occurrence of sensitization in children or adults to codfish. In such cases if vitamin D is needed viosterol can be prescribed in place of the cod-liver oil. Balyeat and Bowen reported several instances of cod-liver oil sensitization, though Walzer and Bowman (1931) found no fish-sensitive patient who could not take cod-liver oil. Freeman (1933) reported desensitization to fish allergens by the rapid hypodermic method.

Studies on allergy to various fishes by Kjell Aas, in 1968, describing immunological methods for study of allergens is important to record.

ALLERGY TO NUTS

Nuts are productive of rather marked and often sudden allergic reactions in patients. They are included in cereal drinks, pastes, candies, and incorporated in many foods. They are ground into meals, flours, and made into milks. Almond oil is used in cosmetics. Wyman (1872) reported a woman who had prickling of the mouth, throat, ears, and eyes with lacrimation, nasal congestion, and watery discharge five minutes after eating chestnuts. Five minutes later a violent cough, slight expectoration, sneezing, obstruction of the throat, and difficult swallowing occurred. Abdominal colic was also present. Similar though milder attacks arose from hazel nuts, filberts, and walnuts. Almonds and hickory nuts produced no trouble. The first clinical report by Smith (1909) of positive skin reactions to buckwheat concerned a patient who also had mild asthmatic symptoms caused by all nuts except almonds and Brazil nuts. Talbot (1917) described nut sensitization of such severity in a child that his mere biting into a cake containing a few walnuts produced so severe a reaction that death was imminent for several hours. In discussing Schloss' paper "Allergy to Common Foods," Talbot (1917) emphasized skin reactions to nuts, especially to walnuts. Stuart (1923) reported the occurrence of positive reactions to several nuts. These also gave positive reactions in one parent. The child had been fed cocoa but no other nuts during its life. This was suggested as the cause of the group reaction to nuts. The following reactions occurred in one of our patients, age two. She had never been given nuts before the time that the mother discovered the presence of severe clinical reactions to them. The child always spat them out most vigorously, indicating an oral reaction, and it is interesting that the mother was also sensitive to all types of nuts. The child's cutaneous reactions to foods were as follows:

Rice	+	Clam	+
Rye	+	Sole	++
Wheat globulin	+	Almond	+
Whole egg	++++	Brazil	+
Egg white	++++	Chestnut	+
Egg yolk	++	Cocoanut	+
Egg mucoid	+++	Hazel nut	+
Cantaloupe	+	Hickory nut	++++
Beef	+	Peanut	++++
Veal	+	Pecan	++++
Beet	+	Walnut, English	++++
Cauliflower	+	Walnut, black	++
Soybean	+	Pine nut	++
Turnip	++	Pistachio	++

Stuart and Farnham (1926) stated that "fish and nut sensitizations tend to persist" late into life. De Besche (1923) reported the record of a woman forty years old, who for four years had had paroxysmal attacks of asthma associated with swelling of the eyes from apples, pears, and nuts. Brown (1927) recorded a sensitization to cocoanut and coffee. Rackemann (1928) described the case of a boy sixteen years of age who had asthma from eggs and nuts. Urticaria from eggs, peanuts, and walnuts was reported in a child 4½ years old by Blackfan (1920). Ratner (1928) reported a case of asthma from nuts in a child, age five. The mother had eaten large amounts of nuts during pregnancy and had thus sensitized the fetus. Other instances of sensitizations to nuts are recorded in the literature, especially by Cooke, Duke, Balyeat, Alexander, and Eyermann. Vaughan (1933) reported cramping and indigestion from black and not from English walnuts. Pistachio nuts and flavor are used in ice creams, candies, and in some cosmetics.

That peanuts are not nuts has been previously stated. Peanut oil is used in soaps, salad oil, and in canned foods requiring oil. Many marked clinical allergies to peanuts exist. Eyermann told of a patient who gained seven pounds overnight from one peanut. Vaughan emphasized the fact that almonds, cherries, apricots, plums, and peaches are all related, belonging to Drupacae. Botanically he also showed the other relations of the various nuts, as already summarized. Almond produces asthma in a child and is an ingredient of cosmetics which may produce dermatitis. As an allergen almond was reported by Schloss (1912) and Eyermann (1928).

Some clinical notes in our own experience are of interest. A man had soreness on the sides of the tongue and urticaria from walnuts. A woman forty years of age had severe itching of the mouth from almonds. Walnuts caused soreness of the gums, cheeks, and tongue in a young girl. A child had a marked asthmatic reaction from walnuts, which she violently disliked. Almonds and peanuts were well tolerated. Canker sores from walnuts occurred in the mouth of a woman. A doctor had generalized urticaria and canker sores from the hulls of almonds or walnuts. One patient had swelling of the tongue, lips, and throat from walnuts and Brazil nuts. Nausea and asthma immediately arose and lasted one-half hour. Another patient had gastric distress and tachycardia from walnuts. A girl had marked spasm in the rectum many hours after eating walnuts. A physician had wheezing from walnut ingestion. Hulled nuts were well tolerated. During youth he had much urticarial swelling in his hands. This reaction was so severe when nuts were first taken at the age of four that he became unconscious. A physician in Spokane had migraine from walnuts and another from peanuts. A child gave reactions to almonds and peanuts, both of which definitely disagreed with the mother. Another boy had itching of his mouth only from pine nuts. Puckering and burning of the mouth from nuts occurred in a woman forty-five years of age.

Cocoanut occasionally produces allergic manifestations. Its uses in candies, on cakes and pastries, and the use of the oil in margarines, lard, soaps, ointments, shampoos, and cosmetics must be kept in mind.

ALLERGY TO COTTONSEED

Cottonseed sensitization may be very severe and exclusion of its products from the diet is often necessary, especially when skin reactivity with the intradermal method is present. One patient who gave a four plus reaction to cottonseed could not take the oil or any shortening made from the seeds and nearly choked to death when she chewed a cotton seed before she was aware of her sensitization. Another boy had asthma if cottonseed oil even in minute amounts was surreptitiously included in his diet. Cottonseed oil is used extensively in cooking and in manufactured substitutes for lard such as Crisco and Snowdrift. Wesson oil and Primrose oil are cottonseed products and many imported olive oils are adulterated with cottonseed or other oils such as peanut, sesame, or sunflower seed oil. Cottonseed oil also is incorporated at times in frostings, candies, cookies, and used in nut pastes and in blanching nuts. It is also used in soaps, salves, cosmetics, and emulsions at times. A flour made of the seed, called Allison's flour, is prescribed for diabetics. It is important to remember that severe clinical allergy occurs to cottonseed oil without skin reactions to cottonseed, as stated in the following discussion.

COTTONSEED OIL

That a nonskin-reacting allergen in cottonseed oil can produce various manifestations of allergy was reported by Randolph and Sisk in 1950, confirming the occurrence of such allergy without skin reactions in our patient, whose history is summarized below.

Since the allergenic allergen in cottonseed is not necessarily present in its oil, Bernton, Spies, and Steven's opinion, in 1940, is justified that it is not always necessary to eliminate cottonseed oil and its products, as such or in prepared foods, because of large scratch reactions to the water-soluble protein in the cottonseed. Loveless and Mitchell made similar comments.

That clinical allergy often results to small amounts of cottonseed oil as such or in shortenings and margarine with or without scratch reactions to the protein allergen in the seed has been confirmed in our patient for thirty years, as evidenced in the following case summary:

Case 225: A woman forty-seven years of age was first seen in May of 1938. She had developed nasobronchial symptoms without fever in November of 1934 with increasing bronchial asthma in February, necessitating treatment at the Walter Reed Hospital for four months. Moderate asthma continued especially in the fall and winter.

Our study revealed no previous illnesses. Skin testing gave no reactions to inhalant and food allergens including cottonseed. Laboratory and x-ray examinations were negative.

The perennial history indicated recurrently activated food allergy confirmed by good relief with our CFE diet in two weeks. Corticoids were not available in 1938. Individual food tests with wheat, corn, rice, eggs, chocolate, and cottonseed oil and shortening reactivated the asthma.

Allergy to cottonseed oil in three months was confirmed as follows: A spoonful of the oil was included in her meals made from her relieving elimination diet for one day. Nausea and headache developed in the evening and coughing and wheezing in the early morning around 4 A.M.

In the last twenty years asthma has been absent except when formerly determined allergenic foods including traces of cottonseed oil or shortening have been eaten with or without the patient's realization.

Clinical allergy to cottonseed in patients with negative scratch reactions to its protein also has been reported, especially by Randolph, being exemplified in the following case records:

Case 226: A man thirty-eight years of age had had perennial nasal allergy and especially fatigue for twelve years associated with sore and painful joints, insomnia, and epigastric distress, especially in the last six years.

Diet history revealed increased digestive distress from peaches, oranges, coffee, chocolate, and especially from lemon and tea.

Individual feeding tests according to Rinkel's technique with corn increased fatigue and epigastric distress and with potatoes, chilliness, sneezing, and rhinorrhea developed. Since satisfactory relief with the elimination of these foods persisted, suspicion of allergy to cottonseed oil indicated a feeding of 15 cc of the oil, which resulted in prompt headache, indigestion, and definite reduction in leukocytes in one hour. With the total elimination of suspected foods and of cottonseed oil, to which a scratch reaction was negative, excellent relief gradually occurred. As in our patient (Case 225), scratch reactions to soluble cottonseed allergen were negative. Reactivation of symptoms occurred with a small amount of shortening containing cottonseed oil even though other allergenic foods continued to be entirely eliminated from the menus.

Case 227: A woman fifty-four years of age had had constant headaches, dizziness, myalgia in the posterior cervical muscles and upper back, weakness and eczema of the hands. Elimination of foods to which allergy was indicated by individual feeding tests did not give desired complete relief until cottonseed oil was entirely excluded from her ingested foods. Symptoms were activated by a feeding test with 15 cc of cottonseed oil. Allergy was also indicated by a reduction of leukocytes in forty minutes.

As in the preceding case reported by Randolph, scratch tests with the soluble cottonseed allergen were negative.

Comment: Our study of allergy to cottonseed oil has always been routine with its exclusion in our elimination diets during the last forty years. Though this exclusion has always been indicated by a large reaction to the water-soluble protein in the seed, exclusion is justified by the occurrence of clinical allergy to an allergen in the oil, even though skin reactions to cottonseed are negative. to cottonseed

This is emphasized by Randolph and by our reported case.

As emphasized by Randolph, clinical allergy to cottonseed oil justifies its elimination from our CFE diet or its modification we have long advised for the immediate study of probable food sensitization. To expedite this decision about possible allergy to cottonseed oil, Rinkel's individual food test modified by Randolph may be advisable. This test, as already stated on page 31, usually yields information more rapidly than from a provocation test with the oil to determine allergy to additional foods after relief of clinical food allergy is obtained from our standardized CFE diet. Individual food tests as advised by Rinkel, rather than provocation feeding tests, are not necessary to determine specific allergies to individual foods as evidenced by our determination of allergy to cottonseed oil with feeding tests as we have advised since 1928 in our patient, as summarized on page 582. The recognition of specific food allergies, especially to sugars and oils, with the technique advised by Rinkel and Randolph, however, will probably be used more frequently than in the past.

ALLERGY TO BEVERAGES

1. Chocolate sensitization is common. It is discussed under beverages, though it is used extensively in other ways in the diet. It is productive of marked as well as acute reactions in certain patients. Sneezing from chocolate was reported by Gould and Pyle (1900). Chocolate sensitization was mentioned by Brown (1920, 1925) and by Van Leeuwen (1925). Hazen (1928) reported dermatitis from chocolate. Spain (1925) described a severe case of perennial hay fever in a woman thirty-five years of age from chocolate, to which skin reactions were persistently negative. Eyermann gave it fourth place on his table of foods productive of nasal allergy.

Deamer *et al.* recently have emphasized chocolate as we have long realized by always keeping it out of the initial elimination diets.

In our own cases marked sensitization to chocolate occurred in twenty-three patients in one series of five hundred, but positive reactions have been present in very few. These negative reactions do not rule out possible food allergy, justifying exclusion of chocolate as well as coffee from all elimination diets. Some of the clinical effects of chocolate which we have observed follow. In one woman it caused marked flushing of the face and neck and also nervousness. Another patient had nasal congestion and sneezing upon smelling chocolate in food. One of our patients had asthma from chocolate for years. One man sneezed if he tasted it. A boy had corneal ulcers from it. Two women became very dizzy and nauseated from it. A man had an itching rash on his face and shoulders from chocolate. Severe migraine occurred from it in a woman fifty-five years of age who could not bear even the smell of this food. A man with migraine from many foods had frequent urination resulting from chocolate. Another man had severe lumbar pain after the ingestion of it.

The presence of cocoa allergen in cocoa butter and in salves, creams, soaps, cosmetics, and suppositories must be remembered. Chocolate in small amounts enters many foods and drinks, and liquid and pill medicines.

2. Tea sensitization along with that from eggs was described by Hutchinson in his interesting book *Idiosyncrasies*, in 1895. Such allergy came to our notice in a few patients, notably in one who had a peculiar irritation and a mild cramping and throbbing distress in the perineum together with a burning at the end of his penis whenever he drank tea. A young girl had an immedi-

ate hot surging sensation in her head and aching of the eyes when she took tea. It produced abdominal cramping in a father and daughter and a sour stomach, abdominal pain, and constipation in another man.

3. Coffee is also a cause of allergic reactions. In our experience several skin reactions have been obtained, though marked clinical reactions are a little hard to differentiate from those resulting from the stimulating effect of the caffeine. In one patient an inevitable diarrhea has always resulted from drinking a cup of coffee. No other ascertainable cause, after careful diagnostic studies, has been discovered. Two patients had severe migraine from, among other foods, coffee. Coffee sensitization of the inhalant type producing perennial hay fever established itself in a man who had been in the coffee roasting business for three years. Ingestion of coffee also produced nasal symptoms, possibly through the allergen-laden aroma. Rosenbloom (1920) and Rackemann (1931) reported asthma from coffee inhalation. Gutmann's (1933) suggestion that various allergic manifestations arising from coffee are due in part to the stimulating effect of the caffeine and other substances such as aldehyde, furfural, acetone, pyridine, and ammonia is not especially apparent. Various adulterants of coffee include chicory, carrots, parsnip, turnip, dandelion, various seeds, acorns, figs, sugar, and molasses. Postum and similar coffee substitutes are made of roasted cereals and dried fruits. A fair substitute for coffee can be made by roasting soybeans in the oven.

4. *Miscellaneous beverages.* Gutmann (1933) discussed allergic reactions to various beverages. He noted the common conclusion that alcohol exacerbates allergic symptoms but probably does not cause allergy itself. Allergy to yeast and hops in beer may be responsible for urticaria, gastric symptoms, diarrhea, colic, asthma, migraine, or coryza arising in certain patients. One beer will agree at times when another does not because of the kind of grain or yeast used. The grapes, grain, or other ingredients used in making wines, whiskey, or other liquors must be kept in mind. Their methods of manufacture must be investigated in susceptible patients. One patient sneezes only when sherry is taken. An Italian has itching dermatitis with new red wine. One physician has allergic coryza for twenty-four hours after drinking wine. His father had identical allergy, more violent, and associated with sneezing.

Likewise, sensitizations to soft drinks necessitates a knowledge of their ingredients. Walzer and Bowman stated that Coca Cola contains caffeine, caramel, essential oils, lime juice, phosphoric acid, and extracts of cocoa leaves or Kola nuts. We have found immunochemical evidence for the presence of chocolate in Coca Cola. Ginger ale contains ginger, lemon juice, and at times capsicum. Root beer contains caramel sugar, various essential oils, sarsaparilla, caramel, cologne, spirits, oils of anise, organe, sassafras, wintergreen, sugar, and water. Further discussion of alcoholic and soft beverages will be found in the book of Coca *et al.* (1931).

ALLERGY TO SPICES AND CONDIMENTS

Possible allergy to spices, condiments, and flavors accounts for their omission from all of our elimination diets. After relief of symptoms is assured for one to two months, those to which marked allergy is assured by history with or without scratch reactions are kept out of the diet, and tolerance to individual desired ones can be determined by provocation tests. Important discussion of these foods and their botanical relationships are on pages 533 to 541.

Sensitization to pepper as revealed by the skin test is quite common. In fact, some of our largest cutaneous reactions have been obtained to black pepper. A patient gave a history of a group sensitization to all types of pepper. This makes it most difficult for her to eat away from home, as the slightest bit produces violent nausea, vomiting, abdominal pain, and collapse. Meyers (1924) reported asthma from pepper sprinkled in a drawer to keep mice away. Paprika and green, red, or black pepper all act alike. Buckwheat sensitization must be remembered in relation to that from pepper, since it is used to adulterate pepper by some concerns.

Mustard sensitization of a marked nature has been studied, especially in three patients. Large cutaneous reactions occurred in all, and any food containing the slightest bit of this seasoning caused acute symptoms. Many patients give large scratch reactions to mustard and have marked gastrointestinal or nasobronchial symptoms from the ingestion of the merest trace. J. A. Clarke (1927) reported edema of the tongue and vomiting for twelve hours or more after eating a trace of mustard. One lad was markedly sensitive to both celery and mustard, both of which caused itching and swelling of the lips but no gastric symptoms if swallowed. It is possible, as is the case with flaxseed, that sensitization may be established at times by applying mustard plasters to the skin.

Vinegar, as recorded by Laroche, Richet, and Saint Girons and as noted in a case of our own, can cause acute gastrointestinal symptoms even in drop doses. The origin of the vinegar must be determined. Apple-sensitive patients should not be given cider vinegar but should use so-called white vinegar which is made from acetic acid. Vinegar douches cause allergic symptoms

in other tissues in sensitive patients (see Chapt. 21).

Various spices may produce allergic reactions. Skin reactions occur from them in some patients as noted in Chapter 2. A physician had asthma from cinnamon for eight years. Those sensitive to *Artemesia* pollens at times cannot tolerate sage seasoning. A child had asthma from sage in dressing. Efron reported asthma, nausea, and cramping from nutmeg. In the "elimination diets" no spices are permitted and are not added until their effects can be carefully determined after the symptoms have been under good control for some weeks.

An interesting case of severe sudden back pain resulting from as little as one drop of Worcestershire sauce was recorded in our former book (1931). The exact ingredient of this sauce to which sensitization existed was never determined.

The dill herb, which is used to make dill pickles, produced a marked nasal allergy in a patient. All other pickles were eaten without sneezing.

Allergic reactions occur to flavors such as peppermint, which caused sneezing in a young girl when taken in any form. In another case marked bladder burning resulted from the taking of any peppermint. Sincke (1934) found vanilla a cause of dermatitis. Peshkin (1924) noted hives from this flavor. Duke has reported the allergic reactions from various essential oils. A young woman developed a marked stinging of the mouth whenever she took cinnamon-flavored gum. Other instances of such sensitizations are to be found in the literature.

When the FFCFE diet is used, all flavors and condiments are excluded, requiring elimination of flavored toothpastes, gargles, mouthwashes, and medicines as advised in our discussion of this diet in Chapter 3.

ALLERGY TO SUGARS AND OILS

Honey allergy, which is frequent, must be remembered. Zenophon, reported by Rolleston, mentioned headache from honey. Hutchinson (1895) noted such idiosyncrasies. Duke described two cases of severe abdominal allergy from this food. One was in a man who at the age of twenty-seven ate an entire cake of honey. Since then the slightest bit of honey has always produced severe abdominal pain. Sticker (1912) recorded urticaria, vomiting, and diarrhea from only the linden blossom honey. Walker (1917) reported asthma from the ingestion only of clover honey, and Menagh (1928) studied a patient whose urticaria was due to honey. Thus sensitization to specific reactions to the pollen from which honey was obtained occurred and was indicated by a query[*] reporting two patients with nausea, vomiting, weakness, generalized numbness, impaired vision, shock, perspiration, and weak pulse. Specific allergy to the bee protein in the honey itself was suggested. Three patients with definite allergy to honey have come under our attention, and the other mild allergies resulting from it have been recorded in our histories. In one case severe migraine always occurred from the eating of honey. Another had severe abdominal, bronchial, and constitutional symptoms from its ingestion. Freeman (1920) reported unconsciousness from honey for seven minutes in a patient! Smith (1909) reported that his buckwheat-sensitive patient could not tolerate honey from bees that fed on buckwheat blossoms but could take other types of honey. The same may also be true of so-called sage honey in *Artemesia*-sensitive patients or for other types of honey from bees that have fed on special types of flowers. Duke reported

[*]*JAMA*, 101:728, 1933.

convulsions, coma, cyanosis and failure of pulse and respiration from ingestion of honey. Another report of edema in the small intestine, with nausea, vomiting, and pain from honey was of interest. Honey is incorporated in some graham crackers and other commercial foods.

Allergy to cane sugar, which belongs to the same subfamily of Gramineae and tribe as corn, has been reported by Duke. We have several patients who develop symptoms best explained by such allergy. It is possible that patients sensitive to cane sugar can tolerate beet sugar. Some patients suspect sugar as a possible cause of allergy. Later when allergenic foods are removed, sugar can be taken as desired. Moreover, ingredients of candy and other sweet foods often are causes. The use of gum arabic, Indian gum, acacia as binders, or in other ways in candies must be remembered. Allergy may arise to artificial dyes, flavors in foods, and to chicle in gum as noted on page 585.

With increasing evidence of clinical allergy to corn glucose in corn-sensitive patients, total elimination of corn sugar, which occurs in Karo syrup, canned fruits, candies, and beverages, is important when cereal grain allergy is being studied and controlled with our CFE diet. Of great importance, moreover, is the use of 5 percent invert sugar by vein instead of 5 percent glucose to relieve dehydration when our CFE diet is used to study and control intractable or severe bronchial asthma, as emphasized in Chapter 8 and also in our discussion of corn allergy on page 546, to which the reader is referred.

Allergy to barley malt syrup in patients sensitive to barley must be suspected, though we can offer no positive evidence for such allergic reactions. Ratner (1935) demonstrated sensitization to malt extracts of barley. Whether patients may be sensitized to the allergens in brown sugar or molasses is also a possibility which needs to be kept in mind.

ALLERGY TO BEET SUGAR

Though Duke first discussed possible allergy to beet sugar in 1925, it was Randolph and Rollins in 1950 who reaffirmed this cause as evidenced in their failure to relieve allergic symptoms by the elimination of allergenic foods demonstrated by individual food tests until allergy to beet sugar was so recognized and controlled. Their studies have demonstrated its occurrence especially when the use of beet sugar predominates over cane sugar as in many countries in Europe and in various areas of the United States. As with cane, allergy to beet sugar is a special challenge when multiple food allergies are not being controlled by our minimal elimination diets or those diets containing foods to which individual food tests, advised by Rinkel and Randolph, have failed to yield desired relief. Possible allergy to beet sugar should be suspected in patients allergic to ingested beets. Allergy to beet pollen or related *Betulaceae* pollens may also occur in patients allergic to beet sugar and justify immunological study.

Demonstrated allergy to monosodium glutamate, as reported by Randolph, must be suspected when clinical allergy to beet sugar exists, since such glutamate used for seasoning many foods is made more often from beets than from wheat, corn, or soy.

The following case record and summaries of two other cases emphasize the important recognition of clinical allergy to beet sugar.

Case 228: A woman forty-three years of age had perennial nasal allergy, much fatigue associated with confusion and poor memory, and at times aphasia and recurrent headaches in varying degrees for fifteen years. Backache and cramping in the legs had increased for fifteen years, being unimproved by spinal fusion. Pulling and pains across the upper back and bouts of torticollis, stiffness, and soreness in many muscles, especially on awakening, had continued.

Individual feeding tests performed by Doctor Randolph showed marked clinical allergy to wheat, corn, eggs and especially potatoes and less to rice, pork, and tomato. Because all of the desired relief failed from the elimination of these foods and because of the history of possible allergy to beets and botanically related spinach in childhood, feeding test with 25 gm of ingested beet sugar was made. In fifty minutes pressure in the frontal area, abdominal cramping and tightness in the muscles in the neck occurred.

Results from the elimination of allergenic foods: After beet sugar and other indicated allergenic foods were eliminated, former fatigue gradually disappeared, and more energy and alertness resulted. Headaches and other symptoms were correspondingly relieved. This enabled resumption of her medical research and more activity away from her home. Ingested beet sugar and other allergenic foods reactivated her symptoms thereafter. In addition, one teaspoonful of powdered monosodium glutamate made from beets caused frontal headaches in two hours and stiffness in the muscles, especially in the neck and shoulders, for two subsequent days. Glutamate from wheat gave no reaction.

Allergy to beet sugar and demonstrated allergy to other individual foods were relieved by elimination of the causative foods in two other cases. Careful perusal of these case reports is advised to the concerned physician.

Monosodium glutamate and glucose made from beets also activated allergic symptoms in these patients. The description of the symptoms resulting from the ingestion of beet sugar should be read, as stated above, by concerned physicians. The last patient demonstrated clinical allergies to both beet and cane sugar.

Production of allergic symptoms by small amounts of allergenic foods, as of cereal grains, cane, and beet sugar and monosodium glutamate and of other allergenic foods emphasizes the importance of accurate labelling of all flavors, condiments, and other ingredients in commercially prepared and distributed food products as emphasized on page 476.

ALLERGY TO CANE SUGAR

Clinical allergy to cane sugar (sucrose) ingested by mouth or given intravenously has received too little consideration, as emphasized by Randolph and Rollins since 1950. It was first noted by Duke in 1925 and later confirmed by Coca in 1943. It has been evidenced in the diet history and by clinical symptoms resulting from its ingestion in our practice for many years and is especially frequent in patients with multiple food allergies requiring our minimal elimination diet for relief. Allergy to corn sugar and less often to beet sugar may also occur, as reported on pages 587 to 588.

As Randolph states, it must be studied in patients with multiple food allergies by its complete elimination for two or three weeks along with the elimination of other allergenic foods. For possible expedition of information about allergy to beet sugar, the individual feeding tests advised by Rinkel and also by Randolph may be advisable.

The importance of considering possible allergy to cane sugar must be remembered when allergy to cereal grains with our CFE diet is receiving consideration. Allergy to corn sugar also requires consideration in such study, as discussed on page 587. The necessity of considering possible allergy to cane sugar is emphasized when it is remembered that sugar cane belongs to the Gramineae family and to the tribe Andropogoneae in the species *officinarum*, closely related to the species of corn. This is shown in our botanical classification of the Gramineae, which is brought to the attention of physicians on page 535. Neill *et al.*

have shown the presence of an antigen, presumably from microbiological infestation of the cane, in some batches of sugar with a Type II pneumococcal specificity.

Definite or slight allergy to allergens in cane sugar may explain some slight or definite uncontrolled allergic symptoms in spite of the CFE diet until cane sugar is also excluded from the menus. This possibility can be studied with the replacement of cane sugar by beet sugar, which is now being advised in the routine preparation of our CFE diet.

The importance of recognizing and controlling possible allergy to cane sugar is evidenced in the following case reports by Randolph and Rollins in 1950.

Case 229: A woman thirty-six years of age had had recurrent sick headaches all of her life associated with nervous tension and extreme fatigue. In addition, lacrimation, edema of the face, abdominal distention, diarrhea, pulling and tautness in the posterior cervical muscles, aches, and cramps in other muscles, along with nasal allergy had occurred. Nasal symptoms and fatigue had continued between the exaggerated attacks, resulting in chronic illness and inability to care for her six children.

"Conversion hysteria" had not been relieved by psychiatric treatment.

Diet history only suggested possible allergy to chocolate.

Study of food allergy with individual feeding tests indicated sensitization to wheat, corn, and to a lesser degree to lettuce, pork, and onions.

In spite of the temporary elimination of these foods, satisfactory relief did not occur until cane sugar allergy was considered. Then, an individual feeding test with cane sugar produced in twenty-five minutes belching, distention, marked dizziness, and scotomata followed by chilling and a generalized severe headache.

Later, slight amounts of cane sugar by mouth caused loginess, extreme fatigue, and abdominal distention all in five minutes.

Comment: Continued elimination of cane sugar and other incriminated foods determined by individual feeding tests relieved the headaches, indigestion, drowsiness, and fatigue, especially on arising, and also relieved her inability to do housework and care for her six children.

A second patient with mental confusion, apprehension, fatigue, muscular aching, and pruritus vulvae required elimination of cane sugar and other demonstrated food allergies before satisfactory relief occurred.

In this and also in a third patient, who was allergic to cane sugar as well as to other food allergens, the intravenous injection of 25 cc of 5 percent invert sugar derived from cane sugar in a pyrogen-free preparation produced in eight minutes dullness, somnolence, chilling, and other symptoms from clinical allergy. This necessitates consideration of allergy to cane sugar when invert sugar is given to patients on our CFE diet to prevent possible exaggeration of allergic symptoms from the intravenous injection of invert sugar as well as corn sugar (glucose).

ALLERGY TO DRUGS

Allergy to drugs and other medicaments has been discussed in this volume. In this place further notes on drug allergy, particularly on ingestants, are desirable. Allergy to ingested and to injected glandular products, especially to insulin, thyroid, and pituitary extracts was considered on page 577.

Hypersensitiveness to organic drugs as quinine, morphine, or senna arises to their specific allergens. Allergy to arsenic, mercury, aspirin, or other chemical medicaments must be explained by Landsteiner's crystalloid theory that the active substances combine with a body protein to which specific sensitization is established. In other chapters allergy to aspirin, quinine, ipecac, podophyllin, rhubarb, pokeroot, senna, belladonna, arsenic, nickel, bismuth, gold, iodides, mercury, opium derivatives, coal tar antipyretics, and cincophen has been discussed. Vallery-

Radot *et al.* (1930) reported urticaria as noted in the French literature and in his practice from quinine, antipyrine, aspirin, emetine, bismuth, and opium with its derivatives. Abrami and Joltrain reported dermatitis in a pharmacist four to five hours after going into a laboratory where emetine was present. After the ingestion of an infinitesimal dose severe edema, pruritus, cough, vomiting, and fever arose for two hours thereafter. Sterile abscesses after injections of certain drugs suggest the possibility of an Arthuslike phenomenon. Sensitizations to any other ingested medicament such as other alkaloids and digitalis are possible. Massive or prolonged administration is usually necessary, and a period of cessation of medication longer than two or three weeks or a gastrointestinal or possibly a severe illness often initiates the allergy. Cooke and Vander Veer noted occasional apparent inheritance toward the tendency to drug sensitizations.

Allergy at times exists to the medium in which medicines are dispensed. Thus allergy to allergens in corn or cottonseed oils in which viosterol is held may occur. One patient had asthma from the allergen in peanut oil in which bismuth was suspended. The ingredients of other vehicles for drugs such as acacia and various syrups are possible causes in sensitized individuals. There was a report* of sensitization to corn oil in which amniotin was contained.

Medications in tablet form frequently contain starch. This starch is usually in the ungelatinized, crystalline form which is least easily dissolved by enzymes and most easily phagocytized after persorption, leading to eventual allergy to starch.

Squire and Madison (1934) reported fifty-two cases of agranulocytosis or granu-

---

JAMA, 104:626, 1935.

locytopenia from amidopyrine. This and other reports have prevented its continued use. Skin sensitivity was shown by the patch test in two patients, which was accompanied by fever and a systemic reaction. To test possible allergy, a patch test and later the giving of one tablet of the drug with subsequent careful counting of the white cells were suggested. Sink suggested allergy as a cause in two cases in 1930. Other manifestations of allergy to amidopyrine have occurred. Schumacher (1910) encountered swelling of lips, erythematous papules on the skin, petechiae, and circumscribed concentric lesions in front of the ears from pyramidon idiosyncrasy. Kammerer (1934) described pruritus, urticaria, erythema, rhinitis, conjunctivitis, edema of the lips, joint pains, dyspnea, low temperature and even collapse, and at times mucous membrane hemorrhages, nasal and renal bleeding, and icterus after such drugs as antipyrin, pyramidon, salipyrin, and antifebrin. Benjamin and Biederman (1936) published an article on agranulocytosis arising from a drug related to amidopyrine.

Unger (1931) reported swelling of the eyelids, cheeks, and lips and blotches on the forehead and palms of hands. Kutz and Traugott (1925) described porphyrin formation from sulfonal. Ortolph (1931) discussed allergic manifestations from barbiturates. Sensitization to Allonal®, Sommacetin®, and other proprietary analgesics, sedatives, or soporifics may be due to the frequently contained amidopyrine or other coal tar products or to the various barbiturates such as phenobarbital or Amytal®. Hueber (1919) reported a papulomacular dermatitis later becoming morbilliform after Luminal had been taken in one-half grain doses for forty days.

Phenobarbitol as a cause of dermatitis was reported by Bothe (1924) and Men-

ninger (1928) and is generally recognized. Exfoliative dermatitis occurred in one of our patients. Cincophen allergy in a woman was noted by Stiefler (1919) after three doses. Edema of the eyes, lips, and vulva with burning, itching, and tension of the skin and a dark brown urine developed. Sokolowski (1931) reported an urticarial eruption in the left palm from atophan. Short and Bauer (1933) reported four cases of such allergy. Quick (1934) suggested that such allergy produced Arthuslike lesions in the liver and that similar lesions arose in the heart, lungs, kidneys, and other tissues and vascular structures of the body. Urticaria, anorexia, nausea, headache, toxemia, or fever indicate its immediate cessation and great caution in its future use. Its intermittent administration is unwise.

The many allergic symptoms and tissue changes arising from phenophthalein have long been reported, as summarized in our book in 1938 and in those especially on dermatology. Excruciating pains in the tibias, chills and fever, and urticaria were examples of such allergy reported by Alvarez in 1949.

Quinine as a cause of dermatitis, fever, gastrointestinal, and other symptoms must be remembered, as discussed in the literature and in our book on *Clinical Allergy* in 1938. Gastrointestinal symptoms from allergy to quinine are not uncommon. Vallery-Radot (1930) reported fever, coryza, and asthma from quinine. White (1927) reported dermatitis from quinine in a rectal suppository. Tzanck and Cottet (1934) encountered hemorrhagic nephritis from quinine allergy. Mienicki and Krzywoblocki (1934) described erythema of all the body, slight fever for six days, and edema of the eyelids and face after quinine ingestion. Exfoliation in five days and a return of the skin to normal in thirty-two days occurred. Dawson and Newman

(1931) reported coryzal reactions to quinine but not to quinidine or quitenine. Dawson (1932) published a useful bibliography on quinine and its alkaloids. Quinine as a cause of bladder, kidney, and joint pains was noted.

Allergy to opiate derivatives producing cutaneous and gastrointestinal symptoms has long been recognized. Winans (1930) described erythema, asthma, and cyanosis to Pantopon®. One of my patients had marked pruritus, congestion of the throat and larynx due to allergy to Pantopon and Dilaudid®. Morphine had always produced nausea and vomiting. Codeine gave no allergic disturbances. Tuft also reported Pantopon allergy. Scheer (1934) observed codeine allergy giving rise to a follicular eruption, rapidly coalescing into a scarlatiniform itching rash. The patch test was positive. Kyrle also reported an erythematous rash without pruritus from codeine.

Chloral may produce a dermatitis either as an ingestant or more frequently by skin application. Abramowitz (1933) reported erythematous reactions of scarlatiniform, urticarial or erythematovesicular, or petechial varieties from its ingestion. Kammerer commented on sneezing, watering of the eyes, asthma, pruritus, and later eczema, purpura, pemphigus and cachexia from allergy to chloral and paraldehyde. Dinitrophenol sensitization productive of skin eruptions and urticaria associated with positive skin reactions was reported by Matzger (1934) and Frumess (1934).

Catgut allergy from the sheep intestine from which most catgut is made was reported by Babcock (1935) and Tripp (1935). As a result scars may open up three to four days after surgery, margins separate, and serous discharge occur. Gratia and Gilson (1934) felt that such catgut allergy produced Arthuslike phenomena causing unsuspected postoperative complications. Sensitization to formalin in catgut sutures has come to our attention. This produced generalized dermatitis during convalescence after surgery. It suggests the probability of allergy to other antiseptic and preservative agents used for medicinal and surgical purposes.

Acacia (gum arabic) allergy was noted by Spielman and Baldwin (1933) as a cause of asthma. Acacia is a polysaccharide and is used in candy, lozenges, trochees, intravenously, and in enemas. Allergy to Karaya gum has been noted. Maytum and Magath (1932) observed nasal obstruction, lachrymation, and laryngeal stridor after the intravenous use of acacia, and we and also Gay observed asthma after its use in a barium enema.

Allergy to chlorine and probably to other mineral ingredients of drinking water has been noted. Possible bromine in baking powder used in bakery products may cause allergic symptoms in sensitive patients. One of our patients has diarrhea from any chlorinated water, and chlorine in minute traces in water burns her skin. This is comparable to the long-recognized allergies to arsenic and mercury which arise not only from their injection but also from oral administration.

Kammerer (1934) cited other instances of cutaneous allergy to drugs, such as digalen (which yielded an erythematous rash), thymol, orthoform, Yatren®, casein, metol, resorcin, and Solganal®. In addition to the disturbances from allergy to iodine, he also recorded gastrointestinal symptoms, hemiplegia, and albuminuria. Tremendous erythema, dermatitis, and shock arose from the local application of the slightest bit of iodine in one patient. Such severe constitutional reactivity to the application of iodine to a small skin area was observed in one of our patients. Harmstorf (1933) recorded a patient who had edema of the penis, scrotum, and surrounding skin from its local application. Klaber and Archer (1935) described dermatitis from an iodine locket. Clifford (1926) and Happel (1921) recorded marked dermatitis even of the bullous and pemphigoid type from iodine applied to the skin. Happel's case had only one drop in the ear canal, with a subsequent burning of the entire skin and swelling of the face and hands. Iodoform allergy was also noted by Bloch (1911) and Hartzell (1917).

These comments are only on a few cases in the medical literature of the last thirty years and in previous literature for fifty to seventy-five years which indicate the great diversity of manifestations and the many drugs which may give rise to allergy in man. This is true of most drugs and medicaments made now by the many pharmaceutical companies, as evidenced in the many reactions reported in varying degrees from their use in their directions and warnings of possible reactions in brochures and also in the medical literature.

Realizing these allergies, they must be studied by their entire elimination except for life-sustaining medicaments to consider the possibility of such allergies in the partial or entire causation of the patient's symptoms. It is to be remembered that possible allergy to all local or parenteral medications must be considered as causes of symptoms in patients.

SUMMARY

1. Frequency of allergy to various foods.
2. Limited value and fallibility of skin reactions. Determined by history, trial diet, and provocation feeding tests.
3. Botanical relationship of foods—its influence to clinical allergy.
4. Clinical allergy to foods as reported in the literature and evidenced in our patients.
5. Allergy to wheat and other cereals.
6. Allergy to flaxseed and buckwheat.
7. Allergy to eggs.
8. Allergy to milk—its major importance in infancy continuing during life.
9. Allergy to fruits.
10. Allergy to vegetables.
11. Allergy to meats and fowl.
12. Allergy to ductless gland products.
13. Hormal allergy. Allergens in liver, thyroid, pancreas, and especially to insulin and pituitary extract including ACTH.
14. Allergy to fish and shellfish and allergy to glue of fish origin.
15. Allergy to nuts including peanuts.
16. Allergy to cottonseed and its oil.
17. Allergy to chocolate.
18. Allergy to beverages including tea, coffee, beer, and wines.
19. Allergy to spices, condiments, and flavors, including vinegar.
20. Allergy to sugars, especially to cane, corn, and beet sugar.
21. Allergy to drugs including catgut, chlorine, and bromine.

Chapter 30

Appendix

This chapter contains a discussion of the cereal-free elimination diet with a general rationale for its use, which we distribute to patients to whom the diet has been prescribed. Also presented are reasons which make this diet superior to test-negative diets. While we do not use total fasting as a routine, factors that indicate the advisability of this technique in conjunction with ecological control are discussed.

Other information included are:

1. Diabetic diets.

2. Symptom Record to be distributed to patients.

3. List of allergens for initial scratch testing.

4. Suggested allergens for skin testing in infancy and childhood.

5. Five schedules for the administration of antigens.

6. Methodology employed in the preparation of allergenic extracts.

7. Environmental control.

8. Occupations, symptoms, and likely sensitizers.

9. The role of atopic allergy in the origin and resultant destructive changes in the lungs.

10. Allergy to tobacco in the causation of obstructive emphysema.

11. Aerosol therapy with adrenergic drugs.

12. Allergy to streptococci in multiple sclerosis (Rosenow).

13. Pertinent information found in previous publications of the author.

A DISCUSSION OF THE USE OF THE CEREAL-FREE ELIMINATION DIET (TO BE GIVEN TO THE PATIENT)

This elimination diet excludes all foods which commonly produce allergy. All the cereal grains, including rice, corn, rye, and especially wheat, are out of the diet. All eggs, milk, and all of their products including butter, cheese, cream, and any food containing the slightest trace of milk are excluded. Margarines are not allowed, since they contain milk or milk solids in larger amounts than does butter itself. Willow Run, made of hydrogenated soy oil, containing no milk, is a good butter substitute and is allowed in this diet. In addition, fish, pork as such, a number of vegetables (especially those of the cabbage family), and many fruits (including oranges, apples, bananas, berries, and melons), are excluded. Finally, the only oil allowed is soybean oil. Tea is allowed when we add it.

It is most important that you do not take one drop or trace of any food which is not included in this diet list. If there is any question about any food, look on the list. If it is not there, do not take it. Moreover, you should avoid the odor of any disallowed food. Thus foods not allowed on the diet should be in covered containers in the refrigerator, and eggs should not be fried nor should bakery products, hot cakes, or waffles made of wheat, milk, and eggs be fried or baked when you are in the kitchen or in a nearby room where you can inhale the odor of them.

You will note that chicken is allowed, but hens are not permitted. This is due to the fact that hens may have unlaid eggs in them which often are broken by the dressers. A little egg which gets on the carcass of the hen causes symptoms if eaten by a very sensitive individual.

Breakfast

Five or six ounces of grapefruit juice (fresh or canned) with sugar should be taken. If weight maintenance is important, include several teaspoonsful of sugar. Grapefruit itself can be taken if the amount eaten will yield five or six ounces of juice. This grapefruit contains vitamin C and provides all you need during the day. If grapefruit juice is excluded from your diet, then other suggested juices can be taken, but they do not contain as much vitamin C and extra vitamin C as such may have to be given.

Since all cereals are out of the diet, it becomes necessary to use tapioca pudding as a substitute for cereals. This tapioca or potato caramel pudding is most necessary if weight maintenance is a problem. If it is not liked, then extra white and/or sweet potato must be taken to furnish sufficient calories. For breakfast, freshly shredded or boiled potatoes, fried with or without bacon, can be eaten.

Bakery products are to be made from soy or lima and potato starch flours according to recipes furnished. The soybean muffins are easy to make; the pancakes are very satisfactory, and the cookies and cupcakes are excellent. Soybean oil in the recipes provides many calories and also helps to maintain weight.

You will note that not one drop or trace of any butter or margarine can be used. Willow Run is a good substitute. Specified jams, preserves, and fruits are to be made with cane or beet sugar but no glucose or corn sugar. For the necessary protein intake, meat must be taken twice a day, at lunch and dinner. Chicken, if allowed, also furnishes protein.

Cow's milk contains two important ingredients: animal protein and calcium. Milk is not necessary for nutrition providing adequate animal protein and calcium are included in other ways. Thus ample protein is assured if lamb or beef or chicken or turkey (if allowed) are taken two times a day together with protein in other foods, including legumes. We will also prescribe two-thirds teaspoonful of calcium carbonate in food or water daily which will furnish all the calcium you require.

Lunches and Dinner

For lunch and dinner, soup or salad, as detailed in the menu, may be eaten if desired. You will note that no canned soups and no soups made away from home can be used, since all ingredients in such soups cannot be determined by you. Many cooks prepare soup with macaroni, clear soup with eggs, and add spices and pepper, all of which are forbidden in this diet.

You will note that the kind of meat and the method of cooking is detailed and that vegetables in the diet listed above can be used and prepared as specified in this menu. Bakery products and bread, as discussed above, must be eaten. Only desserts and bakery products allowed in this diet can be used. Tea may be included as a beverage if advised by us. No commercial candy can be used, though candies can be made according to recipes in the booklet. To increase weight and satisfy the desire for sugar, cube sugar can be eaten after meals and at other times.

Box Lunches

If lunches are taken to work or school, they must be prepared according to the printed directions. If increasing weight is important, a jar of fruit tapioca or potato-caramel pudding must be included. A boiled sweet or white potato can be eaten with salt. Cold meat must be included to maintain protein nutrition. No mixed meats such as bologna, weiners, sausage, or Spam are allowed. Cookies and cakes made according to our recipes or purchased from a supervised bakery may be included. Prescribed fruit juice, tea, or water can be used as beverages. A cold drink can be made with one to two ounces of cane sugar syrup with or without the same amount of juice of a fruit in the diet with sparkling carbonated water such as Belfast or Canada Dry cooled in the refrigerator. Extra ice may be added.

Discussion

This diet must be followed carefully and accurately. At times results are not marked or definite for two to four weeks. Allergens from foods eaten before starting the diet remain in the blood and tissues for days and often for several weeks. Thus if a slight mistake is made in the diet, allergens will persist in the blood and tissues, the allergenic reactions in the shock tissues will continue, and the symptoms will never be relieved.

If foods are not available when eating away from home, the prescribed diet can be eaten previously at home or after returning home.

When it is certain that improvement has occurred, we will add other foods gradually to determine possible tolerance or allergy thereto. It will be necessary to include each new food daily for three to five days, as advised by us, before another is tried. If no symptoms arise, the food may be eaten as desired while other foods are being added. Allergic symptoms from food may arise in a few minutes or an hour or so if marked allergy to it exists or in a day or two if moderate allergy exists. Occasionally reactions from new foods do not occur until they have been taken daily for three to five days and rarely for one to two weeks. Moreover, it must be emphasized that foods may be tolerated in the summer which produce allergy in the fall to late spring, especially in the winter.

If it is important to increase weight, caloric intake must be increased as follows: Take as much of the bakery products as tolerated at each meal. Plenty of the tapioca or potato-caramel pudding should be taken with meals, between meals, and on retiring. White and sweet potatoes will add weight. Two to three ounces of sugar should be measured out each day and taken at intervals throughout the day. Cane sugar syrup made by boiling two cups of sugar with one cup of water for 2½ minutes can be used to sweeten drinks, tea, and on pudding, hotcakes, and so forth. Finally, the fat on meat, plenty of bacon, and soy oil will help to increase weight.

DISADVANTAGES OF OTHER TYPES OF TRIAL DIETS

When our elimination diets were first described, we suggested that physicians modify them according to the patient's requirements in various countries or in various regions of our own country. Foods botanically related to others in the routine elimination diets may be more available or less costly. Thus Richet published slight modifications of the diets in France, and various students in America suggested changes. All of these contributions have added in different degrees to the availability and utility of trial diet, and many menus and recipes have been evolved.

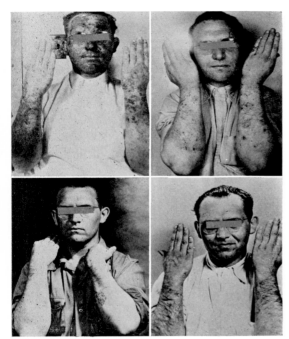

Figure 42. Gradual disappearance of lifelong allergic eczema in one year as a result of food allergy alone, resulting from strict adherence to our cereal-free elimination diet. Photograph 2 in three months, 3 in six months (had worked for the first time in his life for 2 months), 4 complete control in one year. Note the evident change in personality. Strict cooperation for weeks and months is also required for tissue changes in the lungs from severe bronchial asthma to disappear.

However, certain important aims for which our elimination diets were originally suggested have been lost sight of in some of these modifications. It was intended that elimination diets contain as few foods which are infrequent causes of allergy as are required to prepare meals that can be taken for a sufficiently long period to allow adequate study of possible food allergy. It is unwise, therefore, to add extra foods, spices, and beverages until the object of the diet trial has been attained—namely, a definite symptom-free period which is much longer than before diet trial was instituted. Then to such a diet, productive of freedom from symptoms, individual foods may gradually be added for two to three days if tolerated. In order that the allergenicity of each food may be ascertained, five to seven days must intervene between additions. The beneficial effects of summer months (Chapt. 1) must always be remembered. Thereby the degree of allergy and the necessity of continued exclusion of allergenic foods can be determined. In the analysis of the allergenic effect of such additional foods, the physician should keep in mind the varying time of onset and degree of the reactivity of foods, the varying sites of tissue reaction to different foods, the variation in allergic tolerance itself, and the effect of natural desensitization or refractoriness which arises after or during an allergic reaction. These influences are more fully discussed in Chapter 2.

Foods which have been ingested over a period of months or years may have to be entirely omitted from the diet for at least two or three weeks before evidence of clinical relief occurs. This fact is not fully appreciated by physicians who state that food allergy can be ruled out if the symptoms are not relieved by the elimination of suspected foods for three to even ten days. In fact, the persistent and chronic tissue changes arising from food and other allergies which are so evident in atopic eczema and in chronic bronchial and nasal allergy may require many days or weeks of complete freedom from the causative allergens before cellular function and structure are restored (see Fig. 19). Inhalant allergies may also necessitate weeks of hyposensitization or elimination before the tissues return to an approximately normal condition. Thus elimination diets must be so arranged that they can be eaten over a period of days, weeks, or even months without nutritional damage or undesirable weight loss, as discussed in Chapter 3.

Furthermore, the writers have stressed the importance of the exclusion of every trace of the foods that are excluded from the elimination diets during the study of possible food allergy. Until the symptoms are relieved and a subtracted food can be fed to the symptom-free patient in order to determine the degree and severity of its clinical activity, it should be assumed that a maximum degree of allergy to that food exists. This is important, since the sole object of the elimination diets is relief of symptoms without nutritional harm.

Unfortunately in some of the modifications of our elimination diets proposed by others, traces of food have been included which are excluded completely from our diets. For instance, in some diets commercial butter or an oleomargarine has been included. The latter usually contains minute amounts of cow's milk which may be sufficient to prevent relief in patients markedly sensitive to such milk. Even the odor of an allergenic food may produce symptoms in some patients. In certain modifications of our elimination diets, Melba wheat toast or other heated denaturized foods such as canned milk, have been recommended. Here again our experience indicates that patients markedly sensitive to a given food cannot eat it even if it has been subjected to high temperature. Denaturization of these foods is not complete, and symptoms arise from their use even though sensitized guinea pigs will not react to them, as reported by Ratner. In some instances these modified diets have not provided the patients with explicit menus and have not stressed the necessity of the elimination of every trace of a food not included in the diet. The frequent occurrence of pepper allergy is illustrative. Asthma occurred in one patient and angioneurotic edema in another if food containing a trace of pepper was eaten. In another

patient allergy to cottonseed was so great that its allergen in Crisco used in biscuits was enough to perpetuate the disease.

Therefore, as stressed throughout this book, successful diet trial depends on the exclusion of every trace of a food not included in the prescribed diet while possible food allergy is being studied, especially that eaten in friends' homes, in restaurants, or in hotels, as discussed on page 63. This care must be exercised until the symptoms have been relieved or the role of food allergy is excluded. If food allergy is demonstrated, tolerance for the allergenic foods may be determined by further diet trial with provocation tests.

Our elimination diets originally were formulated with these ideas in mind. We have always insisted on the total exclusion of all foods not included in these diets. The proper preparation of meals so that nutritional balance and desired or advisable weight is assured during a period long enough to rule food allergy in or out as a cause of the symptoms is always necessary.

Since allergic or toxic reactions to vitamins and to local oral or parenteral medications occur in varying degrees, their continuation or addition must be critically analyzed and evaluated, as Randolph importantly stresses, by the patient's physician.

DISADVANTAGES OF INITIAL STARVATION COMPARED WITH THE USE OF OUR ELIMINATION DIETS

1. Hospitalization because of necessary supervision and analysis of the results of strict environmental control is not required with our advised study of food allergy with our elimination diets except when it is necessary because of severe bronchial asthma or other invaliding manifestations of allergy.

2. Possible undernutrition or undesirable loss of weight do not occur with elimination diets, vitamins, and calcium carbonate.

3. Since our clinical experience for over three decades indicates that food allergens usually remain in the body for more than four to five days, we have always advised strict adherence to the elimination diets for approximately three weeks so that relief of food allergy is assured before individual food tests with additional foods are done.

4. Drugs and chemicals also usually remain in the body for more than a few days, as long demonstrated in the case of arsenic, mercury, and other chemical medications.

5. Long, persisting tissue changes from food allergy require the elimination of allergenic foods at times for weeks before such tissues return to normal without treatment by corticosteroids.

HOPED FOR ADVANTAGES OF INITIAL TOTAL FASTING AND ACCORDING TO RANDOLPH'S TECHNIQUE CONTROL OF ECOLOGICAL FACTORS

The possible limited use of total initial fasting and necessary hospitalization in an ecologically controlled hospital unit as advised by Randolph in 1965 requires discussion.

1. When multiple food allergies and possible or evident inhalant and drug allergies require study as a cause of the various invaliding symptoms in allergic fatigue and toxemia (see Chapt. 19), which we first reported in 1928, and symptoms are not relieved by the use even of our minimal elimination diets and control of indicated or possible inhalant and drug allergies, initial total fasting for four to five days followed by individual food tests in an ecologically controlled hospital room, as advised by Randolph, may be desirable.

2. When psychological and even psychiatric disturbances in patients usually suffering with the above syndrome or with invaliding illness requiring sanitarium or even institutional care are not relieved with expertized use of our minimal elimination diets and control of possible inhalant and drug allergies, Randolph's complete fasting for four days with subsequent individual food tests for the study of ingestant allergies along with the study of inhalant and other ecological factors in the hospital environment may be advisable.

We agree with Randolph and others that cerebral and neural allergies, especially to foods and also to drugs and chemicals, as discussed in Chapter 18, require increasing recognition and control. Study and control of possible allergic and ecological causes in the chronically ill patient, according to Randolph's methods, we opine, need open-minded consideration because of his long-reported favorable results.

DIABETIC DIETS CONTAINING FOODS IN OUR ELIMINATION DIETS

Various diabetic patients either suffer from definite and obvious food allergies or have symptoms which require a careful study of possible food allergy. We first advised this in our book *Handbook for the Diabetic*, Oxford University Press, 1928. The elimination diet of the diabetic can be formulated so that it contains the foods chosen by the physician for the study of possible food allergy. As with other elimination diets their use must be carefully read and followed, as described in Chapter 3.

A diabetic diet modified from the cereal-free elimination diet is described in our previous publications, including *Bronchial Asthma—Its Diagnosis and Treatment*, 1963, published by Charles C Thomas, Springfield, Illinois.

Insulin therapy, of course, as indicated

by the diabetes must be administered. Similar diets satisfying other food allowances for diabetic patients and containing other foods for the special allergic problem of the patient can be prepared.

SYMPTOM RECORD

A card or sheet of paper can be divided into squares equal to the days of the week and month. In each square can be placed letters indicating symptoms the physician is interested in, with numbers from 0 to 4 to indicate severity. Thus A (Asthma) 3 or B (hay fever) 2, or C (Belching) 1, or D (Epigastric pain) 4, and so on. With a card or sheet for each month, progress can be checked according to desensitization therapy, diet, and seasons. Notes can be inserted by the physician to indicate weather changes, trips, breaks in diet, and so on.

SYMPTOMS

1. Pain	8. Diarrhea
2. Night pain	9. Headache
3. Nausea	10. Dizziness
4. Vomiting	11. Sneezing
5. Gas	12. Nasal symptoms
6. Bloating	13. Cough
7. Constipation	14. Asthma

15. Toxemia	19. Palpitation
16. Hives	20. Dyspnea
17. Eruption	21. Joint pains
18. Itching	22. Bruises

REMARKS

X	Symptoms persist
XX	Symptoms exaggerated
O	Symptoms relieved

Directions

Keep your diet as simple as possible. Chart your important symptoms by number in column indicating hour in which they occur.

Certain foods are causing your illness, whether it is headache, arthritis, peptic ulcer, asthma, or pain. The foods responsible can be determined by a careful diary.

Your cooperation is essential for success. List visits to barber shop, beauty parlor, theater, and so on. List anything unusual. Do not take any medicine not prescribed.

A list of allergens for initial skin testing is given in Table LIV.

TABLE LIV

LIST OF ALLERGENS FOR INITIAL SCRATCH TESTING*

Foods

Cereals:
  Barley*
  Buckwheat*
  Corn*
  Oats*
  Rice*
  Rye*
  Wheat (whole)*
Eggs (whole)*

Eggs (white)
Eggs (yolk)
Cow's milk
  (whole)*
Cow's milk
  (albumin)*
Cow's milk
  (casein)*
Cow's milk
  (cheese)
Goat's milk
Vegetables:
  Artichokes*
  Asparagus*
  Avocados*
  Beans (white)
  Beets*
  Broccoli
  Brussels sprouts
  Cabbage*
  Carrots*
  Cauliflower*
  Celery*
  Cucumber
  Eggplant
  Endive
  Garlic*
  Green peppers
  Kidney beans*
  Leeks
  Lentils
  Lettuce*
  Lima beans*
  Mushrooms*
  Navy beans
  Okra*
  Olives*

TABLE LIV (Cont'd)

Foods (Cont'd)

  Vegetables (Cont'd)

    Onions*
    Parsley
    Parsnips
    Peas*
    Potatoes (sweet)*
    Potatoes (white)*
    Pumpkin*
    Radishes
    Rhubarb*
    Soybeans*
    Spinach*
    Squash*
    String beans*
    Tomatoes*
    Turnips
    Watercress

  Fruits:

    Apples*
    Apricots*
    Bananas*
    Blackberries
    Cantaloupe*
    Casaba melon
    Cherries
    Cranberry
    Currant
    Dates
    Figs
    Grapes
    Grapefruit*
    Honeydew melon
    Lemon*
    Olives*
    Oranges*
    Peaches*
    Pears*
    Pineapples*
    Plums
    Prunes*
    Raisins
    Raspberries
    Strawberries*
    Tangerines
    Watermelon*

  Condiments:

    Anchovies
    Caraway seeds
    Cinnamon*
    Cloves
    Ginger
    Horseradish
    Mints
    Mustard*
    Nutmeg
    Pepper (black)*
    Pepper (white)*
    Pepper (red)
    Paprika
    Pimentos
    Poppy seeds
    Sage*
    Vanilla

Foods (Cont'd)

  Condiments (Cont'd)

    Cocoa*
    Coffee*
    Tea*
    Gelatin
    Tapioca
    Yeast*
    Hops*
    Honey*
    Sago

  Nuts:

    Almonds*
    Brazil nuts
    Cashews
    Chestnuts
    Cocoanuts
    Filberts
    Hickory nuts
    Hazel nuts
    Peanuts*
    Pecans
    Pistachio nuts
    Walnuts (black)*
    Walnuts (English)

  Meats:

    Beef*
    Chicken*
    Deer
    Duck (domestic)*
    Duck (wild)
    Frog's legs
    Goose
    Lamb*
    Liver (calf)
    Liver (lamb)
    Pork*
    Rabbit
    Squab
    Sweetbread (lamb)
    Terrapin
    Turkey
    Veal

  Fish:

    Bass (sea)*
    Blue fish
    Carp
    Catfish
    Clams*
    Codfish*
    Crab*
    Flounder
    Haddock
    Halibut*
    Herring
    Lobster*
    Mackerel
    Oysters*
    Perch
    Pike
    Pickerel
    Red Snapper
    Salmon*
    Sardine

TABLE LIV (Cont'd)

Foods (Cont'd)

Fish (Cont'd)
Scallops
Shad
Shrimp*
Smelts
Sole
Sturgeon
Trout (lake)
Trout (sea)
Tuna fish
White fish*
Epidermals:
Camel hair*
Canary feathers*
Cat hair*
Cattle hair*
Chicken feathers*
Dog hair*
Duck feathers*
Goat hair*
Goose feathers*
Guinea pig hair
Hamster hair
Hog hair
Horse dander*
Human hair
Mouse hair
Ostrich feathers
Parrot feathers
Rabbit hair
Sheep wool*
Turkey feathers
Furs:
Alaska seal
Australian hare
Badger
Beaver
Caracul
Chamois
Fox (gray)
Fox (red)
Fox (silver)
Kilinsky
Leopard
Marmoset
Mink
Mole
Muskrat (Hudson
seal)
Nutria
Otter
Persian Lamb
Raccoon
Skunk
Squirrel
Wolf
Miscellaneous
Inhalants:
Boxwood
Cotton
Cottonseed*
Dust (house)*

Foods (Cont'd)

Miscellaneous
Inhalants (Cont'd)
Feed dusts
(according to
occupation)*
Flaxseed*
Glue*
Henna
Kapok*
Leather
*Lycopodium**
Orris root*
Pyrethrum*
Silk*
Tobacco*
Pollens:
Graminae:
Barley
Bermuda grass
Brome grass
Canary grass
English rye grass
Fescue grass
Johnson grass
Kentucky blue grass
Orchard grass
Red top
Salt grass
Slender wild rye
Timothy
Velvet grass
Walk grass
Wild oats
English plantain
Dock
Chenopodiaceae:
Bractscale
Pickleweed
Rough pigweed
Russian thistle
Spearscale
White goosefoot
Compositae:
Alfalfa
Burweed
Coastal sagebrush
Cocklebur
Dandelion
False ragweed
Giant ragweed
Goldenrod
Marsh elder
Mountain sagebrush
Mugwort*
Short ragweed*
Western ragweed*
Trees:
Birch*
Box elder
Butternut
Cottonwood*
Cypress

Table LIV (Cont'd)

Foods (Cont'd)

  Trees (Cont'd)
    Deodar
    Elm*
    Eucalyptus*
    Hickory*
    Locust*
    Maple
    Acacia*
    Apple*
    Arizona ash
    Black walnut*
    Mountain cedar*
    Oak*
    Olive*
    Peach*
    Pear
    Prune
    Poplar*
    Privet*
    Sycamore*
    Willow*
  Fungi:
    Aspergillus niger
    *A glaucus**
    *Penicillium trichoderma**
    Mucor plumbeus
    *Cladosporium**
    Monilia
    *Alternaria**
    Chactomium
    *Trichophyton**
    Yeasts such as:
    beer*
    baker's*
    brewer's
    distiller's

*The arrangement of this list is similar to that published by Feinberg in 1934. The most important allergens are designated by the asterisk. The pollens for testing depend on the patient's own flora. Botanical names are not printed in Table LII. Other ingestants and pollens are not included; those used for inhalant allergens other than those listed are selected according to the pollens in the published surveys in the state and local living area in which the patient lives, as advised in Chapter 4.

SUGGESTED ALLERGENS FOR SKIN TESTING IN INFANCY AND EARLY CHILDHOOD

Puncture or prick tests (see Chapt. 2) are made through small amounts of the extracts of the allergens dropped on the skin of the back. This method causes minimal discomfort compared with scratch tests. Testing can be completed in ten minutes and reactions determined in another fifteen minutes. Intradermal tests in these patients are contraindicated. Testing with foods may be limited to those ingested or to be eaten by the patient. If allergy to food proteins in the mother's milk is suspected (see page 454), testing may be advisable with additional food allergens in her diet.

Suggested inhalant and food allergens for testing infants and young children follow. The number and variety, especially of the inhalants, vary with the patient's problem, age, and environment. That infants may not react to allergenic foods until the second or third months must be remembered.

TABLE LV

Inhalants	Ingestants
Cat hair	Rice
Dog hair	Corn
Horse hair	Wheat
Cattle hair	Eggs
Mixed feathers	Cow's milk
Wool	Goat's milk
Silk	Beef
Efron	Lamb
Bermuda	Codfish
Timothy	Carrots
Coastal sage	Peas
Western ragweed	Squash
Spearscale	Potatoes
Orris root	Crab
Pyrethrum	Tomatoes
Cottonseed	Soybeans
Kapok	Peanuts
Ray	Peaches
Rough pigweed	Prunes
Acacia	Oranges
Black walnut	Chicken
Live oak	Pork
Sycamore	Bananas
Olive	
Peach pollen	
Alternaria	

Initial testing may be limited to ingested foods and only to inhalants in the infant's environment.

HOUSE DUST EXTRACTS

The procedures advised in Vaughan's text have been followed, the extraction being done with Unger's (D. P.) extracting fluid sterilized with Seitz filtration.

EPIDERMAL AND MISCELLANEOUS EXTRACTS

These have been extracted as advised in Vaughan's text.

STANDARDIZATION OF ALLERGENIC EXTRACTS

Pollen extracts have been standardized by weight–volume or percent. Comparable values of protein nitrogen units follow. Food extracts are utilized for scratch and intradermals as advised by Vaughan. The concentrated house dust extract is used for scratch tests, dilutions in multiples of ten being used for intradermal tests and desensitization. Fungus extracts are standardized, as advised in Sheldon's text.

FIVE SCHEDULES FOR ADMINISTRATION OF ANTIGENS

Our antigens are standard by weight–volume or percent. To simplify the labelling, the 1:50 dilution is labelled #1. The 1:500 is #2, and the weaker dilutions are numbered 3, 4, and 5 and up to 11 or 12 according to the number of 1:10 dilutions required. Thus the 1:5,000,000 is #6, and the 1:5,000,000,000 is #9.

The writer utilizes five schedules for the hypodermic administration of antigens of pollens or other inhalants. Schedule V and IV are advised when it is desired to increase the doses of the weakest dilutions (that is, numbers 7 to 12) as fast as tolerated by the patient. Schedules III and II are used for stronger dilutions (that is, number 6) which must be given less rapidly. Schedule I is substituted for a less rapid schedule if a dose of it has produced too large a local reaction or a reactivation of symptoms or those of a general reaction.

Antigen _____ Patient _____
Dilution _____ Date _____

Schedule I
Give the following doses of Dilution __ every __ days.

1st dose	0.05 cc	6th dose	0.30 cc
2nd dose	0.10 cc	7th dose	0.40 cc
3rd dose	0.15 cc	8th dose	0.50 cc
4th dose	0.20 cc	9th dose	0.60 cc
5th dose	0.25 cc	and so on, as tolerated	

Repeat last tolerated dose every __ days.

Schedule II
Give the following doses of Dilution __ every __ days.

1st dose	0.10 cc	4th dose	0.40 cc
2nd dose	0.20 cc	5th dose	0.50 cc
3rd dose	0.30 cc		

Schedule III
Give the following doses of Dilution __ every __ days.

1st dose	0.1 cc	3rd dose	0.4 cc
2nd dose	0.2 cc	4th dose	0.6 cc

Schedule IV
Give the following doses of Dilution __ every __ days.

1st dose	0.10 cc	3rd dose	0.50 cc
2nd dose	0.25 cc		

Schedule V
Give the following doses of Dilution __ every __ days.

1st dose	0.10 cc	2nd dose	0.30 cc

ADDENDUM FOR EACH DILUTION

This antigen contains pollen dusts, animal emanations, or other allergens prescribed by the physician. Keep refrigerated (not frozen). Inject subcutaneously (not intramuscularly) in alternate outer arms or outer thighs. If local reaction is larger than two or three inches in diameter eight to twelve hours after injection or if symptoms are definitely increased after the injection, reduce the next injection by one or two doses, increasing thereafter as tolerated. The injection should not increase or reactivate symptoms. When the strongest dilutions are injected, the patient should wait in the office for ten to fifteen minutes. If a general reaction occurs, epinephrine 1:1000 should be given as advised. If such symptoms occur after leaving the office, the patient should return immediately for such treatment (see Chapt. 4).

It is important to remember that the smaller the number of the dilution, the stronger its strength.

METHODS FOR MAKING ALLERGENIC EXTRACTS
Pollen Extracts

We have used the glycerine saline extract originally advised by Stier consisting of glycerine 460 cc, NaCl 40 gm, distilled water to make 1,000 cc. With this, 2 percent pollen extracts have been prepared, sterilized by Seitz filtration.

Food Extracts

We have made our food extracts as summarized by Vaughan's text utilizing Unger's extracting fluid (D.P.) containing dextrose 45 gm, sodium bicarbonate 2 gm, phenol 5 gm, and distilled water to make 1000 cc sterilized with Seitz filtration.

Extracts of Fungi

These have been grown in Sabourad's media, being covered with ether and allowed to evaporate as advised in Sheldon's text. Extraction of the pelts has been with Unger's (D.P.) extracting fluid and sterilized with Seitz filtration.

COMPARISON OF UNIT VALUES OF POLLEN EXTRACTS (ACCORDING TO TUFT*)

COMPARABLE VALUES OF POLLEN EXTRACTS

By Weight of Pollen (Noon unit in 0.001 mg pollen)	(Kjeldahl) by Total Nitrogen	Units By Protein Nitrogen (Cooke & Stull)
1 cc of 1:1,000,000 (1 Noon unit)	0.000016	0.64
1 cc of 1:100,000 (10 units)	0.00016	6.4
1 cc of 1:10,000 (100 units)	0.0016	64
1 cc of 1:1,000 (1000 units)	0.016	640
1 cc of 1:100 (10,000 units)	0.16	6400

PERTINENT INFORMATION CONTAINED IN PREVIOUS PUBLICATIONS

Classification of Foods	*Bronchial Asthma—Its Diagnosis and Treatment.* Springfield, Charles C Thomas, 1963.
Regional and local pollen surveys:	*Ibid.*
Serum administration and reactions:	*Ibid.*
Questionnaire for the allergic patient:	*Ibid.*
Nostrums and other empiric therapy advised in bronchial asthma:	*Ibid.*
Literature on manifestations of atopic allergy, especially food allergy, in migraine and sick headaches:	*Clinical Allergy.* Philadelphia, Lea and Febiger, 1937.
Instructions for the establishment of environmental control: 1. In the bedroom 2. In other rooms 3. Pollen air filter (graphic instructions for installation)	*Bronchial Asthma—Its Diagnosis and Treatment.* Springfield, Charles C Thomas, 1963.

Copies of the following summary of the above discussion may be handed patients.

INSTRUCTIONS FOR THE PREPARATION OF A DUST-FREE ROOM

1. Your room should contain only one bed, preferably an iron one. If there is more than one bed in the room it also must be prepared as will be described.

2. All the furniture, rugs, curtains, and drapes must be taken from the room; the clothes closets emptied; and the room cleaned as follows:

a) Seal all of the furnace pipes leading into the room. Clean the wallpaper. Scrub the woodwork and the floors in the room and closets. Wax the floors. Washable scatter rugs may be used.

b) Scrub the bed. Scrub the springs. This must be done outside the cleaned room. If you use box springs, they must be completely encased, as will be described. Cover the mattress, pillows, and box springs with dustproof encasings (covers). The covers must be made of material which is not porous or dust will come through the material. We therefore recommend a cloth which is allergen-proof. These encasings must be sewed on or otherwise closed up so that they are completely air tight. This must be done outside the cleaned room.

---

*Tuft, L.: *Clinical Allergy,* Philadelphia, W. B. Saunders, 1937.

Now set up the cleaned bed in the cleaned room and on it place the cleaned or encased springs and the encased mattress. Make up the bed with the encased pillows and freshly washed bedding. All bedding must be made of material which will stand frequent washing. No quilts or comforter should be used.

c) Wooden chairs which have been scrubbed may be used in this room. Rag rugs washed at least once a week may be used on the floors. Plain light curtains washed once a week may be used on the windows.

d) This room must be cleaned thoroughly once a week.

3. You must sleep in this room. All dressing and undressing must be done elsewhere in the house.

Articles of furniture which contain allergenic dusts should be removed from the house, especially from adjoining halls and rooms, if possible. Otherwise, each article should be vacuum cleaned thoroughly every day at a time when the patient is away from the house. Following the vacuum cleaning the house should be aired thoroughly.

TABLE LVI

OCCUPATIONS, SYMPTOMS AND LIKELY SENSITIZERS

Key: R Respiratory Symptoms—Asthma and Nasal Allergy (hay fever)
      S Skin Symptoms—Eczema and Hives, Angioedema
      C Contact Dermatitis

Occupation	Symptoms	Sensitizers—Allergens
Agricultural	R, S, C	Animal, plant, and mold products. Insecticides, chemicals, drugs, solvents, detergents, and so on
Airplane workers	C	"Dope" solvents, paints, woods, glues, electroplating compounds
Asphalt and pitch workers	C	Pitch, tars, and petroleum products
Autotyper	C	Bichromate form of chromium
Bakers and millers	R, S, C	Flours, conditioners, bleaches, flavoring extracts, vegetable dyes, sugars, eggs, chocolate, mold, and so on
Barbers	C	Cosmetics, depilatories, hair dyes, hair preparations containing mercury, quinine, resorcin, and sulfur
Brewery workers	R, S, C	Barley, grains, hops, malt, yeast, mold, glues, paper products, inks, detergents, and so on
Bricklayers, masons	C	Paints and stains
Bronzers	C	Arsenic and metallic salts
Burnishers	C	Mercurials
Butchers	R, S, C (Hog itch)	Animal hairs and danders, intestinal contents, molds, detergents, insecticides
Cabinet makers and carpenters	R, S, C	Sawdust, resins, glues, lacquers, solvents, varnish, thinners
Candy makers	R, S, C	Nuts, spices, flavorings, fruits, sugars, dyes, vegetable colorings
Canners of fruits and vegetables	C	Fruits, vegetables, juices
Cattlemen	R, S, C	Cottonseed, feeds, grains, hair and danders, molds, pollens, detergents, cleansers, and so on
Chemists	C	Irritants and allergenic substances in common use in the laboratory
Circus workers	R, S, C	Animal hairs and danders; disinfecting, deodorizing and cleansing chemicals; dyes, fabrics, foods, grains, pollens, molds, sawdust
Compositors	C	Chromium compounds
Cooks	R, S, C	Flours, fruits, vegetables, flavorings, vegetable dyes, spices, soaps, detergents, insecticides, mold

possible infection in the etiology of these chronic diseases. In all of these studies the lack of understanding of the underlying cause is expressed as by Mitchell who stated: "The etiology and pathogenesis of chronic bronchitis and emphysema are not understood."

We opine that if allergy to foods had been adequately considered along with possible allergy "to inhaled air pollutants" including tobacco and possible injury from coughing, as suggested by Mitchell, the important major role of food allergy in these chronic respiratory diseases would have been recognized, confirming our reports of good results from its control not only in this volume but in many former publications. Orrie's opinion that there is no fundamental difference between chronic bronchitis and emphysema thus would be elucidated. Other opinions that there is a different etiology in chronic bronchitis and emphysema would have been, in our opinion, reversed. The present treatment consisting of bronchodilators by mouth and by inhalation with hand atomizers and especially IPP therapy and usually continued too often increased doses of corticoids for the control of bronchospasm would be diminished or gradually eliminated by adequate recognition and control of atopic allergy, especially to foods, associated at times with inhalant and drug allergies.

The major responsibility of physicians is to determine and control atopic allergy, especially to foods, responsible for bronchospasm, as advised in Chapter 8. To relieve the bronchospasm and resultant symptoms only for brief periods with drugs given by mouth, parenterally, and by inhalation without adequate study of the allergic causes is comparable to common relief of the symptoms of bronchial asthma with adrenalin hypodermically and too often with the administration of morphine, resulting in uncontrollable addiction, when we first started the study of the causes of bronchial asthma and other manifestations of allergy in 1916.

The major and often the sole role of food allergy in perennial nasal and upper respiratory allergy, in chronic bronchitis, in bronchial asthma, and in obstructive emphysema is depicted according to our experience based on good or excellent results summarized in this volume in the following sequence of their symptoms:

PERENNIAL MANIFESTATIONS OF FOOD ALLERGY RESULTING FROM ITS LOCALIZATION IN SEQUENTIAL AREAS OF THE RESPIRATORY TRACT

| Perennial nasal, sinal, otological, and pharyngeal allergy | Chronic bronchitis or recurrent head and bronchial colds | Bronchial asthma recurrently activated or in recurrent attacks especially in the fall to late spring | Obstructive emphysema with irreversible destruction of alveolar and adjacent tissues and varying degrees of bronchospasm |

The long-recognized localization of atopic allergy, especially to foods, explains its occurrence in single or combined areas of the upper respiratory tract as it does in eczema from food allergy localized in different cutaneous areas of the hands, face, arms, legs, or in other separate areas of the skin.

All of these manifestations of food allergy in the bronchial tract with or without concomitant inhalant and at times drug allergy require study and control of food allergy as advised in this volume. One manifestation may be dominant, others being moderate in degree. Thus the origin of obstructive emphysema is explained by irreversible allergy in the capillaries of the alveolar walls with subsequent thromboses and resultant necroses along with varying degrees of spasm in the bronchial tract with or without evidences of actual bronchial asthma, as discussed in Chapter 11. Bronchial asthma alone with or without moderate obstructive emphysema may occur or symptoms from food allergy may be restricted to the nasal, sinal, aural, or pharyngeal tissues individually or in unison.

ALLERGY TO TOBACCO IN CONTRAST TO IRRITATION OF THE BRONCHIAL MUCOSA AND SMOOTH MUSCLES IN THE CAUSATION OF OBSTRUCTIVE EMPHYSEMA

Important information about the frequency of OE as a result of inhalation of cigarette smoke should be obtained from determination of the frequency and degree of OE in the patients' histories, physical examinations, x-rays of the lungs, routine lung scans, and especially in pathological examinations of lungs removed because of cancer. Its minor role in food allergy, as emphasized in Chapter 8, is important to reread.

If irritation of the bronchial mucosa from cancer producing tar or other chemicals in tobacco smoke is also responsible for the destructive changes of the alveoli and adjacent tissues of OE, definite pathology of OE should usually occur in the lungs of those patients who have inhaled the tar-containing smoke of two to three packs of cigarettes a day for twenty to fifty years.

Our preliminary inquiry of chest surgeons indicates that the frequency of presumptive mild or definite OE by history and physical examination and x-ray of the cancerous lungs is not common.

Pathologists, moreover, have not recorded or suspected emphysema in their routine examination of the lungs for cancer. The challenge, therefore, will be examination of such inflated lungs for evidence of OE supplemented by microscopic examination of tissues in many likely areas to determine the presence and especially the degree of possible emphysema in these lungs removed because of cancer.

Study of possible OE in patients with cancer of the lungs will require pulmonary function tests, repeated if indications of OE after hypodermic injection of epinephrine persist to rule out possible bronchospasm without destructive changes in the lung.

Since chronic bronchitis is usual in OE, inspection and microscopic examination of the walls of medium-sized terminal bronchi also will be important.

If the above clinical, x-ray, and pathological study of patients from whom a lung has been removed because of cancer yield rare or slight evidence of OE which has not been the patient's major complaint for several months or years, the role of cigarette smoke as a major cause of OE will be minimized. This would favor allergy, on the contrary, to tobacco instead of its present commonly assumed irritation as a cause of OE. Allergy to tobacco causing vasculitis, thrombosis, and necrosis of capillaries in the walls of the alveoli which best explain OE resulting from food allergy, as discussed in Chapter 11, would also be the best explanation of destruction of alveoli arising from inhaled tobacco smoke.

Another way in which smoking can produce OE by allergic mechanisms is suggested by the paper of Volkheimer and Schulz (1968) describing stimulation of persorption by smoking. Thus smoking may also act by increasing the amount of exposure of the lungs to particulate food allergens.

Symptoms and evidence of atopic allergy in other tissues, as in the nasobronchial, cutaneous, and neurocerebral tissues also favor predisposition to allergy to tobacco as well as to foods as a cause of OE. Positive skin tests to various types of tobacco would give added support to such allergy, though such tests may be negative as they so often are to foods productive of clinical allergy.

Casting doubt on the frequency of OE resulting either from irritation or even allergy as a common cause are the normal lung scans after intravenous ^{131}I in several of our patients who have smoked two or three packages of cigarettes daily for thirty or forty years and who moreover have no clinical or laboratory evidence of OE. Failure of Aviado to produce tissue changes in mice from inhaled tobacco smoke has been noted in Chapter 11.

Before more definite indications of the role of inhaled tobacco smoke as an irritant or allergic cause of OE can be reported, many more analyses of histories, laboratory, x-ray findings, and lung scans must be obtained in patients who have smoked excessively for many years and who later develop cancer of the lungs.

In our practice lung cancer has developed in only one patient after severe OE had been markedly relieved for two years by strict adherence to our CFE diet.

Case 230: When first seen, he had been in the hospital most of the time for seven months where IPP adrenergic therapy and bronchodilator drugs had been used four times a day, and his wife had been told repeatedly that recovery was not possible.

After excellent relief with our CFE diet minus beef with extra sugar, plus tea to maintain nutrition for 2½ years, increasingly constant cough and x-ray findings of bronchogenic carcinoma developed, confirmed by bronchoscopy. This cancer is best explained by his previous daily smoking of three packages of cigarettes for forty-five years up to four years ago. With strict adherence to our CFE diet plus 2 mg of Aristocort one to three times a week, his SOB had been well controlled with no intermittent positive pressure, adrenergic aerosol therapy. When cancer was found, he stated: "I have no emphysema, only a constant cough with frequent blood in sputum for one month." Roentgen ray treatment along with adherence to his CFE diet plus vitamins was given daily for four weeks, with present relief of his coughing and reduced evidence of cancer in the x-ray of his lungs.

Comment: Extreme OE in a man who had smoked two to three packs of cigarettes daily for forty years was well relieved (drove an automobile to and from Michigan 2 years ago 3 months after our initial control of his SOB) with strict adherence to our CFE diet and no IPP adrenergic aerosol therapy and minimum or no corticosteroids or bronchodilating drugs.

Then 2½ years after OE was so controlled, cancer developed, best explained by his excessive smoking of cigarettes for forty years.

That tobacco was not the primary cause of OE was shown by his excellent control for over two years with strict adherence to our CFE diet. Brief addition of the cereal grains caused SOB in thirty-six hours.

DISCUSSION OF THE COMPLICATIONS OF AEROSOL THERAPY WITH ADRENERGIC DRUGS, ESPECIALLY WITH INTERMITTENT POSITIVE PRESSURE MECHANISMS

The relief of bronchospasm with concomitant decrease or disappearance of bronchorrhea not only in severe bronchial asthma but also in obstructive emphysema resulting from the control of atopic allergy to foods and to a lesser degree to inhalants along with decreasing medications advised in this chapter and in Chapter 8, using a minimum or no inhalation of adrenergic sympathomimetic aerosols, especially with isotroterenol, particularly with intermittent positive pressure mechanisms, must be emphasized.

This is especially important because of increasing recognition of the detrimental results of the inhalation of more than moderate doses of epinephrine which Graeser and we first advised in 1935 for the relief of bronchospasm and of the now advised similar moderate use of isotroterenol.

Such detrimental side effects were first noted by Galiano in 1939 and were emphasized by Benson and Perlman in 1948.

Dautrebande also reported decreased

bronchospasm from the synthetic analogue of epinephrine, isoproterenol (Aleudrin®) in 1946. This benefit was confirmed by Charlier and especially by Segal and Beakey and by Siegmund *et al.* in 1947. Since then it has been known as Isuprel, whose beneficial effect in asthma was again reported by Lowell, Curry, and Scheller in 1949. Presaging the present opinion, they reported relief from its inhalation and also from sublingual doses for self-medication in mild or moderately severe asthma but unsatisfactory relief in severe, prolonged asthma.

Kiegley, in 1966, again emphasized these detrimental effects, reporting increased airway obstruction from continued and excessive inhalation of the aerosol of isotroterenol, with actual causation of iatrogenic asthma in two patients in spite of corticosteroid therapy and the use of other bronchodilating drugs. When this aerosol therapy was stopped, the relief of asthma depending on previously ineffective corticosteroid and bronchodilating drugs other than adrenergic aerosols was enhanced by our control of atopic allergy to inhalants and especially to foods. The asthma recurred, however, with the resumption of the inhalation even of small doses of isoproterenol. This suggests bronchospasm from allergy to this drug comparable to that in the cutaneous tissues after hypodermic injection of epinephrine as reported in former years.

In 1968 Resman reported aggravation of status asthmaticus from prolonged inhalation of adrenergic drugs, even with a hand atomizer, and Brown of England stated that the excessive inhalation of these drugs may produce side effects worse than from large, continued doses of corticosteroids.

Caplin and Haynes, in 1969, confirmed the increase of bronchospasm from the continued inhalation of adrenergic aerosols in spite of indicated desensitization therapy to inhalants and the use of other bronchodilating drugs. This detrimental effect was indicated by the decrease in bronchospasm when the inhalation of these adrenergic drugs was discontinued. We opine that if possible food allergy, which was indicated by the perennial asthma exaggerated in the winter in his patients, had been studied and treated as we advise in this volume, definite decrease in the asthma which would not have impelled the patient to use the excessive inhalation of the adrenergic aerosols would have occurred.

Irritation of the bronchial tissues also occurs from excessive inhalation of these drugs, indicated by inflammation in the trachea with loss of epithelium and leukocytic infiltration of the submucosa in a patient who had used 1 percent epinephrine every two hours for two days before death. Excessive inhalation of these adrenergic drugs also produced tachycardia, pallor, and hyperirritability. Greenberg and Pines, in 1967 in England, suspected death in asthma in part resulting from excessive inhalation of adrenergic pressurized aerosols. Palmer and Diamet also reported increased arterial hypoxemia in varying degrees in twenty patients who had inhaled such aerosol.

In an excellent article on the adverse effects of inhalation of excessive amounts of nebulized isotroterenol in thirty patients with status asthmaticus, Van Metre, in 1969, reported excessive use in nine of the seventeen patients dying of asthma in Johns Hopkins Hospital. That such therapy was probably detrimental was indicated by the decrease in symptoms with discontinuance of its excessive use in thirty patients whose asthma was resistant to all forms of therapy (including corticosteroids in recent years).

As in the articles of Kiegley, Caplin,

and Haynes, evidence that Van Metre's study and therapy had adequately considered perennial food allergy as we advise is not apparent. Our persistent adequate study of inhalant and especially of food allergy, in our opinion, largely explains why intractable asthma and status asthmaticus have been controlled with minimal fatalities compared with other reports, depending, in our opinion, on treatment as advised in this chapter and throughout this volume. Our minimal fatalities also depend on our disuse of sedatives, including barbitals and chlorpromazine, especially morphine, and other opium derivatives as well as of our disuse of IPP aerosol therapy in status asthmaticus and as reported during the last three years, in obstructive emphysema. Van Metre approves of therapeutic small doses of adrenergic aerosols, which we first advised in 1935, but presents irrefutable evidence that excessive inhalation is harmful, at times leading to the "locked-lung" syndrome and death. Its conservative use must be insisted on by allergists and other physicians, preventing its excessive use by the patient whose asthma usually increases because of failure to control atopic allergy to inhalants and especially to foods.

Thus the discontinuance of limited use of inhalation aerosol therapy with adrenergic drugs in perennial bronchial asthma and especially in obstructive emphysema is important for the following reasons:

1. Detrimental effect of more than moderate inhalation of adrenergic aerosol, especially by IPP mechanisms, as summarized above in this chapter, has been increasingly realized in the past thirty years.

2. Good and excellent relief of bronchospasm and resultant shortness of breath from perennial asthma and obstructive emphysema has increasingly occurred in the last five years from a control of allergy to inhalants and especially to foods, as we advise in this chapter and in Chapters 6, 8, and 25.

3. In considering the use of intermittent positive pressure therapy, it is also important to take cognizance of the findings of Dain *et al.* that very large amounts of starch, indeed, with associated cellular reactions are found in the lungs of premature infants after treatment with these breathing devices. This starch appears to have originated from the gloves of the therapists. Because of the evidence we have accumulated that allergy to starch is a major etiological factor in emphysema, it is most clear that iatrogenic introduction of starch into patients' lungs must be absolutely avoided.

We mailed four hundred and fifty-five queries to hospitals taken at random from a directory of United States hospitals. Three hundred and twenty-eight answers were received. These hospitals had 60,671 beds and 1878 IPP machines. The directory stated 1,671,125 beds as the total in all its hospitals so there are some 68,000 IPP machines in these hospitals. Where technicians were assigned full-time to these machines there was an average of 1.48 machines serviced by each full-time technician, for a total of 46,000 technicians. Discontinuance of use of IPP aerosol therapy for emphysema patients better treated by food allergy techniques would reduce the investment needed for these machines and also monies paid to technicians and other personnel administering aerosol therapy and caring for the IPP mechanisms in hospitals, clinics, sanitariums, medical offices, and homes.

This logical study and control of atopic allergy with decreasing use or elimination of corticosteroids and bronchodilating drugs would replace in this way the temporary relief and the too often detrimental results from aerosol adrenergic therapy.

ALLERGY TO STREPTOCOCCI IN MULTIPLE SCLEROSIS*

Because of the good or excellent control and relief of the symptoms of multiple sclerosis (MS) from desensitizing doses of a special streptococcus antigen by vein along with study of food allergy, reported in Chapter 18, the summary of the provocative and excellent report by Rosenow on the possible role of streptococcus in MS is reprinted below.

Summary and Comments

The results of a bacteriologic study of multiple sclerosis made by special methods is reported, and the mechanism by which an infective agent may cause a disease in which the usual manifestations of an infectious etiology are largely lacking is discussed. A green-producing or alpha type of streptococcus was consistently isolated from nasopharynx, tonsils, and infected teeth of patients with definite MS. The cardinal symptoms of this disease were reproduced or closely simulated on appropriate intracerebral inoculation in mice, guinea pigs, rabbits, and monkeys with saline suspensions of the streptococcus obtained directly from the patient with pure cultures of the freshly isolated strains, with strains after twenty or more rapidly repeated subcultures in dextrose brain broth, and with strains after one or more passages through animals.

The "spotty" distribution of the lesions in the white matter of the brain and cord, hemorrhage, edema, demyelinization and infiltration by round cells immediately surrounding blood vessels, and other lesions in relation to vascular beds and their similarity to the early lesions of multiple sclerosis

*As discussed by E. C. Rosenow, 1948.

have been reproduced or simulated. Partial or complete occlusion of vessels by thrombosis or endovascular and perivascular proliferation of or infiltration by lymphocytes and other cells occurred in these experiments quite as these occur in relation to the lesions of multiple sclerosis and the lesions of other diseases of the nervous system.

Lesions of the lungs in rabbits and mice developed not infrequently following inoculation of the streptococcus, which is in accord with the fact that the onset of the disease and especially exacerbations or extensions often follow attacks of influenza or other respiratory infections.

The different strains isolated during the active stage of the disease were agglutinated specifically by the serums of persons stricken by antiserums prepared with closely related streptococci, such as those from encephalitis, and by thermal antibody prepared *in vitro* from streptococci isolated in studies of multiple sclerosis.

Specific streptococcic antigen was demonstrated in skin or blood of persons in the active stage of the disease by intradermal injection of solutions of the respective closely related "natural" and specific streptococcal thermal antibodies, and specific streptococcal antibody was demonstrated by intradermal injection of streptococcal antigen. Cutaneous reactions indicating antigens were greatest during the active stage of the disease, became less marked as active symptoms subsided and as antibodies increased, and both became slight or absent during the quiescent stage.

Intravenous therapeutic injections of histamine and especially of histamine and thermal antibody as given under Dr. Horton's supervision and the thermal antibody and antigen or vaccine without histamine caused a diminution of antigen and an increase in antibody and apparently a concomitant improvement in symptoms in persons during the active stage of multiple sclerosis. A nonspecific and specific means for treatment seem at hand. Regard for the prevention of respiratory infection and for a consideration of foci of infection, especially in teeth and tonsils, is indicated.

The cause of death in animals in which cultures of the brain revealed the streptococcus seemed clear, but in those that died after the streptococcus was no longer isolable from the brain or blood and no longer demonstrable in the lesions simulating in this respect what occurs in multiple sclerosis, the cause of death was obscure. Attempts were made to explain this phenomenon. The evidence adduced indicates that fatalities in the experimental and naturally occurring disease in the absence of living streptococci may be due to the formation of a streptococcic neurotoxin having predilection for vital nerve centers, and to which vital centers become allergic, and perhaps to the formation of an autogenous sensitizing streptococcal-nerve-tissue complex which may function in a manner similar to the wholly foreign adjuvant-nerve-tissue complexes used successfully by others in the production of "allergic" encephalomyelitis.

The possibility of a virus etiology has not been sufficiently studied. The data obtained indicate that a green-producing or alpha streptococcus of low general virulence, having specific localizing, toxicogenic and antigenic properties, is etiologic in multiple sclerosis.

Bibliography

Aas, Kjell: *Studies of Hypersensitivity to Fish.* Universitets-Forlagets Trykneng Ssentaal, Oslo, 1968.

Aas, Kjell, and Elsayed, S.M.: Characterization of a major allergen (Cod). *J Allerg, 44*:333, 1969.

Aas, Kjell, and Jebsen, J.W.: Studies of hypersensitivity to fish. Partial purification and crystallization of a major allergenic component of Cod. *Int Arch Allerg, 32*:1, 1967.

Abramowitz, E.W., and Noun, M.N.: Eczematous dematitis due to exposure to chloral. *J Allerg, 4*:338, 1933.

Abt, I.A.: Asthma in children. *Med Clin N Amer, 1*:1425, 1918.

Ackroyd, J.F.: Allergic purpura, including purpura due to foods, drugs, and infections. *Amer J Med, 14*:605, 1953.

Agar, J.S., and Cazort, A.: Pathologic nasal conditions affecting clinical allergy. *Southern Med J, 32*:1063, 1939.

Albracht, K.: Beitrag zur Therapie des Oedema Fugax (Quincke's). *Deutsch Z Nervenheilk, 47*:833, 1913.

Alderson, V.G.: Personal Verbal Communication. Cited in Rowe, A.H.: *Food Allergy, Its Manifestations, Diagnosis and Treatment.* Philadelphia, Lea and Febiger, 1931, p. 276.

Alexander, H.L.: *Reactions with Drug Therapy.* Philadelphia, Saunders 1955.

Alexander, H.L., and Eyermann, C.H.: Food allergy in Henoch's purpura. *Arch Derm Syph, 16*:322, 1927.

Alexander, H.L., and Eyermann, C.H.: Cited by Graham, E.A., Cole, W. H., Copher, G.H., and Moore, S.: *Diseases of the Gall Bladder and Bile Ducts.* Philadelphia, Lea and Febiger, 1928.

Alexander, H.L., and Eyermann, C.H.: Allergic purpura. *JAMA, 92*:2092, 1929.

Allan, F.N., and Scherer, L.R.: Insulin allergy. *Endocrinology, 16*:417, 1932.

Allan, W.: Relationship of allergy to migraine. *Int Clin, 3*:78, 1935.

Allansmith, M.: Vernal conjunctivitis as an atopic disease. *Calif Med, 95*:163, 1961.

Vernal conjunctivitis. *EENT Digest,* Nov. 1969, p. 37.

Allansmith, M., and Frick, O.L.: Antibodies to grass in vernal catarrh. *J Allerg, 34*:535, 1963.

Allen, T.D., and Seidelman, O.F.: Allergic retrobulbar neuritis. *Illinois Med J, 96*:106, 1949.

al-Mondhiry, H., Marcus, A.J., and Spaet, T.H.: On the mechanism of platelet function inhibition by acetylsalicylic acid. *Proc Soc Exp Biol Med 133*:632, 1970.

Althausen, T.L., Deamer, W.C., and Kerr, W.J.: The false "acute abdomen". II. Henoch's purpura and abdominal allergy. *Ann Surg, 106*: 242, 1937.

Alvarez, W.C.: Food sensitiveness and conditions that may be confused with it. *Med Clin N Amer, 12*:1589, 1929.

Present day treatment of migraine. *Proc Staff Meeting Mayo Clin, 9*:22, 1934.

Pseudocholecystitis apparently caused by food sensitivities. *Proc Staff Meeting Mayo Clin, 9*: 680, 1934.

What is wrong with the patient who feels tired, weak and toxic? *New Eng J Med, 212*:96, 1935.

Ways of discovering foods that are causing indigestion. *Proc Staff Meeting Mayo Clin, 12*: 88, 1937.

A new treatment for migraine. *Proc Staff Meeting, Mayo Clin, 14*:173, 1939.

Violent Reaction to Phenolphthalein. *Calif Med 71*:38, 1949.

Ancona, G.R., Ellenhorn, M.J., and Falconer, E.H.: Purpura due to food sensitivity. *J Allerg, 22*:487, 1951.

Andersen, D.H.: Cystic fibrosis of the pancreas and its relationship to celiac disease. *Amer J Dis Child, 56*:344, 1938.

Andersen, D.H., and di Sant'Agnese, P.A.: *The Celiac Syndrome in Bonnemann's Practice of Pediatrics.* Hagerstown, Prior, 1952, vol. 1, chapt. 29, p. 1.

Anderson, J.M.: Dermatitis from grapes. *Arch Derm Syph, 31*:658, 1935.

Andogsky, A.: Cataracta dermakogenes. *Klin Mbl Augenheilk, 52*:824, 1914.

Andresen, A.F.R.: Discussion of Rowe's article on gastrointestinal allergy. *JAMA, 97*:1444, 1931. Gastro-intestinal manifestations of food allergy. *Med J Rec, 122*:271, 1925.

Andresen, A.F.R.: The treatment of ulcerative colitis. *Med Times, 41*:299, 1933. Migraine, allergic phenomenon. *Amer J Dig Dis, 1*:14, 1934. Gastro-intestinal manifestations of food allergy. *J Med Soc New Jersey, 31*:402, 1934. The surgeon and colonic allergy. *Amer J Surg, 50*:281, 1940. Ulcerative colitis—allergic phenomenon. *Amer J Dig Dis, 9*:91, 1942.

Andresen, A.F.R.: The ulcerative colitis problem. *NY State J Med, 49*:1793, 1949.

Andresen, A.F.R.: Allergy of the gastrointestinal tract. *Rev Gastroenterology, 18*:779, 1951. *Office Gastroenterology.* Philadelphia, Saunders, 1958.

Andrews, G.C.: *Diseases of the Skin: A Textbook for Practitioners and Students.* Philadelphia, Saunders, 1930.

Andrews, G.C., Birkman, F.W., and Kelly, R.J.: Recalcitrant pustular eruptions of palms and soles. *Arch Derm Syph, 29*:548, 1934.

Andrews, G.C., and McNitt, C.W.: Glue sensitivity. *J Allerg, 3*:30, 1931.

Anneberg, A.R.: Corneal reaction due to weed pollen. *Amer J Ophthal, 21*:1265, 1938.

Appelbaum (1940): Cited by Bothman, L.: In *Clinical Manifestations of Allergy in Ophthalmology Year Book of Eye, Ear, Nose and Throat.* Chicago, Year Book Publishers, 1941.

Appelbaum, E., Greenberg, M., and Nelson, J.: Complications following antirabies vaccination. *JAMA, 151*:188, 1953.

Archer, B.H.: Chronic non-specific arthritis, etiology and treatment with special reference to vaccine therapy. *JAMA, 102*:1449, 1934.

Arthur, A.B., Clayton, B.E., Cottom, D.G., Seakins, J.W.T., and Platt, J.W.: Importance of disaccharide intolerance in the treatment of celiac disease. *Lancet, 1*:172, 1966.

Ashby, H.T.: Acute sensitization in infant to cow's milk protein. *Arch Dis Child, 4*:264, 1929.

Ashton, N.: Allergic factors in the etiology of uveitis. *Trans XVIII Int Congr Ophthal, 2*:124, 1955.

Atkinson, M.: Observations on the etiology and treatment of Meniere's syndrome. *JAMA, 116*:1753, 1941.

Auer, John: The influence of systemic changes on local and tissue reactions. *Proc Soc Exp Biol Med, 17*:93, 1919.

Auer, J: Local autogenous inoculation of the sensitized organisms with foreign proteins as a cause of abnormal reaction. *J Exp Med, 32*:427, 1920.

Auer, J.: The functional analysis of anaphylaxis, in George Blumer edition of Billings—Forchheimer's Therapeutics of Internal Diseases, 2:80, 1925.

Auer, J., and Lewis, P.A.: Acute anaphylactic death in guinea pigs. Its cause and prevention; a preliminary note. *JAMA, 53*:458, 1909.

Auer, J., and Lewis, P.A.: Physiology of immediate reaction of anaphylaxis in guinea pigs. *J Exp Med, 12*:151, 1910.

Austen, K.F., and Scheffer, A.L.: Detection of heredity angioneurotic edema by demonstration of a reduction in second component of human complement. *New Eng J Med, 272*:649, 1965.

Austrian, C.R.: Angioneurotic edema, a preliminary report. *Southern Med J. 12*:348, 1919.

Avery, G.B., Villavicencio, O., Lilly, J.R., and Randolph, J.G.: Intractable diarrhea in early infancy. *Pediatrics, 41*:712-722, 1968.

Aviado, D.M., Sadavongvivad, C., and Carrillo, L.R.: Cigarette smoke and pulmonary emphysema. *Arch Environ Health, 20*:483, 1970.

Avit-Scott, J.: A case of orange dermatitis. *Brit J Dermatol, 46*:378, 1934.

Baage, K.H.: Hypersensitiveness to flour as cause of vasomotor rhinitis and asthma. *Ugesk laeger, 95*:513, 1933. Abstr. Mehlidiosynkrasie als Ursache von vasomotorischer Rhinitis und Asthma, *Klin Wschr, 12*:792, 1933. Allergic vasomotor rhinitis in bakers. *Ugesk laeger, 97*:897, 1934.

Babcock, W.W.: Catgut allergy. *Amer J Surg, 27*:67, 1935.

Baer, H.L.: Dermatitis due to aniline dye in food product, report of case. *JAMA, 103*:10, 1934.

Baer, R.L., and Harber, L.C.: Reactions to light, heat, and trauma. In Samter, M. (Ed.): *Immunological diseases.* Boston, Little, Brown, & Co., 1965.

Bailey, L.H.: *Manual of Cultivated Plants.* New York, Macmillan, Rev. Ed., 1949, Tenth Printing 1968.

Baker, H.F.: Incidence of protein sensitization in the normal child. *Amer J Dis Child, 19*:114, 1920.

Balyeat, R.M.: The hereditary factor in allergic diseases. *Amer J Med Sci, 176*:332, 1928.

Perennial hay fever: Diagnosis and treatment, based on the study of 441 cases. *Southern Med J, 22*:492, 1929.

Allergic migraine, based on the study of fifty-five cases. *Amer J Med Sci, 180*:212, 1930.

Migraine: Diagnosis and Treatment. Philadelphia, J.B. Lippincott, 1933.

Complete retinal detachment (both eyes) with special reference to allergy as a possible primary factor. *Amer J Ophthal, 20*:58, 1937.

Complete retinal detachment in both eyes in neuro-dermatitis. *Amer J Ophthal, 20*:550, 1937.

Balyeat, R.M., and Bowen, R.: Cod liver oil sensitivity in children. *Amer J Dis Child, 47*:529, 1934.

Allergic conjunctivitis. *Southern Med J, 28*:1005, 1935.

Balyeat, R.M., and Pounders, C.M.: Pylorospasm due to allergy simulating infantile pyloric stenosis. *Southern Med J. 26*:436, 1933.

Balyeat, R.M., and Rinkel, H.J.: Further studies in allergic migraine: Based on a series of 202 consecutive cases. *Ann Int Med, 5*:713, 1931.

Episcleritis due to allergy. *JAMA, 98*:2054, 1932.

Headaches due to specific hypersensitiveness, history taking an etiology. *Southwestern Med, 16*:5, 1932.

Cited by: Fries, J.H., and Jennings, K.: Recurrent vomiting in children. *J Pediat, 17*:458, 1940.

Banks, B.M., Zetzel, L., and Richter, H.S.: Morbidity and mortality in regional enteritis. Report of 168 cases. *Am J Dig Dis, 14*:369, 1969.

Banyai, A.L.: Bronchial asthma as cause of obstructive emphysema. *Ann Allerg, 23*:457, 1965.

Barach, A.L., and Segal, M.S.: Growing mortality from emphysema and bronchitis. *Ann Allerg, 26*:353, 1968.

Barber, H.W.: Chronic urticaria and angioneurotic edema due to bacterial sensitization. *Guy Hosp Rep, 73*:1, 1923.

Barkan, H.: Ocular angioneurotic edema and glaucoma. *Amer J Ophthal, 2*:800, 1919.

Barnathan, L.: Alimentary Anaphylaxis, Clinical and Experimental Studies, Theses de Paris, 1910-1911.

Barnes, M.H.: Linseed dermatitis. *J Indust Hyg, 13*:49, 1931.

Barrie, H.J., and Anderson, C.J.: Hypertrophy of the pylorus in an adult with massive eosinophil infiltration and giant cell reaction. *Lancet, 2*:1107, 1948.

Barthelme, F.L.: Allergic purpura. *J Allerg, 1*:170, 1929.

Barthelme, F.L. (1930): Cited by Ackroyd, J.F.: Allergic purpura, including purpura due to foods, drugs, and infections. *Amer J Med, 14*:605, 1953.

Bass, Harry, Whitcomb, John F., and Forman, Robert: Exercise training: Therapy for patients with chronic obstructive pulmonary disease. *Chest, 57*:116, 1970.

Bassler, A.: Medical treatment of enteric granulomata (ileitis) and colitis. *Rev Gastroenterol, 5*:150, 1938.

Bassoe, P.: Discussion of Kennedy, F.: *Arch Neurol Psychiat, 15*:28, 1926.

Angioneurotic edema of the brain. *Med Clin N Amer, 16*:409, 1932.

Migraine. *JAMA, 101*:599, 1933.

Bastedo, W.C.: Mucous colitis. *Med Clin N Amer, 1*:675, 1917.

Baum, J.L., and Levene, R.Z.: Corneal thickness after topical corticosteriod therapy. *Arch Ophthal, 79*:366, 1968.

Baxter, W.D., and Levine, R.S.: Evaluation of intermittent positive pressure breathing in prevention of postoperative pulmonary complications. *Arch Surg, 98*:795, 1969.

Bayer, L.M.: Desensitization to insulin allergy. *JAMA, 102*:1934, 1934.

Beck, O.: Histologische Untersuchungen des Siebbeines bei der rhinogenen, retrobubaren Neuritis Optica. *Monat Ohrenh Med Laryng, 57*:893, 1923.

Becker, R.M.: Allergy to penicillinase. *JAMA, 169*:1148, 1959.

Becker, S.W.: Dermatitis associated with neurocirculatory instability; generalized and localized pruritus, neurodermatitis, dyshidrosis, urticaria and anginoneurotic edema, lichen planus, neurotic excoriations, *alopecia areata,* dermatitis *Herpetiformis* and *Scleroderma. Arch Dermat Syph, 25*:655, 1932.

Bedell, A.J.: Stereoscopic fundus photography. *JAMA, 105*:1502, 1935.

Beecher, W.L.: Allergic mucous colitis. *Clin Med Surg,* Aug., 1929.

Beetham, W.P.: Atopic cataracts. *Arch Ophthal, 24*:21, 1941.

Beigelman, M.N.: *Vernal Conjunctivitis*. Los Angeles, Univ. of S. Calif. Press, 1950.

Benjamin, J.E., and Biedermann, J.B.: Agranulocytic leukopenia induced by a drug related to aminopyrine. *JAMA, 107*:493, 1936.

Benson, R.L., and Perlman, F.: Clinical effects of epinephrine by inhalation. *J Allergy, 19*:129, 1948.

Bentolila, L., Ortiz, J.M.V., and Bertotto, E.V.: Allergic cataract. *Ann Allerg, 10*:36, 1952.

Berens: Discussion of Woods, A.C.: *Allergy and Immunity in Ophthalmology*. Baltimore, Johns Hopkins Press, 1933. Cited by Rowe, A.H.: *Clinical Allergy, Manifestations, Diagnosis and Treatment*. Philadelphia, Lea and Febiger, 1937, p. 526.

Berg, Wilhelm: Uber Tieranaphylaxie und Anaphylaktische Migraine. *Klin Wschr, 7-1*:844, 1928.

Berger, A.J., and Eisen, B.: Feasibility of skin testing for penicillin sensitivity. *JAMA, 159*:191, 1955.

Berger, H.: Cause of drug induced thrombocytopenia purpura indentified by passive transfer. *Ann Int Med, 50*:618, 1962.

Berger: Cited by Schloss, O.M.: Allergy in infants and children. *Amer J Dis Child, 19*:433, 1920.

Berneaud, G.: Allergische Augenerkrankungen. *Z Augenheilk, 78*:193, 1932.

Bernoulli, E.: Die Bestimmung der pharmakologischen Wirkungsweise der Digitalis-Präparate. *Cor-Bl f Schweiz Aertze, 40*:896, 1910.

Bernton, H.S., Spies, J.R., and Stevens, H.: Significance of cottonseed sensitiveness. *J Allerg, 11*:138, 1940.

Bettman, J.W.: Allergic retinosis. *Amer J Ophthal, 26*:1323, 1945.

Bettman, Ralph B., and Kobak, Mathew, W.: Relative frequency of evisceration after laporatory in recent years. *JAMA, 172*:1764, 1960.

Bigler, J.: Diarrhea, vomiting and colic in the young infant due to milk allergy. *Pediat Clin N Amer*, May, 503, 1955.

Black, J.H.: Some pressing problems in allergy. *JAMA, 99*:1, 1932.

Black, J.H.: Development of sensitiveness in allergic person; case report. *J Allerg, 4*:24, 1932.

Black, W.C.: Flax hypersensitiveness. *JAMA, 94*:1064, 1930.

Blackfan, K.D.: Cutaneous reactions from proteins in eczema. *Amer J Dis Child, 11*:441, 1916.
A consideration of certain aspects of protein hypersensitiveness in children. *Amer J Med Sci, 160*:341, 1920.

Blackford, J.M., King, R.L., and Sherwood, K.K.: Cholecystitis, study based on follow-up after from five to fifteen years of 200 patients not operated on. *JAMA, 101*:910, 1933.

Blank, P.: Sensitivity to oral administration of castor oil. *Ann Allerg, 3*:296, 1945.

Blankstein, S.S.: Transitory myopia. *Amer J Ophthal, 24*:895, 1941.

Blatt, N.H., and Lepper, M.H.: Reaction following antirabies prophylaxis. *Amer J Dis Child, 86*:395, 1953.

Bleumink, E., and Berrens, L.: Synthetic approaches to the biological activity of beta-lactoglobulin in human allergy to cow's milk. *Nature, 212*:541, 1966.

Bleumink, E., and Young, E.E.: Identification of the atopic allergen in cow's milk. *Int Arch Allerg, 5*:521, 1968.
Studies on the atopic allergen in hen's egg I. Indentification of the skin reactive fraction in egg white. *Int Arch Allerg, 35*:1, 1969.

Bloch, B.: Experimentelle Studien über das Wesen der Jodoformidiosynkrasie. *Ztsch exp Path Therap, 9*:509, 1911.

Blumstein, G.I.: Buckwheat sensitivity. *J Allerg, 7*:74, 1935.

Blumstein, G.I., and Johnson, J: Gastrointestinal allergy simulating regional enteritis. *JAMA, 147*:1441, 1951.

Blumstein, G.I., and Tuft, L.: Allergy treatment in recurrent nasal polyposis: Its importance and value. *Am J Med Sci, 234*:269, 1957.

Bogart, A.H.: The surgical significance of intestinal angioneurotic edema. *Ann Surg, 61*:324, 1915.

Bookman, R.: Allergic parotitis. *Calif Med, 72*:179, 1950.

Booth, B.H., and Patterson, R.: Electrocardiographic changes during human anaphylaxis. *JAMA, 211*:627, 1970.

Bostock, J.: A case of periodical affection of eyes and chest. Read before Medical Society, London, March 16, 1819. Reprint in Coca, A.F., Walzer, M., Thommen, A.: *Asthma and Hay Fever*. Springfield, Charles C Thomas, 1931.

Bothman, L.: Allergic Retinitis: Preretinal Hemorrhage Following Injection of Anti-Tetanic Serum. *Year Book of Eye, Ear, Nose and Throat*. Chicago, Year Book Publishers, 1940, pp. 7-58.
Clinical Manifestations of Allergy in Ophthal-

mology. *Year Book of Eye, Ear, Nose and Throat.* Page 7, The Year Book Publishers, Chicago, 1941.

Bowen, R.: Allergic conjunctivitis. *Southern Med J,* 34:184, 1941.

Bowie, E.J., and Hagedorn, A.B.: Purpura. *Minn Med,* 47:1329, 1964.

Boyden, S.V.: Absorption of proteins on erythrocytes treated with tannic acid and subsequent hemagglutination by antiprotein sera. *J Exp Med,* 93:101, 1951.

Bramigk, F.W.: High rectal pain relieved by elimination and also by "test-free" diets, *Amer J Dig Dis,* 1:899, 1935.

Bray, G.W.: Enuresis of allergic origin. *Arch Dis Child,* 6:251, 1931.
Recent Advances in Allergy. Philadelphia, P. Blakiston's Son, 1934.
Recent advances in the treatment of asthma and hay fever. *Practitioner,* 133:368, 1934.
Some unusual examples of allergic reaction. *Practitioner,* 134:610, 1935.

Brazis: Cited by Larochie, G., Richet, F.C., and Saint Girons, F.: *Alimentary Anaphylaxis,* Transl. by Rowe, U.C. Los Angeles, U. Calif. Press, 1930, French ed., Paris, 1919.

Brem, W.V., Zeiler, A.H., and Hammock, R.W.: Use of fasting donors in blood transfusions: Preliminary report. *Amer J Med Sci,* 175:96, 1928.

Bricker, R.: Cited in Discussion of Kennedy, F.: *J Nerv Ment Dis,* 88:103, 1938.

Briggs, J.: Two-year follow-up study of treatment of asthma with intermittent corticosteriod dose schedule. *Arizona Med,* 25:971, 1968.

Briggs, W.A.: Fulminating pelvic-abdominal edema simulating rupture tubal pregnancy. *JAMA,* 50:528, 1908.

Brille, Denise: In *Bronchitis. An International Symposium, April, 1960.* University of Groningen, Holland. Charles C Thomas, 1961, p. 61.

Brown, A.: Henoch-Schonlein purpura and acute nephritis due to food allergy. *Glasgow Med J,* 27:84, 1946.

Brown, A., and Brown, F.R.: Gastrointestinal allergy. *Med Clin North America,* 26:737, 1942.

Brown, A.L.: Ocular manifestations in serum sickness. *Amer J Ophthal,* 8:614, 1925.

Brown, A.L.: (Cincinnati) Consideration underlying experimental production of uveitis. *Amer J Ophthal,* 15:19, 1932.

Brown, A.L., and Dummer, C.: Experimental iritis

associated with ocular sensitization. *J Med,* 13:238, 1932.

Brown, C.H., and Daffner, J.E.: Regional enteritis. II. Results of medical and surgical treatment in 100 patients. *Ann Int Med,* 49:595, 1958.

Brown, E.A.: The treatment of pollinosis by means of a single annual injection of emulsified extract preparation, standardization and administration. *Ann Allerg,* 17:334, 1959.

Brown, G.T.: Multiple sensitization in bronchial asthma. *JAMA,* 88:1693, 1927.
The treatment of urticaria and angioneurotic edema. *Ann Int Med,* 3:591, 1929.
Cottonseed and kapok sensitization. *JAMA,* 93:5, 1929.
Linseed meal sensitization. *Ann Int Med,* 4:601, 1930.

Brown, H.M., and Fler, J.H.: Role of mites in allergy to housedust. *Brit Med J,* 3:646, 1968.

Brown, H.M., and Wilson, R.N.: Chronic Bronchitis in industry. *Brit Med J,* 1:263, 1959.

Brown, O.H.: Theory, etiology, symptoms and treatment of food sensitization. *Southwest Med,* 12:388, 1928.
Food sensitization and its treatment. *Southwest Med,* 13:210, 1929.
Food allergy. *Southwest Med,* 18:109, 169, 206, 1934.
Allergy: Problem of immunity, digestion, endocrines and metabolism. *Southwest Med,* 20:184, 1936.

Browning, W.H.: Ringworm of extremities due to allergic imbalance. *New Orleans Med Surg J,* 87:747, 1935.

Brunsting, L.A.: Atopic dermatitis of young adults and report of 10 cases with juvenile cataracts. *Arch Dermat Syph,* 34:935, 1936.

Brunsting, L.A., Reed, W.B., and Bair, H.L.: Occurrence of cataracts and keratoconus with atopic dermatitis. *Arch Derm,* 72:237, 1955.

Brunton, T.L.: Poisons formed from food and their relation to biliousness and diarrhea. *Practitioner,* 35:112, 1885.

Bryan, Wm. T.K., and Bryan, Marian P.: The application of *in vitro* cytotoxic reactions to clinical diagnosis of food allergy. *Laryngoscope,* 70:810, 1960.

Buffard, P.: Contribution à l'étude de la valeur de la radiologie dans le diagnostic des affections allergiques à l'intestine grêle. *Lyon med,* 186:18, 19, 1952.

Buffard, P., and Crozet, L.: Zur Dünndarmallergie. *Fortsch Geb Röntgen Ver Röntgenprax,* 76:497, 1952.

Bullock, J.D., and Bodenbender, J.G.: A simple laboratory aid in diagnosing food allergy. *Ann Allerg,* 28:127, 1970.

Bunker, J.P.: Surgical manpower. A comparison of operations and surgeons in the United States and in England and Wales. *New Eng J Med,* 282:135, 1970.

Burchard, H.: Beiträge zum Problem des Säuglingsekzems. *Dermat Ztschr,* 69:149, 1934.

Burk, Alice M., and Bryant, D.J. Precipitating antibodies in asthma: A preliminary communication. *New Zealand Med J,* 72:28, 1970.

Burky, E.L.: Experimental endophthalmitis phacoanaphylactica in rabbits. *Arch Ophthal, 12:* 536, 1934.

Production of lens sensitivity in rabbits by action of staphylococcus toxin. *Proc Soc Exp Biol Med,* 31:445, 1934.

Personal Communication—Cited by Rowe, A.H.: *Clinical Allergy, Manifestations, Diagnosis and Treatment.* Philadelphia, Lea and Febiger, 1937, p. 526.

Burky, E.L., and Woods, A.C.: Lens extract, its preparation and clinical use. *Arch Ophthal, 6:* 548, 1931.

Burrows, B., and Earle, R.H.: Course and prognosis of obstructive lung disease. *New Eng J Med,* 280:308, 1969.

Burton-Fanning, F.W.: Periodic swelling of the salivary glands. *Brit Med J,* 2:517, 1925.

Cade, A., Barral, P., and Roux, J.: L'Anaphylaxie a l'insuline et la pathogénie de certains accidents d'intolérance a l'insuline. *Bull Acad Méd Paris,* 105:575, 1931.

Callaghan, W.C.: Allergic uveitis. *Trans Indiana Acad Ophth Otolaryng,* 38:35, 1955.

Campbell, Berry, and Vogel, Phillip, J.: The allergic mechanisms of multiple sclerosis. *JAMA,* 208:1484, 1969.

Campbell, G.A.: Allergic diseases of childhood. *Canad Med Ass J,* 16:1070, 1926.

Further observation on asthma and eczema with special reference to treatment. *Canad Med Ass J,* 17:1498, 1927.

Campbell, H.B.: Neurological allergy. *Rev Allerg,* 22:80, 1968.

Campbell, J.V.: A report of the toxemias of late pregnancy. *Calif West Med,* 46:226, 1937.

Campbell, M. Brent: Neurological allergy. *Rev Allerg,* 22:80, 1968.

Caplin, Irvin, and Haynes, John T.: Complica-

tions of aerosol therapy in asthma. *Ann Allerg,* 27:65, 1969.

Caputi, S., Sr.: An anaphylactic-type reaction attributed to penicillinase. *New Eng J Med,* 260:432, 1959.

Carr, J.G.: Hypersensitiveness to milk complicating the treatment of duodenal ulcer. *Med Clin North Amer,* 9:1409, 1926.

Casparis, H.: Gastrointestinal allergy in children. *Ann Int Med,* 7:625, 1933.

Caulfeild, A.H.W.: Sensitization and bronchial asthma and hay fever. *JAMA,* 76:1071, 1921. Trypsin and ephedrine dissolved in Gomenol as therapeutic agents in allergic conditions. *Canad Med Ass J,* 20:498, 1929.

Cavanaugh, J.A., and Berman, B.A.: Learning disability, allergy, and hearing loss. Presented at Am Coll Allergists meeting March, 1968.

Cecil, R.L.: Rheumatoid arthritis, a new method of approach to the disease. *JAMA,* 100:1220, 1933.

Chaffee, F.H., and Settipane, G.A.: Asthma caused by F.D. and C. approved dyes. *J Allerg,* 40:65, 1967.

Chambers, J.V.: Heterophile ophthalmic anaphylaxis. *Proc Soc Exp Biol Med,* 30:874, 1933.

Chao, I.T., Wang, W.Y., and Hsu, C.H.: Chronic arthritis associated with erythema and other symptom complex due to sensitivity to common foods. *Chinese Med J,* 11:310, 1964.

Charlier, R.: Therapeutic studies in bronchial asthma with areosol Aleudrin. *Med Times,* 75: 277, 47.

Chen, J.L., Moore, N., Norman, P.S., and Van Metre, T.E., Jr.: Disodium cromoglycate, a new compound for the prevention of exacerbations of asthma. *J Allerg,* 43:89, 1969.

Chernvach, R.M.: Home care of chronic respiratory disease. *JAMA,* 208:821, 1969.

Chiray, M., and Baumann, J.: Colite et Anaphylaxie. *Paris Méd,* 1:299, 1933.

Christian, H.A.: Visceral disturbances in patients with cutaneous lesions of the erythema group. *JAMA,* 69:325, 1917.

Clarke, J.A.: Pulmonary atelectasis as a complication of bronchial asthma. *Arch Int Med,* 45: 624, 1930.

Clarke, T.W.: Epilepsy of allergic origin. *New York J Med,* 34:647, 1934.

Allergic manifestations in the central nervous system. *New York J Med,* 39:1498, 1939.

Neuro-allergy in childhood. *New York J Med,* 48:393, 1948.

Clarke, T.W.: The relation of allergy to character problems in children. *Ann Allerg,* 8:175, 1950.

Clearkin, J.M.: A case of anaphylactic shock due to alimentary absorption. *Lancet,* 205:1080, 1923.

Clein, N.W.: Cow's milk allergy in infants. *Ann Allerg,* 9:195, 1951.

Clifford, S.H.: Iodine hypersensitization. *Boston Med Surg J,* 195:931, 1926.

Cobb, S.: Concerning fits. *Med Clin North Amer,* 19:1583, 1936.

Coca, A.F.: On dialyzability of proteins. *J Immunol,* 19:405, 1930.
Familial Non-reagenic Food Allergy. Springfield, Charles C Thomas, 1943.

Coca, A.F., and Grove, E.F.: A study of atopic reagins. *J Immunol,* 40:455, 1925.

Coca, A.F., Walzer, M., and Thommen, A.A.: *Asthma and Hay Fever in Theory and Practice.* Springfield, Charles C Thomas, 1931.

Cohen, A.E.: Allergy. *Kentucky Med J,* 31:206, 1933.
Bronchial asthma and other allergic conditions. *Kentucky Med J,* 32:209, 1934.

Cohen, M.B.: Pruritis of anaphylactic origin. *JAMA,* 76:377, 1921.

Cohen, M.B.: Hay fever, asthma and other allergic diseases. *Kentucky Med J,* 29:319, 1931.

Cohen, M.B., and Breitbart, J.: Infantile pyloric obstruction. *Amer J Dis Child,* 38:741, 1929.

Cohen, S. S.: On some angioneural arthrosis (periarthroses parthroses) commonly mistaken for gout or rheumatism. *Amer J Med Sci,* 147:228, 1914.

Cohen, S.G.: Immune sera in the study of food antigens. *J Allerg,* 30:250, 1959.

Cohen, V.L., and Osgood, H.: Disability due to inhalation of grain dust. *J Allerg,* 24:193, 1953.

Coke, F.: Sensitization to wheat. *Practitioner,* 129:408, 1932.
Asthma. Wm. Wood & Co., New York.

Coleman, M.: Silk antigen as a contaminant in biological agents from silk filters. *J Allerg,* 28:494, 1957.

Coles, Robert S.: *Ocular Allergy.* Baltimore, Williams and Wilkins, 1958.

Colldahl, H.: Allergy and certain diseases in relation to the digestive tract—some observations on the effect of elimination diets. *Acta Allerg,* 84:20, 1965.

Collens, W.S., Lerner, G., and Fialka, S.M.: Insulin allergy, treatment with histamine. *Amer J Med Sci,* 188:528, 1934.

Collins, E.M., and Pritchett, C.P.: Allergy as a factor in disturbances of the gastrointestinal tract. *Med Clin N. Amer,* 22:417, 1938.

Collins, V.J.: Inhalation therapy education and training progress—a medical specialty. *JAMA,* 207:329, 1969.

Collins-Williams, C.: Acute allergic reactions to cow's milk. *Ann Allerg,* 13:415, 1955.

Collins-Williams, C.: The incidence of milk allergy in pediatric practice. *J Pediat,* 48:39, 1956.

Collins-Williams, C., and Ebbs, J.H.: The use of protein skin tests in the celiac syndrome. *Ann Allerg,* 12:237, 1954.

Collins-Williams, and Vincent, J.: Sensitivity reactions to penicillin in children. *Ann Allerg,* 11:454, 1953.

Colmes, A., Guild, T., and Rackemann, F.M.: Influence of occupation on sensitization in man as determined in a study of 32 bakers. *J Allerg,* 6:539, 1935.

Conlin, F.A.: Conjunctivitis due to food anaphylaxis. *Amer J Ophthal,* 2:486, 1919.

Conway, D.J.: A congenital factor in bronchiectasis. *Arch Dis Child,* 26:253, 1951.

Cooke, R.A.: Protein sensitization in the human with special reference to bronchial asthma and hay fever. *Med Clin N Amer,* 1:721, 1917.
Hay fever and asthma: The uses and limitations of desensitization. *New York J Med,* 107:577, 1918.
Cutaneous reactions in human hypersensitiveness, *Proc New York Path Soc,* 21:1, 1921.
Delayed type of allergic reactions. *Ann Int Med,* 3:658, 1929-1930.
On the constitutional reactions, dangers of the diagnostic cutaneous tests and therapeutic injections of allergens. *J Immunol,* 7:119, 1922.
Gastrointestinal manifestations of allergy. *Bull Ny Acad Med,* 9:15, 1933.
Allergy in clinical medicine. *New Jersey Med Soc J,* 32:15, 1935.
Protein derivatives as factors in allergy. *Ann Int Med,* 16:71, 1942.
Allergy in Theory and Practice, Philadelphia, Saunders, 1947.

Cooke, R.A., and Stull, A.: Preparation and standardization of pollen extracts for treatment of hay fever. *J Allerg,* 4:87, 1933.

Cooke, R.A., and Vander Veer, A.: Human sensitization. *J Immunol,* 1:201, 1916.

Cordes, F.C., and Cordero-Moreno, R.: Atopic cataracts. *Amer J Ophthal*, 29:402, 1946.

Cormia, F.E.: Urinary proteose, allergic dermatoses and eczema-asthma-hay fever complex. *Arch Dermat Syph*, 27:745, 1933.

Cornbleet, T., and Kaplan, M.A.: Urinary proteose in eczema. *Arch Dermat Syph*, 30:497, 1934.

Corper, F.J.: Protein sensitivity in infantile eczema. *Amer J Dis Child*, 29:355, 1925.

Courtney, R.H.: Endophthalmitis phacoanaphylactica with secondary glaucoma; Case. *Amer J Ophthal*, 16:530, 1933.

Cowan, A., and Klauder, J.V.: Frequency of occurrence of cataract in atopic dermatitis. *Arch Ophthal*, 43:759, 1950.

Crawford, W.L.: Allergic diseases in childhood. *Illinois Med J*, 66:534, 1934.

Creazzo, A.: Pathogenesis of gastro-duodenal ulcer; role of anaphylaxis; frequency and significance in patients. *Policlinico*, 42:870, 1935.

Criep, L.H.: Electrocardiographic studies of effect of anaphylaxis on cardiac mechanism. *Arch Int Med*, 48:1098, 1931.

Criep, L.H.: Allergy to pancreatic tissue extract. *J Allerg*, 12:154, 1940.
Cited by Bothman, L.: Clinical Manifestations of Allergy, in Ophthalmology. *Year Book of Eye, Ear, Nose and Throat*. Chicago, Year Book Publishers, 1941.
Allergy in identical twins. *J Allerg*, 13:591, 1942.
Allergy of Joints. *J Bone Joint Surg*, 28:276, 1946.

Criep, L.H., and Friedman, H.: Allergy to penicillin. *New Eng J Med*, 263:891, 1960.

Criep, L.H., and Ribiero, C de C: Procaine allergy., *JAMA*, 151:1185, 1953.

Crispin, E.L.: Visceral crises in angioneurotic edema. *Collected Papers of the Mayo Clinic*, 8:823, 1915.

Critchley, M., and Ferguson, F.R.: Migraine. *Lancet*, 123:182, 1933.

Crohn, B.H., and Yarnis, H.: *Regional Enteritis*, 2nd ed., New York, Greene & Stratton, 1958.

Crowther, C., and Raistreck, H.: Comparative study of proteins of colostrum and milk of cow and their relations to serum proteins *Biochem J*, 10:434, 1916.

Culmone, G.: Anafilassi ed ulcera dello stomaco. *Policlinico* [Chir], 40:297, 1933.

Cursch, Ann, H.: Zur Frage der Allergischen Migraine. *Nervenarzt*, 4:71, 1931.

Curtis, J.K., Liska, A.R., Rasmussen, H.K., and Cree, E.M.: IPPB therapy in chronic obstructive pulmonary disease. *JAMA*, 206:1037, 1968.

Curtis-Brown, R.: The protein of foodstuffs as a factor in the cause of headache. *Wisconsin Med J*, 19:337, 1920.
Protein poison theory: Its application to the treatment of headache and especially migraine. *Brit Med J*, 1:155, 1925.

Cutler, O.I.: Antigenic properties of evaporated milk. *JAMA*, 92:964, 1929.

Czerny: Cited by Schultz, S.W., and Larsen, W.T.: Anaphylaxis and its relation to some diatheses common to infancy and childhood. *Arch Pediat*, 35:705, 1918.

Dain, D.W., Randall, J.L., and Smith, J.W.: Starch in the lungs of newborns following positive pressure ventilation. *Am J Dis Child*, 119:218, 1970.

Daniel R.K.: Allergy and cataracts. *JAMA*, 105:481, 1935.

Danysz, J.: Origine, évolution, et traitement des malades chroniques non contagieuses, théorie de l'immunité, de l'anaphylaxie et de l'antianaphylaxie. Baillière, 1920.

Darling, R.C., di Sant'Agnese, P.A., Perera, G.A., and Andersen, D.H.: Electrolyte abnormalities of the sweat in fibrocystic disease of the pancreas. *Am J Med Sci*, 225:67, 1953.

Dattner, B.: Ueber nervose erschneinungen alimentarer Ueberempfindlichkeit. *Nervenarzt*, 4:573, 1931.

Davidoff, L.M., and Kopeloff, N.: Local cerebral anaphylaxis in the dog. *Proc Soc Exp Biol Med*, 31:980, 1934.

Davidson, M.T.: Case of urticaria due to insulin sensitization. *J Allerg*, 4:74, 1932.
Insulin allergy, review of recent literature and report of case. *J Allerg*, 6:71, 1934.

Davidson, M., and Burnstein, R.: Steatorrhea related to a factor in cow's milk. *Amer J Dis Child*, 93:45, 1957.

Davis, C.M.: Self selection of diet by newly weaned infants: Experimental study. *Amer J Dis Child*, 36:561, 1928.

Davis, D.M.: Allergy in relation to the urogenital tract. *Southwest Med*, 18:9, 1934.

Davis, Ruth, S.: Personal verbal communication.

Davis, S.D., Bierman, C.W., Pierson, W.E., *et al.*: Clinical nonspecificity of milk coproantibodies in diarrheal stools. *N Engl J Med*, 282:612, 1970.

Davis, W.T.: The relation of the eye and certain skin diseases. *Southern Med J.* 14:237, 1921.

Davis: Cited by Drysdale, H.H.: Acute circumscribed edema. *JAMA,* 89:1390, 1927.

Davison, H.M.: Cerebral allergy. *Southern Med Ass J,* 42:712, 1949.
Allergy of the nervous system. *Quart Rev Allerg,* 6:157, 1952.

Davison, H.M., and Thoroughman, J.C.: Cardiovascular allergy, *Southern Med J,* 36:560, 1945.

Dawson, W.T., and Newman, S.P.: Acquired allergic coryzal reaction to quinine, but not to quinidine or quitenine. *JAMA,* 97:930, 1931.

Dean, A.M., Dean, F.W., and McCutcheon, G.R.: Interstitial keratitis caused by specific sensitivity to ingested foods. *Arch Ophthal,* 38:48, 1940.

Dean, L.W.: Laboratory investigations as aids in otolaryngological diagnoses. *JAMA,* 99:542, 1932.
Discussion. *Arch Otolaryng,* 19:142, 1934.

De Besche, A.: Studies on the reactions of asthmatics and on passive transference of hypersusceptibility. *Amer J Med Sci,* 66:265, 1923.

Dederding, D.: Drei Falle von Gehorsbesserung nach diuretischer Behandlung bei schwehörigen Syphilitikern. *Arch Ohr Nas Kehlkopfheilk,* 126:117, 1930.

Dees, S.C.: Asthma in Infants and young children. *JAMA,* 175:365, 1961.

Dees, S.C., and Lowenbach, H.: Allergic epilepsy. *Ann Allerg,* 9:446, 1951.

Dees, S.C., and Simmons, E.C.: Allergy of the urinary tract. *Ann Allerg,* 9:714, 1951.

De Gowin, E.L.: Allergic migraine, review of 70 cases. *J Allerg,* 3:557, 1932.

de Loeper: Cited by Chiray, M., and Baumann, J.: Colite et Anaphylaxie. *Paris Méd,* 1:299, 1933.

Demel, A.C.: La teoria anafilattica dell'ulcera rotunda. *Pathologica,* 15:128, 1923.

Dennis, J.L., Palmer, M., and Cleveland, R.W.: Bronchiolitis in infants. *JAMA,* 172:688, 1960.

Deraney, M.F.: A periodic syndrome due to milk hypersensitivity. *Ann Allerg,* 25:332, 1967.

Derbes, V.J., Dent, G.H., and White, R., Jr.: Intrinsic (non-allergic) bronchial asthma as a manifestation of fibrocystic disease of the pancreas. *J Allerg,* 28:287, 1957.

Derlachi, E.L.: Allergy and otology. *Ann Allerg,* 23:288. 1965.

De Veer, J.A.: Bilateral endophthalmitis phacoanaphylactica; pathologic study of the lesion in eye first involved and, in one instance, the secondarily implicated, or "sympathizing," eye. *Arch Ophthal,* 49:607, 1954.

Diamond, J.S.: Liver function in migraine, with report of 35 cases. *Amer J Med Sci,* 174:695, 1927.

Diamond, J. (1936): Cited by Ackroyd, J.F.: Allergic purpura, including purpura due to foods, drugs and infections. *Amer J Med,* 14:605, 1953.

Dickey, L.B.: Kartagener's syndrome in children. *Dis Chest,* 33:657, 1953.

Diethelm, Hans: Uber Akutes Universelles Angioneurotisches Odem. Inaug. Diss., Zurich, 1905.

Diner, W.C., Kniker, W.T., and Heiner, D.C.: Roentgenologic manifestations in the lungs in milk allergy. *Radiology,* 77:564, 1961.

di Sant'Agnese, P., Darling, R.C., Perara, G.A., and Shea, A.: Abnormal electrolyte composition of sweat in cystic fibrosis of the pancreas. *Am J Dis Child,* 86:618, 1953.

Donnolly, H.H.: The question of the elimination of foreign protein (egg-white) in woman's milk. *J Allerg* (Abstr.), 1:78, 1929.
The question of the elimination of foreign protein (egg-white) in woman's milk. *J Immun,* 19:1, 1930.

Dorst, S.E., and Hopphan, E: Angioneurotic edema: Its relation to bacterial hypersensitivity. *J Lab Clin Med,* 18:7, 1932.

Dowling, G.B.: Allergy in relation to diseases of the skin. *Practitioner,* 134:610, 1935.

Doyle, J.B.: Neurologic complications of serum sickness. *Amer J Med Sci,* 185:484, 1933.

Drueck, C.J.: Pruritus ani and perinei (with reference to food allergy). *Urol Cutan Rev,* 39:490, 1935.

Drusin, Lewis, Engle, M., Allen, Mary, Hagstrom, W.C., and Schwartz, M.S.: The postpericardiotomy syndrome. *New Eng J Med,* 12:272, 598, 1965.

Drysdale, H.H.: Acute circumscribed edema. *JAMA,* 89:1390, 1927.

Dubo, S., McLean, J.A., Ching, A.Y., Wright, H. L., Kauffman, P.E., and Sheldon, J.M.: A study of relationships between family situation bronchial asthma and personal adjustment in children. *J Pediat,* 59:402, 1961.

Duke, W.W.: Food allergy as a cause of abdominal pain. *Arch Int Med, 28:*151, 1921.

Food allergy as a cause of bladder pain. *Ann Clin Med, 1:*117, 1922.

Food allergy as a cause of irritable bladder. *New York Med J, 114:*505, 1922.

Specific hypersensitiveness as a common cause of illness. *JAMA, Ann Clin Med, 1:*178, 1922.

Ménière's syndrome caused by allergy. *JAMA, 81:*2179, 1923.

Food allergy as a cause of illness. *JAMA, 81:* 886, 1923.

Chronic illness often due to common articles of a diet. *Arch Int Med, 32:*298, 1923.

Urticaria caused specifically by action of physical agents (light, cold, heat, freezing, burns, mechanical irritation and physical and mental exertion). *JAMA, 83:*349, 1924.

Soy bean as possible important source of allergy. *J Allerg, 5:*300, 1924.

Allergy, Asthma, Hay Fever, Urticaria and Other Manifestations of Allergy. St. Louis, C. V. Mosby, 1925.

Mental and neurological reactions of the asthma patient. *J Lab Clin Med, 13:*20, 1927.

Allergy as cause of gastro-intestinal disorder. *Southern Med J, 24:*363, 1931.

Also *Amer J Surg, 12:*249, 1931.

Clinical manifestations of heat and effort sensitiveness and cold sensitiveness (relationship to heat prostration, effort syndrome, asthma, urticaria, dermatoses, non-infectious coryza and infections). *J Allerg, 3:*257, 1932.

Also *Arch Int Med, 45:*206, 1930.

And *J Allerg, 3:*408, 1932.

Wheat millers asthma. *J Allerg, 6:*568, 1935.

Dunlap, H.F., and Lemon, W.S.: Hereditary type of angioneurotic edema. *Amer J Med Sci, 177:* 259, 1929.

Dutta, P.C.: Allergy and dysmenorrhea. *J Obstet Gynec Brit Comm, 42:*309, 1935.

Dutton, L.O.: The place of allergy in modern medicine. *Southwest Med, 18:*5, 1934.

Drinking water as a cause of eczema. *J Allerg, 6:*477, 1935.

Personal Communication. Cited by Rowe, A.H.: *Clinical Allergy, Manifestations, Diagnosis and Treatment.* Philadelphia, Lea and Febiger, 1937.

Edwards, E.G.: Transient synovitis of the hip joint in children. *JAMA, 148:*30, 1952.

Edwards, Walton M., 1st Lt. M.C., and Helming, Oscar, 1st Lt., M.C.: A case of severe allergy to pea. *J Allerg, 13:*420, 1942.

Efron, B.G.: Gastro-intestinal manifestations in allergy. *New Orleans Med Surg J, 84:*540, 1932.

Eggleston, E.S.: Colitis, spastic type. *JAMA, 91:* 2049, 1928.

Eiselsberg, K.P.: Gaelenkoliken auf nutritiv-allergischer Grundlage, ihre Diagnostik und Spezifische Therapie. *Klin Wschr, 12:*1174, 1933.

Angina pectoris und allergie. *Klin Wschr, 13:* 619, 1934.

Eisenstaedt, J.S.: Allergy and drug hypersensitivity of the urinary tract. *J Urol, 65:*154, 1951.

Elia, J.C.: The dizzy patient. Springfield, Charles C Thomas, 1968.

Elliott, F.A.: Treatment of herpes zoster with high doses of prednisone. *Lancet, 2:*610, 1964.

Elliot, R.W.: Subcutaneous and pneumothorax in bronchial asthma. *Lancet, 1:*1104, 1928.

Ellis, R.V.: Rational grouping of food allergens. *J Allerg, 2:*246, 1931.

Elschnig, A.: Studien zur sympathischen Ophthalmie. II. Die antigenische Wirkung des Augenpigmentes der Augenpigmenten. *Arch Ophthal, 76:*509, 1910.

Cited by Coles, Robt. S.: *Ocular Allergy,* Baltimore, Williams and Wilkins, 1958.

Studien zur sympathischen Ophthalmie: III. Grafe. *Arch Ophthal, 78:*549, 1911.

Emery, E.S.: Disordered function of the colon. *Med Clin North Amer, 8:*1765, 1925.

Emirgil, C., Sobol, B.J., Norman, J., Moskowitz, E., Goyal, P., and Wadhwani, B.: A study of the long-term effect of therapy in chronic obstructive pulmonary disease. *Am J Med, 47:*367, 1969.

Emmett, J.L., and Logan, A.H.: Urticaria of 17 years' duration: Report of case treated successfully, *JAMA, 101:*1966, 1933.

Engman, M.F., and Wander, W.G.: The Application of cutaneous sensitization to diseases of the skin. *Arch Dermatol Syph, 3:*223, 1921.

Eyermann, C.H.: X-ray demonstration of colonic reactions to food allergy. *Missouri State Med Ass, 24:*129, 1927.

Food allergy as a cause of nasal symptoms. *JAMA, 91:*312, 1928.

The diagnosis of allergy. *Missouri State Med Ass, 26:*481, 1929.

Food allergy and nasal symptoms. *J Allerg, 1:* 350, 1930.

Allergic headache, *J Allerg, 2:*106, 1931.

Allergic purpura. *Southern Med J, 28:*341, 1935.

Eyermann, C.H., and Strauss, A.E.: Malarial urticaria and allergy. *J Allerg*, 1:130, 1929.

Fagerhol, M.K., and Hauge, H.E.: Serum PI types in patients with pulmonary diseases. *Acta Allerg (Copenhagen)*, 24:107, 1969.

Fällström, S.P., Winberg, J., and Anderson, H.J.: Cow's milk induced malabsorption as a precursor of gluten intolerance. *Acta Paediat Scand*, 54:101, 1965.

Farber, S.: Some organic digestive disturbances in early life. *J Mich Med Soc*, 44:587, 1945.

Farrington, J.: Modifications of the Goldman technique for contact testing of the buccal mucosa. *J Invest Derm*, 8:59, 1947.

Faulkner, W.B., Jr., and Wagner, R.I.: Fatal spontaneous pneumothorax and subcutaneous emphysema in an asthmatic. *J Allerg*, 8:267, 1937.

Fein, B.T.: Repeated rib fractures by cough in bronchial asthma. *J Allerg*, 29:209, 1958.

Fein, B.T., and Kamin, P.B.: Allergy, convulsive disorders, and epilepsy. *Ann Allerg*, 26:241, 1968.

Feinberg, S.M.: *Allergy in General Practice*. Philadelphia, Lea and Febiger, 1934.

Feinberg, S.M., and Avies, P.L.: Asthma from food odors. *JAMA*, 98:2280, 1932.

Feingen, George A., and Prager, Denis, J.: Experimental cardiac anaphylaxis. *Amer J Cardiol*, 24:474, 1969.

Fenster, E.: Ileitis ulcerosa. *Burns Beitr Klin Chir*, 164:462, 1936.

Fenwick, *et al.*: *The Health of the Child of School Age*. New York, Oxford Press, p. 76.

Ferguson, L.K.: Concepts in the surgical treatment of regional enteritis. *New Eng J Med*, 264:748, 1961.

Ferraro, A.: Pathology of demyelinating diseases as an allergic reaction of the brain. *Arch Neur Psychiat*, 52:443, 1944.

Field, C.E.: Bronchiectasis in childhood. I. A. clinical survey of 160 cases. *Pediatrics*, 4:21, 1949.
Bronchiectasis in childhood. II. Aetiology and pathogenesis, including a survey of 272 cases of doubtful irreversible bronchiectasis. *Pediatrics*, 4:231, 1949.
Bronchiectasis in childhood. III. Prophylaxis, treatment and progress with a follow-up study of 202 cases of established bronchiectasis. *Pediatrics*, 4:355, 1949.

Fielding-Reid, F.: Allergic manifestation to insulin (letter). *JAMA*, 98:1320, 1932.

Figley, K.D.: Food allergy. *Ohio State Med J*, 28:848, 1932.

Fincher, E.F., and Dowman, C.E.: Epileptiform seizures of Jacksonian character: Analysis of 130 cases. *JAMA*, 97:1375, 1931.

Finder, J.G.: Transient synovitis of the hip joint in children. *JAMA*, 107:3, 1936.

Finizio (1911): Cited by Laroche, G., Richet, Fils. C., and Saint Girons, F.: *Alimentary Anaphylaxis*. Transl. by Rowe, U.C. Press, 1930, French ed., Paris, 1919.

Fink, A.I.: Cincophen poisoning in allergic individuals: Report of 2 cases. *J Allerg*, 1:280, 1930.

Finkelstein, L.O. (1905): Cited by Laroche, G., Richet, Fils. C., and Saint Girons, F.: *Alimentary Anaphylaxis*. Transl. by Rowe, U. C. Press, 1930, French ed., Paris, 1919.

Finkelstein, L.O.: Mohnmilch as Säuglingsnahrung. *Z. Kinderheilk*, 48:522, 1930.

Fishberg, A.M.: Anatomical findings in essential hypertension. *Arch Int Med*, 35:650, 1925.

Fisher, A.A.: Allergic sensitization of the skin and oral mucosa to acrylic denture materials. *JAMA*, 156:238, 1954.

Fitzsimmons, J.S.: Uncommon complication of anaphylactoid purpura. *Brit Med J*, 41:431, 1968.

Flatz, G., Saengudom, C.H., and Sanguanbhok, Hai T.: Lactose intolerance in Thailand. *Nature*, 221:758, 1969.

Fletcher, A.A.: Dietetic treatment of chronic arthritis and its relationship to the sugar tolerance. *Arch Int Med*, 30:106, 1922.
Nutritional aspects of chronic arthritis. *Med J Rec*, 138:363, 1933.

Fletcher, A.A., and Graham, D.: Large bowel in chronic arthritis. *Amer J Med Sci*, 179:91, 1930.
Also: *Trans Ass Amer Physicians*, 44:231, 1929.

Fletcher, C.M.: Chronic bronchitis: Its prevalence, nature and pathogenesis. *Amer Rev Resp Dis*, 80:483, 1959.

Floyer, Sir John: Treatise on Asthma. London. (1698).

Fontana, V.J.: Steroid therapy in childhood asthma. *Clin Pediat*, 7:439, 1968.

Fontana, V.J., Fort, A.F., and Brown, E.: Corticosteroid therapy in asthma. *J Allerg*, 41:58, 1968.

Fontana, V.J., Spain, W.C., and Desanctis, A.G.:

The role of allergy in nephrosis. *New York J Med,* 56:3007, 1956.
Practical Management of the Allergic Child. Appleton-Century-Crofts, Meredith Corporation, New York, 1969.

Ford, R. Muro: Corticosteroids in the treatment of chronic asthma. *Med J Australia,* 1:508, 1968.

Forman, J.: Migraine-like headache due to allergy. *Ohio State Med J,* 29:28, 1933, Atopy as cause of epilepsy. *Arch Neurol Psychiat,* 32:517, 1934.

Foubert, E.L., and Stier, R.A.: Antigenic relationships between bees, wasps, hornets and yellow jackets. *J Allerg,* 29:1, 1958.

Francis, R.S., and Spicer, C.C.: Chemo-therapy in chronic bronchitis. *Brit Med J,* 1:297, 1960.

Frankland, Dr.: St. Mary's Hospital, London, England. Personal Reference.

Frantz, A.: Discussion of Kennedy, F.: *J. Nerv Ment Dis,* 88:98, 1938.

Frazer, A.C., Fletcher, R.F., Ross, C.A.C., Shaw, B., Sammon, H.G., and Schneider, R.: Gluten-induced enteropathy. The effect of partially digested gluten. *Lancet,* 2:252, 1959.

Freeman, J.: Toxic idiopathies: The relation between hay fever and other pollen fevers, animal asthmas, food idiosyncrasies, bronchial and spasmodic asthmas. *Lancet,* 199:229, 1920.
Grass pollen antigen for hay fever desensitization. *Lancet,* 573:630, 1933.

Frick, O.L.: Hemagglutination in sera from egg-sensitive individuals. *Ann Allerg,* 20:794, 1962.

Friedenwald, J.S.: Allergy theory of sympathetic ophthalmia. *Amer J Ophthal,* 17:1008, 1934.

Friedenwald, J., and Morrison, S.: Food Allergy and Its Relation to Gastrointestinal Disorders. *Amer J Dig Dis,* 1:100, 1934.

Friedlaender, S., and Feinberg, S.M.: Aspirin allergy; its relationship to chronic intractable asthma. *Ann Int Med,* 26:734, 1947.

Friedman, H.J., Bowman, K., et al.: Severe allergic reaction caused by silk as a contaminant in typhoid-paratyphoid vaccine. *J Allerg,* 28:489, 1957.

Friedman, T.B., and Molony, C.J.: Role of allergy in atelectasis in children. *Amer J Dis Child,* 58:237, 1939.

Fries, J.H.: Roentgen studies of allergic children with disturbances of pylorus resulting from food allergy. *J Allerg,* 23:39, 1952.

Fries, J.H., Borne, S., and Barnes, H.L.: Varicelliform eruption of Kaposi due to vaccinia virus complicating atopic eczema. *J Pediat, 32:*532, 1948.

Fries, J.H., and Jennings, K: Recurrent vomiting in children. *J Pediat,* 17:458, 1940.

Fries, J.H., Mogil, M.: Roentgen observations on children with gastro-intestinal allergy to foods. *J Allerg,* 14:310, 1942.

Fritz, M.H., Thygeson, Phillips, and Durham, D.G.: Phylyctenular keratoconjunctivitis among Alaskan natives. *Amer J Ophthal, 34:*177, 1951.

Frost, L.C.: A case of intense food anaphylaxis. *Med Rec,* 88:483, 1915.

Frumess, G.M.: Allergic reaction to dinitrophenol; report of case. *JAMA,* 102:1219, 1934.

Fry, L., McMinn, R.M., Cowan, J.D., et al.: Gluten-free diet and reintroduction of gluten in dermatitis herpetiformis. *Arch Derm, 100:*129, 1969.

Fuchs, A., (1895): Cited by Bothman, L.: Clinical Manifestations of Allergy in Ophthalmology, *Year Book of Eye, Ear, Nose and Throat.* Chicago, Year Book Publishers, 1941.

Fukushima, I., Kuroume, T., and Matsumura, T.: Examination of several conditions on the provocative test with causative food. *Jap J Allerg,* 16:866, 1967.
Significance of food allergy in the etiology of orthostatic albuminuria found in "healthy" school children. *Jap J Allerg,* 16:609, 1967.

Funck, C.: Allergy in hypertension and arteriosclerosis (Abstr.). *JAMA,* 39:249, 1926.
Regarding allergic factor in hypertonic and arteriosclerotic diseases. *Arch Veranderungsk,* 39:249, 1926.

Fustenberg, A.C., Lashmet, F.H., and Lathrop, F.: Ménière's symptom complex: Medical treatment. *Ann Otol,* 43:1033, 1934.

Gairdner, D.: The Schönlein-Henoch syndrome (anaphylactoid purpura). *Quart J Med, 17:*95, 1948.

Gallerani, G.: Fenomeni allergici per alimentazione lattea: amaurosi transitoria da Scotoma scintillanti, e cardiopalmo accessionale. *Ann Ottal,* 60:249, 1932.
Cited by Theodore and Schlossman: *Ocular Allergy,* Baltimore, Williams and Wilkins, 1958.

Galloway, J. (1903): Cited by Ackroyd, J.F.: Allergic purpura including purpura due to foods, drugs and infections. *Amer J Med, 14*: 605, 1935.

Gandevia, B.: The changing pattern of mortality from asthma in Australia. *Med J Austral, 1*: 747, 1968.

Gary, N.E., Mazzara, J.T., and Holfelder, L.: The Schönlein-Henoch syndrome. *Ann Int Med, 72*:229, 1970.

Garot, L.: Néphrite Chronique Hypertensive Avec Hypotrophie Migraines, Crises abdominales douloureuses et éclampsie mortelle chez une fillette du huit ans et demi. *Arch Med Enf, 38*:91, 1935.
Also *Liege Med, 28*:297, 1935.

Garver, W.P.: The transference of reagins in blood transfusions. *J Allerg, 11*:32, 1939.

Gault, (1933): Cited by Bothman, L.: Clinical Manifestations of Allergy in Ophthalmology. *Year Book of Eye, Ear, Nose and Throat.* Chicago, Year Book Publishers, 1941.

Gay, L.N.: Treatment of hay fever and pollen asthma by air-conditioned atmosphere. *JAMA, 100*:1382, 1933.

Gay, L.N.: *The Diagnosis and Treatment of Bronchial Asthma.* Baltimore, Williams and Wilkins, 1946.

Gay, L.P.: Personal verbal communication.
Allergy in internal medicine: The acute allergic abdomen. *J Missouri MA, 31*:385, 1934.
Gastrointestinal allergy: The duodenal ulcer syndrome. *Southern Med J, 28*:1153, 1935.
Mucous colitis complicated by colonic polyposis relieved by allergic management: Report of instance. *Amer J Dig Dis, 3*:326, 1936.
Food allergy as a factor in habitual hyperthermia. *J. Allerg, 8*:412, 1936.
Gastrointestinal allergy. *JAMA, 106*:969, 1936.

Gehring, J.H.: Macular edema following cataract extraction. *Arch Ophthal, 80*:626, 1968.

Gelfand, H.H.: Allergenic properties of vegetable gums: Case of asthma due to tragacanth. *J Allerg, 14*:203, 1943.

Gerlach, F.: Treatment of angioneurotic edema. *Med Klinik, 19*:1198, 1923.

Gerlach, F., and Kappis, M.: Hemoclastic crisis. *Med Klinik, 20*:1031, 1924.

Gerrard, J.W.: Familial recurrent rhinorrhea and bronchitis due to cow's milk. *JAMA, 198*:605, 1966.
Personal communication.

Gerrard, J.W., Heiner, O.C., Ives, E.J., and

Hardy, L.W.: Milk allergy, recognition, natural history, Management. *Clin Pediat, 2*: 634, 1963.

Gerrard, J.W., and Lubos, M.C.: The malabsorption syndrome. *Pediat Clin N Amer, 14*:73, 1967.

Gerrard, J.W., Lubos, M.C., Hardy, L.W., Holmlund, B.E., and Webster, D.: Milk allergy: Clinical picture and familial incidence. *Canad Med Ass J, 97*:780, 1967.

Gerson, M.: (Letter) from "Dr. Gerson's address on diet therapy" (salt-free and protein low diet in T.B., dermatoses, asthma, migraine, etc.). *JAMA, 98*:1829, 1932.

Gill: Cited by Zerfoss, K.S.: The relation of allergy to ophthalmology. *Tennessee Med Ass J, 28*:93, 1935.

Glaser, J. (1937): Cited by Fries, J.H., and Jennings, K.: Recurrent vomiting in children. *J. Pediat, 17*:458, 1940.

Glaser, J.: *Allergy in Childhood.* Springfield, Charles C Thomas, 1956.

Glaser, J.: Dietary prophylaxis of allergic disease in infancy. *J Asthma Res, 3*:199, 1966.

Glaser, J., and Lerner, M.L.: Cyclic vomiting of ocular origin. *Amer J Dis Child, 53*:1237, 1937.

Golden, Ross: *Radiologic Examination of the Small Intestine.* Philadelphia, J.B. Lippincott, 1945.

Goldman, A.S., Anderson, D.W., Sellers, W.A., et al.: Oral challenge with milk and isolated proteins in allergic children. *Pediatrics, 32*: 425, 1963.

Goldman, A.S., Sellers, W.A., Halpern, S.R., Anderson, D.W., Furlow, T.E., Johnson, C.H., and collaborators: Milk Allergy. II. Skin testing of allergic and normal children with purified milk proteins. *Pediatrics, 32*:572, 1963.

Goltman, A.M.: Unusual cases of migraine with special reference to treatment. *J Allerg, 4*:51, 1932.
Discussion of headache due to allergy. *J Allerg, 5*:319, 1934.
The Mechanism of Migraine. *J Allerg, 7*:351, 1936.

Good, O.: Discussion in Yale University clinical conference, Nov. 13, 1953. *Amer J Ophthal, 39*:247, 1955.

Goodale, J.L.: Diagnosis and management of vasomotor disturbances of the respiratory air passages. *Amer Laryng Ass,* p. 82, 1916.

The diagnosis and management of vasomotor disturbances of the upper air passages. *Boston Med Surg J*, 175:181, 1916.

Goodman, E.L.: Endophthalmitis phaco-anaphylactica; clinical study. *Arch Ophthal*, 14:90, 1935.

Goslings, W.R.O.: Participant in *Bronchitis, An International Symposium*. April, 1960, University of Groningen, Holland, Charles C Thomas, 1961.

Gould, Frank W.: *Grass Systematics*. New York, McGraw-Hill, 1968.

Gould, G.M., and Pyle, W.L.: *Anomalies and Curiosities of Medicine*. Philadelphia, W.B. Saunders, 1900.

Gracie, J.: Henoch's purpura. *Practitioner, 113*: 419, 1924.

Graeser, J.B., and Rowe, A.H.: Inhalation of epinephrine hydrochloride for relief of asthmatic symptoms. *J Allerg*, 6:415, 1935.
Inhalation of epinephrine hydrochloride for relief of asthma in children. *Amer J Dis Child*, 52:92, 1936.

Graham, E.A., Cole, W.H., Copher, G.H., and Moore, S.: *Diseases of the Gall Bladder and Bile Ducts*. Philadelphia, Lea and Febiger, 1928.

Graham, E.A., and Macky, W.A.: Consideration of stoneless gall bladder. *JAMA, 103*:1497, 1934.

Grant, L.R.: Report of 6 cases of flaxseed sensitization with review of literature. *J Allerg, 3*: 469, 1932.

Gratia, A., and Gilson, O.: Le phénoméne d'Arthus au Catgut Cause Insoupconnée d'accidents Post-operatoires. *Bull Acad Roy Med Belg, 14*:125, 1934.

Gray, I., Harten, M., and Walzer, M.: The allergic reaction in the passively sensitized mucous membrane of the ileum and colon in humans. *Ann Int Med, 13*:2050, 1940.

Graykowski, Edward A., Barile, M.F., Lee, W.B., and Stanley, H.R., Jr.: Recurrent aphthous stomatitis. *JAMA, 196*:637, 1966.

Greenberg, and Pines, A.: Pressurized aerosols in asthma. *Brit Med J*, 1:562, 1967.

Greer, Allen E.: Mucoid impaction of the bronchi. *Arch Int Med, 46*:506, 1957.

Greer, D.: The treatment of food allergy in young infants. *Texas State J Med*, 29:370, 1933.

Grieff: Zur Behandlung der Uberempfindlichkeit gegen Insulin. *Klin Wschr, 10*:1955, 1931.

Grishaw, W.H.: Allergic manifestation to insulin. *JAMA, 97*:1885, 1931.

Gross, P.: The concept of the Hamman-Rich syndrome. A critique. *Am Rev Resp Dis, 85*: 828, 1962.

Grove, R.C.: Surgical Treatment of Sinusitis Associated with Asthma. In Prigal, S.J.: *Fundamentals of Modern Allergy*. New York, McGraw-Hill, 960.

Grulee, C.G., and Bonar, B.E.: Precipitins to egg-white in the urine of new-born infants. *Amer J Dis Child, 21*:89, 1921.

Grün, G.: Hypersensitivity to parenterally administered liver preparation in case of pernicious anemia. *Wien Klin Wschr, 47*:751, 1934.

Gryboski, Joyce D.: Gastrointestinal milk allergy in infants. *Pediatrics, 40*:354, 1967.

Gryboski, J.D., Katz, J., Reynolds, D., and Herskovic, T.: Gluten intolerance following cow's milk sensitivity: Two cases with coprantibodies to milk and wheat proteins. *Ann Allerg, 26*:33, 1968.

Gudmand-Höyer, E., and Jarnum, S.: Milk intolerance following gastric surgery. *Scand J Gastr, 4*:127, 1969.

Gudzent, F.: Testung und Heilbehandlung von Rheumatismus und Gicht mit spezifischen Allergenen. *Deutsch Med Wschr, 61*:901, 1935.

Guglielmini, T., and Molinari, E.: Ascariasis, causing epileptiform syndrome: Case. *Pediat Prat, 12*:163, 1935.

Gutmann, M.J.: Die allergischen Erkrankungen. *Med Welt, 4*:730, 766, 1930.

Gutmann, M.J.: Les Intolerances Digestives; les Troubles Digestifs a type d'anaphylaxie. *Presse Méd, 40*:1654, 1932.
Allergische Erscheinungen durch Genussmittel und deren Beseitigung. *Deutsch Med Wschr, 59*:1281, 1933; 1429, 1933.
Rund um die Pollenallergie (Heuschnupfën, Heuasthma). *München Med. Wschr, 80*:258, 1933.

Gutmann, M.J.: Cited by Urbach, E., and Gottlieb, P.M.: *Allergy*. New York, Grune and Stratton, 1943.

Halberstadt, R. (1911): Ueber Idiosynkrasie der Säulinge gegen Kuhmilch. *Arch Kinderheilk, 55*:105, 1911.
Cited by Laroche, G., Richet, Fils, C., and Saint Girons, F.: *Alimentary Anaphylaxis*. Transl. by Rowe, U.C. Press, 1930, French ed., Paris, 1919.

Hambresin, M.D.: La Maladie de Quincke et l'oeil. *Bull Soc Belg Ophthal, 106*:148, 1954.

Hamburger, J.: Le Probléme des Migraines Allergiques. *Rev Immunol, 1*:102, 1935.

Hamman, L., and Rich, A.R.: Acute diffuse interstitial fibrosis of the lungs. *Bull Hopkins Hosp, 44*:177, 1944.

Hampton, S.F. (1940) Henoch's purpura based on food allergy. *J Allerg, 12*:579, 1941.
Cited by Ackroyd, J.F.: Allergic purpura including purpura due to foods, drugs and infections. *Amer J Med, 14*:605, 1953.

Handwerck, C.: Kurzdauerndes Oedem der Sehnerven-Papillae eines Auges, eine Lokalisation des Akuten umschriebenen Oedem (Quincke's). *München Med Wschr, 54*:2332, 1907.

Hansel, F.K.: Clinical and histopathologic studies of the nose and sinuses in allergy. *J Allerg, 1*:43, 1929.
Observations on cytology of secretions in allergy, in nose and paranasal sinuses. *J Allerg, 5*:357, 1934.
Allergy of the Nose and Paranasal Sinuses. A Monograph on the Subject of Allergy as Related to Otolaryngology. St. Louis, C.V. Mosby, 1936.

Hansel, F.K.: *Clinical Allergy*. St. Louis, Mosby, 1953.

Hansen, E.W.: Allergy in ophthalmology. *Trans Amer Acad Ophthal Otolaryng, 54*:299, 1950.

Hansen, K.: *Allergie*. Stuttgart, G. Thieme, 1956.

Haritantis, A.: Anaphylaxie Alimentaire a Manifestation Clinique Rare. *Presse Méd, 41*:119, 1933.

Harkavy, J.: Skin hypersensitiveness to extracts of tobacco leaf, tobacco pollen, tobacco seed and to other allergens in 200 normal smokers. *J Allerg, 6*:56, 1934.
Skin reactions to tobacco antigen in smokers and non-smokers. *J Allerg, 5*:131, 1934.
Pathogenesis of bronchial asthma with recurrent pulmonary infiltration and eosinophilic polyseroitis. *Arch Intern Med, 67*:709, 1941.
Vascular Allergy and Its Systemic Manifestations. Washington, Butterworths, 1963.
Tobacco allergy in cardiovascular disease. *Ann Allerg, 26*:447, 1968.
Cardiovascular manifestations due to hypersensitivity. *New York J Med,* p. 2757, Nov. 1969.

Harkavy, J., Hebald, S., and Silbert, S.: Tobacco

sensitiveness in thromboangiitis obliterans. *Proc Soc Exp Biol Med, 30*:104, 1932.

Harrington, F.B.: Angioneurotic edema: Report of a case operated on during an abdominal crisis. *Boston Med Surg J, 152*:362, 1905.

Harris, J., and Vaughan, J.H.: Immunologic reactions to penicillin. *J Allerg, 32*:119, 1961.

Harris, M.C., and Shure, N.: *Practical Allergy*. Philadelphia, F.A. Davis, 1957.

Harter, J.G., and Novitch, A.M.: An evaluation of Gay's solution in the treatment of asthma. *J Allerg, 40*:327, 1967.

Hartsock, C.L.: Migraine. *JAMA, 89*:1489, 1927.

Hartzell, M.B.: Eczema rubrum. *Internat Clin, 27*:100, 1917.

Havener, W.H.: A case report of preventable blindness. *Ohio Med J, 55*:203, 1959.

Hayden, H.C., and Cushman, B.: Problem in nutrition in allergy: Report of a case of optic neuritis of an allergic basis. *Illinois Med J, 80*:500, 1941.

Hazen, H.H.: Severe erythema multiforme with anaphylaxis due to oyster protein. *JAMA, 62*:695, 1914.
Allergic dermatoses. *Arch Dermat Syph, 18*:121, 1928.

Healy, J.C., Gallison, D.T., and Brudno, J.: Gastro-intestinal allergy associated with transient intraventricular block. *Northeast J Med, 210*:123, 1934.

Healey, J.C., Daley, F.H., and Sweet, Marian H.: Medical aspects of periodontoclasia and gingivitis. *J Lab Clin Med, 21*:698, 1936.

Heed, J.W., and Goldbloom, A.A.: Addison-Beirmer's anemia (pernicious anemia); report of case showing allergic-like phenomena to liver extract. *JAMA, 96*:1361, 1931.

Heiner, D.C., Sears, J.W., and Kniker, W.T.: Multiple precipitins to cow's milk in chronic respiratory disease, including poor growth, gastrointestinal symptoms, evidence of allergy, iron deficiency anemia and pulmonary hemosiderosis. A syndrome. *Amer J Dis Child, 103*:634, 1962.

Henry, S.A.: Celery itch: Dermatitis due to celery in vegetable canning. *Brit J Dermat, 45*:301, 1933.

Hench, P.S., and Rosenberg, E.F.: Palindromic rheumatism. *Mayo Clin Proc, 16*:808, 1941.

Hepper, N.G., Black, L.F., Dines, D.E., *et al.*: The concept of an emphysema clinic. *Mayo Clin Proc, 43*:306, 1968.

Hermann, H.: A clinical study of 61 cases of

asthma and eczema in infancy and childhood controlled by intracutaneous protein sensitization tests. *Amer J Dis Child, 24*:221, 1922.

Hers, J.F. PH.: Participant in *Bronchitis. An International Symposium.* April, 1960, University of Groningen, Holland, Charles C Thomas, 1961.

Hers, J.F., and Mulder, J.: Mucosal epithelium of the respiratory tract in mucopurulent bronchitis caused by H. influenza. *J Path Bact, 66*: 103, 1953.

Herxheimer, H.: Participant in *Bronchitis. An International Symposium.* April, 1960, University of Groningen, Holland, Charles C Thomas, 1961. Eosinophiles in sputum of patients with asthma and emphysema. *Excerpta Medica, International Congress Series,* No. 42, 1961.

Herxheimer, H., and Bewersdorff, H.: Disodium cromoglycate in the prevention of induced asthma. *Brit Med J, 2*:220, 1969.

Highman, W.J., and Michael, J.C.: Protein sensitization in skin diseases, urticaria and its allies. *Arch Derm Syph, 2*:544, 1920.

Hill, B.H.R., and Swinburn, P.D.: Death from corticotropin. *Lancet, 1*:1218, 1954.

Hill, L.W.: Infantile eczema with special reference to use of milk free diet. *JAMA, 96*:1277, 1931.
Infantile eczema. *J Pediat, 2*:133, 1933.
Chronic atopic eczema (neurodermatitis) in childhood. *JAMA, 103*:1430, 1934.
Allergy in childhood. *Bull NY Acad Med, 16*:395, 1940.

Hinnant, I.M., and Halpin, L.J.: Food allergy in mild and severe cyclic vomiting. *Med Clin N Amer, 19*:931, 1936 (Cleveland Clinic No.).

Hirschberg, L.K.: Anaphylactia: A phenomenon caused by the proteins of tomatoes, crabs, berries, bivalves, eggs and other foods. *JAMA, 55*:1374, 1910.

Hobart, C.: Protein extract of vitreous humor (bovine): Preliminary report. *Arch Ophthal, 10*:237, 1933.

Hoffman, J.: Ueber ein epidemie von Poliomyelitis Anterior Actua in Der Umgebung Heidelbergs in Somner und Herbst. 1908, und bemerkenswerte beobachtungen aus Früheren Jahren. *Deutsch Z Nervenheilk, 38*:146, 1910.

Hogan, M.J.: Atopic keratoconjunctivitis. *Amer J Ophthal, 36*:937, 1953.

Holder, H.G., and Diefenboch, W.E.: Urticaria, its passive transmission by blood transfusion. *Calif West Med, 37*:387, 1932.

Hollander, L.: Mucous colitis due to food allergy. *Amer J Med Sci, 174*:495, 1927.

Holman, J.: Asthmatic syndrome precipitated by foreign bodies in the lung. *J Allerg, 28*:182, 1957.

Holmes, G.: Analysis of some cases of gastrointestinal allergy associated with organic disease. *South Med J, 34*:634, 1941.

Hoobler, B.R.: Some early symptoms suggesting protein sensitization in infancy. *Amer J Dis Child, 12*:129, 1916.

Hoover, R.E.: Nongranulomatous uveitis, a complication of serum sickness. *Amer J Ophthal, 41*:534, 1956.

Hopkins, J.G., and Kesten, B.M.: Allergic eczema, eczema initiated by sensitization to foods. *Amer J Dis Child, 49*:1511, 1935.

Hopkins, J.G., Waters, I., and Kesten, B.: Elimination diets as aid in the diagnosis and treatment of eczema. *J Allerg, 2*:239, 1931.

Hopps, H.C.: Role of allergy in delayed healing and in disruption of wounds. *Arch Surg, 48*: 438, 1944.

Hopps, H.C.: Effect of specific sensitivity to catgut on reaction of tissues to catgut sutures and of healing of wounds in presence of catgut sutures (Auer phenomenon). *Arch Surg, 48*: 445, 1944. Delayed healing and disruption produced by local allergic reaction (Auer phenomenon). *Arch Surg, 48*:450, 1944.

Horder, T.J.: Pruritus. *Lancet, ii*:287, 1935.

Horesh, A.: Allergy to food odors: Its reaction to management of infantile eczema. *J Allerg, 14*: 335, 1943.
Allergy to odor of white potato (Irish potato). *J Allerg, 14*:147, 1944.

Horton, B.T.: The clinical use of histamine. *Postgrad Med, 9*:1, 1951.

Horton, B.T., Wagener, H.P., Aita, J.A., and Woltman, H.W.: Treatment of multiple sclerosis by the intravenous administration of histamine. *JAMA, 124*:800, 1944.

Horwitz: A case of idiosyncracy to egg white. *München med Wchnschr,* Page 1184, June 2, 1908.

Howell, L.P.: Epilepsy and protein sensitization. *Ohio State Med J, 19*:660, 1923.

Hueber, E.: Ein Fall von Luminalvergiftung mit Tödlichem Ausgang. *München Med Wschr, 66*:1090, 1919.

Hunt, T.C.: Bilious migraine, its treatment with bile salt preparations. *Lancet, ii*:279, 1933.

Hurst, A.F.: Pathogenesis and treatment of asthma. *Brit Med J, 11*:839, 1929.

Hurst, A.F.: Recurrent hernia of the stomach through the hiatus oesophagus of the diaphragm. *Guy Hosp Rep, 84*:43, 1934.

Hutchinson, Jonathon: A clinical lecture on some peculiar eruptions allied to chillblains. *Med Times and Gaz Lond, 1*:169, 1879.

Hutchinson, Jonathan: *The Pedigree of Disease,* 1884.
    Illustrations of exceptional symptoms and examples of rare forms of disease. *Brit Med J,* p. 1018, May 29, 1886.
    Idiosyncrasies as regards the digestion of milk and eggs. *Arch Surg* (London), *6*:179, 1895.

Hutinel, V.: Intolerance for milk and anaphylaxis in nurslings. *La Clinique, 15*:227, April 16, 1908.

Inman, W.H., and Adelsyein, A.M.: Rise and fall of asthma mortality in England and Wales in relation to use of pressurized aerosols. *Lancet,* p. 279, Aug. 9, 1969.

Irons, E.E.: Treatment of chronic arthritis; general principles. *JAMA, 103*:1579, 1934.

Ishizaka, K., and Ishizaka, T.: Human reaginic antibodies and immunoglobulin E. *J Allerg, 42*:330, 1968.

Israels, A.A., Warringa, R.J., and Lowenberg, A.: Bronchiectasis. In *Bronchitis. An International Symposium.* Charles C Thomas, 1961, Royal van Gorcum Publisher, Assen, Netherlands.

Ivy, A.C., and Shapiro, P.F.: Studies on gastric ulcer by local allergy. *JAMA, 85*:1131, 1925.

Jackson, B.B.: Chronic regional enteritis. *Ann Surg, 148*:81, 1958.

Jackson, C.: Diseases of the esophagus, angioneurotic edema, urticaria, serum disease and herpes. *Arch Otolaryng, 11*:397, 1930.

Jackson, D., and Yow, E.: Pulmonary infiltration with eosinophilia: Report of two cases of farmer's lung. *New Eng J Med, 264*:1271, 1961.

Jadassohn, W.F., and Schaaf, F.: Experimentelle Untersuchungen, über den Mechanismus der Urtikariellen Eiklaridiosynkrasie des Ekzemkindes. (Antigennatur, Pluralität der Antigene, Neutralisation des Antigens, Beziehungen zur Anaphylaxie). *Z Immunitäts Exp Therap, 79*:407, 1933.

Jampolsky, A., and Flom, B.: Transient myopia associated with anterior displacement of the crystalline lens. *Amer J Ophthal, 36*:81, 1953.

Jegerow, B.: Die Gesetze der Allergie und Schwangerschaft. *Zbl Gynak, 59*:1455, 1934.

Jillson, O.F., and Piper, E.L.: Inhalant allergenic dermatitis: role in dermatitis of the hands. *Arch Derm, 71*:436, 1955.

Jimenez-Diaz, C., Sanchez Cuenca, B., and Puig, J.: Climatic asthma. *J Allerg, 3*:396, 1932.

Jimenez-Diaz, C.: El Asma y Otras Enfermedadas Alergicas. Editorial Espana, 1932.

Johnston, C.R.K.: Allergy of salivary glands. *Cleveland Clin Quart, 14*:55, 1947.

Johnstone, D.E.: Studies on cystic fibrosis of the pancreas: Role of various diluents and the dilution factor in interpretation of the x-ray film for fecal trypsin. *Amer J Dis Child, 84*:191, 1952.
    The allergic celiac syndrome. *Pediat Clin N Amer, 1*:1007, 1954.
    Rice intolerance in infants—masked food allergy. *Ann Allerg, 17*:350, 1959.
    Pediatric allergy in pediatric practice. *Ann Allerg, 28*:55, 1970.

Joltrain, E.: *Les Urticaires.* Paris, Gaston Doin et Cie., 1930.

Jonckheere, F.: La Myoplastie du Couturier dans le Hernies Inguinales Recedivantes. *J Chir* and *Ann Soc Belge Chir, 34, 32*:221-224, 1935.

Jonckheere, F.: A propos d'un "infarctus inexpliqué" du grêle. *J Chir* and *Ann Soc Belge Chir, 34-32*:236, 1935.

Jones, D.W.C.: Angina pectoris as an allergic manifestation and other observations on the allergic state and its treatment. *Med J Aust, 2*:557, 1932.

Jonez, H.D.: Multiple sclerosis: Treatment with histamine and d-tubocurarine. *Ann Allerg, 6*:550, 1948.
    Multiple sclerosis and allergy management with histamine therapy. Part II. *Ann Allerg, 8*:44, 1950.

Jordan, S.M.: The unstable colon and neurosis. *JAMA, 99*:2234, 1932.

Joseph, M.: Corticosteroids in the treatment of chronic asthma. *Med J Austral, 1*:166, 1968.
    Sympathomimetic drugs and bronchial asthma. *Med J Austral, 2*:752, 1968.

Julianelle, L.A., and Lamb, H.D.: Vascularization of cornea: Histological changes accompanying corneal hypersensitiveness. *Amer J Ophthal, 17*:916, 1934.

Julianelle, L.A., and Morris, M.C.: Study of pannus formation in cornea of rabbits. *Proc Soc Exp Biol Med, 30*:295, 1932.

Kahn, I.S.: Pollen toxemia in children. *JAMA*, 88:241, 1927.

Uterine spasm complicating pollen anaphylactic reaction. *JAMA*, 90:2101, 1928.

Henoch's purpura due to food allergy. *J Lab Clin Med*, 14:835, 1929.

Kaijser, R.: Zur Kenntnis der Allergischen Affectionen des Verdauungskanals vom Standpunkt des Chirurgen aus. *Arch Klin Chir*, 188:36, 1937.

Kammerer, H.: *Allergische Diathese und Allergische Erkrankungen*. München, Bergman, 1934.

Kantor, J.L.: Unstable colon. *Southern Med J*, 25:29, 1932.

Kantor, S.Z., Frank, M., Hoch-Kantor, D., Barkai-Goland, R., Marian, D., Schachnner, E., Kessler, A., and De Vries, A.: Airborne allergens and clinical response of asthmatics in Arad, a new town in a desert area in Israel. *J Allerg*, 37:65-74, 1966.

Kaplan, Ivor: The elusive link in incurable bronchial asthma—food allergy. *S Afr Med J*, 41:1123, 1967.

Kaplan, M.H., and Frengley, J.D.: Autoimmunity to the heart in cardiac disease. Current concepts of the relation of autoimmunity to rheumatic fever, postcardiotomy and post-infarction syndromes and cardiomyopathies. *Am J Cardiol*, 24:459, 1969.

Kappas, A., Soyel, W., and Fukushima, D.K.: Fever producing steroids of endogenous origin in man. *Arch Int Med*, 105:701, 1960.

Karpman, H.L.: Acute allergic colitis presenting the clinical picture of acute appendicitis. *JAMA*, 169:1752, 1959.

Karr, W.G., Scull, C.W., and Petty, O.H.: Insulin resistance and sensitivity. *J Lab Clin Med*, 18:1203, 1933.

Karrenberg, C.L.: Beiträge zur ätiologie, symptomatologie und therapie des allergosen; über eine aussergewöhnliche manifestations einer allergie und übes wechsel des Typus eines allergose. *Derm Ztschr*, 63:169, 1932.

Kartagener, M.: Zur Pathogenese der Bronchiektasien. I. Mitteilung Bronchiektasien. I. Mitteilung: Bronchiektasien bei Situ Viscerum Inversus. *Beitr Klin Erforsch Tuberk*, 83:489, 1933.

Keeney, E.L.: The history of asthma from Hippocrates to Mettzer. *J Allerg*, 35:215, 1964.

Kennedy, Foster: Cerebral symptoms induced by angioneurotic edema. *Arch Neurol Psychiat*, 15:28, 1926.

Certain nervous complications following the use of therapeutic and prophylactic sera. *Amer J Med Sci*, 177:555, 1929.

Nature of fits. *Bull NY Acad Med*, 7:221, 1931.

Migraine, symptom of focal brain edema. *New York J Med*, 33:1254, 1933.

Allergic manifestations in the nervous system. *New York J Med*, 36:469, 1936.

Allergy and its affect on the central nervous system. *J Nerv Ment Dis*, 88:91, 1938.

Kerley, C.G.: 146 cases of recurrent vomiting in private practice. *Amer J Dis Child*, 8:292, 1914.

Allergic manifestations to cow's milk. *New York J Med*, 36:1320, 1936.

Kern, R.A.: Dust sensitization in bronchial asthma. *Med Clin N Amer*, 5:751, 1921.

The interpretation of skin tests in the diagnosis of bronchial asthma. *Atlantic Med J*, 30:290, 1927.

Discussion of functional cardiac disorders. *J Allerg*, 4:67, 1932.

Anaphylactic drug reaction. *JAMA*, 179:19, 1962.

Kern, R.A., and Schenck, H.P.: Allergy, constant factor in etiology of so-called mucous nasal polyps. *J Allerg*, 4:485, 1933.

Importance of allergy in etiology and treatment of mucous polyps. *JAMA*, 103:1293, 1934.

Kern, R.A., and Wimberley, N.A. Jr.: Penicillin reactions: Their nature, growing importance, recognition, management and prevention. *Amer J Med Sci*, 226:357, 1953.

Kern, R.A., and Stewart, S.G.: Allergy in duodenal ulcer. *J Allerg*, 3:51, 1931.

Kerr, P.S., Pascher, F., and Sulzberger, M.B.: *Monilia* and *Trichophyton* extracts: Their combined use in eczematous ringworm. *J. Allerg*, 5:288, 1934.

Kerrebijn, K.S., and De Kroon, J.P.M.: Effect on height of corticosteroid therapy in asthmatic children. *Arch Dis Child*, 43:556, 1968.

Kimura, S.J., Hogan, M., and Thygeson, P.: Uveitis in children. *Arch Ophthal*, 51:80, 1954.

Kirsner, J.B., and Elchlepp, J.: The production of an experimental ulcerative "colitis" in rabbits. *Trans Ass Amer Physicians*, 102:102, 1957.

Kirsner, J.B., and Goldgraber, M.B.: Hypersensitivity, autoimmunity and the digestive tract. *Gastroenterology, 38*:536, 1960.

Kirsner, J.B., and Palmer, W.L.: Ulcerative colitis: consideration of its etiology and treatment. *JAMA, 155*:341, 1954.

Kittler, F.J., and Baldwin, D.G.: The role of allergic factors in the child with minimal brain dysfunction. *Ann Allerg, 28*:203, 1970.

Kittredge, W.E.: Allergic hematuria due to milk. *New Orleans Med and Surg J, 101*:419, 1949.

Klaber, R., and Archer, H.E.: Iodide eruption due to wearing iodine locket. *Lancet, i*:744, 1935.

Klein, Russel, C., Salvaggio, John E., and Kundur, V.G.: The response of patients with "Idiopathic" obstructive pulmonary disease and "Allergic" obstructive bronchitis to prednisone. *Ann Int Med, 71*:711, 1969.

Kline, B.S., Cohen, M.B., and Rudolph, J.A.: Histological changes in allergic and nonallergic wheals. *J Allerg, 3*:531, 1932.

Kline, B.S., and Young, A.M.: Normergic and allergic inflammation. *J Allerg, 6*:247, 1935. Case of reversible and irreversible allergic inflammation. *J Allerg, 6*:258, 1935.

Klinge, F.: Das Gewelsbild des fieberhaften Rheumatis mus, das rheumatische Fruhinfiltrat (akutes degenerativ exsudatives stadium). *Virchow Arch Path Anat, 278*:438, 1930.

Knepper, R.: Allergie und Eklampsie. *Klin Wschr, 13*:2, 1751, 1934.

Knepper, R., and Waaler, G.: Hyperegische arteriitis der Kranz und Lundgengefässe bei Funktionelles Belatung. *Virchow Arch Path Anat, 294*:587, 1935.

Knowles, F.C.: *Diseases of the Skin*. Philadelphia, Lea and Febiger, 3rd ed., 1935.

Kobrak, F.: Ueberempfindlichkersstorungen und Allergie unter Berucksichtigung Otologische Fragen. *Z Hals Nasen Ohrenh, 20*:259, 1928.

Kohn, E.: Relations between eczema and climate, occupation and age. *Arch Derm Syph, 171*:125, 1935.

Kraemer, M.: Chronic interstitial enteritis. *Rev Gastroenterology, 4*:239, 1937.

Kramer, H.F.: Discussion and appraisal of some functional disturbances of the digestive tract. *Amer J Dig Dis Nutr, 1*:614, 1934.

Kruse, F.H.: Syndrome of hypertonic and atonic colopathy. *JAMA, 193*:1366, 1934.

Kulczychi, J.L., Craig, J.M., and Schwachman, H.: Resection of pulmonary lesions associated with cystic fibrosis of the pancreas. *New Eng J Med, 257*:203, 1957.

Kullenkampf: Regional enteritis. *Zbl Chir, 65*:2675, 1938.

Kundstadter, R.H.: Gastrointestinal allergy and the celiac syndrome. *J Pediat, 21*:193, 1942.

Kunstadter, R.H., and Schultz, A.: Gastrointestinal allergy and the celiac syndrome with particular reference to allergy to cow's milk. *Ann Allerg, 11*:426, 1953.

Kutz, A. (1932): Cited by Bothman, L.: Clinical Manifestations of Allergy in Ophthalmology. *Year Book of Eye, Ear, Nose and Throat*. Chicago, Year Book Publishers, 1941.

Kutz, A., and Traugott, C.: Ueber einen mit Hämatoporphrurie unter dem Klinischen Bilde des Schwarzwasserfiebers todlich verlaufenden Fall von Gleichzeitiger Idiosynkrasie gegen Chinin und Veronal. *München Med Wschr, 72*:154, 1925.

Kwit, N.T., and Hatcher, R.A.: Excretion of drugs in milk. *Am J Dis Child, 49*:900, 1935.

LaGrange, H.: Pathogenic problem of so-called critical allergic conjunctivitis: specific sensitization; instability of organic colloids. *Brit J Ophthal, 19*:241, 1935.

LaGrange, H., and Deethill, S.: Allergic reactions of conjunctiva. *Ann Oculist* (Paris), *170*:1009, 1933.

Lain, E.S., and Caughron, G.S.: Electrogalvanic cavity produced by metallic dentures. *JAMA, 100*:717, 1933.

Lain, E. S., and Caughron, G. S.: Electrogalvanic phenomena of the oral cavity caused by dissimilar metallic restorations. *J Am Dent Assn, 23*:1614, 1936.

Laing, G.H.: Migraine types in relation to the gastrointestinal tract. *Med Clin N Amer, 11*:49, 1927.

Lamb, H.D.: Corneal corpuscles in reaction of hypersensitiveness. *Amer J Ophthal, 18*:644, 1935.

Landsteiner, K.J.: Experiments on anaphylaxis to azoproteins. *J Exp Med, 39*:631, 1924.

Laroche, G., Richet Fils, C., and Saint Girons, F.: *Alimentary Anaphylaxis*. Transl. by Rowe, U.C. Press, 1930, French ed., Paris, 1919.

Laubry, C., and Mussio-Fournier, J.C.: Common origin of asthma and paroxysmal tachycardia. *Bull Mem Soc Med Hop Paris, 49*:404, 1925.

Lazarus, J.A.: Idiopathic (Schönlein) purpura associated with hematuria. *J Urol, 62*:354, 1949.

Lederer, Francis L.: The problem of nasal polyps. *J Allerg, 30*:420, 1959.

Lehner, E., and Rajka, E.: Der Nachweis der Allergie beider Urticaria Factitia. *Arch Derm Syph, 159*:172, 1930.

Lehrfeld, L.: Vernal conjunctivitis. *J Allerg, 2*:328, 1931.

Lehrfeld, L., and Miller, J.: Additional research on vernal conjunctivitis. *Arch Ophthal, 21*:639 and 1070, 1939.

Lemoine, A.: Allergies in ophthalmology. *Trans Amer Acad Ophthal Otolaryng, 30*:198, 1925. Ocular anaphylaxis. *Arch Ophthal, 1*:706, 1929.

Lemoine, A.N., and Verhoeff, F.H.: Hypersensitiveness to lens protein. *Amer J Ophthal, 5*:700, 1922.

Leney, F.L.: Neurological manifestations of allergy. *South Med J, 46*:1214, 1953.

Leonard, Donald, W.: Progressive gangrene in an operative wound. *Arch Surg, 48*:457, 1944.

Leonhardt, K.O.: Resuscitation of the moribund asthmatic and emphysematous patient. *New Eng J Med, 264*:785, 1961.

Leopold, I.H.: Ocular complications of drugs. *JAMA, 205*:631, 1968.

Leopold, I.H., and Leopold, H.C.: Allergy. In Sorsby, A (Ed.): *Modern Trends in Ophthalmology.* 3rd Series, New York, Paul B. Hoeber, p. 169, 1955.

Leopold, I.H., and Dickinson, T.: Antihyaluronidase and antistreptolysin titers in uveitis. *Trans Amer Acad Ophthal, 58*:201, 1954.

Lepore, M.J., Collins, L.C., and Sherman, W.B.: Small intestine roentgen studies in food allergy. *J Allerg, 32*:146, 1951.

Lesne, E.: Cited by Laroche, G., Richet, Fils, C., and Saint Girons, F.: *Alimentary Anaphylaxis.* Transl. by Rowe, U.C. Press, 1930, French ed., Paris, 1919.

Lesne, E., and Dreyfus, L.: L'anaphylaxie alimentaire. *J Méd Francais, 6*:5 (Jan.), 1913.

Lesne, E., and Richet, Fils, C.: Les Accidents Seriques et leur Traitment. *J Med Francais, 61*:31, 1913.

Letterer, E.: Über die Wirkung von elektrokolloidalem Kupfer auf das reticuloendotheliale System. *Klin Wchnschr, 12*:597, 1933. Cited by Urbach, E., and Gottlieb, P.M.: *Allergy,* New York, Grune and Stratton, 1943.

Levin, P., Fonkalsrud, E.W., and Barber, W.F.: Surgical treatment for pediatric ulcerative colitis. *Surgery, 60*:201, 1966.

Levin, M.B., and Pinkus, H.: Autosensitivity to D.N.A. *New Eng J Med, 264*:533, 1961.

Levin, S.J.: Allergic epilepsy: Report of case in 3 year old child. *JAMA, 97*:1624, 1931.

Levitt, L.M., and Burbank, B.: Glomerulonephritis as a complication of Schonlein-Henoch syndrome. *New Eng J Med, 248*:530, 1953.

Levy, E.: Allergic background of tinnitus aurium. *Z Laryng Rhinol Otol, 23*:410, 1932.

Lewin, P., and Taub, S.J.: Allergic synovitis due to ingestion of English walnuts. *JAMA, 106*:2144, 1936.

Lewis, E.R.: Otitis media and allergy. *Ann Otol, 38*:185, 1929.

Lewis, J.H., and Hayden, H.C.: Effect of heat on antigenic properties of milk. *Amer J Dis Child, 44*:1211, 1932.

Lewis, M.W.: Disillusionments in nasal surgery. *Minn Med, 17*:323, 1934.

Lewis, T., and Grant, R.T.: Vascular reactions of skin to injury: Liberation of a histamine-like substance in injured skin, the underlying cause of factitious urticaria and of wheals produced by burning; and observations upon nervous control of certain skin reactions. *Heart, 11*:209, 1924.

Lewis, T., and Harmer, I.M.: Vascular reactions of skin to injury, further evidence and release of histamine-like substance from injured skin. *Heart, 14*:19, 1927.

Lichtwitz, L.: Die Arzneitherapie der Funktionsanomalein der Glatten Musculatur. *Klin Wschr, 49*:2353, 1925.

Lichtwitz, L.: Function of liver in relation to its blood supply. *Rev Gastroenterol, 1*:33, 1934.

Lietze, Arthur: Quantitation of food adulterants by multiple radial immunodiffusion. I. Cross-reacting antigen mixtures. II. Wheat in bread sold, as "wheat-free" for the use of allergy patients. *J Ass Official Analytical Chemists, 52*:988, 995, 1969. Laboratory research in food allergy. *J Asthma Res, 7*:25, 127, 1969-1970.

Lietze, Arthur, Rowe, A.H., and Rowe, A., Jr.: Unlisted wheat in hypo-allergenic bread and other bakery products. *Ann Allerg, 25*:175, 1967.

Lietze, Arthur: Allergies and health foods (letter). *Sci Dig,* June, 1969, p. 95.

Lietze, A., Rowe, A.H., and Rowe, A., Jr.: Hypoallergenic breads—wheat content of products available in the San Francisco Bay area. *Calif Med, 107*:500, 1967.

Lietze, Arthur: The role of particulate insoluble substances in food allergy. III. Heat labile antibody to wheat starch in sera of wheat sensitive patients. *Ann Allerg, 27:9, 1969.*

Lietze, A., Rowe, A.H., and Rowe, A., Jr.: An empirical test for corn allergy. *Ann Allerg, 26:587, 1968.*

Die Bedeutung unlöslicher Nahrungspartikel für die Allergie. I. Stärke-Antikörper beim Menschen. *Allergie und Asthma 15:11, 1969.*

Die Bedeutung unlöslicher Nahrungspartikel für die Allergie. II. Antikörper gegen lösliche und unlösliche Weizenantigene in Seren von Nahrungsmittelallergikern. *Allergie und Asthma 15:17, 1969.*

Lietze, A., and Reed, C.E.: Studies on house dust allergens: The separation of closely related allergens of different specificity and their relationship to allergenically inactive antigens. *Int Arch Allerg, 20:344, 1962.*

Lifschitz, M.I., Bowman, F.O., Denning, C.R., Wylie, Robt. H.: Pneumothorax as a complication of cystic fibrosis: Report of 20 cases. *Amer J Dis Child, 116:633, 1968.*

Lindsay, J.C.: Food anaphylaxis. *Canad Med Assn J, 16:58, 1926.*

Lintz, W.: Appendicitis in 300 cases of asthma and other forms of allergy. *NY J Med, 25:368, 1925.*

The diagnosis and treatment of 244 cases of gastrointestinal allergy. *New York J Med, 34:282, 1934.*

Lippard, V.W., Schloss, O.M., and Johnson, P.A.: Immune reactions induced in infants by intestinal absorption of incompletely digested cow's milk protein. *Amer J Dis Child, 51:562, 1936.*

Little, W.T.: Letter—"Immunizing Against Eggs," Queries and Minor Notes. *JAMA, 86:1308, 1926.*

Litzner, S.: Über Kreislauf- und Herzschädigungen bei der Kohlenoxydvergiftung. *Med Klin, 32:630, 1936.*

Cited by Urbach, E., and Gottlieb, P.M.: *Allergy,* New York, Grune and Stratton, 1943.

Liveing, E.: *On megrim and sick headache and some allied disorders.* London, 1873.

Lobos, M.C., Gerrard, J.W., and Buchan, D.J.: Disaccharidase activities in milk-sensitive and celiac patients. *J Pediat, 70:325, 1967.*

Loeffler (1881): Cited by Schoenberg, M.J.: A contribution to the experimental study of ocular anaphylaxis. *Opthalmology, 11:1, 1914-15.*

Loewy, F.F.: Thrombopenic hemorrhagic purpura. *Lancet, i:845, 1934.*

Loffler, W.: Die fuchtige Lungen Infiltrate mit eosinophilie. *Schweiz Med Wschr, 66:1069, 1936.*

Londe, S., and Pelz, M.D.: Chronic sialodochoparotitis with recurrent subacute exacerbation. *J Pediat, 2:594, 1933.*

Longcope, W.T.: Protein hypersensitiveness and its relation to the etiology of disease. *JAMA, 77:1535, 1921.*

Generalized edema associated with disease of gastrointestinal tract. *Int Clin, 2:1, 1934.*

Longobardie, A., Ruggles, D.W., and Burgess, A.M.: Rupture of stomach during oxygen therapy by nasal catheter. *Arch Int Med, 55:1014, 1961.*

Lopez-Majano, V., Tow, D.E., and Wagner, H.N., Jr.: Regional distribution of pulmonary arterial blood flow in emphysema. *JAMA, 197:112, 1966.*

Lopez-Majano, V., and Wagner, H.N., Jr.: Clinical application of lung scanning. *Dis Chest, 54:356, 1968.*

Loveless, M.H.: Immunological studies of pollinosis; passive sensitization of man through transfusion. *J Immunol, 41:15, 1941.*

Loveless, M.H.: The relationship between the thermostable antibody in the circulation and clinical immunity. *J Immunol, 47:165, 1943.* Repository immunization in pollen allergy. *J Immunol, 79:68, 1957.*

Loveless, M.H., and Nall, T.M.: Use of *Polistes* venom in petroleum-argacel repositories to immunize against yellow jacket wasp-sting allergy, *J Immunol, 94:785, 1965.*

Lowell, F.C.: Bronchial asthma. *Amer J Med, 20:778, 1956.*

Lowenstein, A.: Uber die Klinische und histologische Form des innersekretorischen Katarakts. Versuch einer Abgrenzung. *Arch Ophthal, 132:224, 1934.*

Lubbers, H.A.: Migraine en Anaphylaxie. *Nederl T Geneesk, 2:1073, 1921.*

Lundberg, A.: Ein Paar Falle Von Allergischer Conjunctivitis bei Urticaria Patientin. *Acta Ophthal, 15:60, 1937.*

Luria, R., and Wilensky, I.: Kann die Paroxysmale Takykardie als Eine Allergische Krankheit Gelten? *Deutsch Med Wschr, 56:1430, 1930.*

Lust: Cited by Schultz, S.W., and Larsen, W.T.: Anaphylaxis and its relation to some diatheses common to infancy and childhood. *Arch Pediat, 35:705, 1918.*

Lyon, G.M.: Allergy in an infant of three weeks. *Amer J Dis Child,* 36:1012, 1928.

MacBride, W.L., and Schorer, E.H.: Erythematous and uriticarial eruptions resulting from certain foods. *J Cutan Dis,* 34:70, 1916.

MacDonald, W.J.: Etiology of eczema. *New Eng J Med,* 207:940, 1932.

Magendie, F.: *Lectures on the Blood and on the Changes Which It Undergoes During Disease.* Philadelphia, Haswell, Barrington and Haswell, 1839.

Malik, E.B., Watson, W.C., Murray, D., and Cruickshank, B.: Immunofluorescent antibody studies in idiopathic steatorrhea. *Lancet,* 1: 1127-1129, 1964.

Malley, W., Lietze, A.C., and Reed, C.E.: The separation of substances in timothy pollen extract producing allergic skin reactions from those producing hemmaglutination reactions. *J Allerg,* 31:413, 1960.

Mallory, W.J.: Medical aspects of colitis. *JAMA,* 90:601, 1928.

Manwaring, W.H.: The role of hepatic tissues in the acute anaphylactic shock. *JAMA,* 69:772, 1917.
Intestinal and lymphatic reactions in anaphylaxis. *J Amer Med Ass,* 77:849, 1921.

Manwaring, W.H., and Marino, H.D.: The action of the urinary bladder in rabbit anaphylaxis. *J Immunol,* 13:69, 1927.

Mariante, T.: *Toxemia Alergica.* Buenos Aires, Clinica Medica "El Ateneo," 1948.

Marks, A.: Diffuse interstitial pulmonary fibrosis. *Med Clin North Am,* 51:439, 1967.

Marks, M.B.: Allergy in relation to orofacial deformities in children. *J Allerg,* 36:293, 1965.

Marks, R., and Whittle, M.W.: Results of treatment of dermatitis herpetiformis with a gluten-free diet after one year. *Brit Med J,* 4:72, 1969.

Martin, F.J.: Allergic colic in infants in the general practice of pediatrics. *Pediatrics,* 18:832, 1956.

Mason, V.R.: Optic neuritis in serum sickness. *JAMA,* 78:88, 1922.

Masugi, M.: Zur Pathogenese der Diffusen Glomerulonephritis als Allergisches, Erkrankung des Niere. *Klin Wschr,* 14:373, 1935.

Masugi, M., and Sato, T.: Ueber die allergische gewebs reaktion der Niere Zugleich Ein Experimenteller Beitrag zur Pathogenese der diffusen Glomerulonephritis und der Periarteritis Nodosa. *Virchow Arch Path Anat,* 293: 615, 1934.

Mateer, J.S., *et al.*: Colon bacillus vaccine therapy as related to chronic functional diarrhea, chronic headache, chronic toxic vertigo and unstable colon. *Amer J Dig Dis Nutrit,* 11:621, 1935.

Matheson, A.: Personal communication. Cited by Glaser, J.: *Allergy in Childhood.* Springfield, Charles C Thomas, 1956.

Mathieu, E.: Un cas d'urticaire profonde compliquée de paralysie du plexus brachial. *Union Méd du Canada,* 61:377, 1932.

Matsumura, T., Takayoshi, K., and Fukushima, I.: Significance of food allergy in the etiology of orthostatic albuminuria. *J Asthma Res,* 3:325, 1966.

Matsumura, T., Kuroume, T., Mitomo, A., and Kobayashi, K.: Age differences of BDB hemagglutinating antibody titres against milk and egg allergens. *Int Arch Allerg,* 30:341, 1966.

Matzger, E.: Bronchial asthma caused by liver and liver extract diet in a patient suffering from primary anemia. *JAMA,* 96:110, 1931.
Can sensitivity to dinitrophenol be determined by skin tests? *JAMA,* 103:253, 1934.

Mauksch, H.: Pollenallergie als Ursache einer Keratitis Superficialis. *Z Augenheilk,* 91:343, 1937.

Maunsell, K., Pearson, R.S.B., and Livingstone, J.L.: Long term corticosteroid treatment of asthma. *Brit Med J,* 1:661, 1968.

Maunsell, K., Wraith, D.G., and Cunnington, A.M.: Mites and housedust allergy in bronchial asthma. *Lancet,* 1:1267, 1968.

Maxwell, J.: Massive collapse of the lung. *St. Barth Hosp Rep,* 70:183, 1937.

Mayerhofer, E.: Die Biologische Allergie des Neugeborenenziet. *Wien Med Wschr,* 85:57, 1935.

Maytum, C.K., and Magath, T.B.: Sensitivity to acacia. *JAMA,* 99:2251, 1931-1932.

McAllen, M.: National statistics on asthma deaths and side effects of bronchodilators. *J Roy Coll Gen Pract,* 17:212, 1969.

McCarthy, M.P., and Wiseman, J.R.: Pylorospasm, an infantile allergic manifestation. *Med Woman J,* 44:335, 1937.

McClure, C.W., and Huntsinger, M.E.: Observations on migraine. *Boston Med Surg J,* 196: 270, 1927.

McClure, C.W., and Huntsinger, M.E.: Paroxysmal headache. *New Eng J Med, 199*:1312, 1928.

McDonagh, T.J.: Lactose intolerance; a newly recognized cause of gastrointestinal symptoms seen in the practice of occupational medicine. *J Occup Med, 11*:51, 1969.

McIntosh, J.A.: Distinction between appendiceal allergy and appendicitis in 310 appendices. *Southern Med J, 23*:1147, 1930.

McIntyre, F.C.: The quantitative determination of histamine in animal tissues. *J Allerg, 26*: 292, 1955.

McKhann, C.F., Spector, S., and Meserve, E.R.: An association of gastrointestinal allergy with the celiac syndrome. *J Pediat, 22*:362, 1943.

McLean, J.A., Schrager, J., and Stoeffler, V.R.: Severe asthma in children. *Michigan Med, 67*: 1219, 1968.

McNeill, J.H.: Allergic reaction to honey. Queries and minor notes. *JAMA, 101*:728, 1933.

McQuarrie, I.: Some recent observations regarding nature of epilepsy. *Ann Int Med, 6*:497, 1932.
Non-organic convulsive disorders of childhood with special reference to idiopathic epilepsy. *Calif West Med, 41*:1, 1934.

Melli, G.: Klinische Beobachtung über das Asthma Bronchiale. *Seuchenbekämpfung, 7*:177, 1930.

Menagh, F.T.: The results of treatment in bronchial asthma. *Ann Clin Med, 5*:656, 1927.
Etiology and results of treatment in angioneurotic edema and urticaria. *JAMA, 90*:668, 1928.

Mendelsohn, H.V.: Sensitization tests: Their value in dermatology. *Arch Derm Syph, 29*:845, 1934.

Menkin, V.: Studies on inflammation, fixation of foreign protein at site of inflammation. *J Exp Med, 52*:201, 1930.

Menninger, W.C.: Skin eruptions with phenobarbitol (Luminal). *JAMA, 91*:14, 1928.

Messer, J.W., Peters, G.P., and Bennett, W.A.: Causes of death and pathological findings in 304 cases of bronchial asthma. *Dis Chest, 38*: 616, 1960.

Meyer, H. S.: Chronic sialodochitis. *J Pediat, 4*: 248, 2/1934.

Mienicki, M., and Krzwoblocki, B.: Case of hypersensitiveness toward quinine and attempts at transferring this state to animals. *Urol Cutan Rev, 38*:256, 1934.

Miller, J.L.: Evidence that idiopathic epilepsy is a sensitization disease. *Amer J Med Sci, 168*:635, 1924.

Miller, J.L., and Lewin, P.: Evidence of the anaphylactic character of intermittent hydrarthrosis. *JAMA, 82*:1177, 1924.

Minot, G.R.: Three cases of chronic dietary deficiency; features are chronic fatigue, anemia, prolonged coagulation of blood. *Med Clin N Amer, 16*:761, 1933.

Mitchell, R.S.: *Bronchitis. 2nd International Symposium.* April, 1964, University of Groningen, The Netherlands, Charles C Thomas Publisher, 1964. Royal Vangorcum Publisher, Assen, Netherlands, 1964.

Mitchell, W.F., Sivon, I., and Mitchell, J.H.: Vulvo-vaginal pruritus associated with hay fever. *Ann Allerg, 6*:144, 1948.

Mitchell, W.F., Woharton, C.W., Larson, D.G., and Modic, R.: Housedust, mites and insects. *Ann Allerg, 27*:93, 1969.

Mitra, P.N.: Sensitiveness to meat. *Indian Med Gaz, 61*:26, 1926.

Mittelmann, B.: Allergic pruritus neurotic excoriations. *J Allerg, 4*:141, 1933.

Miyamoto, T., Oshima, S., Ishizaki, T., and Sato, S.: Allergenic identity between the common floor mite (*Dermatophagoides farinae*, Hughes, 1961) and house dust as a causative antigen in bronchial asthma. *J Allerg, 42*:14, 1968.

Mogena, H.G.: Le Facteur Allergique dans les Colites. *Arch Mal Appar Dig, 25*:57, 1935.

Moloney, J.C.: Etiology of migraine. *Arch Neurol Psychiat, 19*:684, 1928.

Moore, M.T.: Paroxysmal abdominal pain—a form of focal symptomatic epilepsy. *JAMA, 129*:1233, 1945.

Moore, M.W.: Extra-respiratory tract symptoms of pollinosis. *Ann Allerg, 16*:152, 1958.

Moro, E.: Importance of egg-white reaction in study of infantile eczema. *Derm Wschr*, Sept. 3, 1932.

Moro, E., and Keller, W.: Ueber die parallergie. *Klin Wschr, 14*:1, 1935.

Mueller, H.L., and Lanz, M.: Hyposensitization with bacterial vaccine in infectious asthma. *JAMA*, 1379, May, 1969.

Muncaster, S.B., and Allen, H.E.: Bilateral uveitis and retinal periarteritis as a focal reaction to the tuberculin test. *Arch Ophthal, 21*:509, 1939.

Mussio-Fournier, J.C.: Tachycardie Paroxystique

d'origne Anaphylactic. *Presse Méd, 40*:1225, 1932.

Nakayama, K.: Surgical removal of the carotid body for bronchial asthma. *Dis Chest, 40*: 3595, 1961.

Nater, J.P., and Swartz, J.A.: Atopic allergic reactions due to raw potato. *J Allerg, 40*:202, 1967.

Neff, T.A., and Petty, T.L.: Long-term continuous oxygen therapy in chronic airway obstruction. *Ann Int Med, 72*:621, 1970.

Neill, J.M., Hehre, E.J., Sugg, J.Y., and Jaffe, E.: Serological studies on sugar. I. Reactions between solutions of reagent sucrose and Type II antipneumococcus serum. *J Exp Med, 70*: 427, 1939.

Nelp, W.B.: Pancreatitis induced by steroid therapy. *Arch Int Med, 108*:702, 1961.

New, G.B., and Kirch, W.A.: Permanent enlargement of lips and face secondary to recurring swellings and associated with facial paralysis: Clinical entity. *JAMA, 100*:1230, 1933.

Niles, W.L., and Torrey, J.C.: Clinical significance of *B Coli* Hemolyticus. *Amer J Med Sci, 187*:30, 1934.

Nilsson, D.C.: Sources of allergenic gums. *Ann Allerg, 18*:518, 1960.

No Authors: Symposium on steroids and childhood asthma: Steroid therapy in childhood asthma? *Clin Pediat, 7*:439, 1968.

Noun, L.J.: Chronic otorrhea due to food sensitivity. *J Allerg, 14*:82, 1942.

Novey, H.S., and Meleyco, L.N.: Alarming reaction after intravenous administration of 30 ml. of epinephrine. *JAMA, 207*:2435, 1969.

Oberndorf: Cited by Drysdale, H.H.: Acute circumscribed edema. *JAMA, 89*:1390, 1927.

O'Brien, C.S., and Allen, J.H.: Allergic keratoconjunctivitis. *Arch Ophthal, 29*:600, 1943.

O'Byrne, G.T.: Loefflers syndrome—report of a case in an infant. *Texas J Med, 43*:446, 1947.

O'Keefe, E.S.: Relation of food to infantile eczema. *Boston Med Surg J, 183*:569, 1920.

A dietary consideration of eczema in younger children. *JAMA, 78*:483, 1922.

Protein sensitivity in children with negative cutaneous reactions. *JAMA, 80*:1120, 1923.

Eczema in exclusively breast-fed babies. *Boston Med Surg J, 190*:415, 1924.

O'Keefe, E.S., and Rackemann, F.M.: Studies in eczema. VI. Eczema: Its relation to allergy. *JAMA, 92*:883, 1929.

Oliver, K.S., and Crowe, S.J.: Retrobulbar neu-

ritis and infection of the accessory nasal sinuses. *Arch Otolaryng, 6*:503, 1927.

Olsen, A.M.: Bronchiectasis and dextrocardia: Observations on etiology of bronchiectasis. *Coll Papers Mayo Clinic & Mayo Foundation, 34*:764, 1932.

Olsen, A.M., and Prickman, L.E.: Hypersensitivity to soy beans. *Proc Staff Meet Mayo Clinic, 11*: 465, 1936.

Ordman, D.: Relation of climate to respiratory allergy. *Ann Allerg, 19*:29, 1961.

Orie, N.G.M.: Participant in *Bronchitis. An International Symposium*. April 1960, University of Groningen, The Netherlands, Charles C Thomas, Publisher, 1961. Royal Vangorcum Publisher, Assen, Netherlands.

Orie, N.G.M., and Sluiter, H.J. (Eds.): *Bronchitis. An International Symposium*. April, 1960, University of Groningen, The Netherlands, Charles C Thomas, Publisher, 1961. Royal Vangorcum Publisher, Assen, Netherlands.

Bronchitis, Second International Symposium. April, 1964, University of Groningen, The Netherlands, Charles C Thomas Publisher, 1964. Royal Vangorcum Publisher, Assen, Netherlands.

Ortolph, W.: Ein Schwerer Fall von Ueberempfundlichkeit. *Med Klin, 27*:1929, 1931.

Orton, C.: A case of poisoning by eggs. *Practitioner, 36*:365, 1886.

Osler, W.: Hereditary angioneurotic edema. *Amer J Med Sci, 95*:362, 1888.

On the visceral complications and erythema exudativum multiforme. *Amer J Med Sci, 110*: 628, 1895.

On the visceral manifestations of the erythema group of skin diseases. *Amer J Med Sci, 127*: 1, 1904.

Visceral lesions of purpura. *Brit Med J, 1*:517, 1914.

The Principles and Practice of Medicine. New York, D. Appleton, 1916.

Ott, M.D.: Gastrointestinal allergy and migraine in childhood. *Iowa Med Soc J, 26*:192, 1936.

Overholt, R.H.: Glomectomy for asthma. *Dis Chest, 40*:605, 1961.

Pagniez, P., and Nast, A.: Recherches sur la Pathogenie de le Crise de Migraine. *Presse Méd, 28*, 1920.

Pagniez, P., and Lieutand, P.: Phenomena of the type of anaphylaxis in the pathogenesis of epileptic seizures. *Presse Méd, 27*:693, 1919.

Pagniez, P., Vallery-Radot, P., and Nast, A.: Therapeutique Preventative de Certaines Migraines. *Presse Méd*, 27:172, 1919.

Palm, C.R., Murcek, M.A., Roberts, T.R., *et al.*: A review of asthma admissions and deaths at Children's Hospital of Pittsburgh from 1935 to 1968. *J Allerg*, 46:257, 1970.

Pardee, I.: Allergic reactions in the central nervous system: Report of two cases. *Arch Neurol Psychiat*, 36:1360, 1938.

Pardo-Castello, V.: Allergic cutaneous eruptions after high voltage roentgen therapy. *Arch Dermat Syph*, 33:886, 1936.

Paris, W.E., Barrett, A.M., and Coombs, R.A.: Fatal reaction to cow's milk protein. *Lancet*, 2:1106, 1960.

Park, E.A.: A case of hypersensitiveness to cow's milk. *Amer J Dis Child*, 19:46, 1920.

Parlato, S.J.: Corneal ulcers due to common allergen. *Arch Ophthal*, 14:587, 1935.

Parry, T.G.W.: Ocular reaction to foreign protein. *Brit Med J*, 2:397, 1939.

Paviot, J., Lageze, P., and Naussac, H.: Les Arthropathies Proteinique. *Gaz Hopitaux*, 105:299, 1932.

Pearson, R.B.: Cited by Bray, G.W.: Some unusual examples of allergic reaction. *Practitioner*, 134:610, 1935.
Recurrent swelling of the parotid glands. *Arch Dis Child*, 10:363, 1935.

Pearson, R.S.: Asthma-allergy and prognosis. *Proc Roy Soc Med*, 61:467, 1968.

Peck, George, A., and Moffat, Dean: Allergy to the pollen of the common sugar beet, *Beta Vulgaris*. *J Allerg*, 30:140, 1959.

Pemberton, R.: Some metabolic and nutritional aspects of chronic arthritis. *Amer J Digest Dis Nutrit*, 1:438, 1934.

Pennington, E.S.: *Trichophytin* and *Monilia* extracts in allergic dermatoses. *J Allerg*, 7:54, 1935.

Pepys, J., Chan, M., and Hargreave, F.E.: Mites and house-dust allergy. *Lancet*, 1:1270, 1968.

Perez-Moreno, B.: Sindrome Pseudo-Epileptico De Origen Alergico. *Pediat Espan*, 24:258, 1935.

Peshkin, M.M.: Significance of protein skin reactions in bronchial asthma. *New York Med J* and *Med Rec*, 118:88, 1923.
Bronchial asthma and other allergic manifestations in pharmacists. *JAMA*, 82:1854, 1924.
Asthma in children. I. Etiology. *Amer J Dis Child*, 31:763, 1926.

II. The incidence and significance of eczema, urticaria and angioneurotic edema. *Amer J Dis Child*, 32:862, 1926.

Peshkin, M.M., and Miller, J.A.: Quinine and ergot allergy and thrombocytopenic purpura; report of case. *JAMA*, 102:1737, 1934.

Peterman, M.G.: Convulsions in childhood. *JAMA*, 102:1729, 1934.

Peters, G.: Bronchial asthma due to soybean allergy: Report of a case with audiovisual documentation. *Ann Allerg*, 23:270, 1965.

Phillips, J.M.: Angioneurotic edema. *JAMA*, 78:497, 1922.

Piness, G.: Etiology of 150 cases of bronchial asthma. *Calif J Med*, 19:29, 1921.
Gastro-intestinal food allergy. *J Allerg*, 1:172, 1929.

Piness, G., and Miller, H.: Food factor in allergy. *Colorado Med*, 30:405, 1933.
Allergy of the upper respiratory tract. *JAMA*, 113:734, 1939.

Piness, G., Miller, H., and Sullivan, E.P.: Intelligence rating of allergic children. *J Allerg*, 8:168, 1937.

Plummer, J.S.: Retinal allergy. *Arch Ophthal*, 17:516, 1937.

Porter, L., and Carter, W.E.: *Management of the Sick Infant*. St. Louis, C.V. Mosby, 1927.

Portner, M.M., Thayer, K.H., Kent, J.R., Harter, J.G., and Rayyis, S.: Successful Initiation of Alternate Day Prednisone in Chronic Steroid Dependent Asthmatics (CSDA) Read at Meeting of Academy of Allergy, New Orleans, Feb., 1970.

Posner, A.: Personal communication. As cited in *Ocular Allergy* by Theodore, F.H., and Schlossman, A., Baltimore, Williams and Wilkins, 1958.

Posner, A., and Schlossman, A.: A syndrome of unilateral recurrent attacks of glaucoma with cyclitic symptoms. *Arch Ophthal*, 39:517, 1948.

Potvin, and Bossu, A.: L'Allergie en Ophthalmologie. *Bull Soc Belg Ophthal*, 106:1, 1954.

Pounders, C.M.: Intestinal disturbances in infancy due to allergy. *Arch Pediat*, 49:314, 1932.

Powell, N.B.: Allergies of the genito-urinary tract. *Ann Allerg*, 19:1019, 1961.

Powell, N.Y., Boggs, P.B., and McGovern, J.P.: Allergy of the lower urinary tract. *Ann Allerg*, 28:252, 1970.

Prausnitz, C., and Küstner, H.: Studien über die

Ueberempfindlichkeit. *Centralbl Bakt Abt Originale, 86*:160, 1921.

Preiser, F.M., Donner, M.W., and Van Metre, T.E.: Comparison of midplane, full-chest tomograms, diffusing capacities, sputum eosinophil, and other parameters in patients with asthma and emphysema. *J Allerg, 44*: 154, 1969.

Prewitt, L.H.: Retinal detachment due to allergy. *Arch Ophthal, 18*:73, 1937.

Prickman, L.E., and Buckstein, H.F.: Hypersensitivity of acetyl salicylic acid. *JAMA, 58*: 445, 1937.

Prickman, L.E., and Moersch, J.J.: Bronchostenosis complicating allergic and infectious asthma. *Ann Int Med, 11*:387, 1940,

Prigal, S.J.: Allergy and multiple sclerosis. A critical review. *J Allerg, 27*:170, 1956.

Prigal, S.J.: *Fundamentals of Modern Allergy.* New York, McGraw-Hill, 1960.

Prince, H.E.: Mold fungi in the etiology of respiratory allergic diseases. III. Immunological studies with mold extracts. I. Preparation of experimental extracts. *Ann Allerg, 2*:483, 1944.

Prince, H.E., Selle, W.A., and Morrow, M.B.: Molds in etiology of asthma and hay fever; preliminary report. *Texas J Med, 30*:340, 1934.

Proetz, A.W.: Allergy in middle and internal ear. *Ann Otol, 40*:61, 1931.

Pusey, W.A.: *The History of Dermatology.* Springfield, Charles C Thomas, 1933.
Permanent enlargement of the lips and face (letter). *JAMA, 100*:1626, 1933.

Pusey, W.A. (1911): Cited by Bothman, L.: Clinical Manifestations of Allergy in Ophthalmology. *Year Book of Eye, Ear, Nose and Throat.* Chicago, Year Book Publishers, 1941.

Quick, A.J.: Probable allergic nature of cincophen poisoning, with special reference to Arthus phenomenon and with precautions to be followed in cincophen administration. *Amer J Med Sci, 187*:115, 1934.

Quincke, H.: Circumscribed edema. *Mschr Prakt Derm,* July, 1882.
Ueber meningitis serosa. *Klin Vorträge, N.F.,* Vol. 67, 1893.
Acute circumscribed edema and similar conditions. *Med Klin, 17*:675, 1921.

Rackemann, F.M.: A critical study of 150 cases of bronchial asthma. *Arch Int Med, 22*:517, 1918.
Fatal asthma; report of case with autopsy. *Boston Med Surg J, 194*:531, 1926.
Analysis of 213 cases in which the patients were relieved for more than two years. *Arch Int Med, 41*:346, 1928.
Sensitiveness. *J Allerg, 1*:2, 1929.
Nature of allergy. *J Allerg, 1*:536, 1930.
Clinical Allergy, Particularly Asthma and Hay Fever. New York, Macmillan, 1931.
Skin tests to foods in asthma. *J Allerg, 2*:113, 1931.
Allergy; review of current literature. *Arch Int Med, 55*:141, 1935.
Allergy; a review of the literature of 1936. *Arch Int Med, 57*:184, 1936.

Rackemann, F.M., and Greene, J.E.: Periarteritis nodosa and asthma. *Trans Ass Amer Physicians, 54*:112, 1939.

Rackemann, F.M., and Wille, F.L.: Nasal sinusitis and asthma: A thesis. *Arch Otolaryng, 30*: 1051, 1939.

Ramirez, M.A.: Horse asthma following blood transfusion. *JAMA, 73*:984, 1919.
Protein sensitization in eczema, a report of 78 cases. *Arch Dermatol Syph, 2*:365, 1920.

Ramirez, M.D., and Eller, J.J.: Intradermal, scratch, indirect and contact tests in dermatology. *JAMA, 95*:1080, 1930.

Randolph, H.: Allergic response to dust of insect origin. *JAMA, 103*:560, 1934.
Fatigue and weakness of allergic origin (allergic toxemia) to be differentiated from "nervous fatigue" or neurasthenia. *Ann Allerg, 3*:418, 1945.

Randolph, T.G.: Fatigue syndrome of allergic origin. *Miss Valley Med J, 70*:105, 1948.
Allergy as a cause of acute torticollis. *J. Lab Clin Med, 33*:1614, 1948.
Allergy as a cause of acute torticollis. *Amer Practitioner Dig Treatment, 1, No. 10,* 10/ 1950.

Randolph, T.G.: Allergic myalgia. *J Michigan Med Soc, 50*:487, 1951.
Clinical sensitivities to petroleum, coal, pine and their derivatives. *J Allerg, 25*:81, 1954.
Food Susceptibility (Food Allergy) Current Therapy. H. Conn (Ed.), Philadelphia, Saunders, pp. 418-423, 1960.
Human ecology and susceptibility to the human environment. *Ann Allerg, 518*:657, 1961.
Ecologic orientation in medicine. Comprehensive environmental control in diagnosis and

therapy. *Ann Allerg*, 23:7, 1965.

Clinical ecology as it affects the psychiatric patient. *Int J Soc Psychiat*, 12:245, 1966.

Randolph, T.G., and Hettig, R.A.: Coincidence of allergic disease, unexplained fatigue and lymphadenopathy: Possible confusion with infectious mononucleosis. *Amer J Med Sci*, 209: 306, 1945.

Randolph, T.G., and Rollins, J.P.: Allergic reactions from the ingestion or intravenous injection of cane sugar (sucrose). *J Lab Clin Med*, 36:242, 1950.

Allergic reactions from the ingestion of beet sugar (sucrose) and monosodium glutamate of beet origin. *J Lab Clin Med*, 36:407, 1950.

Randolph, T.G., and Sisk, W.N.: Cottonseed protein versus cottonseed oil sensitivity; case of cottonseed oil sensitivity. *Ann Allerg*, 8:5, 1950.

Randolph, T.G., and Walter, C.K.: Allergic reactions following the intravenous injection of corn sugar (dextrose or glucose). *Arch Surg*, 61:554, 1950.

Rappaport, B.Z.: In Discussion of Squier, T.L., and Madison, F.W.: Thrombocytopenic purpura due to food allergy. *J Allerg*, 8:143, 1937.

Rappaport, E.M., Alper, Abe, and Rappaport, E.O.: Failure of surgery to relieve symptoms in prolapse of the gastric mucosa through the pylorus. *Ann Int Med*, 38:224, 1953.

Rasmussen, H.: Iodide hypersensitivity in the etiology of periarteritis nodosa. *J Allerg*, 26: 394, 1955.

Ratner, B.: Certain aspects of eczema and asthma in infancy and childhood from the standpoint of allergy. *Med Clin N Amer*, 6:815, 1922.

Eczema in infancy due to protein sensitization. *Med Clin N Amer*, 9:817, 1925.

Pulmonary tuberculosis in early infancy simulating bronchial asthma. *Med Clin N Amer*, 9: 826, 1925.

Possible cause of food allergy in certain infants. *Amer J Dis Child*, 26:277, 1928.

Allergy in children. *Med Clin N Amer*, 12: 847, 1928.

Possible causal factors of food allergy in certain infants. *Abstr Bull NY Acad Med*, 4:523, 1928.

Possible explanation for horse serum anaphylaxis in man. *JAMA*, 94:2046, 1930.

Diagnosis and management of allergic children. *JAMA*, 96:571, 1931.

(Discussion) Deaths in asthma usually due to morphine. *JAMA*, 97:982, 1931.

Ratner, B.: Treatment of milk allergy and its basic principles. *JAMA*, 105:934, 1935.

Allergy, Anaphylaxis and Immunotherapy. Baltimore, Williams and Wilkins, 1943.

Abdominal pain in children due to allergy. *JAMA*, 127:696, 1945.

Allergic manifestations in the central nervous system. *Amer J Dis Child*, 75:747, 1948.

Ratner, B., and Greenburgh, J.E.: Congenital protein hypersensitiveness, protein hypersensitiveness transmitted from allergic mother to child. *J Allerg*, 3:149, 1932.

Ratner, B., and Gruehl, H.L.: Passage of native proteins through normal gastrointestinal wall. *J Clin Invest*, 13:517, 1934.

Anaphylactogenic properties of milk: Immunochemistry of purified proteins and antigenic changes resulting from heat and acidification. *Amer J Dis Child*, 49:287, 1935.

Anayphylactogenic properties of malted sugars and corn syrup. *Amer J Dis Child*, 49:307, 1935.

Ratner, B., Jackson, H.C., and Gruehl, H.L.: Transmission of protein hypersensitiveness from mother to offspring; passive sensitization *in utero*. *J Immunol*, 14:291, 1927.

Rattner, H.: Dermatitis of the penis from rubber. *JAMA*, 105:1189, 1935.

Rattner, H., and Pusey, W.A.: Neurodermatitis or irritant dermatitis? Report of a case. *JAMA*, 99: 1934, 1932.

Ravdin, S., and Johnston, C.G.: Regional ileitis; a summary of the literature. *Amer J Med Sci*, 198:269, 1939.

Reimann, H.A.: *Periodic Diseases*. Philadelphia, F.A. Davis, 1963.

Reisman, R.E., and Arbesman, C.E.: Systemic allergic reactions due to inhalation of penicillin. *JAMA*, 203:986, 1968.

Remington, J.S., Vosti, K.L., Lietze, A., and Zimmerman, A.L.: Serum proteins and antibody activity in human nasal secretions. *J Clin Invest*, 43:1613, 1965.

Report: Sensitization to corn oil in which amniotin was contained. *JAMA*, 104:626, 1935.

Report: Drug Committee of the American Academy of Allergy, 1967.

Rich, A.R.: Sensitization in vasomotor rhinitis. *Laryngoscope*, 32:510, 1922.

The role of hypersensitivity of periarteritis nodosa as indicated by seven cases during serum sickness and sulfonamide therapy. *Bull Hopkins Hosp,* 71:123, 1942.

Additional evidence of the role of hypersensitivity in the etiology of periarteritis nodosa. Another case associated with a sulfonamide reaction. *Bull Hopkins Hosp,* 71:375, 1942.

Role of hypersensitivity in pathogenesis of rheumatic fever and periarteritis nodosa (Lewis Linn McArthur lecture) *Proc Int Med Chicago,* 15:270, 1945.

Richet, C.: *Anaphylaxis.* Transl. by J.H. Bligh, 1913, London. Original in French, 1911, Alcan, Paris.

Riehm, W.: Allergic mechanisms and the eye. *Med Klin,* 40:1317, 41:1353, 1934.

Riesman, D.: Vascular crises. *Amer J Med Sci,* 185:29, 1933.

Riley, H.A.: Migraine and its treatment. *Bull NY Acad Med,* 8:717, 1932.

Rinkel, H.J.: Headaches due to allergy (abstract). *J Allerg,* 5:318, 1933-1934.

Gastro-intestinal allergy. II. Concerning the mimicry of peptic ulcer syndrome by the symptoms of food allergy. *Southern Med J,* 27:630, July, 1934.

Food allergy. *J Kansas Med Soc,* 37:177, May, 1936.

The leucopenic index. II. Concerning the nature of food sensitization in intractable allergic diseases. *J Lab Clin Med,* 21:814, 1936.

The leucopenic index in allergic diseases. *J Allerg,* 7:356, 1936.

Food allergy. II. The technique and clinical application of individual food tests. *Ann Allerg,* 2:504, 1944.

Rinkel, H.J.: Food allergy. The role of food allergy in internal medicine. *Ann Allerg,* 2:115, 1944.

Rinkel, H.J., and Balyeat, R.M.: Pathology and symptomatology of headaches due to specific sensitization. *JAMA,* 99:806, 1932.

Rinkel, H.J., and Gay, L.P.: The leucopenic index: Technic and interpretation. *J Missouri Med Ass,* 33:182, 1936.

Rinkel, H.J., Lee, C.H., Brown, D., Jr., Willoughby, J.W., and Williams, J.M.: The diagnosis of food allergy. *Arch Otolaryng,* 79:71, 1964.

Rinkel, H.J., Randolph, T.G., and Zeller, M.: *Food Allergy.* Springfield, Charles C Thomas, 1951.

Roberts, H.J.: Gastrointestinal wheat allergy. *J Allerg,* 27:523, 1956.

Robinson, E.M.: Report of case of uterine spasm

caused by orris root. *Med J Rec,* 129:139, 1929.

Robinson, G.H., and Grauer, R.C.: Use of autogenous fungus extracts in the treatment of mycotic infections. *Arch Derm Syph,* 32:787, 1935.

Robinson, H.: Eczema. *Arch Derm,* 16:638, 1927.

Roch, M., and Scheff: Crises Asthmatiformes par Idiosyncrasie a legard de la Pomme de Terre, Choc. Hémoclasique et cutireaction. *Soc Méd Hop,* p. 883, 1921.

Rohrbach, H.O.: Supervision of the dairy herd is necessary to prevent analyphylactic symptoms in infant feeding. *Atlantic Med J,* 28:670, 1925.

Rohrer (1915): Cited by Vaughan, W.T., in *Practice of Allergy* (Third Edition), St. Louis, Mosby, 1954, p. 1033.

Rolleston, H.: *Idiosyncrasies.* London, 1927. *Report on the Work of the Asthma Research Council.* 1927-1934.

Rosenau, M., and Anderson, J.: Further studies upon phenomenon of anaphylaxis. *Bull Hyg Lab U.S.P.H.S.,* #50, 1909.

Rosenbloom, J.: Report of a case showing the relation between occupation and a certain case of bronchial asthma. *Amer J Med Sci,* 160:414, 1920.

Rosenblum, A.H.: An unusual case of pyloric stenosis. *Amer J Dis Child,* 80:356, 1950.

Rössle, R.: Die Geweblichen Asserungen der Allergie, Wien. *Klin Wschr,* 45:609, 1932.

Allergy and pathergy. *Fortschr Med,* 51:359, 1933.

Rose, B.: The cryopathies. In Samter, M. (Ed.): *Immunological Diseases,* Boston, Little, Brown & Co., 1965.

Rose, S.J.: Bronchial asthma and arsphenamine. *JAMA,* 90:405, 1928.

Rosenow, E.C.: Bacteriological studies of multiple sclerosis. *Ann Allerg,* 6:271, 1948.

Rothmund, A.: Über Cataracta in Verbindung mit einer eigentümlichen Haut degeneration. *Arch Ophthal,* 14:159, 1868.

Rowe, A.H.: Recent advances in the diagnosis and treatment of hay fever and asthma. *Calif State J,* 20:94, 1922.

The treatment of bronchial asthma. *JAMA,* 84:1902, 1925.

Allergy in the etiology of disease. *J Lab Clin Med,* 1:13, 1927.

Food allergy: A common cause of abdominal

symptoms and headache. *Food Facts,* 3:7, 1927.

Food allergy: Its control by elimination diets. *West Hosp Nurses' Rev, 13, Nos. 1 and 2,* 1928.

Food allergy, its manifestations, diagnosis and treatment. *JAMA,* 91:1623, 1928.

Abdominal food allergy: Its treatment with elimination diets. *Calif West Med,* 29:5, 1928.

Rowe, A.H.: *A Handbook for the Diabetic,* New York, Oxford University Press, 1928.

Allergic toxemia and migraine due to food allergy. *Calif West Med,* 33:785, 1930.

Food Allergy. Its Manifestations, Diagnosis and Treatment, Philadelphia, Lea and Febiger, 1931.

Desensitization to foods with reference to propetanes. *J Allerg,* 3:68, 1931.

Elimination diets for diagnosis and treatment of food allergy. *J Allerg,* 2:92, 1930, 1931.

Gastro-intestinal allergy. *JAMA,* 97:1440, 1931.

Uterine allergy. *Amer J Obstet Gynec,* 24:333, 1932.

Food allergy in the differential diagnoses of abdominal symptoms. *Amer J Med Sci, 183:* 529, 1932.

Allergic migraine. *AMA,* 99:912, 1932.

Roentgen studies of patients with gastrointestinal food allergy. *JAMA, 100:*394, 1933.

The present status of food allergy. *Northwest Med,* 32:217, 1933.

An evaluation of skin reactions in food sensitive patients. *J Allerg,* 5:135, 1934.

Revised "elimination diets" for the diagnosis and treatment of food allergy. *Amer J Dig Dis Nutr, 1:*6, 1934.

The challenge of allergy in medical practice. *Calif West Med,* 40:5, 1934.

Food allergy: A common problem in practice. *Southern Med J,* 28:261, 1935.

Protection of nutrition during the use of "elimination diets." *Amer J Dig Dis Nutr, 2:* 306, 1935.

Gastro-intestinal allergy. *Lancet,* 56:120, 1936.

Clinical Allergy. Manifestations, Diagnosis and Treatment. Philadelphia, Lea and Febiger, 1937.

Bronchial asthma. *JAMA,* 111:1827, 1938.

Pine pollen allergy. *J Allerg,* 4:10, May, 1939.

The elimination diets in the diagnosis and treatment of food allergy. *J Amer Diet Ass,* 16:3, 1940.

Seasonal and geographic influences on food allergy. *J Allerg,* 13:55, 1941.

Elimination diets for the study and treatment of food allergy. *J Lancet LXII,* 8:307, 1942.

Chronic ulcerative colitis—allergy in its etiology. *Ann Int Med,* 17:83, 1942.

Clinical allergy in the nervous system. *J Nerv Ment Dis,* 99:834, 1944.

Elimination Diets and the Patient's Allergies. 2nd ed. Philadelphia, Lea and Febiger, 1944.

Delayed healing of an abdominal wound due to food allergy. *West J Surg Obstet Gynec,* 54:313, 1946.

Atopic dermatitis of the hands due to food allergy. *Arch Dermat Syph,* 54:683, 1946.

Rowe, A.H.: Dermatitis of the hands due to atopic allergy to pollen. *Arch Dermat Syph,* 53:437, 1946.

Fever due to food allergy. *Ann Allerg,* 6:252, 1948.

Canker sores. *JAMA,* 138:1288, 1948.

Bronchial asthma in infants and children—its diagnosis and treatment. *Calif Med, 69, No. 4,* Oct., 1948.

Chronic ulcerative colitis—an allergic disease. *Ann Allerg,* 7:727, 819, 1949.

Elimination diets (Rowe). *Quart Rev Allerg,* 4:227, 1950.

Management of food allergy. *Postgrad Med,* 8:1, 1950.

Obscure fever in a child. *JAMA, 142:*398, 1950.

Allergic toxemia and fatigue. *Ann Allerg,* 8:72, 84, 1950.

Botannical survey of Northern California. *Ann Allerg,* vol. 3, 1952. (P. Kallos, 1952. S. Karger, Basel, Switzerland.)

Multiple food allergies and allergic toxemia. *JAMA,* Dec. 4, 1952.

Botannical survey of Northern California. *Ann Allerg,* 10:605, 1952.

Regional enteritis—its allergic aspects. *Gastroenterology,* 23:553, 1953.

Food allergy. Reasons for delayed recognition and control by physicians. *Quart Rev Allerg Appl Immunol,* 8:391, 1954.

Strained meat formulas in allergic diseases of infants and children. *Calif Med,* Oct., 1954.

Chronic ulcerative colitis. *JAMA, 156:* 1218, 1954.

Chronic ulcerative colitis and regional enteritis

—their allergic aspects. *Ann Allerg, 12*:387, 1954.

Allergic bronchial asthma and rhinitis. *Calif Med, 85*:33, 1956.

Diarrhea caused by food allergy. *J Allerg, 27*, 5:424, 1956.

La Alergia Alimenticia Y Sus Manifestaciones Clinicas. *Rev Clin Espan, XVII, LXII*:6, Sept., 1956.

Allergic toxemia and fatigue. *Ann Allerg, 17*: 9, 1959.

Chronic ulcerative colitis and regional enteritis responding to anti-allergic therapy. *Gastroenterologia, 91*:6, 1959.

Zur Klinik und Therapie von Nahrungsmittelallergien. *Allerg Asthma* (Leipzig), 8:256, 1962.

The Manifestations and Control of Food Allergy, Read by Invitation at First Congress on Food Allergy, Vichy, France, July, 1963. Les Regimes d'elimination dans le Traitement des Allergies Alimentaires. *Med Hyg, 21*:789, 1963.

Bronchial Asthma—Its Diagnosis and Treatment. Springfield, Charles C Thomas, 1963. Eczema of the hands due to food and pollen allergy. *Ann Allerg, 23*, Aug., 1965.

Elimination Diets (Rowe)—A Booklet with Diets, Menus and Recipes. 1965, 8th ed., Sather Gate, Berkeley, Calif.

Rowe, A.H., and Fong, J.: Specificity of graminae pollens as evidenced by precipitin reactions. *Proc Soc Exp Biol Med, 40*:570, 1939.

Rowe, A.H., and Mauser, C.L.: The cereal-free elimination diets and the soybean emulsion for the study and control of infantile eczema. *J Allerg, 13*:166, 1942.

Rowe, A.H., and Richet Fils, C.: Chronic nervous manifestations of alimentary anaphylaxis. *J Med Francaise, 19*:170, 1930.

Rowe, A.H., and Rowe, A., Jr.: Bronchial Asthma in patients over the age of fifty-five years—diagnosis and treatment. *Ann Allerg, 5*:509, 1947.

Local cutaneous allergy (Arthus phenomenon) from epinephrine. *J Allerg, 19*:62, 1948.

Bronchial asthma in adults—causes and treatment. *Calif Med, 72*:228, 1950.

Allergy and infection. *JAMA, 151*:846, 1953.

Seasonal and geographic influences on food allergy. *Int Arch Allerg, 13*:233, 1958.

Rowe, A.H., and Rowe, A., Jr.: Bronchial asthma

—its treatment and control. *JAMA, 172*:1734, 1960.

Rowe, A.H., and Rowe, A., Jr.: Unusual extra-respiratory manifestations of pollen allergy. *Ann Allerg, 19*:1004, 1961.

Food allergy: Its role in emphysema and chronic bronchitis. *Dis Chest, 48*:609, 1965.

Bronchial asthma—food, inhalant, drug and chemical allergies in its etiology, *Minnesota Med, 50*:1321, 1967.

Rowe, A.H., Rowe, A., Jr., and Sinclair, C.: Bronchial asthma in infants and children due to food and inhalant allergies. *J Asthma Res, 4*:189, 1967.

Rowe, A.H., Rowe, A., Jr., and Uyeyama, K.: The allergic epigastric syndrome. *J Allerg, 25*:464, 1954.

Rowe, A.H., Rowe, A., Jr., and Uyeyama, K.: Chronic ulcerative colitis due to pollen allergy with six case reports. *Acta Med Scand, 152*: 139, Fasc. II, 1955.

Rowe, A.H., Rowe, A., Jr., and Young, E.J.: Bronchial asthma due to food allergy alone in ninety-five patients. *JAMA, 169*:1158, 1959.

Rowe, A.H., Rowe, A., Jr., Young, E.J., and Uyeyama, K.: Chronic ulcerative colitis—atopic allergy in its etiology. *Amer J. Gastroent, 34*:49, 1960.

Atopic allergy in chronic ulcerative colitis. *JAMA, 184*:429, 1963.

Rowe, A.Jr.: Atopic dermatitis due to sensitivity to pollen. *Calif Med, 91*:341, 1959.

Rubin, M.I.: Allergic intestinal bleeding in the newborn. *Amer J Med Sci, 200*:385, 1940.

Rubin, M.I.: The intestinal manifestations of milk allergy in the newborn period. *Penns Med J, 45*:711, 1942.

Rudy, A.: Urticaria and insulin resistance with reference to relation of skin to carbohydrate metabolism; report of case and review of literature. *New Eng J Med, 204*:791, 1931.

Ruedemann, A.D.: Ocular allergy. *Ohio State Med J, 30*:304, 1934.

Ruiz-Moreno, Guido: Toxemia Alergica. *El Dia Medico, Ano XII, #47*:1092, 1940.

Ruiz-Moreno, G.: Sueno, sonmolencia, sed e impotencia sexual de origen alergico. *Rev Assoc Med Argent, 56*:483, 1942.

Toxaemia alergica. Capitulo de libro "Compendio de alergia clinica," de Henry I. Shahon. (Traduccion castellana). Buenos Aires: Libreria Hachette. S.A., 1943.

Consideraciones sobre un posible caso historico

de toxemia alergica. *Prensa Med Argent, 30:* 687, 1943.

Un caso mas de toxemia alergica. *Prensa Med Argent,* 31:90, 1944.

Sachs, O. (1916): Cited by Ackroyd, J.F.: Allergic purpura, including purpura due to foods, drugs and infections. *Amer J Med,* 14:605, 1953.

Salen, E.B.: Allergische Reaktion der Harnwege. *Acta Med Scand,* 88:197, 1932.

Salen, E.B.: Ist die Sensibilizerung bei der Allergie ubiquitär? Allergische Reaktion der Harnwege. *Acta Med Scand,* 78:197, 1932.

Salicus, O.: Allergic pancreatitis. *Bol Ass Med P Rico,* 52 #6, June, 1960.

Salter, H.H.: *On Asthma: Its Pathology and Treatment.* London, 1868.

Samitz, M., Dance, A., and Rosenberg, P.: Cutaneous vasculitis in association with Crohn's disease. *Cutis,* 6:51, 1970.

Sammis, F.E.: Dermatitis herpetiformis associated with food allergy. *Arch Derm Syph,* 32:798, 1935.

Sanarelli, G.: Hemorrhagic allergies (Sanarelli-Schwartzman phenomenon) in human and experimental pathology. *Schweiz Med Wschr,* 65:904, 1935.

Sanders, T.E.: Intermittent occlusion of the central retinal artery. *Amer J Ophthal,* 22:8, 1939.

The ocular Schwartzman phenomenon. *Amer J Ophthal,* 22:10, 1939.

Sanford, A.H.: Protein sensitization in asthma and hay fever. *Minnesota Med,* 3:174, 1920.

Sattler, C.H.: Untersuchungen über die Wirkung von Blutserum nach Einspritzungin's Auge. *Arch Augenheilk,* 64:390, 1909.

Scadding, J.G.: Chronic Diffuse Interstitial Fibrosis of the Lungs. *Brit Med J,* 5171:443, 1960.

Schachne, L.: Personal communication. Cited by Theodore, F.C., and Schlossman, A.: Ocular Allergy. Baltimore, Williams and Wilkins, 1958.

Schaffer, N., Mulomut, N., and Center, J.G.: Studies on allergenic extracts. I. A new method for preparation of mold extracts using a synthetic medium. *Ann Allerg,* 17:380, 1959.

Scheer, M., and Keil, H.: The skin eruptions of codeine. *JAMA,* 102:908, 1934.

Schenk, H.P., and Kern, R.A.: An evaluation of the therapeutic effect of the Caldwell-Luc

operation on bronchial asthma. *J Allerg,* 3:296, 1932.

Schepers, G.W.H.: The pathology of regional enteritis. *Amer J Dig Dis,* 12:97, 1945.

Schers (1929): Cited by Fries, J.H., and Jennings, K.: Recurrent vomiting in children. *J Pediat,* 17:458, 1940.

Schlessinger, L.: Acute relapsing edema of eyelids and exophthalmos. *München Med Wschr,* No. 5., 1899.

Schloss, O.M.: A case of allergy to common foods. *Amer J Dis Child,* 3:341, 1912.

Allergy to common foods. *Trans Amer Pediat Soc,* 27:62, 1915.

Allergy to common foods. *Arch Pediat,* 32: 349, 1915.

Allergy in infants and children. *Amer J Dis Child,* 19:433, 1920.

Incubation studies in intestinal allergies. *Amer J Med,* 7:155, 1949.

Schloss, O.M., and Anderson, A.: Allergy to cow's milk in infants with severe malnutrition. *Proc Soc Exp Biol Med,* 20:5, 1922.

Treatment of milk allergy. *JAMA,* 106:1025, 1936.

Schloss, O.M., and Worthen, T.W.: The permeability of the gastro-enteric tract of infants to undigested protein. *Amer J Dis Child,* 11:342, 1916.

Schlossman, Abraham: *Ocular Allergy.* Baltimore, Williams and Wilkins, 1958.

Schoenberg, M.J.: A contribution to the experimental study of ocular anaphylaxis. *Ophthalmology,* 11:1, 1914-1915.

Schofield, A.T.: A case of egg poisoning. *Lancet,* i:716, 1908.

Scholtz, H.G.: Schwerste Stomakake, Kojunktivitis, Rhinitis and Bronchitis bei Allergischer Diathese. *München Med Wschr,* 79:916, 1932.

Scholtz, W.: Allergic skin diseases. *Deutsch Med Wschr,* 59:519, 1933.

Schorer, G.: Unusual phenomena with angioneurotic edema. *Schweiz Med Wschr,* 55:340, 1925.

Schultz, S.W., and Larsen, W.T.: Anaphylaxis and its relation to some diatheses common to infancy and childhood. *Arch Pediat,* 35:705, 1918.

Schumacher: Verbal personal communication. Cited by Rowe, A.H.: *Clinical Allergy, Manifestations, Diagnosis and Treatment.* Philadelphia, Lea and Febiger, 1937.

Schwartz, L.: Skin hazards in American industry.

U.S. Public Health Bull. 215. U.S. Treasury Department, Washington, 1934.

Sensitivity to external irritants in industry. *New York J Med,* 36:1969, 1936.

Dermatitis from wrist straps. *Public Health Rep,* 51:423, 1936.

Allergic Dermatitis: Extrinsic. Cooke, R.A. (Ed.): *Allergy in Theory and Practice.* Philadelphia, W.B. Saunders, 1947, p. 263.

Sedan, J., and Guillot, P.: Uvéites medicamenteuses. *Bull Soc Franc Ophthal,* 11:145, 1955.

Seegal, B.C., and Seegal, D.: Local organ hypersensitiveness: Indirect method for its production in rabbit eye. *J Immunol,* 25:221, 1933.

Seegal, B.C., Seegal, D., and Khorazo, D.: Local organ hypersensitiveness, fate of antigen and appearance of antibodies during development of hypersensitiveness in rabbit eye. *J Immunol,* 25:207, 1933.

Seegal, D., and Seegal, B.C.: Local organ hypersensitiveness; experimental production in rabbit eye. *Proc Soc Exp Biol Med,* 27:390, 1930.

Segal, M.S., Attinger, E.O., and Goldstein, M.M.: Mechanical aids and drugs. Bronchial obstruction and bronchospasm. *Ann Allerg,* 17:413, 1959.

Segal, M.S., Beakey, U.F., Bresnick, E., and Levinson, L.: A comparative study of the action of various sympathomimetic amine aerosols in encountering the dyspnea and bronchospasm induced by histamine and by acetyl-beta-methylcholine. *J Allerg,* 20:97, 1949.

Seinfeld, B.M., and McCombs, R.P.: Skin window, an aid in the diagnosis of drug allergy. *J Allerg,* 28:156, 1966.

Seitz, L.: Beruhen die Schwangerschaft auf Einem Allergischen Zustand? *Zbl Gynaek,* 59:1207, 1935.

Senger, H.A.: Colon disorders simulated by urolithiasis. *Med Clin N Amer,* 12:193, 1928.

Serio, F.: La Sintomatologia Radiologica della Anafilassi. *Gastro-intestinale Riforma Med,* 48:1742, 1932.

Shannon, W.R.: Demonstration of food reactions in human breast milk by anaphylactic experiments in guinea-pigs. *Amer J Dis Child,* 22:223, 1921.

Eczema in breast-fed infants as a result of sensitization to foods in the mother's dietary. *Amer J Dis Child,* 23:392, 1922.

Neuropathic manifestations in infants and children as a result of anaphylactic reactions to foods contained in the dietary. *Amer J Dis Child,* 24:89-94, 1922.

Anaphylaxis to food proteins in breast-fed infants and its probable relation to certain diseases of the nursing infant, especially exudative diathesis. *Minnesota Med,* 5:137, 1922.

Anaphylaxis: Its part in the diseases of infancy and childhood. *Lancet,* May 1, 1924.

Sheard, L., Caylor, H.D., and Schlotthauer: Photo-sensitization of animals after the ingestion of buckwheat. *J Exp Med,* 47:1012, 1928.

Shearer, R.V., and Dubois, E.L.: Ocular changes induced by long-term hydroxychloroquine therapy. *Amer J Ophthal,* 64:245-252, 1967.

Sheldon, J.D.: Serious meningitis of allergic nature with report of case. *Lancet,* i:798, 1933.

Sheldon, J.M., Lovell, R.S., and Mathews, K.P.: *A Manual of Clinical Allergy.* Philadelphia, W. B. Saunders, 1953.

Sheldon, J.M., and Randolph, T.G.: Allergy in migraine-like headaches. *Amer J Med Sci,* 190:232, 1935.

Sheldon, J.M., and Robinson, W.D.: Subcutaneous emphysema in asthma. *JAMA,* 107:1884, 1936.

Shelmire, B.: The etiology of eczema. *Southwest Med,* 17:297, 1933.

Sherrick, J.: Personal communication. Cited by Rowe, A.H.: *Manifestations, Diagnosis and Treatment.* Philadelphia, Lea and Febiger, 1937.

Shookhoff, C., and Lieberman, D.L.: Hypersensitiveness to acetyl salicylic acid expressed by angina pectoris syndrome with and without urticaria. *J Allerg,* 4:506, 1933.

Angina pectoris syndrome, activated by ragweed sensitivity in patient with coronary vessel sclerosis: Case report. *J Allerg,* 4:513, 1933.

Short, C.L., and Bauer, W.: Cincophen hypersensitiveness, report of four cases and review. *Ann Int Med,* 6:1449, 1933.

Siegel, S.C., Levin, B.J., Ely, R.S., and Kelley, V.C.: Adrenal function in allergy. III. Effect of prolonged intermittent steroid therapy in allergic children. *Pediatrics,* 24:434, 1959.

Simon, F.A.: Species non-specific antigenic factor in mammalian serums; preliminary report. *J Allerg,* 6:1, 1934.

Simon, F.A., and Ryder, C.F.: Hypersensitiveness to pituitary extracts. *JAMA,* 106:512, 1936.

Simonds, J.P.: A study of the simultaneous changes in the blood pressure in the carotid artery and jugular and portal veins in anaphylactic and peptone shock in the dog. *Amer J Physiol,* 65:512, 1923.

Simonds, J.P., and Brandes, W.W.: Effect of the obstruction of the hepatic veins on the systemic circulation. *Amer J Physiol,* 72:320, 1925.
Smooth muscle in hepatic veins. *J Immunol,* 13:1, 1927.

Sincke, G.E.: Hypersensitivity to vanilla. *Derm Wschr,* 99:1480, 1934.

Singer, G.: Leber-Gallenkrisen-alimentäre Schädigung-anaphylaktischer Chok. *Arch f Verdauungskr, 42:*322, 1928.

Sison, A.B.M.: Ophthalmic migraine of allergic origin. *J Philip Med Ass,* 13:250, 1933.

Sluiter, H.J.: Participant in *Bronchitis. An International Symposium.* April, 1960, University of Groningen, The Netherlands, Charles C Thomas, 1961. Royal Vangorcum Publisher, Assen, Netherlands.

Small, J.C.: Streptococci in relation to rheumatic disease. *Med Clin N Amer,* 13:857, 1930.

Small, J.C., and Small, J.C., Jr.: Treatment of rheumatic diseases by desensitization with an aqueous extract of streptococci. *Ann Allerg,* 12:409, 1956.

Small, W.S.: Allergy in Southern California due to fertilizer. *J Allerg,* 23:406, 1952.

Smith (1937): Cited by Fries, J.H., and Jennings, K.: Recurrent vomiting in children. *J Pediat,* 17:458, 1940.

Smith, D.R.: Essential dysmenorrhea and allergy. *J Missouri Med Ass,* 28:382, 1931.

Smith, H.C.: Buckwheat poisoning. *Arch Int Med,* 3:350, 1909.

Smith, P.S.: Cyclic vomiting and migraine in children. *Virginia Med Monthly,* 60:591, 1934.

Smith, Dutton, and Tallerman (1934): Cited by Fries, J.H., and Jennings, K.: Recurrent vomiting in children. *J Pediat,* 17:458, 1940.

Sokolowski, A.: Ein Fall von Ueberempfindlichkeit gegen atophan mit Fixem Exanthem. *Wien Klin Wschr, 44:*108, 1931.

Solow, I.A., and Updegraff, W.C.: Serous otitis media—symposium. II. Allergic serous otitis media; treatment and results. *Ann Allerg,* 23:281, 1965.

Spain, W.C.: The diagnosis and treatment of atopic coryza (perennial hay fever). *Ann Otol,* 34:1093, 1925.
Food hypersensitiveness. *New York J Med,* 33:1100, 1933.

Spector, H.I.: Loeffler's syndrome (transient pulmonary infiltration with eosinophilia) report of a case and review of the available literature. *Dis Chest, 11:*380, 1945.

Speer, F.: The allergic tension—fatigue syndrome. *Pediat Clin N Amer,* 1:1029, 1954.

Speer, F.: Food allergy in childhood. *Arch Pediat,* 75:363, 1958.
Colic and allergy—a ten year study. *Arch Pediat,* 75:271, 1958.

Speer, F.: The allergic tension-fatigue syndrome in children. *Int Arch Allerg,* 12:207, 1958.
Allergy of the Nervous System, Springfield, Thomas, 1970.

Speizer, F.E., Doll, R., Heaf, P., and Strang, L.B.: Investigation into use of drugs preceding death from asthma. *Brit Med J,* 1:339, 1968.

Speizer, F.E., Doll, R., and Heaf, P.: Observations on recent increase in mortality in asthma. *Brit Med J,* 1:335, 1968.

Spieksma, F. Th. M., *et al.*: The mite fauna of housedust. *Acarologia,* 9:226, 1967.

Spielman, A.D., and Baldwin, H.S.: Atopy to acacia (gum arabic). *JAMA,* 101:444, 1933.

Spies, J.R., Stevan, M.A., Stein, W.J., and Coulson, E.J.: The chemistry of allergens. XX. New antigens generated by pepsin hydrolysis of bovine milk products. *J Allerg,* 45:208, 1970.

Squier, T.L., and Madison, F.W.: Primary granulocytopenia due to hypersensitivity to amidopyrine. *J Allerg,* 6:9, 1936.
Thrombocytopenic purpura due to food allergy. *J Allerg,* 8:143, 1937.

Ssolowjew, A., and Ariel, M.D.: Experimentelle Untersuchungen uber die hypergische Hirhautenzundung. *Virchow Arch Path Anat,* 295:201, 1935.

Stack, B.H., Grant, I.W., Irvine, W.J. *et al.*: Idiopathic diffuse interstitial lung disease. A review of 42 cases. *Am Rev Resp Dis,* 92:939, 1965.

Stack, B.H., and Grant, I.W.: Rheumatoid interstitial lung disease. *Brit J Dis Chest,* 59:202, 1965.

Staffiere, D., Dentiolila, L., and Levit, L.: Hemiplegra and allergic symptoms following ingestion of certain foods. *Ann Allerg,* 10:38, 1952.

Starck, Von Z.: Primary specific allergy and idiosyncratic shock. *Mschr Kinderheilk,* 32:119, 1926.

Stavitsky, A.B., and Arquilla, E.R.: Micromethods for the study of proteins and antibodies. III.

Procedure and applications of hemagglutination and hemagglutination inhibition reactions with bis-diazotized benzidene and protein-conjugated red blood cells. *J Immunol,* 74: 306, 1955.

Stein, I., and Wecksell, I.: Cardiac disease accompanying allergic drug reactions. *J Allerg,* 45:48, 1970.

Stein, M., and Cassara, E.L.: Pre-operative pulmonary evaluation and therapy in surgery. *JAMA, 211*:787, 1970.

Sterling, Alexander: Food allergy or gastro-intestinal anaphylaxis. *Med J Rec, 129*:610, 1929.

Stevens, F.A.: Chronic infectional edema. *JAMA, 100*:1754, 1933.

Sticker: *Das Heufieber und verwandte Störunger.* Wien-Leipzig, Hölder, 1912.

Stiefler, G.: Ein Fall von Angioneurotischem Oedem nach Atophangebrauch. *Med Klin,* 73:927, 1919.

Stier, R.F., and Hollister, G.L.: A comparative study of pollen antigens as determined by the skin reactions. *J Lab Clin Med, 12*:1139, 1927.

Stoesser, A.V.: Recent observations in study of asthma due to food allergy. *J Allerg, 3*:332, 1932.

Stokes, J.H.: Eczema problem. *Amer J Med Sci, 179*:69, 1930.
West Virginia Med J, 26:159, 1930.

Stokes, J.H.: The complex of eczema, diagnostic and etiologic analysis. *JAMA,* 98:1127, 1932. Functional neuroses as complications of organic disease: An office technic of approach with special reference to the neuro-dermatoses. *JAMA, 105*:1087, 1935.

Strebel, J.: Über Allergiebedingte Lidödome und ihre Uraschen. *Klin Mbl Augenheilk,* 97:644, 1936.

Stremple, J.F., Polacek, M.A., and Ellison, E.H.: The acute non-surgical abdomen of Henoch-Schonlein syndrome in the elderly patient. *Amer J Surg, 115*:870, 1968.

Strickler, A., and Goldberg, J.M.: Anaphylactic food reactions in dermatology. Preliminary report. *JAMA, 66*:249, 1916.

Stroud, C.M.: Allergic dermatitis. *J Allerg,* 2:118, 1931.
Allergic dermatitis. *Southern Med J,* 28:665, 1935.

Strümpell, A. von: Ueber das Asthma Bronchiale und Seine Bezierhungen zur sogenannten exsudativen Diathese. *Med Klin,* 6:889, 1910.

Stuart, G.J.: A simple method for preparing strained meat formulas. *J Allerg,* 16:253, 1945.

Stuart, H.C.: The excretion of foreign proteins in human milk. *Amer J Dis Child,* 25:135, 1923.

Stuart, H.C., and Farnham, M.: Acquisition and loss of hypersensitiveness in early life. *Amer J Dis Child, 32*:341, 1926.

Sulzberger, M.B.: Studies in tobacco hypersensitivity; comparison between reactions to nicotine and to denicotinized tobacco extract. *J Immunol,* 24:185, 1933.

Sulzberger, M.B., and Goodman, J.: The relative importance of specific skin hypersensitivity in adult atopic dermatitis. *JAMA, 106*:1000, 1936.
Description of a technic for the study of allergy in eczematous and eczematoid dermatoses. *Lancet,* 56:134, 1936.

Sulzberger, M.B., and Kerr, P.: Trichophytin hypersensitiveness of urticarial type with circulatory antibodies and passive transference. *J Allerg, 2*:11, 1930.

Sulzberger, M.B., and Simon, F.A.: Arsphenamine hypersensitiveness in guinea-pigs; experiments demonstrating (A) regional geographic variability in susceptibility to sensitization, (B) chemical specificity of hypersensitivity, and (C) variation in sensitizing proclivities (sensitization index) of different brands. *J Allerg,* 6:39, 1934.

Sutton, I.C.: Acute dermatitis from wearing of "horn-rim" spectacles. *JAMA,* 89:1059, 1927.

Sweet, Clifford: My child won't eat. *Arch Pediat,* 47:582, 1930.
Voluntary food habits of normal children. *JAMA, 107*:765, 1936.

Sweetser, H.B.: The allergic factor in migraine. *Minn Med,* 17:31, 1934.

Swift, and Derick (1928 & 1930): Cited by Woods, A.C.: *Allergy and Immunity in Ophthalmology.* Baltimore, Johns Hopkins Press, 1933.

Swinny, Boen: A filter adapter for small quantities of solutions. *J Lab Clin Med, 23*:1098, 1938.

Synder, R.A.: Allergic purpura. *Ann Allerg,* 26: 328, 1968.

Talbot, F.B.: Idiosyncrasy to cow's milk in relation to anaphylaxis. *Boston Med Surg J, 175*:409, 1916.
Role of food idiosyncrasies in practice. *New York J Med,* 17:419, 1917.

Role of food idiosyncrasies in practice. *Med Rec,* 91:875, 1917.

Relation of food idiosyncrasies to the diseases of childhood. *Boston Med Surg J,* 179:285, 1918.

Eczema in childhood. *Med Clin N Amer, 1*: 985, 1918.

Treatment of Epilepsy. New York, Macmillan Company, 1930.

Tallant, E.J., O'Neill, H.A., Urbach, F., and Price, A.M.: Gastrointestinal food hypersensitivity, roentgenographic demonstration. *Nutrition, 16*:40, 1949.

Tallerman, K.H.: Recurrent vomiting attacks in childhood. *British Med J,* 2:766, 1934.

Tallroth, A.: On regional enteritis with special reference to its etiology and pathogenesis. *Acta Chir Scand,* 88:407, (Suppl. 77), 1943.

Taub, S.J.: Allergy due to silk. *J Allerg,* 1:539, 1930.

Local allergy to the eye. *J Allerg,* 8:75, 1936.

Taub, S.J., and White, C.J.: Urticaria due to grass pollen. *J Allerg,* 2:186, 1931.

Taylor, D.M., Thomson, D.C., and Truelove, S.C.: Immunological study of celiac disease and idiopathic steatorrhea. *Brit Med J,* 2:727, 1961.

Taylor, K.B., and Truelove, S.C.: Circulating antibodies to milk proteins in ulcerative colitis. *Brit Med J,* 2:924, 1961.

Templeton, H.J.: Tricophytin—its use according to allergic principles. *J Allerg,* 5:521, 1934.

Templeton, H.J., and Lunsford, C.J.: Eczema solare and porphyria. *Arch Dermat Syph,* 25: 691, 1932.

Tenani, O.: Spora Un Caso di Edema Angioneurotico di Quincke in Rapporto Con La Malaria. *Atti Acad Sci Med Nat Ferrara,* 85:193, 1911-1912.

Theodore, Frederick H., and Schlossman, A.: *Ocular Allergy.* Baltimore, Williams and Wilkins, 1958.

Theodore, F.C., and Lewson, A.C.: Bilateral iritis complicating serum sickness. *Arch Ophthal,* 21:82, 1939.

Thomas, J.W.: The treatment of severe allergic reactions to insect bites and stings. *Virginia Med Monthly,* 85:415, 1958.

Thomas, J.W., and Wicksten, V.P.: Allergy in relation to the genitourinary tract. *Ann Allerg,* 2:396, 1944.

Thomas, T.F.: Thrombocytopenia secondary to sulfamethoxpyridazine. *New York J Med,* 63: 2554, 1963.

Thomas, W.A., and Post, W.E.: Paroxysmal tachycardia in migraine. *JAMA,* 84:569, 1925.

Thomas, W.S.: Generalized edema occurring only at the menstrual period. *JAMA, 101*:1126, 1933.

Thommen, A.A. (1931): See Coca, A.F., Walzer, M., and Thommen, A.A.

Tileston, W.: Migraine in childhood. *Amer J Dis Child,* 16:312, 1918.

Todd, L.C.: Food allergy with special reference to migraine. *Southern Med Surg,* 95:587, 1933.

Todd, L., and Tkach, S.: Synovectomy of knee in rheumatoid arthritis. *Southern Med J,* 62: 1093, 1969.

Tomasi, T.B., Jr.: *Disease of the Liver, Immunological Diseases.* Boston, Little, Brown and Company, p. 880, 1965.

Tow, D.E., and Wagner, H.N., Jr.: Lung scanning in pulmonary diseases. *New York J Med,* 276: 1053, 1967.

Tripp, H.D.: Catgut allergy. *Indiana Med Ass,* 28:383, 1935.

Tudor, R.B.: Gastrointestinal allergy to cow's milk in the neonatal period. *Lancet,* 76:245, 1956.

Tuft, Louis: Fatalities following reinjection of foreign serum; report of unusual case. *Amer J Med Sci,* 175:325, 1928.

Insulin hypersensitiveness; immunologic considerations and case reports. *Amer J Med Sci,* 176:707, 1928.

Allergic migraine. *Pennsylvania Med J,* 39: 162, 1935.

Clinical Allergy. Philadelphia, W.B. Saunders, 1937.

Clinical Allergy. 2nd ed. Philadelphia, Lea and Febiger, 1949.

Problems of the geriatic asthmatic and their clinical management. *JAMA,* 145:1480, 1951.

Letter to editor on atopic dermatitis due to food and inhalant allergy. *J Allerg,* 26:293, 1956.

Tuft, Louis, and Blumstein, G.I.: Studies in food allergy. II. Sensitization to fresh fruits: Clinical and experimental observations. *J Allerg,* 13:574, 1942.

Tuft, L., and Girsh, L.S.: Buccal mucosal tests in patients with canker sores (aphthous stomatitis). *J Allerg,* 29:502, 1958.

Tumpeer, I.H.: The allergic nature of infantile

diathesis and associated frequency of widened mediastinal shadow (thymus?). *Arch Pediat,* 51:407, 1934.

Turnbull, J.A.: Food allergens in connection with arthritis. *Boston Med Surg J,* 191:438, 1924.

Turrettini, M.G.: Maladie de Quincke par Sensibilization Tardive au Pain et Aux Autres Farineaux. *Bull Soc Méd Hôp Paris,* 46:811, 1922.

Tynes, B., Mason, K.N., Jennings, A.E., *et al.*: Variant forms of pulmonary cryptococcus. *Ann Int Med,* 69:1017, 1968.

Tzanck, A.: Les Intolerances Gastriques a Forme Hemorragique (le Probleme des Hémorrhagies dites "essentielles"). *Bull Soc Méd Hôp Paris,* 48:585, 1932.

Tzanck, A., and Cottet, J.: Les Intolérances Rénales. *Presse Mèd,* 42:415, 1934.

Uhlenhuth, P.: Zur Lehre von der Unterscheidung verschiedener Eiweissarte mit Hilfe spezifischer Sera. In Festschrift zum 60. Geburtstage von Robert Koch, Jena: *Gustav Fischer.* p. 49, 1903.

Ullmann, K.: Ein Fall zirkumskripten angioneurotischen Oedemen mit Konsecutiven Epileptiformen Anfällen. *Arch Schiffs Tropen Hyg,* 3:176, 1899.

Unger, D.L., and Unger, L.: Migraine as an allergic disease. *J Allerg,* 23:426, 1952.
Allergic reactions to ACTH. *Dis Chest,* 40:359, 1961.

Unger, L.: Food sensitization in bronchial asthma. *Illinois Med J,* 44:40, 1923.
Drug idiosyncrasy. *J Allerg,* 3:76, 1931.
Discussion: Eggs causing acne and epilepsy. *JAMA,* 103:129, 1934.
Bronchial Asthma. Springfield, Charles C Thomas, 1945.

Urbach, E.: Oral method of desensitization toward certain foods. *JAMA,* 95:214, 1930.
Oral desensitization in dermatoses due to food allergy by means of specific peptones. *Klin Wschr,* p. 2046, 1930.
Idiosyncrasy to food as occasional cause of vasomotor rhinitis and asthma. *Mschr Ohrenheilk,* 66:160, 1932.
Wohnungsallergene als Ursache Chronischer Dermatosen und Mykosen. *Münich Med Wschr,* 80 (1):212, 1933.
Skin Diseases and Nutrition Including the Dermatoses of Children. Transl. by Schmidt, Maudrich, 1933.

Parallergie und Metallergie. *Klin Wschr,* 13:1417, 1934.
Methods for diagnosis and treatment of nutritive allergic dermatoses. *Dermat Ztschr,* 70:214, 1934.

Urbach, E.: Odors (osmyls) as allergenic agents. *J Allerg,* 13:387, 1942.

Urbach, E., and Fasal, P.: Vasoallergie oder Vasoneuropathie als Ursache von Költe-Wärme und Druckurtikaria? Ein Beitrag zur Pathogenese und Therapie der Sogenannten Physikalischen Allergien der Haut. *Wien Klin Wschr,* 46:1069, 1100, 1933.

Urbach, E., and Gottlieb, P.M.: *Allergy,* 2nd ed., New York, Grune and Stratton, 1946.

Urbach, E., and Wilder, J.: Allergisch bedingter Ménièrescher Symptomenkomplex. *Med Klin,* 30:1420, 1934.

Vail (1938): Personal communication.

Vallery-Radot, Pasteur: Pathogenesis of migraines. *Rev Neurol,* 1:881, 1925.
Les Phénomenes de choc dans l'urticaria. Paris, 1930.

Vallery-Radot, P.: A propos de la communication de M. Ch. Flanden: "Un cas d'anaphylaxie alimentaire chez l'homme". *Bull et mem soc med hop de Paris,* 54:980, 1930.

Vallery-Radot, Pasteur, and Blamoutier, P.: Un Cas Mortel de Maladie de Quincke avec Crises Douloureuses Abdominales Accompagnées de Spasmes Vasculaires. *Bull Soc Mèd Hôp Paris,* 47:459, 1931.

Vallery-Radot, Pasteur, and Hamburger, J.: *Les Migraines: Etude Pathoginique Clinique et Therapeutique.* Paris, Masson et Cie, 1935.

Vallery-Radot, Pasteur, and Heimann, V.: Hypersensibilitiés Specifiques dans les Affections Cutanées. Paris, Masson et Cie, 1930.

Vallery-Radot, Pasteur, Ledoux-Lebard, Hamburger, J., Hugo, A., and Calderon, G.: Arteriography in anaphylactic shock of rabbit. *Presse Med,* 43:1057, 1935.

Vallone, D.: Anafilassi e ulcera gastrica. *Arch Ital Chir,* 25:535, 1930.

van Bronswijk, J.E.M.H., and Sinha, R.N.: Pyroglyphid mites (Acari) and house dust allergy. *J Allerg,* 47:31, 1971.

Van Leeuwen, W.S.: *Allergic Diseases.* Philadelphia, Lippincott, 1925.

Van Metre, T.E., Jr.: Role of the allergist in diagnosis and management of patients with uveitis. *JAMA,* 195:167, 1966.
Adverse effects of inhalation of excessive

amounts of nebulized isoproterenol in status asthmaticus. *J Allerg, 43*:101, 1969.

Van Metre, T.E., Jr., Cooke, R.E., Gibson, L.E., and Winkenwerder, W.L.: Evidence of allergy in patients with cystic fibrosis of the pancreas. *J Allerg, 31*:141, 1960.

Van Metre, T.E., Jr., and Maumenee, A.E.: Specific ocular uveal lesions in patients with evidence of histoplasmosis. *Arch Ophthal, 71*: 314-324, 1964.

Van Metre, T.E., Jr., and Pinterton, H.L., Jr.: Growth suppression in asthmatic children receiving prolonged therapy with prednisone and methyl prednisone. *J Allerg, 30*:103, 1959.

Vanselow, Neal, A.: The status of hyposensitization therapy in allergic disease. *Univ Mich Ctr Bull, 34*:137-142, 1968.

Vaughan, W.T.: Diseases associated with protein sensitization. *Virginia Med Monthly,* Sept. 1922.

Allergic Migraine, *JAMA,* 88:1383, 1927.

Allergic eczema. *J Lab Clin Med,* 13:24, 1927.

Allergic factor in mucous colitis. *Southern Med J,* 21:894, 1928.

The effect of allergic reactions on the course on non-allergic diseases. *J Lab Clin Med, 15*: 726, 1930.

Food allergens. I. A genetic classification with results of group testing. *J Allerg,* 1:385, 1930.

Food allergy as common problem. *J Lab Clin Med,* 19:53, 1933.

Allergic migraine: Analysis of a follow-up after 5 years. *Amer J Med Sci,* 185:821, 1933.

Food allergens: Leucopenic index; preliminary report. *J Allerg,* 5:601, 1934.

Further studies on leucopenic index in food allergy. *J Allerg,* 6:78, 1934.

Allergy and Applied Immunology, 2nd ed. St. Louis, C.V. Mosby Company, 1934.

Some observations on food allergy. *Amer J Dig Dis,* 1:384, 1934.

An analysis of the allergic factor in recurrent paroxysmal headaches. *J Allerg,* 6:365, 1935.

The leucopenic index as a diagnostic method in the study of food allergy. *J Lab Clin Med,* 21:1278, 1936.

Practice of Allergy. St. Louis, C.V. Mosby Company, 1939.

Palindronic rheumatism among allergic persons. *J Allerg,* 14:256, 1943.

Antral gastritis: Roentgenological and gastroscopic findings. *Radiology,* 44:531, 1945.

Vaughan, W.T., and Fowlkes, R.E.: Allergic reactions associated with cohabitation. *JAMA, 105*:955, 1935.

Vaughan, W.T., and Hawke, E.K.: Angioneurotic edema with some unusual manifestations. *J Allerg,* 2:125, 1931.

Vaughan, W.T., and Sullivan, C.J.: Pressure episodes after ingestion of allergenic foods—indicated in 3 of 24 food sensitive patients. *J Allerg,* 8:572, 1937.

Venger, N.: Fatal reaction to sulfobromophthalein sodium in a patient with bronchial asthma. *JAMA, 175*:506, 1961.

Verhoeff, F.H., and Lemoine, A.N.: Endophthalmitis phacoanaphylactica. *Int Congr Ophthal,* Washington, p. 234, 1922.

Vogt, A.: Weitere Ergebrisse der Spaltlampmikroskopie. *Arch Ophthal, 109*:97, 1922.

Volkheimer, G.: Durchlässigkeit des Darmes und der Placenta für grosskorpusculäre Elemente. *Allergie und Asthma,* 9:133, 1963.

Volkheimer, G.: Das Phänomen der Persorption von Stärkekörnern. *Die Stärke, 20*:117, 1968.

Volkheimer, G., and Schulz, F. H.: Persorption of vegetable food particles. *Qualitas Plantarum et Materiae Vegetabilies,* 17:17, 1968.

Volkheimer, G., Schulz, F.H., Wendland, H., and Hausdorf, E.D.: Le Phénomène de la Persorption et son Importance En Allergologie. *Extrait du Maroc-Médical,* 506:47, 1967.

Von Pirquet, C., und Schick, B.: *Die Serumkrankheit.* Leipzig Und Wien, Franz Deuticke, 1905, Berlin.

Von Szily, A.: *Die Anaphylaxie in der Augenheilkunde.* Stuttgart, Ver. Ferdinand Enke, 1914.

Voorhurst, R., Spieksma, F. Th. M., Varekamp, H., Leupen, M.J., and Lyklema, A.W.: The housedust mite and the allergen it produces. *J Allerg,* 39:325, 1967.

Wagner, H.C., and Rackemann, F.M.: Kapok: Its importance in clinical allergy. *J Allerg,* 7:224, 1936.

Waldbott, G.L.: Asthma due to local anesthetic. *JAMA,* 99:1942, 1932.

"Allergic" shock from substances other than pollen and serum. *Ann Int Med,* 7:1308, 1934.

The types of human hypersensitiveness (letter). *JAMA, 102*:1631, 1934.

Waldbott, G. L., and Shea, J.J.: Allergic parotitis. *J Allerg, 18*:51, Jan., 1947.

Waldmann, T.A., Wochner, K.D., Laster, L., and Gordon, R.S.: Allergic gastroenteropathy. A cause of excessive gastrointestinal protein loss.

New Eng J Med, 276:761, 1967.

Walker, I.C.: Studies on the sensitization of patients with bronchial asthma to the different proteins in wheat and the whole protein of wheat, corn, rice, barley, rye and oat. *J Med Res,* 35:509, 1917.

Studies on the sensitization of patients with bronchial asthma to proteins in animal, fruit and vegetable foods. *J Med Res,* 36:231, 1917.

The treatment of patients with bronchial asthma with subcutaneous injections of the proteins to which they are sensitive. *J Med Res,* 36:423, 1917.

A comparison between the cutaneous and the intradermal tests in the sensitization of asthmatic and hay fever patients. *J Med Res,* 37: 287, 1917.

Studies on the cause and treatment of bronchial asthma. *JAMA,* 39:363, 1917.

Causation of eczema, urticaria and angioneurotic edema by proteins other than those derived from food. *JAMA,* 70:897, 1918.

Treatment of bronchial asthma. *Med Clin N Amer,* 1:1177, 1918.

A clinical study of 400 patients with bronchial asthma. *Boston Med Surg J,* 179:288, 1918.

Treatment of bronchial asthma with vaccine. *Arch Int Med,* 23:220, 1919.

Frequent causes and the treatment of perennial hay fever. *JAMA,* 75:782, 1920.

Walker, V.: In allergy in ophthalmology; discussion. *Proc Roy Soc Med,* 40:582, 1947.

Wallen-Lawrence, Z., and Koch, F.C.: Relative digestibility of unsweetened evaporated milk, boiled milk and raw milk by trypsin *in vitro. Amer J Dis Child,* 39:18, 1930.

Wallis, R.L.M., Nicol, W.D., and Craig, M.: Importance of protein hypersensitivity in diagnosis and treatment of epileptics. *Lancet, ii:* 741, 1923.

Walstad, P.M., and Conklin, W.S.: Rupture of the normal stomach after therapeutic oxygen therapy. *New Eng J Med,* 264:1201, 1961.

Walzer, M.: Direct method of demonstrating absorption of incompletely digested proteins in normal human beings; preliminary report. *J Immunol,* 11:249, 1926.

Allergy of the abdominal organs. *J Lab Clin Med,* 26:1867, 1941.

Walzer, M., and Bowman, K.B.: Passive local sensitization in atopic individuals. *Proc Soc Exp Biol Med,* 28:425, 1931.

Walzer, M., *et al.:* Allergic reaction in gall-bladder; experimental studies in rhesus monkey. *Gastroenterology,* 1:565, 1943.

Walzer, M., Gray, I., and Harten, M.: Gallbladder allergy. *Gastroenterology,* 1:565, 1943.

Ward, J.F.: Protein sensitization as a possible cause of epilepsy and cancer. *New York Med J, 115:*592, 1922.

Protein sensitization in epilepsy—a study of 1000 cases and 100 normal controls. *Arch Neurol Psychiat,* 17:4237, 1927.

Wason, J.M.: Angioneurotic edema. *JAMA,* 86: 1332, 1926.

Watson, D.W.: The lymphocyte and ulcerative colitis. *Gastroent,* 56:385, 1969.

Immune responses and the gut. *Gastroent,* 56: 944, 1969.

Watson, T.J.: Identification and follow up of children with exudative otitis media. *Proc Roy Soc Med,* 62:455, 1969.

Way, Stuart: Eczema. *Calif West Med,* 37:255, 1932.

Weatherford, H.L.: Pathology, influence of anaphylactic shock on liver structure of liver in dog. *Amer J Pathol,* 11:611, 1935.

Weekers, L.: Nouvelle pathogénie des phlyctènes. *Bull Acad Roy Med (Belgique),* 23:577, 1909.

Weekers, L.: Cited by Bothman, L.: Clinical Manifestations of Allergy in Ophthalmology. In *The Year Book of Eye, Ear, Nose and Throat.* Chicago, Year Book Publishers, p. 7, 1941.

Weekers, L., and Barrac, G.: Les Manifestations Oculaires de l'oedème de Quincke. L'oedème allergique paroxystique intra-oculaire. *Arch Ophthal,* 54:193, 1937.

Weil, H.I.: Angioneurotic edema (a "series" of cases with clinical observations). *JAMA* 58: 1246, 1912.

Weil, R.: Articles on hepatic allergy. *J Med Res* and *J Immunol,* 1913-1917.

Weill, O.: Tachycardie Paroxystique et Anaphylaxie. *Presse Med,* 40:376, 1932.

Weinstein, P.: Beiträge zur Aetiologie und Therapie des Frehjährskatarrhs. *Klin Mbl Augenheilk,* 86:802, 1931.

Weisenburg, T.H., Yaskin, J.C., and Pleasants, H., Jr.: Neuropsychiatric Counterfeits of Organic Visceral Disease. *JAMA,* 97:1751, 1931.

Weiss, R.C., and Crepea, S.B.: Development of sensitization to penicillinase following its use in penicillin reaction. *J Allerg,* 16:209, 1945.

Weizenblatt, S.: Allergic ocular reactions to

tuberculin (bilateral cyclitis and neuroretinitis). *Arch Ophthal,* 41:436, 1949.

Wells, H.G.: Studies on the chemistry of anaphylaxis. *J Infect Dis,* 5:1908.
The present status of the problems of anaphylaxis. *J Physiol,* 1:44, 1921.
The Chemical Aspects of Immunity, 2nd ed., The Chemical Catalog Company, 1929.

Wells, H.G., and Osborne, T.B.: Anaphylaxis reactions with the purified proteins from milk. *J Infect Dis,* 29:200, 1921.

Werley, G.: Is allergy a factor in angina pectoris and cardiac infarct? *Med J Rec,* 136:417, 1932.
Food allergy and other food factors in angina pectoris. *Southern Med J,* 28:1156, 1935.

Wesseley, K.: Über anaphylaktische Erscheinungen an der Hornhaut (experimentelle Erzeugung einer parenchymatösen Keratitis durch artfremdes Serum). *München Med Wschr,* 58:1713, 1911.
Das Problem der Keratitis Parenchymatosa. *München Med Wschr,* 43:1673, 1933.

Westcott, F.H.: Migraine headaches, recent advances in classification, diagnosis and treatment. *J Allerg,* 5:624, 1933-1934.

Westphal, Von C.: Eosinophile cystitis. *Deutsch Arch Klin Med,* 173:104, 1932.

White, C.J.: Allergy in diseases of the skin. *Med Clin N Amer,* 18:1252, 1935.

White, C.J., and Taub, S.J.: Sensitization dermatoses of non-fungous nature following superficial fungus infections (ringworm) of the extremities. *JAMA,* 98:524, 1932.

White, P.J.: The relation between colic and eczema in early infancy. *Amer J Dis Child,* 38:935, 1929.

Whitfield: Cited by Dowling, G.B.: Allergy in relation to diseases of the skin. *Practitioner,* 134:610, 1935.

Whitfield, A.G.W.: Steroid therapy in pulmonary fibroses. *Brit J Dis Chest,* 53:28, 1959.

Wiener, H.J.: Ueber eosinophilie des darmschleims. *Berlin Klin Wschr,* 49:258, 1912.

Wilder, J.: Kälturticaria. *Wien Klin Wschr,* 47:1458, 1932.

Wilder, W.M., and Davis, W.D., Jr.: Duodenal enteritis. *Southern Med J,* 59:884, 1966.

Williams, D.A., and Leopold, J.G.: Death from bronchial asthma. *Acta Allerg,* 14:83, 1959.

Williams, J.R.: Allergic insulin reactions. *JAMA,* 94:1112, 1930.

Second case of gastro-intestinal allergy due to insulin. *JAMA,* 100:658, 1932.

Williams, M. Henry, Jr., and Kane, Cecelia: Treatment of bronchial asthma with Cromolyn. *JAMA,* 209:1882, 1969.

Williamson, J., and Dalakos, T.G.: Posterior subcapsular cataracts and macular lesions after long-term corticotrophin therapy. *Brit J Ophthal,* 51:839, Dec., 1967.

Willoughby, J.W.: Provocative food test technique. *Ann Allerg,* 23:543, 1965.

Wilmer, H.B., and Miller, M.M.: A case of epilepsy presenting unusual manifestations. *J Allerg,* 5:628, 1934.

Wilson, G., and Hadden, S.B.: Neuritic and multiple neuritis following serum therapy. *JAMA,* 98:123, 1932.

Wilson, S.J., and Walzer, M.: Absorption of unaltered egg protein in infants and in children. *Amer J Dis Child,* 50:49, 1935.

Winans, H.M.: Reaction to Pantopon (pantopopium hydrochloricum) simulating protein sensitization. *JAMA,* 95:199, 1930.

Winkelman, N.W., and Moore, M.T.: Allergy and the nervous diseases. *J Nerv Ment Dis,* 93:736, 1941.

Winkelmann, R.K.: Chronic urticaria. *Proc Mayo Clin,* 32:329, 1957.

Wintrobe, M.M.: *Clinical Hematology,* 5th ed. Philadelphia, Lea and Febiger, 1961.

Wise, F., and Sulzberger, M.B.: *The 1934 Year Book of Dermatology,* p. 94.

Wise, F., and Wolf, J.: Dermatophytosis and dermatophytids. *Arch Derm Syph,* 34:1, 1936.

Wiseman, R.D., and Moore, D.E.: Allergy as a cause of glaucoma. *J Allerg,* 25:355, 1954.

Withers, O.R.: Gastrointestinal allergy with special reference to the esophagus. *Southern Med J,* 32:838, 1939.

Wittig, H.J., and Glaser, J.: The relationship between bronchiolitis and childhood asthma: a follow up study of 100 cases of bronchiolitis. *J Allerg,* 30:19, 1959.

Wittig, H.J., and Goldman, A.S.: Nephrotic syndrome associated with inhaled allergens. *Lancet,* 1:542, 1970.

Wolkowicz, M.J.: Central serous retinopathy (clinical and experimental studies). *Amer J Ophthal,* 42:531, 1956.

Woltman, H.W.: Headaches. *Med Clin N Amer,* 8:1319, 1925.

Wood, Clarke T.: *The Relation of Allergy to Character Problems in Children.* Utica, Psychiatric Quarterly State Hospitals Press, New York, Jan., 1950.

Woods, A.C.: Ocular anaphylaxis. I. The reaction to perfusion with specific antigen. *Arch Ophthal, 45*:557, 1916.

Immune reactions following injuries to the uveal tract. *JAMA, 77*:1312, 1921.

The application of immunology to ophthalmology. *Arch Ophthal, 53*:321, 1924.

Allergy and Immunity in Ophthalmology. Baltimore, Johns Hopkins Press, 1933.

Allergy in relation to sympathetic ophthalmia. *New York J Med, 36*:67, 1936.

Clinical problems of allergy in relation to conjunctivitis and iritis. *Arch Ophthal, 17*:1, 1937.

Woods, A.C., and Guyton, J.S.: Role of sarcoidosis and brucellosis in uveitis. *Arch Ophthal, 31*: 469, 1944.

Woringer, P.: L'allergie au Blanc d'oeuf chez le nourisson. *Compt Rend Soc Biol, 108*:6, 1931.

L'epeuve de Prausnitz et Küstner dans l'allergie au blanc d'oeuf du nourrisson. *Compt Rend Soc Biol, 108*:8, 1931.

L'allergie au blanc d'oeuf chez le nourisson. *Presse Med, 40*:1383, 1932.

Abst. Nouvelles recherces sur l'allergie au blanc d'oeuf chex le Nourrisson. *Bull Soc Pediat Paris, 30*:419, 1932.

Wright, R., and Truelove, S.C.: Circulating antibodies to dietary proteins in ulcerative colitis. *Brit Med J, 2*:142, 1965.

Wyman, M.: *Autumnal Catarrh (Hay Fever).* Cambridge, 1872.

Wynn, J.: Senile pruritus due to hypersensitiveness. *J. Lab Clin Med, 13*:16, 1927.

Yandell, H.: What orris powder may do in a labyrinth storm. *Southwest Med, 17*:257, 1933.

Zeller, M.: Rheumatoid arthritis—food allergy as a factor. *Ann Allerg, 7*:200, 1949.

Zerfoss, K.S.: The relation of allergy to ophthalmology. *Tennessee State Med Ass J, 28*:93, 1935.

Zucker, A., and Bendo, D.: Anaphylactic reactions to ACTH. *New York J Med, 61*:623, 1961.

Zuelzer, W.W., and Apt, L.: Disseminated visceral lesions associated with extreme eosinophilia. Pathologic and clinical observations on syndrome of young children. *Amer J Dis Child, 78*:153, 1949.

Zussman, B.M.: Food hypersensitivity simulating rheumatoid arthritis. *Southern Med J, 59*:935, 1966.

Zybell: Cited by Laroche, G., Richet, Fils, C., and Saint Girons, F.: *Alimentary Anaphylaxis.* Transl. by Rowe, U.C. Press, 1930, French ed., Paris, 1919.

Index